FOURTH EDITION

COMPREHENSIVE
Respiratory Therapy Exam
Preparation Guide

Albert J. Heuer, PhD, MBA, RRT-ACCS, RPFT, FAARC
Professor, Rutgers School of Health Professions
Associate Course Director, RTBoardReview,Net
Strategic Learning Associates, LLC
Lead Therapist, Adult Intensive Care
Morristown Medical Center
Morristown, New Jersey

Narciso E. Rodriguez, BS, RRT, RRT-NPS, RRT-ACCS, RPFT
Course Director, RTBoardReview.net
Strategic Learning Associates, LLC
Staff Therapist
Saint Barnabas Medical Center
Livingston, New Jersey

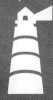

JONES & BARTLETT
LEARNING

World Headquarters
Jones & Bartlett Learning
5 Wall Street
Burlington, MA 01803
978-443-5000
info@jblearning.com
www.jblearning.com

Jones & Bartlett Learning books and products are available through most bookstores and online booksellers. To contact Jones & Bartlett Learning directly, call 800-832-0034, fax 978-443-8000, or visit our website, www .jblearning.com.

18452-5

Production Credits
VP, Product Management: Amanda Martin
Director of Product Management: Cathy L. Esperti
Product Specialist: Rachael Souza
Senior Project Specialist: Dan Stone
Digital Project Specialist: Angela Dooley
Marketing Manager: Suzy Balk
Composition: S4Carlisle Publishing Services
Cover Design: Kristin E. Parker
Senior Media Development Editor: Troy Liston
Rights Specialist: Rebecca Damon
Cover Image (Title Page, Part Opener, Chapter Opener): © David Zydd/Shutterstock
Printing and Binding: CJK Group Inc.

Library of Congress Cataloging-in-Publication Data

Library of Congress Control Number: 2019919761

6048

Printed in the United States of America

24 23 22 21 20   10 9 8 7 6 5 4 3 2 1

Dedication

We have been blessed in many ways and one of them has been to have the privilege to have had a teacher, colleague, mentor, and friend like Craig L. Scanlan, a previous editor of this textbook. Though we all had many positive influences in our life, Craig is credited for shaping our professional development as respiratory care educators and scholars. Though he is gone from this earth, his sustained and substantial contributions to respiratory care will always be felt for decades to come. This textbook is dedicated to his memory and the profound mark he has left on our profession and our personal lives.

—Al Heuer, PhD, MBA, RRT-ACCS, RPFT, FAARC

—Narciso E. Rodriguez, BS, RRT, RRT-NPS, RRT-ACCS, RPFT

Contents

Contents

Contents

Contents

Contents

New to This Edition

- An updated introduction that provides the content and layout of the most up-to-date information about the **Therapist Multiple-Choice (TMC)** and **the Clinical Simulation Examination (CSE)** according to the new Detailed Content Outlines for both examinations effective on January 15, 2020, and how to use this book to succeed in it.
- Chapters that are organized in the same sequence as the content areas for the **2020 TMC examination matrix**.
- Chapter content updated to reflect the current standard of care and the practices used in the "**NBRC Hospital**" and the **2020 NBRC Detailed Content Outlines** for the TMC and CSE.
- Updated content on preparing for and taking the TMC and CSE.
- **Updated CSE Case Management Pearls**, which provide relevant details including the etiology, manifestations, and treatment of over 35 respiratory diseases and dysfunctions that are most likely to appear in the CSEs.
- **New questions** added to pre-post chapter testing regarding new topics for the TMC/CSE examinations.
- Five new **CSE Practice Problems** added to the ones already available in the Navigate 2 Premier Access companion website.

Introduction

USING THIS BOOK AND ONLINE RESOURCES: YOUR ROAD MAP TO SUCCESS

Albert J. Heuer and Narciso E. Rodriguez

To become a Certified Respiratory Therapist (CRT), you currently must pass the National Board for Respiratory Care (NBRC) Therapist Multiple-Choice (TMC) Examination at the CRT level (lower cut score). To become a Registered Respiratory Therapist (RRT), you must pass the TMC at the higher RRT cut score and pass the NBRC Clinical Simulation Exam (CSE). Preparing for and passing these exams is no small task. Each year, despite intensive schooling, many candidates fail one or both exams, often requiring multiple attempts to achieve their goal. Moreover, because most states require that you pass the CRT exam to become licensed (with many more mandating the RRT credential), you simply cannot afford to do poorly on your board exams.

To accomplish any major task, you need the *right plan* and the *right tools*. This book and the Navigate 2 Premier Access digital product provide you with both. Our plan is based on decades of experience in helping candidates pass their board exams. Underlying our plan is a set of tried-and-true tools that have helped thousands of candidates become licensed and get registered. Follow our program, and you, too, can obtain the NBRC credentials you desire!

BOOK OVERVIEW

This book and its online resources provide you with everything you need to pass the 2020 NBRC exams. Following this introduction, Section I provides 17 chapters covering the *topical content* tested on both the TMC and CSE exams. Each chapter in Section I covers the corresponding NBRC exam topic as listed in the detailed content outline. This approach lets you concentrate on the exact knowledge tested in each area. Organizing these chapters by NBRC topic also is helpful if you have to retake the TMC examination. The best way to ensure success when retaking the TMC examination is to focus your efforts on those topics where you previously did poorly. To do so, simply review your NBRC written exam score report to identify the major topics where you scored lowest, and then focus your work on the corresponding text chapters. Due to new changes effective in 2020 you may need to contact your program faculty to access a detailed report of your performance in any NBRC examination.

Because the same 17 major topics underlie the CSE exam, Section I also is useful in preparing for that portion of the NBRC test battery. However, due to the CSE's unique structure and case-management approach, this text provides a separate three-chapter section on preparing for and taking the CSE exam.

Section I: Shared Topical Content (Chapters 1–17)

Chapter Objectives and What to Expect

Each chapter begins with a set of *Objectives* and a brief description of *What to Expect* on the corresponding section of the NBRC exams. Chapter objectives delineate the specific knowledge you need to master. The *What to Expect* descriptions specify the number and level of questions you will encounter on the current exams. This information is intended to help you set your study priorities. For example, with 18 questions (the largest section on the TMC examination) topic III-E—Ensure Modifications Are Made to the Respiratory Care Plan—is almost 10 times larger than topic II-B, Ensure

Infection Prevention (2 questions). Based on this knowledge, you would logically give much more attention to the larger/more important topic when preparing for the TMC/CSE exams. And because the length of our chapters roughly corresponds to the topical emphasis on the NBRC exams, you also can gauge the needed exam prep time by the relative length of the chapters.

Topical Content Areas Covered on the NBRC TMC and CSE Exams

I. PATIENT DATA
- A. Evaluate Data in the Patient Record
- B. Perform Clinical Assessment
- C. Perform Procedures to Gather Clinical Information
- D. Evaluate Procedure Results
- E. Recommend Diagnostic Procedures

II. TROUBLESHOOTING AND QUALITY CONTROL OF DEVICES, AND INFECTION CONTROL
- A. Assemble and Troubleshoot Devices
- B. Ensure Infection Prevention
- C. Perform Quality Control Procedures

III. INITIATION AND MODIFICATION OF INTERVENTIONS
- A. Maintain a Patent Airway Including the Care of Artificial Airways
- B. Perform Airway Clearance and Lung Expansion Techniques
- C. Support Oxygenation and Ventilation
- D. Administer Medications and Specialty Gases
- E. Ensure Modifications Are Made to the Respiratory Care Plan
- F. Utilize Evidence-Based Practice
- G. Provide Respiratory Care in High-Risk Situations
- H. Assist a Physician/Provider in Performing Procedures
- I. Conduct Patient and Family Education

What You Need to Know: Essential Content

The Essential Content section is the "meat" of each Section I chapter. We have distilled this content down to what we consider the essential need-to-know information most likely to appear on the NBRC exams, with an emphasis on bulleted outlines and summary tables.

T^4—Top Test-Taking Tips

Each chapter includes our unique T^4 feature, where we provide specific tips regarding key topical knowledge frequently tested on the NBRC TMC examination (over 350 tips in total). Our insight for these tips derives from both feedback that recent candidates have provided to us and our own experience in taking these exams for voluntary recredentialing.

Chapter Post-Tests and Mock TMC Exams

To confirm your mastery of each chapter's topical content, you should create a content post-test, available online via the *Navigate 2 Premier Access for Comprehensive Respiratory Therapy Exam Preparation Guide, Fourth Edition*, which contains Navigate TestPrep (access code provided with every new text). You can create multiple topical content post-tests varying in length from 10 to 20 questions, with each attempt presenting a different set of items. You can select questions from all three major NBRC TMC sections: Patient Data; Troubleshooting and Quality Control of Devices, and Infection Control; and Initiation and Modification of Interventions. A score of at least 70–80% indicates that you are adequately prepared for this section of the NBRC TMC examination. If you score below 70%, you should first carefully assess your test answers (particularly your wrong answers) and the correct answer explanations. Then return to the chapter to review the applicable content. Only then should you re-attempt a new post-test. Repeat this process of identifying your shortcomings and reviewing the pertinent content until your test results demonstrate mastery.

A word of warning: Some candidates try to memorize as many questions and answers as possible in hopes that doing so will help them pass the NBRC exams. *This is a huge mistake and a waste of your time.* The likelihood of seeing the exact same questions from any source on the NBRC exams is very small to none.

In order to prepare for the TMC practice exams, you can generate a TMC-like exam online using the *Navigate 2 Premier Access for Comprehensive Respiratory Therapy Exam Preparation Guide, Fourth Edition,* via Navigate TestPrep. This exam is randomly generated from a pool of over 600 questions, so—as with the chapter post-tests—each attempt will be different. You can easily customize the exam topics (Patient Data; Troubleshooting and Quality Control of Devices, and Infection Control; and Initiation and Modification of Interventions) and the number of questions you want in the exam in order to mimic the NBRC TMC exam.

Section II: Clinical Simulation Exam (CSE) Preparation (Chapters 18–20)

Most candidates know that the CSE has a unique structure. What most candidates fail to appreciate—and the reason why so many do not pass the CSE—is that the skills assessed on this exam also differ significantly from those tested on the TMC. Yes, the CSE shares the same topical content with the TMC. However, mastering topical content alone will not get you a passing score on the CSE because the CSE also tests your *case-management abilities.*

Section II of the text helps you prepare for the CSE by emphasizing case-management preparation. Chapter 18 reviews the seven disease categories from which current CSE cases are drawn and outlines a specific review strategy that focuses on disease management skills. Chapter 19 discusses the different reasoning needed to do well on the information gathering and decision-making sections of CSE problems, while also recommending both general *Do's* and *Don'ts* and specific choices likely to help you boost your scores. Chapter 20 completes the CSE section with over 30 case-management pearls covering the clinical problems most likely to appear on the CSE.

Appendices Available on the Navigate 2 Premier Access

There are two supplemental appendices available on the Navigate 2 Premier Access. Appendix A provides a set of *Test-Taking Tips and Techniques,* designed to help you improve your multiple-choice test "wiseness" and boost your TMC scores. For those needing a review of common formulas and computations that can appear on the TMC exam, Appendix B provides a comprehensive summary of common *Cardiopulmonary Calculations.*

TEST PREPARATION STRATEGY

TMC Test Preparation

Figure 1 outlines the strategy we recommend that you follow to prepare for the TMC examination. Based on our experience in guiding candidates, *you should devote at least 4 weeks to this process.* One of the most common reasons why candidates fail the TMC examination is hasty or last-minute preparation. Do yourself a favor and follow a deliberate and unhurried process. Remember—it was the slow-and-steady tortoise who won the race, not the hurrying hare!

Some of you will implement this strategy on your own, whereas others may be guided in their preparation while still in a respiratory therapy program. In either case, it is important to proceed systematically through each chapter and not to move forward until you have mastered the relevant content.

For Those Who Have Not Been Successful

If you purchased this text because you failed an NBRC exam, you are not alone. For example, approximately one in four candidates is unsuccessful in passing the TMC examination the first time around, with only about a third of repeaters passing on subsequent attempts. Although you likely are unhappy with your test results, such an event gives you an advantage over those who have never taken the exam. First, you know what to expect regarding the testing procedures. Second, your score report can help you identify where you did well and where you did poorly.

The current NBRC TMC score report provides your overall score and the scores for each of the three major content sections (i.e., Patient Data; Troubleshooting and Quality Control of Devices and

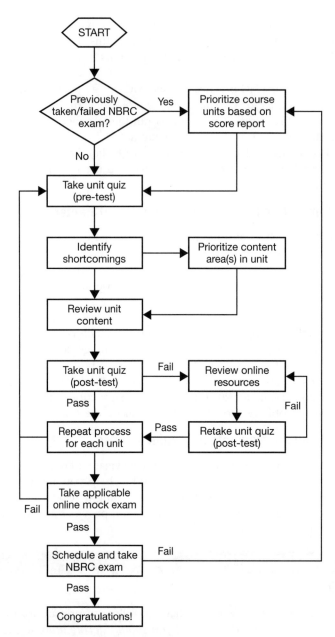

Figure 1 Recommended Preparation Strategy for the TMC Examination.

Infection Control; and Initiation and Modification of Interventions). Due to new changes effective in 2020 you may need to contact your program faculty to access a detailed report of your performance in any NBRC examination. Based on this information from your school, we recommend that you compute the percentage of correct questions for each of the three content areas on your NBRC score report. For example, if you correctly answered 10 of the 20 questions on Section II of the TMC examination (Troubleshooting and Quality Control of Equipment, and Infection Control), you would compute your percentage correct as 10/20 = 0.50 or 50%. *We recommend that you flag any major section on which you scored less than 75%.* You should then focus your attention on these flagged sections and their corresponding book chapters in preparing to retake the exam. Of course, you should still review chapters in the major content areas where you scored more than 75%—*but only after attending to your high-priority needs.*

Topical Chapter Review Process

For this strategy to succeed, it is essential that you proceed systematically through each chapter. This normally involves the following steps:

1. Review the applicable chapter content.
2. Take the chapter post-test to assess your mastery of that topic.
3. Repeat steps 1 to 2 for each chapter until the mastery level is achieved.

Regarding step 3, we recommend that you set a goal of achieving at *least 70–80% correct as the measure of chapter mastery*. In addition, if you follow our advice, your chapter post-test scores generally should rise with each new attempt, which confirms that you are indeed learning and moving toward mastery.

Take a Mock TMC Examination on the Navigate 2 Premier Access

Mock TMC exams created in the Navigate 2 Premier Access TestPrep are intended to simulate the corresponding NBRC test. Like the chapter post-tests, this online exam gives you feedback on every question, including the correct answers and their corresponding explanations.

With this feedback, these mock exams serve as an additional learning tool in your path to success on the TMC exams. First, your overall score on the mock exams will tell you how well you have mastered the content covered in the book. Second, a careful review of the question explanations should enhance your understanding of the concepts likely to be tested on the NBRC TMC examination. Finally, review of these explanations can help you identify any remaining areas of weakness you need to address before scheduling your exam date.

Because a mock TMC examination serves as a bridge between the book and the actual NBRC TMC examination, we recommend that you take it only *after* mastering all 17 of the book's topical content chapters, as indicated by a "passing" score of at least 70–80% on each of their post-tests. We also recommend that you complete a mock TMC examination *at least a week* before you are scheduled to take the actual NBRC TMC examination. This way, you will have enough time to review any persistent areas of misunderstanding and can avoid the anxiety that last-minute cramming always creates.

We also recommend that you track your time when taking a mock TMC examination. *Based on the number of questions included and the NBRC time limits, you will need to complete approximately one question per minute.* If you find yourself taking significantly longer on each question, you will need to increase your testing pace before taking the actual NBRC exam.

What if you do not score well on our mock TMC exams? If you carefully follow the strategy we outline here, it is highly unlikely that you will do poorly on this test. In the unusual case where you score less than 70%, it's "back to the books." In this case, a careful review of the test items you got wrong on our mock TMC exam should help you identify the content areas and book chapters that need additional review.

Schedule and Take the Exam

After successfully mastering all topical chapters and passing a mock TMC examination, it is time to schedule and take the real thing. If you have not already done so, we strongly recommend that you use some of the time you have set aside to review the *Test-Taking Tips and Techniques* guidance in Appendix A. Also, consider taking a practice trip to and from your NBRC testing center, ideally at the same time at which your exam is scheduled. This run-through can help you gauge travel time and iron out little details, such as where you will park and where you can get a cup of coffee before the exam.

What if you do not pass the NBRC TMC examination? There are several Do's and Don'ts associated with a failed attempt on the exam. First, the Don'ts:

- Don't get disheartened or give up.
- Don't immediately reschedule a retake.

Instead, take a proactive approach. Do the following:

- Do carefully analyze your NBRC score report. This report can be obtained from your former school or program.

- Do use your score report to prioritize content areas needing further study.
- Do revisit the key-content-area resources we provide in the book and online.
- Do give yourself adequate time to implement your new study plan (at least 3–4 weeks).

CSE Test Preparation

To be eligible to take the CSE, you must first score at the RRT level (uppercut score) on the NBRC TMC examination. Although there currently is no "published" RRT-level cut score, you should strive to achieve a TMC score of at least 67–70% if you expect to qualify for the CSE.

If you achieve the RRT cut score on the TMC, you can then go ahead and schedule the CSE exam. *Don't make the mistake of immediately attempting the CSE!* As emphasized in Chapter 18, we strongly recommend that you also devote at least 3 to 4 weeks to preparing for the CSE. Besides avoiding the anxiety caused by last-minute preparation, this approach lets you apply your TMC results to your study plan.

As previously discussed, the CSE shares the same topical content as is covered on the TMC examination. Consequently, preparation for the CSE should begin with a review of all 17 Section I book chapters. As discussed in Chapter 18, you should use your TMC results you obtained from your program to identify the topics needing the most attention, and then proceed with their review.

However, the topical review should *not* be the primary focus of your CSE preparation. Why? There are three reasons. First, to be eligible for the CSE, you already had to demonstrate topical content mastery by passing the TMC at the RRT level. Second, *the primary focus of the CSE is case management, not topical knowledge*. Third, the CSE's structure requires that you develop and apply special test-taking skills specific to its unique test format.

In terms of case management, we recommend that you devote most of your time to reviewing the management of specific cases likely to appear on the CSE. Chapter 18 applies this important information and outlines our recommendations on the resources you should use to strengthen your case-management knowledge.

In regard to test-taking proficiency, the unique format of the CSE requires a different set of skills from those needed to succeed on multiple-choice exams (the test-taking tips covered in Appendix A). For this reason, we provide a separate chapter designed to help you develop CSE-specific testing proficiency (Chapter 19). You should review these tips before working through the online practice simulation problems.

To give you experience with the CSE format and help you apply the case-management and CSE test-taking skills, the Navigate 2 Premier Access provides several simulation problems to practice. If you score poorly on any individual practice problem or consistently have difficulty with either information gathering or decision making, we recommend that you review the test-taking skills in Chapter 19 and the corresponding case-management "pearls" provided in Chapter 20. Then retake the applicable practice problems until you achieve the required minimum passing scores.

After completing the practice problems and applying their results to your exam preparation, it is time to take the NBRC CSE. The same general guidance we recommend for scheduling and taking the NBRC TMC applies to the CSE.

SECTION I

**Shared Topical Content
TMC and CSE Exams**

CHAPTER 1

Evaluate Data in the Patient Record (Section I-A)

Narciso E. Rodriguez

The patient medical record contains vital information on the patient's past medical history, physical examinations, lab and imaging test results, and other respiratory-related monitoring data—all of which are needed to support sound decision making. For this reason, the NBRC exams will evaluate your ability to assess relevant patient information in the record and apply it to optimize care.

OBJECTIVES

In preparing for this section of the NBRC exams (TMC/CSE), you should demonstrate the knowledge needed to evaluate the following documentation found in the patient record:

1. Patient history
2. Physical examination relative to the cardiopulmonary system
3. Lines, drains, and airways (chest tubes, vascular lines, artificial airways)
4. Laboratory results
5. Blood gas analysis and hemoximetry (CO-oximetry) results
6. Pulmonary function testing results
7. 6-minute walk test results
8. Imaging study results
9. Maternal and perinatal/neonatal history
10. Sleep study results
11. Trends in monitoring results in fluid balance, vital signs, intracranial pressure, ventilator liberation parameters, pulmonary mechanics, noninvasive measures of gas exchange and cardiac monitoring (i.e., ECG, hemodynamic parameters, cardiac catheterization, and echocardiography)
12. Determination of a patient's pathophysiologic state

WHAT TO EXPECT ON THIS CATEGORY OF THE NBRC EXAMS

TMC exam: 10 questions; 4 recall, 6 application
CSE exam: indeterminate number of questions; however, section I-A knowledge is a prerequisite to succeed on the CSE, especially on Information Gathering sections.

WHAT YOU NEED TO KNOW: ESSENTIAL CONTENT

Evaluate Data in the Patient Record

Table 1-1 lists the major sections of the typical patient record and the information that may be found in each section.

Patient History

Table 1-2 summarizes areas to emphasize when reviewing a patient's medical history. Section I-B provides more details on occupational and environmental exposure history.

Table 1-1 Typical Contents Found in the Patient Record*

Section of Record	Information Located in That Section
Admitting sheet/face sheet	Patient's next of kin, address, religion, and employer; health insurance information
Informed consent	Consent forms signed by the patient (and witness) for various diagnostic and therapeutic procedures, such as bronchoscopy, blood transfusions, and surgery
Advance directives and do-not-resuscitate (DNR) orders	Properly signed and witnessed DNR, do-not-intubate (DNI), and advance directives
Medication reconciliation sheet	List of current medications at admission (including respiratory medications taken at home) to prevent medication discrepancies, medication errors, and drug interactions during patient management and discharge
Patient history	Past/present family, social, and medical history; medications and demographics
Prescribing provider's orders	Doctor's (or nurse practitioner's/physician assistant's) diagnostic and therapeutic orders, including those pertaining to respiratory care
Laboratory results	WBC/RBC counts, ABGs, electrolytes, coagulation studies, and culture results (e.g., sputum, blood, urine)
Imaging studies	X-ray, CT, MRI, PET, V/Q scan reports; may also include ultrasound and echocardiography results
Electrocardiograms (ECGs/EKGs)	The results of ECG/EKGs
Other specialized studies	Often separate reports for PFTs, sleep, metabolic, and exercise testing
Progress notes	Discipline-specific notes on a patient's progress and treatment plan by physicians and other caregivers
Therapy (respiratory)	Respiratory therapy charting; may include ABGs, PFT results
Nurses' notes and flow sheet	Nurses' subjective and objective record of the patient's condition, including vital signs, fluid I/O, and hemodynamic and ICP monitoring trends
Lines, drains, and airways	Central lines such as pulmonary artery catheter (PAP), femoral venous lines, arterial lines, and PIC lines. Oropharyngeal/nasopharyngeal gastric tube and feeding tubes. Chest tubes and wound drainage systems. Endotracheal or tracheostomy airway tubes. Cranial drainage systems

*A neonate's medical record may have a section dedicated to birth history, or it may be included in the patient history section.

ABG, arterial blood gas; CT, computed tomography; ICP, intracranial pressure; I/O, intake/output; MRI, magnetic resonance imaging; PIC, peripherally inserted catheter; PET, positron emission tomography; PFT, pulmonary function test; RBC, red blood cell; V/Q, ventilation-perfusion; WBC, white blood cell.

Prescribing Provider's Orders

All respiratory care normally is provided by order of the patient's doctor or other licensed providers with prescribing authority, such as nurse practitioners or physician assistants. You cannot accept orders transmitted to you via unauthorized third parties, such as registered nurses. If an order is communicated to you via a third party, you must verify that the order has been entered in the patient's record before proceeding. You also should not accept blanket orders, such as "continue previous medications" or "resume preoperative orders."

Regarding verbal or telephone orders, if "the doctor is in the house" and the situation is not an emergency, you should secure a regular written order or a computerized provider order entry (CPOE). If a verbal order is required and you are authorized to take it, you must document that you read the order back to the originator and that the originator confirmed the accuracy of the order as read back.

Table 1-2 Key Record Elements Related to Patient History

Element	Importance
Demographic data	Factors such as a patient's place of residence and age may be relevant in that some respiratory conditions tend to be more common in certain age groups, in specific geographic locations, and among certain ethnic groups.
History of present illness (HPI)	The patient's chief complaint, description of symptoms, frequency, duration, quality, severity, onset, and features that aggravate or alleviate discomfort are often important in diagnosis and treatment.
Past medical history (PMH)	Surgeries, treatments for cancer and heart disease, history of asthma and COPD, and congenital and childhood conditions also may be relevant.
Past/current medication history	Complete knowledge of medications that the patient has been taking is essential when implementing new prescriptions, and for medication reconciliation, including their dosages and frequencies. Previous medical tests and procedures history may be found here.
Family disease history	The health status of blood relatives may be useful in considering diseases with hereditary tendencies (e.g., cardiovascular conditions, diabetes).
Occupational history and environmental exposures	Work history (e.g., mining, chemical production, and work involving asbestos) and past environmental exposures (including in the home) may be linked to respiratory dysfunction.
Social history	Smoking, tobacco use, and vaping may contribute to respiratory disorders and should be noted along with alcohol or drug use, social activities, hobbies, recreational activities, and pets.
Patient education history	Knowledge of prior patient/caregiver education regarding the medical condition and treatment can help in planning future efforts.

You also must ensure that all orders are accurate and complete. A complete order generally includes the following information:

- Date and time of order (often with an expiration date)
- Name of therapy or diagnostic test being prescribed
- Requisite details for therapy (e.g., ventilator settings, drug concentration) or conditions for diagnostic testing
- Frequency of therapy or testing (if intermittent)
- Name, signature, and credentials of the originator

If the order is for a drug (including oxygen), it must also contain the drug name, administration route, and dose/concentration (for O_2, the liter flow or Fio_2). If the order is for mechanical ventilation, it should include at least one and ideally both of the following:

- Desired range for $Paco_2$ and desired range for Pao_2 or oxygen saturation
- Ventilator settings to achieve the desired blood gas results

Should any of these elements be missing, the order is incomplete, and you should contact the originator for clarification. The same procedure applies if the order falls outside institutional standards and protocols. For example, if the order specifies a drug dosage higher than that recommended for your patient or includes a ventilator mode or setting not normally applied in similar cases, you should contact the originator for clarification before proceeding.

Advance Directives and DNR Orders

Unless otherwise informed, you should presume that your patients want lifesaving treatment. Indeed, *whenever in doubt or when written orders are not present, you should always initiate emergency life support when needed.* However, to ensure that your actions match your patients' desires, you should always determine whether advance directives have been established.

Advance Directives

- Specify the healthcare choices patients want if they are unable to make informed decisions
- Usually obtained upon admission to the hospital
- Legally oblige all healthcare providers to abide by the patient's choices
- May include one or both of the following:
  ○ A living will: document specifying the level of care that patients desire should they become incapacitated
  ○ A durable power of attorney (aka a *proxy directive*): a document giving another individual (the *surrogate*) legal authority to make decisions for a patient

Do-Not-Resuscitate (DNR) Orders

- A DNR order is a special type of advance directive whereby patients choose to forego resuscitation should they suffer a cardiorespiratory arrest.
- A DNR request can come from the patient or a surrogate, but a written order must be placed in the record by the attending physician.
- A patient or surrogate can change or revoke a DNR order at any time, either in writing or orally.
- A DNR order is occasionally referred to as a Do Not Attempt to Resuscitate (DNAR) order

Should a patient or surrogate ask you to change or revoke an advance directive or DNR order, you must *immediately* notify the attending physician, who is obliged to document the new request in the patient record.

Additional elements of the physical examination relative to the cardiopulmonary system as well as assessment of lines, drains and the airway will be covered in detailed in Section I-B.

Laboratory Results

Pertinent laboratory data that you need to assess include both hematology and clinical chemistry test results. **Table 1-3** lists common lab reference ranges for adult patients for the tests likely to appear on NBRC exams as well as the significance of their results.

Below are common examples of abnormal findings likely to appear on NBRC exams:

- Elevated overall white blood cell (WBC) count and differential WBC values such as neutrophils and bands suggest an acute bacterial infection.
- Abnormal red blood cells (RBCs) impact the O_2 carrying capacity of the blood. Increased RBCs (polycythemia) may be associated with chronic hypoxemia, whereas decreased levels may be related to bleeding or anemia.
- Low serum potassium (hypokalemia) may lead to dysrhythmias such as premature ventricular contractions (PVCs) and may be associated with respiratory muscle weakness. Certain respiratory medications, such as albuterol, may lower serum potassium.
- Low platelet count or abnormally long prothrombin time (PT), International Normalized Ratio (INR), and partial thromboplastin time (PTT) indicate a potential for excessive bleeding with invasive procedures causing tissue or blood vessel trauma, such as ABG sampling, thoracentesis, suctioning or bronchoscopy.
- Cardiac markers such as creatine kinase isoenzyme (CK-MB) and troponin I can help confirm the occurrence of acute myocardial infarction, whereas B-type natriuretic peptide (BNP) levels can help diagnose congestive heart failure (CHF).
- Sputum culture and sensitivities, together with gram staining, are used to identify the causative agent in bacterial pneumonia. Samples that grow ≥ 106 colony-forming units (CFU) per milliliter of a respiratory pathogen are considered positive. Inadequate collection methods or recent antibiotic administration can cause false-positive and false-negative results. Therefore, results must be interpreted cautiously.

Table 1-3 Reference Ranges and Significance of Selected Laboratory Tests (Adult Values)

Test	Reference Ranges*	Significance
Hematology		
Red blood cells (RBCs)	M: 4.6–6.2 × 10⁶/mm³ F: 4.2–5.4 × 10⁶/mm³	• Oxygen transport • Response to hypoxemia • Degree of cyanosis
Hemoglobin	M: 13.5–16.5 g/dL F: 12.0–15.0 g/dL	• Oxygen transport • Response to hypoxemia • Degree of cyanosis
Hematocrit	M: 40–54% F: 38–47%	• Hemoconcentration (high) or polycythemia (high) • Hemodilution (low)
White blood cells (WBCs)	4500–11,500/mm³	• Infection (high)
Platelets	150,000–400,000/mm³	• Slow blood clotting (low) • Check before arterial blood gas puncture (ABG)
Prothrombin time (PT)	12–14 seconds	• Slow clotting (high) • Check before ABG
International Normalized Ratio (INR)	0.8–1.2 (2.0–3.0 for patients on anticoagulants)	• Slow clotting (high) • Check before ABG
Partial thromboplastin time (PTT)	25–37 seconds	• Slow clotting (high) • Check before ABG
Clinical Chemistry		
Sodium (Na)	136–145 mEq/L	• Acid–base/fluid balance
Potassium (K)	3.5–5 mEq/L	• Metabolic acidosis (high) • Metabolic alkalosis (low) • Cardiac arrhythmias (low)
Chloride (Cl)	98–105 mEq/L	• Metabolic alkalosis (low)
Blood urea nitrogen (BUN)	7–20 mg/dL	• Renal failure (high)
Creatinine	0.7–1.3 mg/dL	• Renal disease (high)
Glucose	70–105 mg/dL	• Diabetes/ketoacidosis (high)
Total protein	6.3–7.9 g/dL	• Liver disease; malnutrition (low)
Albumin	3.5–5.0 g/dL	• Liver disease; malnutrition (low)
Cholesterol	150–220 mg/dL	• Atherosclerosis (high)
Lactate acid	0.4–2.3 mEq/L	• Tissue hypoxia, shock (high)
Cardiac Biomarkers		
Total creatine kinase (CK)	50–200 U/L	• Acute myocardial infarction (AMI)/various skeletal muscle disorders (high)
Creatine kinase isoenzyme (CK-MB)	< 4–6% total CK	• AMI (rises 4–6 hours after insult, peaks at 24 hours, returns to normal in 2–3 days)
Troponin I	< 0.4 µg/L	• AMI/acute coronary syndrome (rises 3–6 hours after insult, peaks at 12 hours, can persist 7 days)
B-type natriuretic peptide (BNP)	< 20 pg/mL	• < 100 pg/L rules out diagnosis of congestive heart failure (CHF) • > 500 pg/mL helps rule in diagnosis of CHF

*Reference ranges vary by institution and specific sources. However, exam candidates should be fine in using these ranges for the NBRC exams.
F, female; M, male

Blood Gas Analysis and Hemoximetry (CO-oximetry) Results

Analysis of arterial blood gas (ABG) samples provides precise measurement of acid-base balance and of the patient's ability to oxygenate and ventilate (remove CO_2 from the blood). The following are some considerations you should keep in mind while reviewing ABG results.

Normal Ranges

To review ABG results, you first need to know the adult reference ranges as listed in **Table 1-4**. We recommend that you first interpret the acid-base status, then evaluate oxygenation separately.

Interpreting Primary Acid-Base Disturbances

To quickly asses the primary acid-base status, you need to consider only two parameters: pH and $Paco_2$.

As indicated in **Figure 1-1**, you first determine whether the pH is normal (7.35–7.45), low (< 7.35; acidemia), or high (> 7.45; alkalemia). After judging the pH, you then assess the $Paco_2$ and determine the primary disturbance causing the abnormality as follows:

- Normal pH, normal $Paco_2$: Normal acid-base balance.
- Low pH/acidemia (< 7.35)
  - $Paco_2$ > 45 torr: Primary disturbance is *respiratory acidosis*.
  - $Paco_2$ ≤ 45 torr: Primary disturbance is *metabolic acidosis*.
- High pH/alkalemia (> 7.45)
  - $Paco_2$ < 35 torr: Primary disturbance is *respiratory alkalosis*.
  - $Paco_2$ ≥ 35 torr: Primary disturbance is *metabolic alkalosis*.

You confirm metabolic involvement (either *primary* or *compensatory*) by assessing the base excess (BE). Values greater than +2 indicate *metabolic alkalosis* (base gain), and values less than –2 indicating *metabolic acidosis* (base deficit). Chapter 4 provides details on the advanced assessment of acid-base balance.

Interpreting the Severity of Hypoxemia (Basic)

The severity of hypoxemia (in room air) is classified as follows:

- Mild: Pao_2 60–79 torr
- Moderate: Pao_2 40–59 torr
- Severe: Pao_2 < 40 torr

Of course, *this interpretation depends in part on whether the patient is breathing supplemental O_2.* For example, if a patient's Pao_2 is less than 60 torr when breathing a high Fio_2 (≥ 0.60), most clinicians would categorize this level of hypoxemia as severe. Chapter 4 provides details on the advanced assessment of oxygenation.

Table 1-4 Arterial Blood Gas Reference Ranges

Parameter	Normal Range
pH	7.35–7.45
$Paco_2$	35–45 torr
Pao_2	80–100 torr*
HCO_3^-	22–26 mEq/L (mmol/L)
BE	0 ± 2
Sao_2	95–98%*
*Breathing room air.	

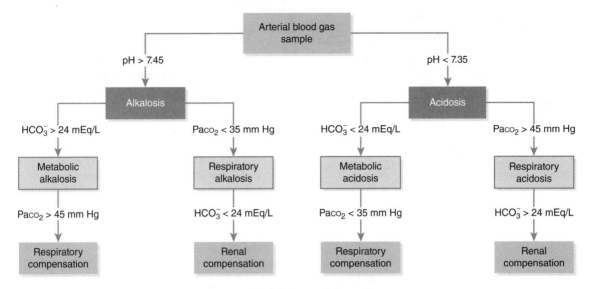

Figure 1-1 Interpretation of Basic Acid-Base Disturbances.

Common Abnormal Patterns

Table 1-5 Describes several common abnormal ABG patterns frequently appearing on the NBRC exams.

Hemoximetry (CO-oximetry)

Hemoximetry is indicated when accurate measures of any hemoglobin (Hb) parameters are needed and when you need to calibrate a pulse oximetry reading (SpO_2) against the actual arterial saturation.

Below are common examples of measured Hb findings and their interpretation likely to appear on NBRC exams:

- Carboxyhemoglobin (COHb):
    - Normal CO levels are < 1.5%. For smokers, inner-city dwellers, and those living near industrial areas normal CO levels of 3–6% can be found.
    - To assess smoke inhalation/CO poisoning COHb levels of at least 3–4% in nonsmokers and at least 10% in smokers can be considered outside the expected physiologic range. If due to smoke inhalation, 100% via non-rebreather mask is required to treat the inhalation. If dangerous levels are detected and the patient is symptomatic (confusion or altered mental status), hyperbaric oxygen administration may be necessary to treat the symptoms.
- To assess methemoglobinemia (metHb) during inhaled nitric oxide (INO) delivery.
    - Normal metHb level in a healthy subject usually is < 1.5% of the total Hb%
    - INO can combine with hemoglobin to form nitrosylhemoglobin, which is rapidly oxidized to methemoglobin. Tissue hypoxia results when there is excessive metHb due to an increased affinity of the Hb to oxygen.
    - During INO delivery metHb should be assessed by CO-oximetry in a 4 to 6 h interval according to institutional protocol and dose delivered.

Pulse oximetry (SpO_2) accuracy can be affected by many factors such as artifacts and physiologic conditions. When in the presence of low readings, abnormal waveforms or CO exposure suspicion, a CO-oximetry test must be done to assess for SpO_2 accuracy.

Table 1-5 Common ABG Abnormalities

Underlying Disorder	Typical ABG Result	Interpretation
Moderate to severe chronic obstructive pulmonary disease (COPD) with CO_2 retention	pH = 7.36 $Paco_2$ = 58 torr Pao_2 = 62 torr (in room air) HCO_3^- = 34 mEq/L BE = +7	Fully compensated respiratory acidosis with mild hypoxemia (acute-on-chronic respiratory acidosis)
Pneumonia, asthma attack, pulmonary emboli, or any other condition associated with moderate or severe hypoxemia	pH = 7.53 $Paco_2$ = 27 torr Pao_2 = 53 torr (2 L/min cannula) HCO_3^- = 22 mEq/L BE = −7	Uncompensated respiratory alkalosis with moderate hypoxemia; alkalosis is the result of hyperventilation due to the hypoxemia
Uncontrolled diabetes with ketoacidosis	pH = 7.32 $Paco_2$ = 28 torr Pao_2 = 108 torr (in room air) HCO_3^- = 14 mEq/L BE = −10	Partially compensated metabolic acidosis with normal oxygenation
Cardiopulmonary arrest	pH = 7.05 $Paco_2$ = 60 torr Pao_2 = 39 torr (in room air) HCO_3^- = 16 mEq/L BE = −8	Combined *respiratory and metabolic acidosis* with severe hypoxemia (likely causing lactic acidosis)

Pulmonary Function Test Results

Pulmonary function tests (PFTs) include spirometry, static lung volumes and capacity measures, and diffusion studies. PFT results provide information useful in diagnosing the category of disease, the degree of impairment, and the likely prognosis.

Most pulmonary diseases are categorized as restrictive, obstructive, or mixed. **Table 1-6** summarizes the primary features of these categories. Predicted PFT values are primarily a function of a patient's height, sex, and age. The degree of impairment is determined by comparing actual PFT results with predicted values, expressed as percent predicted. Although severity classifications vary by specific test, in the NBRC exams, hospital results generally are categorized as follows:

- Normal: 80–120% of predicted
- Mild: 70–79% of predicted
- Moderate: 50–69% of predicted
- Severe: < 49% of predicted

For obstructive disorders, reversibility is assessed by bronchodilator pre-/post-testing. An increase in flows of 12–15% or more after bronchodilator therapy suggests significant reversibility.

In addition to measures of flow and volume, the patient record may include carbon monoxide diffusing capacity (DLco) test results. In patients with healthy lungs, the normal reference range is 25–30 mL/min/mm Hg. A low DLco is observed in disorders such as pulmonary fibrosis and emphysema due to the thickening and destruction of alveolar surface, whereas higher-than-normal values may occur in polycythemia.

Table 1-6 Restrictive Versus Obstructive Disease

Category of Disorder	Examples	Impact on Flows and Volumes	Typical Measurements
Restrictive	Neuromuscular disorders, obesity, pulmonary fibrosis	↓ Volumes	FVC, IRV, ERV, RV, TLC
Obstructive	Asthma, chronic obstructive pulmonary disease (COPD)	↓ Flows	FEV_1, FEV_1% (FEV_1/FVC), PEFR, FEF_{25-75}
Mixed (combined restrictive and obstructive)	Cystic fibrosis	↓ Volumes ↓ Flows	As above

Table 1-7 6-Minute Walk Test (6MWT)

Indications/why ordered	To assess overall functional capacity or changes in capacity due to therapy in patients with moderate to severe heart or lung disease.
Basic procedure	Measures distance a patient can walk on a flat surface in 6 minutes (i.e., the 6-minute walking distance [6MWD]).
Key findings	*Screening*: 6MWD < 500–600 meters indicates abnormal functional capacity (may require further evaluation). *Treatment effect*: Pre-/post-Tx gain of ≥ 10–20%.

6-Minute Walk Test Results

The NBRC expects you to be familiar with the 6-minute walk test (6MWT). **Table 1-7** outlines the indications for this test, basic procedures, and key findings. Chapters 3 and 4 provide more details on performing and assessing the results of this test.

Imaging Studies

The most common imaging study for patients with respiratory disorders is the chest x-ray. Chapter 2 details the review and interpretation of the chest film.

Table 1-8 provides a summary of the findings associated with the most common pulmonary conditions that are likely to appear in the patient record and NBRC exams.

In addition to the chest x-ray, the NBRC expects candidates to be familiar with other selected imaging test results, as summarized in **Table 1-9**.

Key points related to these imaging modalities include the following:

- MRI imaging:
  - Support of mechanically ventilated patients undergoing MRI requires an FDA-approved ventilator.
  - Applicable ventilators typically are labeled as either "MR Safe" or "MR Conditional."
  - If MR Conditional, you *must* follow the manufacturer's operational protocol, which usually includes *at least* locking the device a safe distance from the MRI magnet.
- Thoracic ultrasound:
  - Provides a two-dimensional cross-sectional view of underlying structures ("B mode")
  - Pneumothorax detected by the *absence* of the *gliding sign* (a normal finding visible as a shimmering of the parietal/visceral pleural line during breathing)
  - Interstitial/alveolar syndrome (e.g., pulmonary edema, pneumonia) detected via the proliferation of B lines (aka "lung rockets" or "comet tails"), bright vertical bands arising from pleural line and coursing down into the lung tissue
  - Pleural effusion detected as an echo-free or dark zone in a scanned dependent region, especially at or near the costophrenic angle

Table 1-8 Radiographic Findings Associated with Common Respiratory Disorders

Condition	Radiograph Findings
Abnormalities of the chest wall	• Broken ribs: possible flail chest • Kyphoscoliosis/lordosis: causes lung restriction and decreases lung volumes
Acute respiratory distress syndrome (ARDS)	• Nonhomogeneous bilateral lung opacities (white-out) and infiltrates with normal heart size consistent with pulmonary edema
Airway complications	• Right (common) or left mainstem intubation: tendency for the opposite lung to collapse • Tracheal narrowing (stenosis) or tracheal dilation (tracheomalacia) • Tracheal edema and inflammation: croup ("steeple sign" on anteroposterior [AP] film) and epiglottitis ("thumb sign" on lateral neck x-ray) • Mucus plugging causes affected lung, lobe, or segment to collapse
Atelectasis	• Increased radiopacity (whiteness) in the film • Air bronchograms due to tissue collapse around opened airways • Elevated hemidiaphragm on the affected side • Shift of trachea and mediastinum toward the affected side
Consolidation or infiltration	• Air bronchograms: airways silhouette surrounded by collapsed tissue • Increased radiopacity (whiteness) of the affected area
Congestive heart failure (CHF)	• Increased vascular markings • Cardiomegaly: increased heart size (cardiothoracic ratio > 50%) • Presence of pleural effusions/Kerley B lines
Emphysema (chronic obstructive pulmonary disease [COPD])	• Lowered, flattened diaphragms • Decreased lung and vascular markings (hyperaeration, radiolucency) • Increased retrosternal air space (lateral film) • Presence of bullae/blebs (pockets of air in the lung parenchyma) • Narrow mediastinum
Pleura effusion	• Homogeneous areas of increased density that are position dependent, confirmed by a lateral decubitus chest x-ray • Loss of sharp costophrenic angles • Presence of a meniscus at the fluid-air interface
Pneumothorax	• Loss of peripheral lung markings • Air between the lung margin and chest wall (radiolucent space) • Mediastinal shift to the opposite side • Possible depression of diaphragm on the affected side • Sulcus sign (deepening of the costophrenic angles observed on supine films)
Pulmonary edema	• Fluffy or patchy densities in the perihilar areas and gravity-dependent lower lung fields • May be accompanied by cardiomegaly, pleural effusions, and air bronchograms

- Pulmonary angiography:
  - Pulmonary angiography is now performed in conjunction with CT scan and is replacing V/Q scans as the gold standard for diagnosis of pulmonary embolism.
  - Usually, the contrast media fills the pulmonary vessels, appearing as bright white "tree branches"; emboli will appear dark and block any further distal flow of the contrast media.

Table 1-9 Specialized Imaging Studies

Imaging Test	Description
Computed tomography (CT) scan	Facilitates evaluation of abnormalities of the lungs, mediastinum, pleura, and chest wall as well as diagnosis of pulmonary emboli (CT angiography)
Magnetic resonance imaging (MRI)	Highly detailed imaging for identifying the pathology of the heart, major vessels, mediastinum, lungs, and chest wall
	Contraindicated in morbidly obese patients and those with implanted metallic devices
Positron emission tomography (PET)	Creates "metabolic images" of body tissue via uptake of a radioactive tracer injected into the patient
	Detects cellular metabolic changes and can identify abnormal cell growth such as those found in lung cancer
Thoracic ultrasound	Use of high-frequency sound to rapidly detect pneumothorax or pleural effusion or to guide thoracentesis and insertion of central lines and chest tubes
	Also used to assess for trauma to the ribs, diaphragm, heart, and large thoracic blood vessels
Pulmonary angiography	By injection of contrast medium, permits evaluation of arterial abnormalities such as an arterial aneurysm or pulmonary embolism
Ventilation-perfusion (V/Q) scan	Angiography to examine lung perfusion and an image of the distribution of ventilation via inhalation of radiolabeled gas (xenon-133)

- Ventilation-perfusion scans:
  - For the ventilation scan, the patient inhales a xenon gas or a technetium-tagged aerosol; for the perfusion scan, technetium is injected intravenously.
  - A high probability of pulmonary embolism is indicated if multiple segmental perfusion defects are visible without corresponding ventilation defects.
  - V/Q scans are being replaced by high-resolution CT (HRCT) angiography.

Maternal and Perinatal/Neonatal History

Maternal Data

The medical record of a pregnant woman typically includes assessment of factors in the history that may place the mother or neonate at risk. Common factors associated with high-risk pregnancies that you should look for in the record include the following:

- Socioeconomic factors:
  - Low income and poor housing
  - Unwed status, especially adolescent (younger than 16 years)
  - Minority status
- Obstetric history:
  - History of infertility
  - History of infant malformation or birth injury
  - History of miscarriage, stillbirth, or ectopic pregnancy
  - High parity (many children)
  - History of premature or prolonged labor
  - History of a low-birth-weight infant
- Maternal medical history:
  - Obese or underweight before/during pregnancy
  - Cardiac, pulmonary, or renal disease
  - Diabetes or thyroid disease
  - Gastrointestinal or endocrine disorder
  - History of hypertension or seizures
  - History of venereal and other infectious diseases
  - Weight loss greater than 5 pounds

- Current obstetric status:
  - Surgery during pregnancy
  - The absence of prenatal care
  - Rh sensitization or maternal anemia
  - Excessively large or small fetus
  - Preeclampsia or premature labor
  - Premature membrane rupture or vaginal bleeding
  - Postmaturity
- Habits:
  - Smoking, vaping and tobacco use.
  - Regular alcohol intake
  - Drug use or abuse

The record also may include information used to estimate the fetal age, such as time since last menses, ultrasound measurement of the fetus's crown-to-rump length, and biochemical analysis of amniotic fluid to obtain levels of chemical indicators of fetal lung maturity. See Chapter 2 for details on interpreting these and other measures of gestational age.

Perinatal and Neonatal Data

A separate medical record is established for neonates, which includes birth and delivery information such as the delivery position, presence of meconium, the 1- and 5-minute Apgar scores, and any significant interventions immediately following the birth, such as intubation, resuscitation, and positive pressure ventilation after delivery. The Apgar score is an assessment of the infant's color, heart rate, reflex irritability, muscle tone, and respiratory effort, each rated from 0 to 2. Scores thus range from 10 for a stable, responsive neonate to 0 if stillborn.

Sleep Studies Results

Sleep disorders or **dyssomnias** are widespread, with obstructive sleep apnea (OSA) being the most common form. Common to all dyssomnias is the symptom of excessive daytime sleepiness, usually assessed using the Epworth Sleepiness Scale (ESS). The ESS is a simple, eight-item questionnaire that evaluates the likelihood of a patient dozing off in several everyday situations. Scores range from 0 to 24, with the threshold value of 10 indicating the need for further evaluation.

In addition to the assessment for daytime sleepiness, the record may include information relevant to assessing the patient's risk for sleep disorders. A simple tool and helpful mnemonic used to assess these risk factors is the STOP-BANG Questionnaire, as depicted in **Table 1-10**. A "Yes" answer to three or more questions indicates a high risk of OSA.

Table 1-10 STOP-BANG Questionnaire*

STOP		
S (*snore*)	Do you snore loudly (louder than talking or loud enough to be heard through doors)?	Yes No
T (*tired*)	Do you often feel tired, fatigued, or sleepy during the daytime?	Yes No
O (*observed*)	Has anyone observed you stop breathing during sleep?	Yes No
P (blood *pressure*)	Do you have or are you being treated for high blood pressure?	Yes No
BANG		
B (*body mass index [BMI]*)	BMI > 35 kg/m²?	Yes No
A (*age*)	Age > 50 years old?	Yes No
N (*neck circumference*)	Neck circumference > 40 cm?	Yes No
G (*gender*)	Male gender?	Yes No

*Republished with permission of Oxford University Press from Chung et al. High STOP-Bang score indicates a high probability of obstructive sleep apnoea. *Br J Anaesth.* 2012;108(5):768–775. Permission conveyed through Copyright Clearance Center, Inc.

Date: 3/19/2013	Patient: Jane Doe	Patient ID: 1234567

Exam: Standard attended laboratory PSG measuring 2 EEG channels, 2 EOG channels, chin EMG, ECG, leg activity, O_2 saturation, thoraco-abdominal movements, and nasal airflow

Summary Data	
Bedtime: 22:38 Time in bed (min): 465.5 Total sleep time (min): 387.5 Sleep efficiency: 83.4% Wake before sleep (min): 15 Wake during sleep (min): 59.5 Wake after sleep (min): 3 Number of arousals: 8 % Stage wake: 16.6%	% Stage 1: 4.3% % Stage 2: 63.7% % Stage 3–4: 4.9% % Stages REM: 27.1% Latency to stage 1 (min): 10 Latency to stage 2 (min): 19 Latency to persistent sleep (min): 16.5 Latency to stage REM (min): 104

ECG: Usual heart rate in wake was 76, in sleep 70.

EEG: Percentage of REM sleep was increased versus normal, and REM latency was longer than normal.

EMG: There were occasional increases in muscle activity in sleep with abnormal respiratory events.

Respiration: There were 110 abnormal respiratory events (17/hour sleep), with 70% being primarily obstructive apneas/hypopneas and the rest respiratory effort-related arousals (RERAs). Waking O_2 saturation was 95%. During apnea/hypopnea events the Spo_2 declined to 89% in NREM sleep and 86% in REM sleep. Audio monitoring revealed snoring during REM respiratory events. Sao_2 was below 88% for < 2 min/hour sleep.

Medications: None.

Interpretation: Moderate obstructive sleep apnea syndrome (OSAS) (ICD Code: 780.53-0).

Figure 1-2 Sample Polysomnography Report.

For patients at risk for sleep disorders such as OSA, tests such as overnight oximetry or the more definitive polysomnogram (sleep study) may be ordered to help make the diagnosis. A polysomnogram is a continuous recording of variables that measure sleep stages and cardiopulmonary function during sleep. Variables typically measured include the electroencephalogram (EEG); the electro-oculogram (EOG); the electromyogram (EMG); Spo_2; nasal airflow; and chest, abdominal, and leg movements. **Figure 1-2** provides a sample polysomnography report similar to that usually found in the patient record.

Full interpretation of a sleep study report requires the expertise of a physician trained in sleep disorders. However, the application of the basic definitions provided in **Table 1-11** can help you assess the presence and severity of a patient's sleep disorder.

Based on generally accepted guidelines, the severity of the disorder is judged according to the frequency of either apnea-hypopnea index (AHI) or respiratory disturbance index (RDI) events as follows:

- 0–4/h = Normal range
- 5–14/h = Mild sleep apnea
- 15–30/h = Moderate sleep apnea
- > 30/h = Severe sleep apnea

If a patient is diagnosed with a sleep disorder, several treatment options are available. Chapter 4 contains more details on the treatment of sleep disorders.

Trends in Monitoring Results

Fluid Balance (Intake and Output)

Fluid balance is the relationship between fluid intake, mainly from drinking and IV infusion, and output, primarily from urination. Usually, intake equals output, with each being about 2–3 liters per day in adults. A positive fluid balance results from excessive intake or decreased output and may contribute to pulmonary or peripheral edema and hypertension. A negative fluid balance is generally due to insufficient hydration and excessive urine output due to diuretics administration or due

Table 1-11 Definitions Related to Sleep Studies

Term	Definition
Obstructive apnea	A cessation of airflow (> 80% reduction in flow) for at least 10 seconds, during which there is *a continued effort to breathe*
Central apnea	A cessation of airflow (> 80% reduction in flow) for at least 10 seconds, during which there is *no effort to breathe*
Hypopnea	A reduction in airflow of at least 30% from baseline lasting at least 10 seconds and associated with significant oxygen desaturation (> 3–4%)
Apnea-hypopnea index (AHI)	The average number of apneas and hypopneas occurring per hour of sleep
Respiratory effort–related arousal (RERA)	A 10-second or longer sequence of breaths with increasing respiratory effort leading to an arousal from sleep
Respiratory disturbance index (RDI)	The average number of apneas, hypopneas, and RERAs occurring per hour of sleep

to excessive vomiting and diarrhea (most common in children). **Table 1-12** outlines the common causes, clinical signs, and lab values associated with abnormal fluid gain and loss. In assessing output, you should note that urine is usually 60% of the total (1200–1500 mL/day), equivalent to a rate of at least 50 mL/h. Values below 25 mL/h are considered abnormal and termed **oliguria**. Chapter 13 covers recommendations related to adjusting fluid balance.

Vital Signs

In regard to vital signs, the NBRC expects you to know the normal reference ranges by major age group, as delineated in **Table 1-13**. **Table 1-14** outlines the common causes of abnormal trends in vital signs and possible corrective actions.

Intracranial Pressure

Intracranial pressure (ICP) is the pressure inside the skull and thus in the brain tissue, blood, and cerebrospinal fluid (CSF), as measured by either an intraventricular catheter or intraparenchymal probe. ICP commonly is monitored in patients with traumatic brain injury (TBI), intracranial hemorrhage, or cerebral edema.

In supine healthy adults, the ICP ranges between 10 and 15 mm Hg. An ICP > 20 mm Hg for more than 5 to 10 minutes is considered abnormally high in an adult. Pressures > 25 mm Hg for a prolonged period of time are associated with poor patient outcomes.

Decreased ICP may result from the following:

- Head elevation
- Decrease in CSF volume
- Severe arterial hypotension
- Hyperventilation/hypocapnia

Increased ICP may result from the following:

- Increased volume of the following:
  - Brain (edema or tumor)
  - Blood inside the skull (hemorrhage/hematoma)
- Restricted venous outflow (central venous pressure [CVP] > ICP)
- Right heart failure/cor pulmonale
- High intrathoracic pressure (positive end-expiratory pressure [PEEP], recruitment maneuvers)
- Severe arterial hypertension
- Hypoventilation/hypercapnia
- Hypoxia

Note also that the following procedures can cause a rise in ICP and should be performed with great care or avoided in affected patients:

- Moving/positioning the patient (especially Trendelenburg position)
- Flexion and hyperextension of the neck

Table 1-12 Common Causes, Clinical Signs, and Lab Values Associated with Abnormal Fluid Gain and Loss

Abnormal Fluid Gain (Fluid Overload)	Abnormal Fluid Loss (Fluid Depletion)
Common Causes	
Congestive heart failure	Diarrhea
Renal failure	Vomiting
High sodium intake	Sweating/fever
Cirrhosis of the liver	Hemorrhage
Over-infusion of fluids, TPN, blood products	Diuretics
	Excessive urination
Clinical Signs	
CNS: Confusion, tremors, ataxia, convulsions	CNS: sleepy, apathy, stupor, coma
CV: ↑ CVP, venous distension	CV: rapid/thready pulse, collapsed veins, ↓ BP
Respiratory: copious secretions, crackles, orthopnea	Respiratory: thick, inspissated secretions
Skin: pitting edema, anasarca	Skin: decreased skin turgor, atonia
Face/mouth: Periorbital edema, moist tongue,	Face/mouth: sunken eyes, dry tongue,
weight gain, bulging fontanelle (neonates/infants)	weight loss, sunken fontanelle (neonates/infants)
Lab Values	
↓ Hematocrit	↑ Hematocrit
↓ BUN	↑ BUN
↓ Serum osmolality	↑ Serum osmolality
↓ Urine specific gravity	↑ Urine specific gravity
BP, blood pressure; BUN, blood urea nitrogen; CNS, central nervous system; CV, cardiovascular; CVP, central venous pressure; ↓, decreased; ↑, increased; TPN, total parenteral nutrition.	

- Intubation
- Suctioning/coughing
- Ventilator related
  - Asynchrony
  - High PEEP/high mean airway pressure (MAP)
  - Recruitment maneuvers

Ventilator Liberation Parameters

Bedside respiratory monitoring data usually are recorded for patients at risk for developing respiratory failure or those being assessed for liberation from mechanical ventilation. **Table 1-15** summarizes the commonly cited adult reference ranges for these measures, as well as the critical threshold values that indicate a patient's inability to maintain adequate spontaneous breathing.

Among these measures, the respiratory rate and rapid shallow breathing index (RSBI) are the best indicators of whether a patient being considered for weaning can tolerate spontaneous breathing. The maximal inspiratory pressure (MIP)/negative inspiratory force (NIF) and vital capacity (Vc) measures are less frequently obtained, being used primarily to monitor spontaneously breathing patients with neuromuscular disorders for changes in respiratory muscle strength and function. Actual

Table 1-13 Reference Ranges for Vital Sign Measurements

Vital Sign	Adult	Child	Infant
Temperature	98.6°F (37°C)	37.5°C	37.5°C
Pulse	60–100/min	80–120/min	90–170/min
Respiratory rate	12–20/min	20–25/min	35–45/min
Blood pressure	< 120/80 mm Hg	94/52 mm Hg	84/52 mm Hg

Table 1-14 Abnormal Trends in Vital Signs

Trend	Possible Cause	Possible Corrective Actions
Increased heart rate (tachycardia)	• Anxiety/pain • ↓ PaO_2, ↓ or ↑ $PaCO_2$ • Medications • Trauma • Fever • Failure to wean from mechanical ventilation • Ventilator asynchrony	• Relieve anxiety; treat pain • Stabilize blood gases • Treat the fever and the cause of the fever • If failure to wean, return to previous settings • Check patient-ventilator synchrony; obtain and evaluate ABG • Negative chronotropic agents (e.g., calcium channel blockers, beta-blockers)
Decreased heart rate (bradycardia)	• Hypothermia • Medications • Cardiac disease • Cardiopulmonary arrest	• Provide a warm blanket and fluids • Evaluate cardiac status (ECG, cardiac enzymes) • Positive chronotropic agents (e.g., atropine, epinephrine, dopamine) • Perform cardiopulmonary resuscitation (CPR) if needed
Irregular heart rate (atrial fibrillation [A-fib], atrial flutter [A-flutter] with variable block, PVCs, type I [Wenckebach] second-degree AV block)	• Hypoxemia • Electrolyte imbalances • Coronary artery disease • Mitral valve insufficiency • Congenital heart defects • Medications • Caffeine • Thyrotoxicosis	• Treat underlying cause (e.g., hypoxemia, electrolyte imbalance) • Antiarrhythmic drugs • Cardioversion (A-fib/A-flutter) • Radiofrequency ablation • Pacemaker
Increased blood pressure (hypertension)	• Anxiety/pain • Response to ↓ PaO_2, ↓ $PaCO_2$ • Medications • Cardiovascular disease • Trauma (sympathetic response)	• Reassure; alleviate fear; relieve and treat pain • Obtain and evaluate ABG • Assess for cardiovascular events • Evaluate patient for cardiovascular risk factors • Antihypertensive medication
Decreased blood pressure (hypotension)	• Hypovolemia • Trauma (bleeding) • Medications • Cardiovascular collapse	• Fluid resuscitation • Surgical intervention to stop the hemorrhage • Vasoactive drugs to increase BP (e.g., dopamine) • Provide CPR if necessary
Fever	• Infection • ↑ Metabolic rate caused by ↑ work of breathing • Overheated humidifier	• Treat infection; review precautions • Check for mucus plugs; assess ETT position • Check sensitivity and patient-ventilator settings • Check the temperature of humidifier heater

Trend	Possible Cause	Possible Corrective Actions
Increased respiratory rate (tachypnea)	• Anxiety/pain • Altered ventilator settings • ↓ Pao_2 or ↑ $Paco_2$ • Failure to wean during mechanical ventilation • Ventilator asynchrony • ↑ Metabolic rate (fever, infection)	• Reassure; alleviate fear; relieve/treat pain • Check patient–ventilator settings • Obtain and evaluate ABG • If failure to wean return to previous settings • Check patient–ventilator settings; adjust settings or recommend sedation • Evaluate the patient's metabolic rate
Decreased respiratory rate (bradypnea)	• Sleep • Oversedation • ↓ $Paco_2$ • ↓ Metabolic rate • Respiratory failure/arrest • Hypothermia	• Normal observation during sleep • Reverse sedation or provide support • Restore normal ventilatory status • Provide airway and ventilatory support if necessary • Warm blanket and fluids
Irregular Breathing		
Kussmaul: deep and fast respirations	• Metabolic acidosis (e.g., diabetic ketoacidosis)	• Treat underlying cause
Biot: clusters of rapid breaths interspersed with periods of apnea	• Damage to medulla by stroke or trauma • Brain herniation/↑ ICP	• Treat underlying cause • Lower ICP
Cheyne-Stokes: cycles of progressive rise/fall in V_T followed by periods of apnea	• CNS diseases • Congestive heart failure (CHF)	• Treat underlying cause • Bilevel or adaptive servo-ventilation
Agonal: gasping, labored, and sometimes noisy respirations	• Cerebral ischemia • Cerebral hypoxia/anoxia	• Treat underlying cause

ABG, arterial blood gas; AV, atrioventricular; BP, blood pressure; CNS, central nervous system; CPR, cardiopulmonary resuscitation; ↓, decreased; ECG, electrocardiogram; ETT, endotracheal tube; ICP, intracranial pressure; ↑, increased; PVC, premature ventricular contraction; V_T, tidal volume.

Table 1-15 Adult Respiratory Monitoring Thresholds

Parameter	Reference Range	Critical Threshold*
Tidal volume (V_T)	5–7 mL/kg PBW†	< 4–5 mL/kg PBW or < 300 mL
Respiratory rate/frequency (f)	12–20/min	< 6/min or > 30–35/min
Minute volume/ventilation ($\dot{V}E$)	5–10 L/min	< 4 L/min or > 10 L/min
Rapidshallow breathing index (RSBI) ($f/V_{T[L]}$)	< 50	> 105
Deadspace fraction (V_D/V_T)	0.25–0.35	> 0.6–0.7
Vital capacity (Vc)	70 mL/kg PBW	< 10–15 mL/kg PBW
Maximal inspiratory pressure (MIP)/negative inspiratory force (NIF)	80–100 cm H_2O (negative)	< 20–25 cm H_2O (negative)

PBW, predicted body weight; SB, spontaneous breathing.

*Indicating possible inability to maintain adequate spontaneous ventilation.

†PBW for males (kg) = 50 + 2.3 (height [in] − 60)

†PBW for females (kg) = 45.5 + 2.3 (height [in] − 60)

Table 1-16 Common Causes of Abnormal Pulmonary Mechanics

Decreased Lung Compliance	Decreased Thoracic Compliance	Increased Airway Resistance
Pulmonary fibrosis (C)	Kyphoscoliosis (C)	Bronchospasm (I + E)
Pulmonary edema/ARDS (A)	Obesity (C)	Small airway closure (E)
Atelectasis/mainstem intubation (A)	Pectus excavatum (C)	Increased secretions (I + E)
Pneumothorax (A)	Fibrothorax (C)	Airway edema (I + E)
Large pleural effusion (A or C)	Chest wall tumor (C)	Airway tumors (I + E)
Surfactant deficiency (A)	Circumferential chest burns (A)	Artificial airway occlusion (I + E)
A, acute; C, chronic; I, inspiratory; E, expiratory.		

measurement of the deadspace fraction (V_D/V_T) ratio (via the Bohr equation) is uncommon; however, this parameter can be estimated via volumetric capnography.

Pulmonary Mechanics and the Work of Breathing

Pulmonary mechanics data include measures of respiratory system compliance and airway resistance. Although some ICU ventilators automate the measurement of these parameters, the NBRC expects candidates to be able to make these computations at the bedside manually. Chapters 3 and 4 detail the measurement procedures and assessment of compliance and resistance during mechanical ventilation.

As measured via body plethysmography, respiratory system compliance (lung + thoracic) normally is about 100 mL/cm H_2O. Normal values obtained during mechanical ventilation usually are lower, in the range of 40–80 mL/cm H_2O. During volume-controlled (VC) ventilation, a reduction in compliance is indicated by rising plateau pressures. **Table 1-16** outlines the common causes of decreased lung and thoracic compliance, both acute and chronic. Note that due to loss of elastic tissue, lung compliance typically increases in patients with emphysema.

Normal airway resistance measured via plethysmography ranges from 1 to 3 cm H_2O/L/sec in a healthy subject. During mechanical ventilation, the artificial airway adds at least 4–6 cm H_2O/L/sec to the total resistance. Thus, levels significantly above 5–9 cm H_2O/L/sec are associated with airway obstruction (see Table 1-15). During VC ventilation, an increase in airway resistance is related to a widening of the difference between the peak and plateau pressures.

Work of breathing (WOB) is a measurement of the energy used to breathe. The normal reference range for healthy adults is 0.5–0.7 joules/L, obtained by computing the area of an esophageal pressure-volume curve during spontaneous breathing. Any condition that decreases overall compliance or increases airway resistance will also increase WOB (see Table 1-15).

Estimates of the WOB can be obtained during mechanical ventilation using the pressure-volume graphics display. Alternatively, you can estimate the inspiratory work of breathing during volume ventilation using the area under the airway pressure curve (the pressure-time product). More commonly, you can conclude that a patient likely is experiencing increased WOB based on the clinical signs of tachypnea and accessory muscle use.

Noninvasive Monitoring Data

Pulse Oximetry

Pulse oximetry (Spo_2) measures hemoglobin saturation in the blood during peak systolic pulsation. The reference range for adults breathing room air is 95–98%, with values below 88–90% on any Fio_2 indicating arterial hypoxemia. Drops in Spo_2 are usually the result of cardiac, pulmonary, or combined cardiopulmonary disease. Significant declines (more than 4–5%) during exercise or sleep are abnormal.

Because the relationship between Spo_2 and Pao_2 is often misunderstood, we recommend application of the "40–50–60/70–80–90" rule of thumb—that is, *Pao$_2$ values of 40, 50, and 60 torr roughly correspond to saturation values of 70%, 80%, and 90%, respectively.*

Also critical in assessing Spo_2 values is the knowledge that standard pulse oximetry is *not* accurate in victims of carbon monoxide (CO) poisoning and the understanding that readings may be affected by movement artifacts, skin pigmentation, and peripheral circulation.

Table 1-17 Conditions Associated with Changes in Petco$_2$

	Rise in Petco$_2$	Fall in Petco$_2$
Sudden change	• A sudden increase in cardiac output (e.g., return of spontaneous circulation [ROSC] during CPR) • A sudden release of a tourniquet • Injection of sodium bicarbonate • Tracheal intubation	• Sudden hyperventilation • A sudden drop in cardiac output/cardiac arrest* • Massive pulmonary/air embolism • Circuit leak/disconnection* • Esophageal intubation* • Endotracheal (ET)/trach tube obstruction or dislodgement*
Gradual change	• Hypoventilation • Increased metabolism/CO$_2$ production (fever) • Rapid rise in temperature (malignant hyperthermia)	• Hyperventilation • Decreased metabolism/CO$_2$ production • Decreased pulmonary perfusion • Decrease in body temperature

*Can result in a Petco$_2$ of 0 torr.

Data from Gentile MA, Heuer AJ, Kallet RH. Analysis and monitoring of gas exchange. In Kacmarek RM, Stoller JK, Heuer AJ, eds. *Egan's Fundamentals of Respiratory Care* (11th ed.). St. Louis, MO: Mosby; 2017.

Transcutaneous Monitoring

The transcutaneous partial pressure of O$_2$ (Ptco$_2$) and CO$_2$ (Ptcco$_2$) can be monitored continuously via the application of a heated sensor on the skin. Although initially used in neonates, Ptco$_2$/Ptcco$_2$ monitoring also can be used in older children and adults. In assessing these data, candidates need to know that the Ptcco$_2$ closely approximates the arterial Pco$_2$ under most conditions, making it a useful measure in evaluating real-time changes in ventilation during mechanical ventilation. On the other hand, the Ptco$_2$ is equivalent to the arterial Pao$_2$ only in well-perfused patients and when Pao$_2$ is less than 100 torr. The Ptco$_2$ value underestimates the Pao$_2$ value in perfusion states causing vasoconstriction (e.g., low cardiac output, shock, dehydration) and when Pao$_2$ is greater than 100 torr. Ptco$_2$ also tends to underestimate Pao$_2$ in children and adults, due to their thicker skin.

Capnography

Capnometry measures carbon dioxide concentration in expired gases. Capnography is the measurement and *graphical display* of CO$_2$ levels, usually the end-tidal Pco$_2$, or Petco$_2$. Chapter 5 outlines the indications for capnography, and Chapter 6 provides details on the setup and calibration of capnographs.

In patients with healthy lungs, the Petco$_2$ provides a reasonable estimate of the arterial Pco$_2$, typically running 2–5 torr below the normal ABG value, or between 30 and 43 torr. **Table 1-17** differentiates between the causes of sudden and gradual changes in Petco$_2$ readings. Chapter 4 provides additional detail on interpreting capnography data, including analysis of the real-time graphic display of Petco$_2$.

Comparing the Petco$_2$ to the Paco$_2$ via the difference between the two measures (the Paco$_2$ – Petco$_2$ gradient) also can help spot changes in patient status. Specifically, a rise in the Paco$_2$ –Petco$_2$ difference indicates an increase in physiologic deadspace, most commonly associated with decreased perfusion to ventilated areas of the lung, as occurs in acute pulmonary embolism.

Cardiovascular Evaluation and Monitoring Data

Key cardiovascular monitoring data with which the NBRC expects candidates to be familiar include electrocardiograms (ECGs), hemodynamic parameters, and cardiac catheterization and echocardiogram reports.

ECG Rhythms

Cardiac dysrhythmias can be classified as being lethal (causing death) and nonlethal. Here we provide a brief discussion of common nonlethal dysrhythmias, along with example ECG rhythm strips. Chapter 15 covers the identification and protocol-based (Advanced Cardiac Life Support [ACLS]) management of lethal rhythms.

Tachycardia (Figure 1-3) is identified in the ECG rhythm strip as follows:

- Rate of 100–180 beats/min (adults)
- PR interval usually < 0.2 sec
- A P wave for every QRS complex
- Shortened R-R interval (< 0.60 sec) with normal QRS complexes

For common causes and treatment recommendations, review the previous section on vital signs.

Bradycardia (Figure 1-4) is identified in the ECG rhythm strip as follows:

- Rate < 60 beats/min (adults)
- Regular rhythm with a normal PR interval
- Normal P waves followed by regular QRS complexes
- A prolonged (> 1 sec) R-R interval

For common causes and treatment recommendations, review the previous section on vital signs.

Atrial fibrillation (Figure 1-5) is identified in the ECG rhythm strip as follows:

- Irregular rhythm
- Variation in interval and amplitude in the R-R interval (more than 10% variation)
- Absent P wave with "fibrillatory" baseline

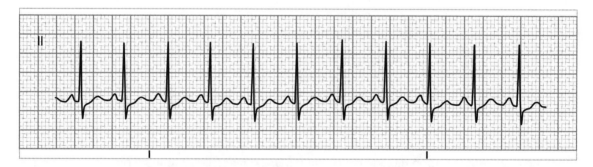

Figure 1-3 Example of Sinus Tachycardia (Rate ≈ 130/min).

Reproduced from Garcia T, Miller GT. *Arrhythmia recognition: The art of interpretation.* Sudbury, MA: Jones and Bartlett; 2004.

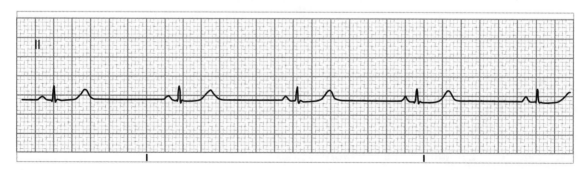

Figure 1-4 Example of Sinus Bradycardia (Rate ≈ 45/min).

Reproduced from Garcia T, Miller GT. *Arrhythmia recognition: The art of interpretation.* Sudbury, MA: Jones and Bartlett; 2004.

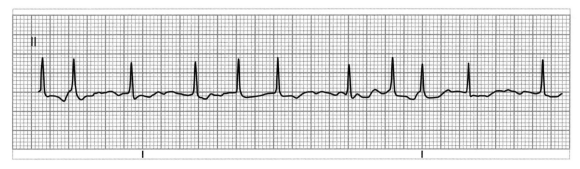

Figure 1-5 Example of Atrial Fibrillation.

Reproduced from Garcia T, Miller GT. *Arrhythmia recognition: The art of interpretation.* Sudbury, MA: Jones and Bartlett; 2004.

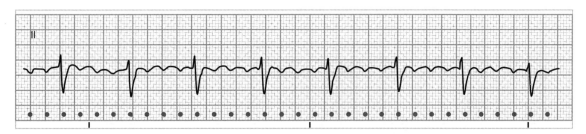

Figure 1-6 Example of Atrial Flutter with 4:1 Conduction Ratio.

Reproduced from Garcia T, Miller GT. *Arrhythmia recognition: The art of interpretation.* Sudbury, MA: Jones and Bartlett; 2004.

Atrial fibrillation can be a side effect of β-agonist drugs (e.g., albuterol). If it occurs during treatment, stop the treatment, stabilize the patient, and notify the physician. If this rhythm was already present before the therapy, assess the patient's baseline heart rate and history, and consult with the patient's nurse and physician before administering treatment.

Atrial flutter (Figure 1-6) is identified in the ECG rhythm strip as follows:

- Classic "sawtooth" pattern seen in between the QRS complexes
- Absence of a PR interval

Causes and treatment recommendations are the same as with atrial fibrillation.

Premature ventricular contractions (PVCs) (Figure 1-7) are identified in the ECG rhythm strip as follows:

- Abnormal QRS complexes (> 0.12 sec in width)
- Underlying rhythm usually regular but becomes irregular with a PVC
- No P wave present before the PVC
- T waves deflected in the opposite direction following the PVC

PVCs can be caused by anxiety, caffeine, tobacco, alcohol, and certain drugs, such as β-agonists and theophylline. PVCs also can be caused by myocardial ischemia, acidosis, electrolyte imbalance, hypoxia, and direct myocardial stimulation. Many respiratory procedures can cause hypoxemia or myocardial stimulation. If PVCs occur while you are performing any respiratory procedure, stop what you are doing, provide supplemental O_2 to stabilize the patient, and notify the physician immediately.

Hemodynamic Parameters

Hemodynamic measures are often obtained on critically ill patients to assess cardiovascular function, monitor/adjust fluid balance, or titrate drug administration. **Table 1-18** lists the most common

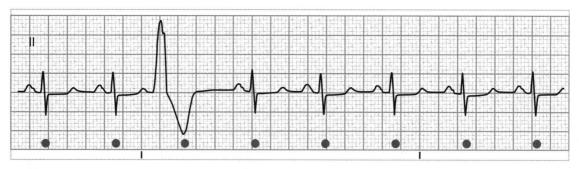

Figure 1-7 Example of a Sinus Rhythm with a Premature Ventricular Contraction.

Reproduced from Garcia T, Miller GT. *Arrhythmia recognition: The art of interpretation.* Sudbury, MA: Jones and Bartlett; 2004.

Table 1-18 Common Hemodynamic Parameter Reference Values (Adults)

Parameter	Reference Values*
Systolic blood pressure	< 120 mm Hg
Diastolic blood pressure	< 80 mm Hg
Mean arterial blood pressure (MAP)	70–105 mm Hg
Central venous pressure (CVP)	2–6 mm Hg
Right atrial pressure	2–6 mm Hg
Right ventricular pressure, systolic	15–30 mm Hg
Right ventricular pressure, diastolic	2–8 mm Hg
Pulmonary artery (PA) pressure, systolic	15–30 mm Hg
PA pressure, diastolic	8–15 mm Hg
PA pressure, mean	9–18 mm Hg
PA wedge pressure (PAWP)	6–12 mm Hg
Cardiac output (CO)	4.0–8.0 L/min
Cardiac index (CI)	2.5–4.0 L/min/m^2
Stroke volume (SV)	60–130 mL/beat
Stroke index (SI)	30–50 mL/m^2
Ejection fraction (EF)	65–75%
Systemic vascular resistance (SVR)[†]	900–1400 dynes-sec/cm^5
Pulmonary vascular resistance (PVR)[†]	110–250 dynes-sec/cm^5

* Reference ranges vary by institution and specific sources. However, exam candidates should be fine in using these ranges for the purposes of the NBRC exams.

[†] To convert resistance measures from dynes-sec/cm^5 to mm Hg/L/min, divide by 80.

hemodynamic measures and their adult reference values. Details on the interpretation of hemodynamic data are provided in Chapter 4.

Cardiac Catheterization

Cardiac catheterization helps to diagnose structural abnormalities of the heart and its chambers or valves via measurement of chamber and vessel pressures, as well as visualization of chamber volumes and flows, also via contrast media imaging (ventriculography). For patients diagnosed with coronary artery disease (CAD), cardiac catheterization also provides several treatment options, including coronary angioplasty (aka balloon dilatation or percutaneous transluminal coronary angioplasty [PTCA]), coronary artery stenting, or coronary artery atherectomy (plaque removal).

Generally, at least a 50–70% reduction in the diameter of a blocked artery must occur before there is a severe decrease in the blood flow to the surrounding myocardium. Typically, this is the point at which a doctor will recommend treatment, either by catheterization or by coronary artery bypass graft (CABG) surgery.

Echocardiography

Echocardiography provides noninvasive indices of cardiac performance (e.g., ejection fraction, cardiac output) and estimates of flows and pressures in the great vessels. The following sections provide a summary of expected echocardiography findings for the disorders most commonly seen by respiratory therapists (RTs).

Persistent Pulmonary Hypertension of the Newborn (PPHN)

- Presence of right-to-left shunting (especially during systole) at the ductus arteriosus and possibly the foramen ovale
- Absence of congenital heart disease (e.g., partial/total anomalous pulmonary venous return)
- High-pressure gradient across tricuspid valve with regurgitation (insufficiency)
- High pulmonary artery pressure
- Enlargement of the right ventricle (RV), right atrium (RA), and pulmonary artery (PA)
- Flattening or bowing of the interventricular septum toward the left

Pulmonary Arterial Hypertension (PAH)

- High velocity of tricuspid regurgitation
- Estimated systolic PAP > 36 mm Hg without evidence of obstruction to right-sided flow (e.g., pulmonic valve stenosis)
- Enlarged pulmonary artery
- Pulmonic valve regurgitation
- Possible dilated right ventricle with reduced systolic function
- Possible displacement of the interventricular septum to the left
- Possible right atrial enlargement
- Possible pericardial effusion
- Normal left ventricular systolic and diastolic function
- Absence of left-sided valvular or congenital heart disease

Heart Failure

- Systolic failure (decreased left ventricular [LV] contractility)
    - Increased LV end-diastolic volume
    - Increased LV end-diastolic pressure
    - Decreased LV ejection fraction (< 45%)
- Diastolic failure (abnormal LV filling, high filling pressures)
- Normal or decreased LV end-diastolic volume
- Increased LV end-diastolic pressure (lessened by Valsalva maneuver)
- Normal LV ejection fraction (> 50%)
- Enlarged left atrium, with possible bulging of the interatrial septum to the right
- Evidence of slow LV relaxation, early filling, and decreased chamber compliance
- Increased PA pressures
- Absence of valvular heart disease, intracardiac shunts, cardiac tamponade, or pericardial constriction

Determination of a Patient's Pathophysiologic State

Success on the NBRC exams (especially on the CSE) requires proficiency in case and disease management. In the NBRC "hospital," RTs are expected to be broadly experienced in diagnosing and managing a large variety of conditions and disorders, including those affecting various organ systems and patient age categories, as well as different levels of acuity.

Traditionally, the model of clinical practice recommends a diagnosis, prognosis, and treatment approach to manage the most common diseases. However, to use this approach, RTs must have a working knowledge of the clinical manifestations associated with a particular respiratory disease or condition. A cornerstone of this working knowledge is the ability to evaluate the data gathered from the medical record and patient examination. If the correct data are not gathered, and interpreted properly the ability to effectively manage the patient is lost.

By having this knowledge you will be in a better position to (1) gather and evaluate the clinical data relevant to the patient's respiratory status, (2) assess the severity of the disease or condition, and (3) select and implement a treatment plan that is based on the data gathered and disease severity assessment.

By understanding this approach, you will be able to determine a patient's pathophysiology state and succeed in both the TMC and the CSE, especially on the decision-making sections of the exam.

T⁴—TOP TEST-TAKING TIPS

You can improve your score on this section of the NBRC exam by reviewing these tips:

- Factors such as a patient's place of residence and age may be relevant in that some respiratory conditions tend to be more common in certain age groups, in specific geographic locations, and among certain ethnic groups.
- If an order for respiratory care is incomplete or falls outside institutional standards, contact the originator for clarification.
- Smoking, tobacco use, and vaping may contribute to respiratory disorders and should be noted along with alcohol or drug use, social activities, hobbies, recreational activities, and pets.
- Do not initiate resuscitation on a patient with a DNR order or comparable advance directive; however, if in doubt, *always proceed with resuscitation.*
- List all current medications at admission (including respiratory medications taken at home) to prevent medication discrepancies, medication errors and drug interactions during patient management and discharge.
- During physical examination, assess for central lines such as pulmonary artery catheter (PAC), femoral venous lines, arterial lines, and PIC lines; oropharyngeal/nasopharyngeal gastric tube and feeding tubes; chest tubes and wound drainage systems; endotracheal or tracheostomy airway tubes; cranial drainage systems.
- Be sure to know the normal vital signs for children and infants in addition to the adult norms.
- Elevated overall white blood cell (WBC) count and differential WBC values such as neutrophils and bands suggest an acute bacterial infection.
- Increased RBCs may be associated with chronic hypoxemia (secondary polycythemia).
- Cardiac markers such as troponin can help confirm the occurrence of acute myocardial infarction, whereas BNP levels can help diagnose CHF.
- The hematocrit (Hct) is affected by fluid volume (i.e., inadequate fluid volume/hemoconcentration [high Hct] or excessive fluid volume/hemodilution [low Hct]).
- Potassium levels typically run high in metabolic acidosis and low in metabolic alkalosis; low chloride levels are associated with metabolic alkalosis.
- Sputum culture and sensitivities, together with gram staining, are used to identify the causative agent in bacterial pneumonia.
- High lactic acid levels indicate tissue hypoxia, usually due to poor perfusion/shock.
- Identify the primary acid-base disturbance using the pH and $Paco_2$:
  - ↓ pH, $Paco_2 > 45$ torr = respiratory acidosis
  - ↓ pH, $Paco_2 \leq 45$ torr = metabolic acidosis

- ○ ↑ pH, $Pa_{CO_2} < 35$ torr = respiratory alkalosis
- ○ ↑ pH, Pa_{CO_2} normal = metabolic alkalosis
- When judging the degree of hypoxemia, *always consider the Fio₂*—a P_{O_2} of 65 torr on room air is mild hypoxemia; a P_{O_2} of 65 torr on 70% O_2 indicates a severe disturbance in arterial oxygenation.
- The most common acid-base disturbance in acute conditions causing hypoxemia (e.g., asthma, pneumonia) is uncompensated respiratory alkalosis; the alkalosis is caused by hyperventilation due to hypoxemia.
- Hemoximetry is indicated when accurate measures of any hemoglobin (Hb) parameters are needed.
- COHb levels of at least 3–4% in nonsmokers and at least 10% in smokers can be considered outside the expected physiologic range.
- 100% O_2 via non-rebreather mask is required to treat smoke inhalation.
- Prolonged cardiopulmonary arrest results in a combined respiratory and metabolic/lactic acidosis with severe hypoxemia.
- Normal PFT values typically are within the range of 80–120% of predicted values; values below 50% predicted are progressively more and more severe.
- Most pulmonary diseases are categorized as restrictive, obstructive, or mixed.
- Judge the reversibility of an obstructive disorder by bronchodilator pre-/post-testing; an increase in flows ≥ 12–15% after bronchodilator therapy confirms reversibility.
- The normal reference range for DL_{CO} is 25–30 mL/min/mm Hg; a low DL_{CO} is observed in disorders such as pulmonary fibrosis and emphysema, whereas higher-than-normal values may occur in polycythemia.
- A 6MWD < 500–600 meters indicates an abnormal functional capacity.
- The chest x-ray of a patient with ARDS typically reveals bilateral lung opacities and infiltrates ("white-out") with *normal heart size.*
- The chest x-ray of a patient with emphysema typically shows low, flat diaphragms, decreased lung and vascular markings (hyperaeration, radiolucency), and increased retrosternal air space (lateral film).
- On ultrasound exam, a pneumothorax is detected by the *absence* of the gliding sign (a normal finding visible as a shimmering of the parietal/visceral pleural line during breathing).
- On a normal pulmonary angiogram, the pulmonary vessels appear as bright white "tree branches"; emboli appear dark and block any further distal flow of the contrast media.
- There is a high probability of pulmonary embolism if a V/Q scan reveals multiple perfusion defects without corresponding ventilation defects.
- Poverty, minority status, obesity, complicated obstetric history, comorbidities, and absence of prenatal care all place the mother or neonate at risk for perinatal problems.
- Obstructive apnea is defined as the cessation of airflow for at least 10 seconds, during which there is *continued effort to breathe*; central apnea also causes a cessation of airflow for at least 10 seconds, during which *no breathing effort occurs.*
- The number of apneas + hypopneas occurring per hour of sleep (the apnea-hypopnea index or AHI) determines the severity of sleep apnea: normal 0–4/h, mild 5–14/h, moderate 15–30/h, and severe > 30/h.
- Normal adult fluid intake and output are each about 2–3 liters per day; urine is the major contributor to output, averaging 1200–1500 mL/day (at least 50 mL/h); adult urine output < 25 mL/h is abnormally low (*oliguria*).
- Signs of fluid overload include weight gain, ↑ CVP, venous distention, crackles on auscultation, pitting edema, and lab values indicating hemodilution (e.g., Hct).
- Signs of dehydration include weight loss, stupor, rapid/thready pulse, collapsed veins, ↓ BP, thick secretions, sunken eyes, and lab values indicating hemoconcentration (e.g., ↑ Hct).
- Whenever vital signs are abnormal, review the patient's medications to see if they may be the cause.
- Kussmaul breathing suggests diabetic ketoacidosis, Biot breathing indicates brain damage/↑ ICP, Cheyne-Stokes breathing can occur in patients with CNS disease or CHF, and agonal breathing is a sign of cerebral hypoxia/anoxia.

- A normal adult ICP is 10–15 mm Hg, a sustained ICP > 20 mm Hg is unsafe, and an ICP > 25 mm Hg is critical; common RT procedures (suctioning, high PEEP) can elevate ICP.
- A vital capacity < 10–15 mL/kg PBW indicates limited ventilatory capacity and is associated in some patients with the need for ventilatory support or difficulty weaning.
- During volume ventilation, reduced compliance causes the plateau pressure (P_{plat}) to rise; acute decreases commonly are due to pulmonary edema, atelectasis, or pneumothorax.
- During volume ventilation, an increase in airway resistance widens the difference between PIP and P_{plat}; common causes of acute increases include bronchospasm, increased secretions, and airway edema.
- Pao_2 values of 40, 50, and 60 torr roughly correspond to saturation values of 70%, 80%, and 90%, respectively.
- The transcutaneous Po_2 ($Ptco_2$) corresponds to the Pao_2 only in well-perfused patients, and when Pao_2 is less than 100 torr; otherwise, it tends to underestimate the Pao_2.
- The end-tidal Pco_2 ($Petco_2$) typically runs 2–5 torr *below* the $Paco_2$, or about 30–43 torr; sudden decreases in $Petco_2$ can be caused by a sudden fall in cardiac output, large pulmonary embolism, circuit leak/disconnection, or ET tube obstruction or dislodgement.
- On an ECG, atrial fibrillation (A-fib) is characterized by an irregular rhythm, absent P waves, and an undulating baseline; A-fib can be a side effect of β-agonist bronchodilators; if it occurs during treatment, stop and notify the physician.
- PVCs indicate irritability of the myocardium (due to many causes, including hypoxemia); if PVCs occurs during treatment, stop, give supplemental O_2, and notify the physician.
- Normal PA systolic pressure is 15–30 mm Hg; normal PA wedge pressure (PAWP or PCWP) is 6–12 mm Hg.
- For patients with coronary artery disease, treatment by catheterization or coronary artery bypass graft is indicated if the diameter of any coronary artery is reduced by > 50–70%.
- Heart valve stenosis increases pressures behind the valve ("back" pressure) but decreases pressures ahead of it; valve regurgitation/insufficiency also can cause the pressure behind a "leaking" valve to increase.
- The echocardiogram of a patient with systolic heart failure (decreased LV contractility) will reveal a low ejection fraction (< 45%); in diastolic failure (abnormal LV filling, high filling pressures), the ejection fraction often is normal (> 50%).

POST-TEST

To confirm your mastery of each chapter's topical content, you should create a content post-test, available online via the Navigate Premier Access for Comprehensive Respiratory Therapy Exam Preparation Guide, which contains Navigate TestPrep (access code provided with every new text). You can create multiple topical content post-tests varying in length from 10 to 20 questions, with each attempt presenting a different set of items. You can select questions from all three major NBRC TMC sections: Patient Data, Troubleshooting and Quality Control of Devices and Infection Control, and Initiation and Modification of Interventions. A score of at least 70–80% indicates that you are adequately prepared for this section of the NBRC TMC exam. If you score below 70%, you should first carefully assess your test answers (particularly your wrong answers) and the correct answer explanations. Then return to the chapter to re-review the applicable content. Only then should you reattempt a new post-test. Repeat this process of identifying your shortcomings and reviewing the pertinent content until your test results demonstrate mastery.

CHAPTER 2

Perform Clinical Assessment (Section I-B)

Albert J. Heuer

Collecting and interpreting patient data via interview, physical examination, and review of x-rays constitutes the third-largest topic on the TMC exam and is extensively covered in case simulations on the CSE. Thus, proficiency in this area is essential if you want to do well on these exams.

OBJECTIVES

In preparing for the shared NBRC exam content (TMC/CSE), you should demonstrate the knowledge needed to:

1. Interview patients to assess:
   a. Level of consciousness, pain, emotional state, and ability to cooperate
   b. Level of pain
   c. Breathing difficulties, exercise tolerance, and sputum production
   d. Smoking history and environmental exposures
   e. Activities of daily living (ADLs)
   f. Learning needs (e.g., literacy, social/culture, preferred learning style)
2. Assess a patient's overall cardiopulmonary status by inspection, palpation, percussion, and auscultation
3. Review and interpret chest and lateral neck radiographs

WHAT TO EXPECT ON THIS CATEGORY OF THE NBRC EXAMS

TMC exam: 10 questions; 3 recall, 6 application, and 1 analysis
CSE exam: indeterminate number of questions; however, section I-B knowledge is a prerequisite to succeed on the CSE, especially on Information Gathering sections.

WHAT YOU NEED TO KNOW: ESSENTIAL CONTENT

Interviewing the Patient

Interviewing provides essential information about a patient's (1) level of consciousness, emotional state, and ability to cooperate; (2) experience of pain; (3) degree of shortness of breath/dyspnea and exercise tolerance; (4) sputum production; (5) smoking history; (6) environmental exposures; (7) activities of daily living; and (8) learning needs.

Level of Consciousness, Emotional State, and Ability to Cooperate

To quickly assess the level of consciousness or "sensorium," ask patients for the time of day (time), where they are (place), and who they are (person).

- Alert patients are well oriented to time, place, and person—"oriented × 3."
- Common causes of disorientation include the following:
  - Neurologic injury
  - Sedation and analgesics (especially opioid)
  - Severe hypoxemia or hypercapnia
- *In general, only alert patients can fully cooperate and participate in their care.*

You must also assess the emotional state of alert patients. A normal emotional state is evident when patients respond with changing facial expressions suitable to the conversation, describe themselves as appropriately concerned about their condition, and appear either relaxed or moderately anxious. Patients in an abnormal emotional state typically seem depressed, overly anxious, or irritable. They may also have difficulty focusing and exhibit breathlessness, dizziness, trembling, palpitations, or chest pain. *In general, patients in an abnormal emotional state will be difficult to manage until their emotional state can be resolved.*

A more comprehensive but easy-to-apply assessment that includes evaluation of alertness is the AVPU Scale. AVPU stands for **A**lert; response to **V**erbal stimulus; response to **P**ain; **U**nresponsive. The following box (**Box 2-1**) outlines the AVPU Scale criteria:

The Glasgow Coma Scale (GCS) provides the most objective assessment of consciousness (**Table 2-1**). To apply this scale, you assess the patient's eye, verbal, and motor responses and score each component on a numeric scale. You then sum the three values to yield a total score, with the lowest value being 3 (deep coma) and the highest value being 15 (fully alert). Relative impairment is interpreted as follows:

- Mild impairment: 13–15
- Moderate impairment: 9–12
- Severe impairment (coma): ≤ 8

Glasgow component scores are often reported in shorthand. For example, a Glasgow score recorded as "E3, V2, M2" indicates an Eyes rating of 3, a Verbal rating of 2, and a Motor rating of 2, for a total score of 7—indicating severe impairment.

Box 2-1 The AVPU Scale

A	**Alert** and oriented. Signifies orientation to time, place, and person. Reported as "oriented × 1, 2, or 3," noting any disorientation—for example, "oriented × 2, unaware of time."
V	Responds to **Verbal** stimulus. Indicates that the patient only responds when verbally prompted. Note if the response is appropriate or inappropriate—for example, if you ask, "What is your name?" and the answer is unclear or confusing, you have obtained a verbal response, but the patient is not appropriately oriented.
P	Responds to **Pain**. If the patient does not respond to verbal stimuli, firmly pinch the patient's skin and note if there is a response (e.g., moaning or withdrawal from the stimulus).
U	**Unresponsive.** If the patient fails to respond to painful stimulus on one side, try the other. A patient who remains flaccid without moving or making a sound is unresponsive.

Table 2-1 Glasgow Coma Scale

	1	2	3	4	5	6
Eyes	Does not open eyes	Opens eyes in response to painful stimuli	Opens eyes in response to verbal stimuli	Opens eyes spontaneously	N/A	N/A
Verbal	Makes no sounds	Unintelligible speech	Utters inappropriate words	Confused, disoriented	Oriented, converses normally	N/A
Motor	Makes no movements (flaccid)	Extension in response to painful stimuli	Abnormal flexion in response to painful stimuli	Flexion/ withdrawal in response to painful stimuli	Localizes painful stimuli	Obeys commands

Level of Pain

- To determine if an alert patient is experiencing pain, ask, "Are you having any pain or discomfort now?"
- If the answer is yes, then the patient is in pain.
- Have the patient rate severity on a scale of 0 (no pain) to 10 (the worst possible pain).
- Patients can use the same scale to pinpoint their maximum tolerable level of pain.

For young children or those unable to express themselves, you can interview family members to get information about behaviors the patient typically exhibits with pain and activities that may cause or worsen it. Without such information, you may have to rely on observing behaviors such as moaning or facial expressions such as grimacing or tearing.

After you determine the severity of pain, you should assess how much it interferes with the patient's daily activities. To do so, use a similar 10-point scale, with 0 signifying "no interference" and 10 signifying "unable to carry out usual activities." *Whenever you encounter an interference rating greater than 4, report this finding to the patient's physician.*

Breathing Difficulties and Exercise Tolerance

The evaluation of patients' breathing difficulties (shortness of breath/dyspnea, orthopnea, etc.) and exercise tolerance is a critical skill for all respiratory therapists (RTs).

Shortness of breath or *dyspnea* is a patient's sensation of breathlessness. *Orthopnea* is a patient's sensation of uncomfortable breathing when lying down, which typically is relieved by sitting or standing up. Both shortness of breath/dyspnea and orthopnea are associated with a variety of cardiac and pulmonary disorders.

The most common method used to quantify a patient's shortness of breath/dyspnea is the Borg Scale (**Table 2-2**). Like the pain scale, the Borg Scale ranges from 0 to 10, with 0 representing no sensation of shortness of breath/dyspnea and 10 representing maximal sensation. As indicated in Table 2-2, the Borg Scale can be used to assess a patient's shortness of breath/dyspnea *or* degree of exertion and is always applied in association with a predefined level of activity (e.g., exercise test level, end of a 6-minute walk). To administer the Borg Scale, have the patient stop the activity, review the ratings, and select the number corresponding to the breathing difficulty being experienced at that moment.

Usually, in combination with shortness of breath/dyspnea, the following observations indicate that a patient is experiencing an abnormally high work of breathing:

- Tachypnea
- Thoracic–abdominal dyssynchrony or paradox ("seesaw" motion)
- Use of accessory muscles of respiration

Table 2-2 Modified Borg Scale

Rating	For Rating Shortness of Breath/Dyspnea	For Rating Exertion
0	Nothing at all	Nothing at all
0.5	Very, very slight (just noticeable)	Very, very weak (just noticeable)
1	Very slight	Very weak
2	Slight	Weak (light)
3	Moderate	Moderate
4	Somewhat severe	Somewhat strong
5	Severe	Strong (heavy)
6*		
7	Very severe	Very strong
8*		
9	Very, very severe (almost maximal)	Very, very strong (almost maximal)
10	Maximal	Maximal

*It allows the patient to choose a middle level of intensity between the preceding and subsequent level of intensity.

Table 2-3 American Thoracic Society Breathlessness Scale*

Grade	Degree	Description of Breathlessness
0	None	Not troubled with breathlessness except with strenuous exercise
1	Slight	Troubled by shortness of breath when hurrying on level ground or walking up a small hill
2	Moderate	Walks slower than people of the same age on level ground because of breathlessness or has to stop for breath when walking at own pace on level ground
3	Severe	Stops for breath after walking about 100 yards or after a few minutes on level ground
4	Very severe	Too breathless to leave the house or breathless when dressing and undressing

*Essentially the same as the Medical Research Council Breathlessness Scale (UK).

Chris Stenton, "The MRC breathlessness scale", Occupational Medicine, Volume 58, Issue 3, 1 May 2008, Pages 226–227. Used with permission from Oxford University Press on behalf of the Society of Occupational Medicine.

The gold standard for assessing a patient's exercise tolerance is a graded cardiopulmonary exercise test. A less rigorous but very useful alternative for evaluating exercise tolerance is the 6-minute walk test (6MWT). Procedures for these tests are covered in Chapter 3, with their interpretation discussed in Chapter 4.

A more straightforward measure for assessing exercise tolerance is the American Thoracic Society (ATS) Breathlessness Scale (**Table 2-3**). By inquiring as to when a patient first notices breathlessness, you can assign a grade of 0–4 to the symptom, with a descriptive term indicating the degree of impairment.

Sputum Production

Sputum assessment should be included in patient history taking and be conducted whenever secretion clearance takes place. Typically, you evaluate the volume, color, and consistency of sputum, as described later in this chapter.

When asking about sputum volume, use familiar measures such as a teaspoon (5 mL), tablespoon (15 mL), or shot glass full (1 oz or 30 mL). When collecting sputum, use a calibrated sputum cup for measurement. *As a rule of thumb, sputum production greater than 30 mL/day indicates the need for airway clearance.*

Smoking History

You should obtain the smoking history of all patients, including whether the habit involves cigarettes, cigars, pipe smoking, and electronic cigarettes primarily. For former smokers, determine how long ago they quit. For current or former cigarette smokers, quantify their smoking history in *pack-years* as follows:

Pack-years = daily packs of cigarettes smoked × number of years smoking

Example: A 38-year-old patient has been smoking 1-1/2 packs per day for 20 years.

Pack-years = 1.5 × 20 = 30 pack-years

The number of cigarettes smoked per day (1 pack = 20 cigarettes) also is a good indicator of nicotine dependence, along with how soon after waking up the patient begins smoking. Patients who smoke more than one pack a day and those who must have their first cigarette upon waking up are heavily nicotine dependent. Note that nicotine dependence can also occur in individuals who inhale nicotine vapor using electronic cigarettes ("vaping"). However, the long-term health effects of vaping are not yet fully understood.

Environmental Exposure

Due to its importance in diagnosis, the occupational and environmental exposure history is often considered a separate category of the interview. The accompanying box (**Box 2-2**) outlines the key areas for questioning patients regarding their occupational and environmental exposure history.

Box 2-2 Outline of Occupational and Environmental Exposure History

Part 1. Exposure Survey

A. Exposures

- Current and past exposure to metals, dust, fibers, fumes, chemicals, biologic hazards, radiation, or noise
- Typical workday (job tasks, location, materials, and agents used)
- Changes in routines or processes
- Other employees or household members similarly affected

B. Health and Safety Practices at Work Site

- Ventilation
- Personal protective equipment (e.g., respirators, gloves, and coveralls)
- Personal habits (Smoke and eat in work area? Wash hands with solvents?)

Part 2. Work History

- Description of all previous jobs, including short term, seasonal, part-time, and military service
- Description of present jobs

Part 3. Environmental History

- Present and previous home locations
- Jobs of household members
- Home insulating and heating/cooling system
- Home cleaning agents
- Pesticide exposure
- Water supply
- Recent renovation/remodeling
- Air pollution, indoor and outdoor
- Hobbies (e.g., painting, sculpting, ceramics, welding, woodworking, automobiles, gardening)
- Hazardous wastes/spill exposure

Data from Carter W, et al. *Taking an exposure history*. Atlanta, GA: U.S. Department of Health and Human Services, Agency for Toxic Substances and Disease Registry; 2000.

Activities of Daily Living

Activities of daily living (ADLs) represent the basic tasks of everyday life. Measurement of ADLs is important because they are predictive of both healthcare use (such as hospital admissions) and outcomes (such as mortality).

The simplest measure of basic ADLs is depicted in **Table 2-4**, which addresses an individual's degree of independence with everyday self-care activities. Each of the six questions is answered as a "yes" or "no," with the scale score being the number of "yes" answers. A score of 6 indicates full function; 4, moderate impairment; and 2 or less, severe impairment. Patients unable to perform these activities usually require daily caregiver support.

Learning Needs

Patient education fosters healthy behaviors and increases patients' involvement in their healthcare decisions. It is also an essential component of disease management.

Table 2-4 Basic Activities of Daily Living

Category	Description	Independent?	
		Yes	No
1. Bathing	Receives no assistance or assistance in bathing only part of the body	☐	☐
2. Dressing	Gets clothed and dresses without assistance except for tying shoes	☐	☐
3. Toileting	Goes to the bathroom, uses the toilet, and returns without any assistance (may use cane or walker for support and may use bedpan or urinal at night)	☐	☐
4. Transferring	Moves in and out of bed and chair without assistance (may use cane or walker)	☐	☐
5. Continence	Controls bowel and bladder completely by self (without occasional accidents)	☐	☐
6. Feeding	Feeds self without assistance (except for cutting meat or buttering bread)	☐	☐

Reproduced from Katz S, Downs TD, Cash HR, et al. Progress in the development of the index of ADL. *Gerontologist.* 1970;10:20–30.

The first step in patient education is an assessment of the individual's learning needs, abilities, and readiness to learn. Usually, this is performed via a comprehensive educational assessment conducted upon admission to a care unit and documented in the patient's medical record. In performing such an assessment, you first determine whether any language barrier is present. If so, you may need to request a certified medical translator to interview the patient. The use of family members is strongly discouraged due to privacy concerns (among other issues) unless it is an emergency.

You then determine the patient's preferred learning method. To do so, have patients tell you about something they recently learned and how they learned it or how they would have liked to learn it. Hints as to preferred ways of learning also can be gleaned from questions about the patient's work and hobbies.

The next step is to identify any barriers affecting learning, as revealed by a review of the record or via patient interview. **Table 2-5** outlines the most common barriers to learning and suggests ways to address them. Note the importance of gaining family assistance in overcoming many of these barriers.

In terms of health literacy—the ability of a person to understand and act on basic health information—a low educational level (less than high school completion) should raise a red flag. You also should suspect literacy problems in the following situations:

- The patient offers excuses when asked to read (e.g., left eyeglasses at home).
- The patient does not reorient the materials provided so that they are readable (e.g., leaves materials upside down).
- The patient identifies medications by their appearance (e.g., color or shape) rather than by name.
- The patient fails to take medications correctly or cannot describe how to take them.
- The patient has difficulty filling out forms correctly.

Differences in social/culture and religion also may create unique patient needs that providers should identify and address. Key guidelines regarding determining cultural and spiritual needs include the follows:

- Identify the patient's preferred language for discussing health care by:
  - noting the patient's preferred language in the medical record;
  - asking the patient, "In what language do you prefer to discuss your health care?"; or
  - arranging for language services to help identify the patient's preferred language.
- Ask the patient if any cultural or religious practices might affect treatment (e.g., dietary needs, prayer times).
- Determine if there are specific garments or religious items that need to be worn.

Table 2-5 Accommodating Common Barriers to Patient Learning

Barrier to Learning	Accommodations
Age (young child)	Keep teaching/learning episodes short.
	Use a "fun-and-games" approach.
	Enlist family assistance.
Reduced level of consciousness	Postpone until the patient becomes alert.
	Apply methods that don't require cooperation.
Presence of pain	Recommend analgesia.
	Postpone until pain management is effective.
Presence of anxiety	Postpone until anxiety management is effective.
	Enlist family assistance.
	Recommend anxiolytic (anti-anxiety) therapy.
Physical limitations	Ascertain specific limitations.
	Apply methods that circumvent the limitations.
	Enlist family assistance.
Educational level/health literacy	Assess for health literacy problems.
	Adjust language level and presentation (oral, written, visual) as appropriate.
Cultural, language, or religious factors	Ascertain key factors affecting care.
	Modify to accommodate.
	Enlist family assistance.
Vision difficulty	Have the patient wear glasses.
	Emphasize sound and touch.
	Enlist family assistance.
Hearing difficulty	Have the patient use a hearing aid.
	Emphasize visualization and touch.
	Enlist family assistance.

- Determine if anything in the hospital environment conflicts with the patient's cultural or spiritual beliefs (e.g., a crucifix); if so, either remove or cover the items
- Respect the patient's modesty/need for privacy by:
  - arranging for culturally acceptable providers (e.g., by gender or age);
  - respecting any cultural or religious restrictions on touching or personal space;
  - exposing only body areas needed to examine or treat the patient;
  - providing privacy in toileting and other hygiene activities; and
  - using full gowns or robes for ambulation and transport.
- Determine if the patient engages in any alternative health practices (e.g., yoga, exercises for asthma), and, if not contraindicated, recommend that they are included in the care plan.
- If requested, make available a private area for prayer.
- Determine if there are specific times to avoid tests or procedures due to cultural or religious practices.
- Record any cultural or religious needs/preferences you identify in the patient's chart and communicate these to other members of the care team.

After identifying barriers to learning, you should assess the patient's readiness to learn. Especially useful in this regard is the desire of patients to learn more about their condition. When patients are ready to learn, they tend to express discomfort with their current situation.

The last step is to determine the patient's learning needs as related to the care you will provide. To do so, you should ask the following questions, using language appropriate to the patient's ability to understand:

- Does the patient understand his or her current condition?
- Is the patient knowledgeable about his or her medications?
- Is the patient familiar with the procedures you will implement?
- Is the patient familiar with the equipment you plan to use?

If answers to any of these questions indicate a shortcoming or "knowledge gap," you have identified a learning need. In addition to identifying needs, you should determine the patient's "wants"—that is, any specific things the patient desires to learn. In combination, these needs and "wants" provide the basis for setting educational goals.

As outlined in **Table 2-6**, how you evaluate a patient's learning depends on whether your focus was on improving knowledge, developing skills, or changing attitudes.

Like all patient interventions, patient education episodes should be documented in the medical record. Such documentation must include who was taught (patient and family), what was taught, how it was taught, and what relevant outcomes were achieved.

Assess a Patient's Overall Cardiopulmonary Status by Inspection

Regarding inspection, the NBRC expects candidates to be proficient in evaluating a patient's general appearance, examining the airway, and evaluating cough and sputum production. In addition, you should understand the basic procedures used to assess an infant's cardiopulmonary status.

General Appearance

Table 2-7 summarizes the major observations arising from patient inspection.

Table 2-6 Evaluating Patient Learning

Change That You Are Evaluating	Method to Evaluate the Change
Patient knowledge	Teach-back (ask patients to repeat in their own words the information you are trying to get them to understand)
Patient skill level	Return demonstration (ask patients to perform the procedure after you have demonstrated it to them)
Patient attitudes	Discussion with the patient and family or observation of behavioral change

Table 2-7 Signs Observed During Patient Inspection and Their Implications

Sign	Observation	Potential Implications
General		
Body habitus	Weak/emaciated (cachexic)	General ill health/malnutrition
	Obesity (BMI > 30 kg/m²)	Obstructive sleep apnea
		Obesity-hypoventilation syndrome
Position	Sitting/leaning forward	Respiratory distress
	Always elevated with pillows	Orthopnea, congestive heart failure (CHF)
Respiratory rate	Tachypnea	Respiratory distress, restrictive disease
Breathing pattern	Prolonged exhalation	Expiratory obstruction (asthma, chronic obstructive pulmonary disease [COPD])
	Prolonged inspiration	Upper airway obstruction (croup, epiglottitis)
	Rapid and shallow	Loss of lung volume (atelectasis, fibrosis, ARDS, pulmonary edema)

General		
	Kussmaul breathing (deep and fast)	Diabetic ketoacidosis
	Biot breathing (irregular breathing with periods of apnea)	Increased intracranial pressure
	Cheyne-Stokes breathing (waxing and waning)	CNS disease or severe CHF
Speech pattern	Interrupted, unable to speak in full sentences	Respiratory distress
Skin	Diaphoretic (sweating)	Fever, increased metabolism, acute anxiety
	Mottled/acrocyanosis	Poor peripheral perfusion

	Skin integrity	Pressure ulcers/sores
		
		• Buttock & sacrum
		• Facial sores:
		  ○ BiPAP/CPAP mask
		  ○ Ear sores from nasal cannula tubing
		
		Airway skin breakdown
		
		• Tracheostomy: Stoma site
		• Endotracheal tube (ETT): Mouth or lip skin sores

Facial expression	Anxious	Fear, pain
Personal hygiene	Poor	An illness affecting a patient's daily activities
Sensorium	Depressed	Poor cerebral oxygenation, degenerative brain disorders, drug overdose
Head/Neck		
Nose	Nasal flaring (especially in infants)	Increased work of breathing
Lips/oral mucosa	Central cyanosis	Arterial hypoxemia
Lips	Pursed-lip breathing	Expiratory airway obstruction
Jugular veins	Distended	Right heart failure (cor pulmonale)
Trachea	Not in midline	Atelectasis, pneumothorax, pleural effusion (large)
Neck circumference	> 43 cm (17 in.) men; > 37 cm (15 in.) women	Obstructive sleep apnea
Thorax		
Configuration	Barrel chest	COPD
	Kyphoscoliosis	Restrictive lung defect
	Pectus excavatum (sunken sternum)	Restrictive lung defect
Muscle activity	Accessory muscle use	Increased work of breathing, loss of normal diaphragm function
	Abdominal paradox	Diaphragmatic fatigue or paralysis increased work of breathing
	Retractions	Reduced lung volume, decreased lung compliance, increased work of breathing
Extremities		
Digits	Clubbing	Bronchogenic carcinoma, COPD, cystic fibrosis, chronic cardiovascular disease
Capillary beds	Peripheral cyanosis (acrocyanosis)	Poor perfusion

ARDS, acute respiratory distress syndrome; BMI, body mass index; CNS, central nervous system; COPD, chronic obstructive pulmonary disease.

Regarding cyanosis, the NBRC expects you to know the difference between the central and peripheral types:

- Central cyanosis:
  - Indicates low Sao_2 associated with poor oxygenation of the blood by the lungs
  - Usually evident as a bluish tint of the mucous membranes of the lips and mouth
  - With normal Hb content, generally first appears when Sao_2 drops below 80% (Pao_2 45–50 torr)
- Peripheral cyanosis:
  - Due to poor blood flow
  - Tends to appear only in the extremities
  - Can occur with normal Sao_2 saturation
  - When seen together with cool extremities, suggests circulatory failure

Regardless of type, the intensity of cyanosis increases with the amount of Hb in the blood. For this reason, patients with polycythemia can be cyanotic yet still have adequate O_2 content. Conversely, patients with anemia can be severely hypoxic before cyanosis ever appears.

Airway Assessment:

Assessment of the airway can help identify the cause of other findings, such as snoring and sleep apnea. Airway assessment also can help determine whether special procedures or equipment will be needed for artificial airway insertion. To assess the airway, you should follow these steps:

1. Inspect the patient's external nose, noting any asymmetry or deformities.
2. Test for nasal patency by separately occluding each nostril as the patient breathes in.
3. Inspect the nasal cavities (use a nasal speculum and penlight if needed) for a deviated septum, polyps, edema, erythema, bleeding, or lesions.
4. With the patient's mouth open wide and the tongue extended, look for dentures or other dental appliances, and inspect the tongue, hard/soft palate, uvula, and tonsillar pillars.
5. Inspect the neck for length and circumference; have the patient flex and extend the neck as far as possible while you view the motion from the side.

Table 2-8 outlines the potential significance of the most common observations associated with the assessment of a patient's airway.

Patients with Artificial Airways

Particular attention should be paid to examining the skin and airway of patients with artificial airways in place. The stoma site of a patient with tracheostomy tubes or the mouth and lips of those with endotracheal tubes (ETT) should be inspected for skin integrity and evidence breakdown. Likewise, for patients receiving BiPAP or CPAP therapy, the skin on the bridge of the nose, cheeks, and lips should be inspected for evidence of sores or skin irritation.

Overall Skin Integrity

The patient's overall skin integrity should be inspected for evidence of breakdown and or sores. Skin sores can develop in bed-bound patients, especially on the buttock, sacrum, and back. When present, skin sores are rated on a scale from stage 1, which is the least severe and often characterized by skin redness/discoloration but unbroken skin, to stage 4, which are sores affecting multiple layers of tissue, including muscle and bone. It is important for these sores to be quickly identified and treated to help prevent worsening, as they are a potential source of infection and sepsis.

Cough and Sputum

Table 2-9 describes some of the common types of coughs and their likely causes. As indicated in Table 2-9, several conditions are associated with a productive cough, such as chronic bronchitis, infections, bronchiectasis, lung abscess, pertussis, and asthma. Sputum assessment should be included in patient history taking and be conducted whenever secretion clearance takes place. Typically, you evaluate the volume, color, consistency, and odor of sputum.

Table 2-8 Inspection of the Airway

Area	Observation	Significance
Nostrils/nasal cavity	Broken, misshapen, swollen nose; occluded nasal passages; deviated septum	Compromised nasal route for O_2 or airway insertion
Oral cavity and pharynx	Dentures or dental appliances present	Potential aspiration risk; may need to be removed for airway access
	Macroglossia (large tongue)	Associated with difficult intubation and may impair aerosol delivery via the mouth
	Mallampati classification of pharyngeal anatomy (also see Chapter 9): Class I: Full visibility of tonsils, uvula, and soft palate Class II: Visibility of hard and soft palate, the upper portion of tonsils, and uvula Class III: Soft and hard palate and base of the uvula are visible Class IV: Only hard palate visible	Class IV is associated with difficult intubation as well as a high incidence of sleep apnea
Neck	Short/thick (circumference > 43 cm [17 in.] men; > 37 cm [15 in.] women	Difficult endotracheal (ET) intubation; difficult tracheostomy tube fit
	Poor range of motion (patient cannot touch the chest with the tip of the chin and cannot fully extend neck)	Difficult bag-valve-mask (BVM) ventilation; difficult ET intubation

Table 2-9 Common Types of Coughs with Likely Causes

Description	Likely Causes
Acute (< 3 weeks)	Postnasal drip, allergies, and infections (especially common cold, bronchitis, and laryngitis)
Chronic (> 3 weeks) or recurrent (adults)	Postnasal drip, asthma, gastroesophageal reflux, chronic bronchitis, bronchiectasis, COPD, tuberculosis (TB), lung tumor, angiotensin-converting enzyme (ACE) inhibitors, CHF
Recurrent (children)	Viral bronchitis, asthma, allergies
Barking	Epiglottitis, croup, influenza, laryngotracheal bronchitis
Brassy or hoarse	Laryngitis, laryngeal paralysis, laryngotracheal bronchitis, pressure on the laryngeal nerve, mediastinal tumor, aortic aneurysm
Wheezy	Bronchospasm, asthma, cystic fibrosis, bronchitis
Dry/unproductive	Viral infections, inhalation of irritant gases, interstitial lung diseases, tumor, pleural effusion, cardiac conditions, a nervous habit, radiation or chemotherapy
Dry progressing to productive	Atypical pneumonia, Legionnaires' disease, pulmonary embolus, pulmonary edema, lung abscess, asthma, silicosis, emphysema (late phase), smoking, AIDS
Chronic productive	Bronchiectasis, chronic bronchitis, lung abscess, asthma, fungal infections, bacterial pneumonia, TB
Paroxysmal (especially at night)	Aspiration, asthma, CHF
Positional, especially when lying down	Bronchiectasis, CHF, chronic postnasal drip or sinusitis, gastroesophageal reflux with aspiration
Associated with eating or drinking	Neuromuscular disorders affecting the upper airway, esophageal problems, aspiration
Data from from Heuer, Al. Clinical Assessment in Respiratory Care (8th ed.). St. Louis, MO: Mosby; 2013.	

In terms of color, sputum is typically described as being either clear/white, pinkish, red, yellow, or green. Consistency is generally described as being thin/watery, frothy, or thick/viscous. Foul-smelling or *fetid* sputum suggests tissue necrosis. In combination, these characteristics help classify the sputum "type" as being mucoid, mucopurulent, purulent, or bloody and indicate the likely disorder (**Table 2-10**).

Neonatal Inspection

The NBRC expects you to be proficient in basic fetal/neonatal assessment methods, including Apgar scoring, evaluation of gestational age, and transillumination.

Apgar Score

The Apgar score (**Table 2-11**) is used to assess neonates at 1 and 5 minutes after birth. The score's five dimensions (**A**ppearance, **P**ulse, **G**rimace, **A**ctivity, **R**espirations) are rated from 0 to 2, with a maximum score of 10 and a minimum score of 0 (stillborn). An Apgar score of 7–10 is normal. Babies scoring 4–6 typically need more intensive support, and those scoring 0–3 usually undergo resuscitation. *Needed interventions should never be delayed in order to obtain the Apgar score.*

Gestational Age

Normal gestation lasts 38–42 weeks. Knowledge of gestational age can help clinicians anticipate perinatal problems and establish sound care plans. **Table 2-12** summarizes the methods commonly used to estimate gestational age *before* birth. After birth, clinicians determine gestational age by careful assessment of selected neuromuscular and physical characteristics using methods developed by Dubowitz and Ballard. Although RTs normally do not conduct this assessment, you should be familiar with the assessment components.

Table 2-10 Sputum Assessment

	Color and Consistency	Likely Conditions
Mucoid	Clear/white, thin to thick	Asthma
Mucopurulent	Clear to yellowish, thick	Chronic bronchitis, cystic fibrosis, pneumonia (blood streaked)
Purulent	Yellow to green, thick	Aspiration pneumonia, bronchiectasis (fetid/foul-smelling, may separate into layers), lung abscess (fetid/foul-smelling, may separate into layers)
Bloody	Pink to red/dark red, thin (unless coagulated)	Tuberculosis (red), lung cancer (red), pulmonary infarction (red), pulmonary edema (pink, watery, frothy)
Data from MacIntyre NR. Respiratory monitoring without machinery. *Respir Care*. 1990;35:546–553.		

Table 2-11 Apgar Score

Parameter	Apgar Sign	0	1	2
Color	Appearance	Blue or pale	Pink body with peripheral cyanosis (*acrocyanosis*)	Completely pink
Heart rate	Pulse	Absent	< 100 beats/min	> 100 beats/min
Reflex irritability	Grimace	Unresponsive	Grimace when stimulated*	Active movement, crying, coughing
Muscle tone	Activity	Flaccid, limp	Some flexion of extremities	Active movement
Respiratory effort	Respirations	Absent	Slow, irregular, weak, gasping	Crying, vigorous breathing
*Catheter in nares or tactile stimulation.				

Table 2-12 Methods Used to Estimate Gestational Age Before Birth

Method	Measurement	Comments
Time since last menses	Weeks since the end of last normal menstrual period + 2	Traditional but unreliable
Ultrasonography	Crown to rump length up to 14 weeks Fetal head diameter (biparietal diameter) between 14 and 20 weeks' gestation	Accurate and reliable
Biochemical analysis (measurement of amniotic fluid phospholipid levels) *	Lecithin/sphingomyelin (L/S) ratio > 2.0 Presence of phosphatidylglycerol (PG) Lecithin/albumin (L/A) ratio ≥ 40.0 mg/g	Fetal maturity indicated by L/S ratio > 2; presence of PG; or L/A ratio > 40.0 mg/g
*Used primarily to indicate fetal lung maturity and predict infant respiratory distress syndrome.		

Figure 2-1 depicts the Ballard Gestational Age Assessment and scoring system. Scores are summed across both components to yield a composite score. A composite score of 10 or less indicates significant prematurity (≤ 28 weeks' gestation). An infant born at full term (38–42 weeks) typically scores in the 35–45 range, with higher values indicating a post-term baby.

Transillumination of Chest

Transillumination uses high-intensity fiber-optic light applied to the chest wall to detect pneumothoraces in infants. You should recommend transillumination for high-risk infants (especially those receiving mechanical ventilation) with clinical signs of pneumothorax—that is, retractions, tachypnea, cyanosis, hypotension, and asymmetrical chest motion.

The accompanying box (**Box 2-3**) outlines the basic procedure. Normally, a halo of only about 1 cm forms under the light. If the underlying chest broadly "lights up," in an irregular fashion, a pneumothorax is likely. Note that if the test is negative, but the infant still exhibits signs suggesting a pneumothorax, you should recommend an immediate chest x-ray.

Assess a Patient's Overall Cardiopulmonary Status by Palpation

You palpate a patient to (1) evaluate heart rate, rhythm, and intensity; (2) assess accessory muscle activity and tracheal position; (3) evaluate vocal/tactile fremitus; (4) estimate thoracic expansion; and (5) assess the skin and tissues of the chest and extremities.

Heart Rate, Rhythm, and Pulse Strength

To evaluate a patient's heart's rate, rhythm, and intensity, you should palpate both peripheral and apical pulses (over the precordium). You palpate the peripheral pulse to measure a patient's heart rate, typically using the radial artery. You palpate the apical pulse to assess the location and strength of the heart's point of maximum impulse (PMI). Normal references ranges for heart rates by age group are specified in Chapter 1.

Based on this knowledge, you determine whether the rate is normal or whether the patient has tachycardia or bradycardia. **Table 2-13** outlines the most common causes of tachycardia and bradycardia.

To detect if the pulse is regular or irregular, you may need to palpate it for a full minute. Minor irregularities are common, particularly in children (sinus arrhythmia). If you detect an irregularity, repeat your assessment with a second clinician simultaneously measuring the apical rate via palpation or auscultation. If the apical rate exceeds the peripheral rate, a *pulse deficit* exists. A pulse deficit usually indicates a cardiac arrhythmia, such as atrial fibrillation or flutter, premature ventricular contractions (PVCs), or heart block.

Neuromuscular maturity

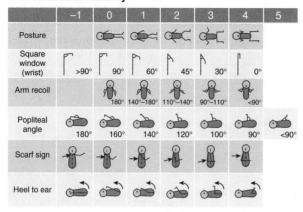

	−1	0	1	2	3	4	5
Posture							
Square window (wrist)	>90°	90°	60°	45°	30°	0°	
Arm recoil		180°	140°–180°	110°–140°	90°–110°	<90°	
Popliteal angle	180°	160°	140°	120°	100°	90°	<90°
Scarf sign							
Heel to ear							

Maturity rating

Score	Weeks
−10	20
−5	22
0	24
5	26
10	28
15	30
20	32
25	34
30	36
35	38
40	40
45	42
50	44

Physical maturity

Skin	Sticky; friable; transparent	Gelatinous; red; translucent	Smooth; pink; visible veins	Superficial peeling and/or rash; few veins	Cracking; pale areas; rare veins	Parchment; deep cracking; no vessels	Leathery; cracked; wrinkled
Lanugo	None	Sparse	Abundant	Thinning	Bald areas	Mostly bald	
Plantar surface	Heel-toe 40–50 mm: −1 <40 mm: −2	>50 mm; no crease	Faint red marks	Anterior transverse crease only	Creases ant. 2/3	Creases over entire sole	
Breast	Imperceptible	Barely perceptible	Flat areola; no bud	Stippled areola; 1–2 mm bud	Raised areola; 3–4 mm bud	Full areola; 5–10 mm bud	
Eye/ear	Lids fused loosely: −1 tightly: −2	Lids open; pinna flat; stays folded	Slightly curved pinna; soft; slow recoil	Well-curved pinna; soft but ready recoil	Formed and firm; instant recoil	Thick cartilage; ear stiff	
Genitals male	Scrotum flat; smooth	Scrotum empty; faint rugae	Testes in upper canal; rare rugae	Testes descending; few rugae	Testes down; good rugae	Testes pendulous; deep rugae	
Genitals female	Clitoris prominent; labia flat	Prominent clitoris; small labia minora	Prominent clitoris; enlarging minora	Majora and minora equally prominent	Majora large; minora small	Majora cover clitoris and minora	

Figure 2-1 Ballard Gestational Age Assessment.

Republished with permission of Elsevier, from Ballard JL, Novak KK, Denver M. A simplified score for assessment of fetal maturation in newborn infants. *J Pediatr.* 1979;95(5):769–774. Permission conveyed through Copyright Clearance Center, Inc.

Box 2-3 Transillumination Procedure

1. Place the infant in the supine position, and switch on the light.
2. Hold the light against the skin along the midaxillary line about halfway down the chest on the affected side.
3. Observe whether or not the chest illuminates (lights up). In a normal chest (no air present), an even, round shadow will be seen around the light ("halo" sign).
4. Repeat the assessment on the same side at the midclavicular line halfway down the chest.
5. Repeat the assessment on the opposite side of the chest to compare the degree of illumination.

Careful assessment of the peripheral pulse also can reveal variation in strength. **Table 2-14** summarizes the most common findings and their likely causes.

For apical pulse assessment, the following guidelines apply:

- Locate/palpate the heart's point of maximum impulse (PMI), normally at or near the fifth intercostal space, midclavicular line.

Table 2-13 Common Causes of Abnormal Heart Rate

Tachycardia	Bradycardia
• Fever	• Vasovagal reflex
• Hypoxemia	• Cardiac arrhythmias
• Pain	• Increased intracranial pressure
• Shock	• Hypothyroidism
• Anemia	• Hypothermia
• Cardiac arrhythmias	• Electrolyte imbalances
• Hyperthyroidism	• Drugs
• Thyrotoxicosis	o Beta-adrenergic blockers
• Drugs	o Calcium-channel blockers
o Beta-agonists	o Digoxin
o Cholinergic blockers (e.g., atropine)	o Antiarrhythmic agents
o Stimulants (e.g., nicotine, caffeine)	
o Illicit drugs (e.g., amphetamines, cocaine)	

Table 2-14 Summary of Pulse Findings

Type	Description	Causes
Strong	Easy to palpate	Increased stroke volume (e.g., exercise); hypertension
Weak or thready	Hard to palpate	Decreased cardiac contractility; decreased blood volume; loss of vascular tone (e.g., septic shock); aortic stenosis
Bounding	Rapid/strong initial pressure rise followed by a quick fall-off	Aortic insufficiency; patent ductus arteriosus; atherosclerosis
Pulsus alternans	Pulse alternates in strength from beat to beat	Left-sided heart failure/congestive heart failure (CHF)
Pulsus paradoxus	Pulsations vary with the breathing cycle (weaker pulses during inspiration)	Severe airway obstruction (status asthmaticus); cardiac tamponade

- A weak impulse may indicate hyperinflation (as with COPD) or decreased cardiac contractility.
- Abnormally strong pulsations or a downward/left shift of the PMI suggests left ventricular hypertrophy.
- The PMI moves when the mediastinum is displaced: *toward* areas of atelectasis and *away from* space-occupying lesions such as pneumothoraces or pleural effusions.

Accessory Muscle Activity

The accessory muscles of inspiration include the sternocleidomastoid, scalenes, upper trapezius, and pectoralis major. Typically, these muscles of the upper thorax and neck are minimally active during quiet breathing. Increased activity at rest is commonly observed in patients with emphysema and any patient experiencing an increased work of breathing. Increased activity at rest also is common in patients with impaired diaphragm function, such as those with spinal cord injury or certain chronic neuromuscular conditions.

Thoracic Expansion/Chest Movements

Palpation can help determine if chest expansion is equal on both sides. Anteriorly, you place your hands over the lower lateral chest wall, with the thumbs extended along the lower rib margins.

Posteriorly, you position your hands over the lateral chest with the thumbs meeting at about the eighth thoracic vertebra. When the patient takes a full, deep breath, each thumb should move equally about 1–2 inches from the midline. Lesser or unequal movement is abnormal. Bilateral reductions in chest expansion are seen in COPD patients and those with neuromuscular disorders. Unilateral reductions in chest movement (on the affected side) occur with lobar pneumonia, atelectasis, pleural effusion, pneumothorax, and unilateral (right or left) phrenic nerve paralysis.

Tracheal Position

Usually, the trachea lies in the midline of the neck, which can be confirmed by palpating it just above the sternum, between the clavicles. Shifts away from the midline can sometimes be felt or seen during bedside patient assessment and confirmed with a chest x-ray. The direction of the shift often suggests the potential causes. In such instances, the trachea will shift either ***toward areas of decreased lung volume*** or ***away from space-occupying pathology***, as follows:

- ***Toward*** areas of reduced lung volume, most notably:
  - Atelectasis
  - Fibrosis
  - Surgical resection
- ***Away from*** space-occupying lesions, such as:
  - Pneumothorax
  - Large pleural effusion
  - Large mass lesions (e.g., tumors)

Tactile Fremitus

- Vibrations that you can feel on the chest wall
- Rhonchial fremitus (also known as tactile rhonchi)
- Associated with excess secretions in the large airways
- Detected by placing the flat of your hand on the chest to either side of the sternum
- Diminishes or clears with coughing or after suctioning/airway clearance therapy

Vocal Fremitus

- Result of voice sounds being transmitted to the chest wall
- Assessed with the patient saying "ninety-nine" while you palpate the chest wall
- Increased in conditions increasing lung tissue density (e.g., pneumonia, atelectasis)
- Decreased in the following conditions:
  - Severe obesity (fat tissue impedes sound transmission)
  - COPD (hyperinflation decreases sound transmission)
  - Pneumothorax or pleural effusion (lungs separated from the chest wall)
  - Lung lobe or segment blocked by a mucus plug or foreign body

Skin and Soft Tissues

You can palpate the skin and soft tissues to determine the temperature and assess for crepitus, edema, capillary refill, and tenderness.

When blood flow is reduced, blood vessels in the extremities constrict to help direct flow to the vital organs. With less blood flow, the extremities tend to cool. For this reason, cold hands and feet usually indicate poor perfusion.

Especially in patients receiving positive-pressure ventilation, gas can leak into the tissues around the head, neck, and chest, forming subcutaneous bubbles, a condition called *subcutaneous emphysema*. When palpated, these bubbles produce a crackling sensation called *crepitus*. Although subcutaneous emphysema itself is harmless, it often occurs in conjunction with a pneumothorax. For this reason, *if you detect crepitus, assess the patient for pneumothorax, and immediately communicate your findings to the patient's physician*. Most clinicians also recommend a chest x-ray whenever crepitus occurs in mechanically ventilated patients.

Many patients with chronic heart failure exhibit gravity-dependent tissue edema, typically in the feet and ankles (pedal edema). Firmly pressing on edematous tissue with a finger causes it to "pit" or indent. The degree of pitting is usually rated on a 3-point scale, with +3 being the most serious. In general, the farther up the legs the edema can be detected, the more severe the heart failure.

You assess capillary refill by pressing firmly on a patient's fingernails, then releasing the pressure and noting how quickly blood flow returns. When cardiac output is reduced, and digital perfusion is poor, the capillary refill is slow, taking 3 seconds or longer.

The chest wall can also be palpated to determine areas of tenderness. The onset, location, and intensity of the tenderness can give valuable insight as to the cause of the pain and treatment options.

Abdomen

In addition to the chest wall, the abdomen can be palpated for evidence of distention and tenderness. Abdominal distention and pain can restrict diaphragmatic movement, impair coughing and deep breathing, and contribute to respiratory insufficiency. Typically, the right upper quadrant of the abdomen is palpated for tenderness and to estimate the size of the liver. Abdominal tenderness and an enlarged liver (hepatomegaly) may be seen in patients with chronic cor pulmonale.

Assess a Patient's Overall Cardiopulmonary Status by Percussion

In a complete thoracic exam, you should percuss the lung fields on both sides of the chest, being sure to avoid bony structures and female breasts. To move the scapulae out of the way for posterior percussion, have the patient raise his or her arms. Key points regarding percussion include the following:

- Percussion over normal, air-filled lung tissue produces a moderately low-pitched sound that is easily heard—*normal resonance*.
- A hollow/loud and low-pitched percussion note is termed *increased resonance* (also known as tympanic or hyperresonant), typically indicating hyperinflation (acute asthma, COPD) or pneumothorax.
- A *dull/flat percussion note* (short, muted, high-pitched) occurs over areas of increased tissue density, as observed in patients with pneumonia, atelectasis, or lung tumors.
- *Decreased resonance* occurs if there is fluid in the pleural space.

Percussion over the lower posterior thorax can help determine the position of the diaphragm and its range of motion. As you percuss downward over the lower lung fields, the sound changes from normal resonance to a dull note, indicating the level of the diaphragm. The difference between the maximum inspiratory and expiratory levels represents the full range of diaphragm motion, which in adults ranges from 5 to 7 cm. Diaphragm motion typically is decreased in patients with neuromuscular disorders and severe hyperinflation.

Assess a Patient's Overall Cardiopulmonary Status by Auscultation

You auscultate the thorax to identify lung and heart sounds. In general, you should use the stethoscope's diaphragm for auscultation of higher-pitched breath sounds, whereas the bell is recommended to listen to lower-pitched heart sounds.

Breath Sounds

Table 2-15 summarizes the characteristics of normal breath sounds, *which are considered normal only if noted at the specified location*. Normal sounds identified at abnormal locations are abnormal! For example, bronchial breath sounds are abnormal when heard over the lung periphery. They tend to replace normal vesicular sounds when lung tissue increases in density, as in atelectasis and pneumonia/consolidation.

Breath sounds are diminished when the patient's breathing is shallow or slow. Decreased breath sounds also occur when airways are obstructed or the lung is hyperinflated, as in asthma or COPD. Air or fluid in the pleural space and obesity can reduce breath sounds as well.

Table 2-15 Normal Breath Sounds

Breath Sound	Description	Normally Heard at (Location)
Vesicular	Low-pitched, soft sounds; heard primarily during inhalation, with only a minimal exhalation component	Periphery of the lungs
Bronchial	High-pitched, loud, tubular sounds with an expiratory phase equal to or longer than the inspiratory phase	Over trachea
Bronchovesicular	Moderate pitch and intensity; equal inspiratory and expiratory phases	Around upper sternum (anterior); between scapulae (posterior)

Table 2-16 Adventitious Breath Sounds

Lung Sounds	Characteristics	Likely Mechanism	Causes
Rhonchi	Coarse, discontinuous	Airflow through mucus	Pneumonia, bronchitis, inadequate cough
Wheezes	High pitched; usually expiratory	Rapid airflow through partially obstructed airways	Asthma, congestive heart failure, bronchitis
Stridor	High pitched, monophonic; commonly inspiratory	Rapid airflow through obstructed upper airway	Croup, epiglottitis, post-extubation edema
Pleural friction rub	Creaking or grating sound heard mainly during inhalation (can occur during both phases of breathing)	Inflamed pleural surfaces rubbing together during breathing	Pleurisy
Crackles: inspiratory and expiratory	Coarse; often clear with coughing	Excess airway secretions moving with airflow	Bronchitis, respiratory infections
Crackles: early inspiratory	Scanty, transmitted to mouth; not affected by cough	The sudden opening of atelectatic bronchi	Bronchitis, emphysema, asthma
Crackles: late inspiratory	Diffuse, fine; occur initially in the dependent regions	The sudden opening of collapsed peripheral airways	Atelectasis, pneumonia, pulmonary edema, fibrosis

Abnormal or *adventitious* breath sounds include rhonchi, wheezes, crackles (rales), and stridor. **Table 2-16** summarizes the characteristics, likely mechanisms, and common causes of these adventitious breath sounds.

Heart Sounds

Heart sounds are generated when the heart valves close. The first heart sound (S_1) signals the closure of the mitral and tricuspid valves, and the second heart sound (S_2) occurs with the closure of the pulmonic and aortic valves. You listen to heart sounds to assess the apical heart rate and to identify gross abnormalities in structure or function:

- Heart sound intensity is diminished in the following conditions:
  - COPD, pleural effusion, pneumothorax, and obesity (reduced transmission of sound to the chest wall)
  - Heart failure, hypotension, and shock (decreased cardiac contractility or blood volume)
- Heart sound intensity is increased in the following patients:
  - Patients with partial obstruction to outflow from the ventricles, as in mitral stenosis (affecting S_1) and pulmonary hypertension (affecting S_2)
  - Children and thin-chested patients (decreased transmission distance)
  - Heart sound intensity (especially S_1) can vary with cardiac arrhythmias that alter ventricular filling, such as atrial fibrillation and complete heart block.

You will sometimes hear a third heart sound (S_3) occurring just after S_2. The presence of this extra sound creates a galloping pattern, often equated with the saying the word "Kentucky." S_3 often can be heard in normal children and well-conditioned athletes. Its presence in older patients usually indicates CHF.

Cardiac murmurs indicate turbulent flow through a heart valve. Systolic murmurs are heard when either an atrioventricular (AV) valve allows backflow (*regurgitation*) or a semilunar valve restricts outflow (*stenosis*). Diastolic *murmurs* occur with semilunar valve regurgitation or AV valve stenosis.

Auscultatory Assessment of Blood Pressure

You also use auscultation to measure blood pressure manually. As you deflate the cuff, you listen for the *Korotkoff sounds*, caused by turbulent flow through the partially obstructed artery. The pressure at which the Korotkoff sounds first appear is the systolic pressure, and the point at which these sounds suddenly become muffled and disappear is the diastolic pressure. **Table 2-17** describes several situations demanding special consideration when auscultating a patient's blood pressure.

Integrating Physical Examination Findings

Table 2-18 summarizes the major physical findings associated with various common clinical disorders.

Review and Interpret the Chest Radiograph

Here we describe the process of reviewing a chest x-ray, including what to look for during assessment. The accompanying box (**Box 2-4**) outlines the basic steps in reviewing a chest x-ray. Chapter 1 outlines the various imaging studies used in the diagnosis and management of respiratory disorders.

Table 2-17 Special Considerations in Manually Measuring Blood Pressure by Auscultation

Problem	Caused by	Solution
Inaudible blood pressure	Poor technique	Use proper technique.
	Severe hypotension or shock	Consider arterial line monitoring.
	Venous engorgement (due to repeated measurements)	Remove the cuff and have the patient raise his or her arm over the head for 1–2 minutes before repeating the measurement. Use the other arm.
Irregular cardiac rhythms	Atrial fibrillation, frequent premature ventricular contractions (PVCs), heart block	Make several measurements and use the average.
Auscultatory gap	A silent interval between systolic and diastolic sounds that can result in underestimating systolic pressure or overestimating diastolic pressure; usually caused by hypertension	Measure and record three pressures: (1) the opening systolic or "snap" pressure, (2) the pressure at which continuous pulses again are heard, and (3) the diastolic pressure.
Paradoxical pulse (*pulsus paradoxus*)	A larger than normal drop (more than 6–8 mm Hg) in systolic pressure during inspiration in patients with severe airway obstruction (such as acute asthma) or conditions that impair ventricular filling (such as cardiac tamponade)	To measure paradoxical pulse, slowly deflate the cuff until you hear sounds only on exhalation (point 1). Then reduce the pressure again until you can hear sounds throughout the breathing cycle (point 2). The difference in pressures between points 1 and 2 is the paradoxical pulse measurement.

Table 2-18 Physical Findings Associated with Various Common Clinical Disorders

Abnormality	Inspection	Palpation	Percussion	Auscultation
Asthma	Use of accessory muscles	Reduced expansion	Increased resonance	Expiratory wheezing
Chronic obstructive pulmonary disease (COPD)	Increased antero-posterior (AP) diameter; accessory muscles use	Reduced expansion	Increased resonance	Diffuse decrease in breath sounds; early inspiratory crackles
Consolidation (pneumonia or tumor)	Inspiratory lag	Increased vocal fremitus	Dull note	Bronchial breath sounds; late inspiratory crackles
Pneumothorax	Unilateral expansion	Tracheal shift away; decreased vocal fremitus	Increased resonance	Absent breath sounds
Pleural effusion	Unilateral expansion	Tracheal shift away; absent vocal fremitus	Dull note	Absent breath sounds
Atelectasis	Unilateral expansion	Tracheal shift toward; absent vocal fremitus	Dull note	Absent breath sounds
Diffuse interstitial fibrosis	Rapid, shallow breathing	Often normal; increased fremitus	A slight decrease in resonance	Late inspiratory crackles
Upper airway obstruction (e.g., croup, foreign body)	Labored breathing	Often normal	Often normal	Inspiratory and expiratory stridor and possible unilateral wheezing (foreign body aspiration)

Box 2-4 Basic Steps in Review of a Chest X-Ray

1. Obtain image; verify identification (patient, date), orientation (using side marker), and image quality.
2. Identify the view of the film (anteroposterior [AP] or posteroanterior [PA]).
3. Review the entire film for symmetry, and identify the following:
   a. Clavicles, scapulae, and ribs
   b. Spinal column (note whether it is midline)
   c. Lungs, right and left
   d. Level of diaphragms and costophrenic angles (sharp or blunted)
   e. Gastric air bubble
   f. Breast shadows
4. Trace the outline of each rib, noting the angle and any fractures or other abnormalities.
5. Observe the tracheal position.
6. Identify the carina and the mainstem bronchi.
7. Examine the hila for size and position.
8. Identify the lung markings.
9. Identify the aortic knob and the heart shadow.
10. Estimate the cardiothoracic ratio.
11. Note the presence and position of any artificial airways or catheters.
12. State an overall impression of the film.
13. Compare with previous films if available.

Image Orientation and Quality

The first step in reviewing an x-ray is to verify the patient and date of the film and assess image orientation and quality. As outlined in **Table 2-19**, you can use the mnemonic R-I-P-E to assess image orientation and quality.

Lung Fields

Because a radiograph is a negative, areas of increased whiteness or *radiopacity* indicate high-density objects, such as bone or consolidated tissue, whereas areas of darkness or *radiolucency* indicate low-density matter, such as air. **Table 2-20** lists the most common causes of radiopacity and radiolucency seen on an x-ray.

Position of Diaphragm

The position of the diaphragm on x-ray can offer clues as to its functioning or the presence of pulmonary disease. For example, a patient with a condition affecting the phrenic nerve, such as quadriplegia, often shows signs of an *elevated* diaphragm. This is due to the inability of the diaphragm to contract (drop) to facilitate lung inflation. In contrast, a properly functioning diaphragm may have

Table 2-19 R-I-P-E Mnemonic for Assessing Chest Radiograph Quality

R	Rotation	The patient's shoulders should be perfectly perpendicular to the x-ray beam (i.e., not rotated left or right). The patient is aligned "straight" if the thoracic spine aligns in the center of the sternum and equally between the medial end of each clavicle.
I	Inspiration	A good inspiratory effort is needed to visualize lung structures, especially at the bases properly. Inspiration is adequate if the diaphragm is at the level of the 10th posterior rib (8th to 9th posterior ribs in anteroposterior [AP] films) or 6th anterior rib on the right.
P	Position	Verify AP versus posteroanterior (PA) view. • The AP view is most common in bedridden patients. In the typical AP view, the medial borders of the scapula are seen in the upper lung fields, the ribs appear more horizontal, and the heart appears more magnified. • In the typical PA view, the borders of the scapula are clear of the upper lung fields, the ribs are angled downward, and the heart appears less magnified. Verify left versus right sides of the film. If not labeled with a side marker, both the gastric bubble (upright posture only) and the apex of a normal heart should appear on the right side of the film (patient's left side). Verify proper angulation (head/toe). In the AP view, the clavicle should be at about the level of the third rib.
E	Exposure	Verify the proper intensity of the x-ray beam passing through the patient. In a good exposure, the intervertebral disks should be barely visible through the heart, and the costophrenic angles should be well defined (assuming proper inspiration and no effusions). Overexposed = too dark; underexposed = too white.

Table 2-20 Common Pulmonary Abnormalities Altering Lung Field Density on Chest X-rays

Increased Radiopacity	Increased Radiolucency
• Atelectasis	• Pulmonary emphysema
• Consolidation	• Pneumothorax
• Interstitial lung disease	• Pneumomediastinum
• Pulmonary infiltrates/edema	• Pneumopericardium
• Pleural effusion	• Subcutaneous emphysema
• Lung/mediastinal tumors	• Pulmonary interstitial emphysema
• Calcification	

Table 2-21 Chest X-ray Abnormalities Associated with Changes in the Diaphragm

Abnormality	Likely Problem
Blunted costophrenic angles (affected side)	Lower-lobe pneumonia, pleural effusion
Flattened diaphragm (affected side)	Hyperinflation (chronic emphysema or acute asthma), tension pneumothorax, large pleural effusion
Elevated diaphragm (affected side)	Phrenic nerve paralysis, hepatomegaly, atelectasis
Air under diaphragms (differentiate from normal gastric air bubble)	Perforated gastrointestinal tract

a *flattened* appearance due to hyperinflation associated with a chronic condition such as severe emphysema or an acute one such as asthma or a pneumothorax or due to a large pleural effusion. **Table 2-21** summarizes key findings related to the position or appearance of the diaphragm.

Heart Size and Position

A chest radiograph can help differentiate heart failure from primary pulmonary disease, especially in patients who present with shortness of breath/dyspnea. Findings suggesting heart failure include the follows:

- Cardiomegaly
- Prominent upper lobe vascular markings
- Kerley B lines
- Pleural effusion(s)

The term *cardiomegaly* most commonly refers to an enlarged heart seen on a chest x-ray. Normally, the heart width is less than 50% of the width of the thoracic cage. Cardiomegaly exists when the ratio of cardiac to thoracic width (CT ratio) exceeds 50% on a posteroanterior (PA) chest radiograph. Note that because the heart lies primarily in the anterior chest, it is magnified on an AP film. Also, factors such as patient rotation or an incomplete inspiration can exaggerate heart size on both PA and AP views.

In terms of position, the heart lies within the mediastinum and normally is visualized primarily to the left of the midline/spine (right side of x-ray), consisting mostly of the lateral border of the left ventricle. A smaller portion of the heart (right atrial border) lies typically to the right of the midline/spine (left side of x-ray). Any lateral movement of the mediastinum away from the midline will also shift the heart position in the same direction.

Position of Endotracheal or Tracheostomy Tubes

An AP chest x-ray is the most common method used to confirm proper placement of an endotracheal (ET) or tracheostomy tube. Ideally, the tube tip should be positioned 4–6 cm above the carina. This normally corresponds to a location between thoracic vertebrae T2 and T4, or about the same level as the superior border of the aortic arch.

Position of Indwelling Tubes, Catheters, and Foreign Objects

Objects visible on a chest radiograph that are not "of" the patient are *foreign bodies*. Foreign bodies include those appearing by accident or trauma—such as an aspirated tooth or bullet—as well as purposefully placed medical devices (e.g., cardiac pacemakers). Aspiration of small objects is the most common source of accidental foreign-body ingestion, especially in children. This possibility always should be considered when encountering airway obstruction in children and justifies recommending both a chest *and* lateral neck and chest x-ray.

Other than some plastics and aspirated food matter, most foreign bodies are denser than human tissues. Thus, these objects appear radiopaque, with their shape often helping to identify their origin. For example, an aspirated coin will appear as a solid white, round object on a radiograph. Likewise, devices such as surgical staples are easily identifiable by their shape and position.

In contrast, low-density plastic devices, such as ET tubes and vascular catheters, are more difficult to visualize on an x-ray. For this reason, radiopaque markers are embedded in these devices. **Table 2-22** outlines common medical devices, airways, lines, and drains that may be visualized on a chest radiograph.

Pulmonary Artery Size

Though not easily visualized, the size of the pulmonary artery can be often be evaluated by trained personnel viewing a chest x-ray. Pulmonary arterial abnormalities associated with congenital cardiovascular defects can be seen. In addition, other abnormalities such as pulmonary artery engorgement and enlargement due to pulmonary emboli or other conditions may manifest themselves on a chest x-ray. If such abnormalities are suspected, another testing is often necessary such as ultrasound, CT scan, and angiography to confirm the abnormality and formulate a treatment plan.

Review Lateral Neck Radiographs

When used together with a chest radiograph, lateral neck x-rays are useful in assessing for upper airway obstruction, especially in children. The most common causes of upper airway obstruction in children are aspirated foreign bodies and infection. As indicated previously, high-density aspirated

Table 2-22 Medical Devices, Airways, and Lines Visualized on the Chest Radiograph

Devices	Comments
Extrathoracic	
Electrocardiogram (ECG) leads	Three electrodes and lead wires typically are visible.
Clamps, syringes, and other instruments	May be on top of or under the patient but can appear to be "inside" the thorax and thus confuse interpretation.
Ventilator circuits, heating wires, temperature sensors	Adult circuits normally exhibit typical corrugated appearance; wires/sensors may be confused with intrathoracic devices such as pacemakers.
Breast implants	Either unilateral or bilateral; shadows can be confused with lung pathology.
Intrathoracic	
Thoracostomy (chest) tubes	To evacuate air (pneumothorax), the tube normally is positioned anterosuperiorly; to evacuate fluid, it is positioned posteroinferiorly.
Endotracheal tubes	The tube tip should be 4–6 cm above the carina, or between T2 and T4.
Nasogastric or feeding tubes	Visualized passing through the mediastinum and diaphragm into the stomach. Misplacement high in the esophagus or the trachea can result in aspiration.
Central venous catheter	Should be seen in the superior vena cava or right atrium.
Pulmonary artery (PA) catheter	The catheter tip should appear in the lower lobe, ideally posteriorly. Improper placement can result in false pulmonary artery wedge pressure (PAWP) readings.
Implanted cardiac pacemakers and cardioverter/defibrillators	The pulse generator is usually visualized below the clavicle; one or two pacing wires should appear coursing through the superior vena cava into the heart chamber(s).
Sternal wires	Appear on the chest radiograph as several opaque "tied" loops running up and down the sternum (in patients after median sternotomy for cardiac surgery).
Metallic heart valves	Appear in the same location as what they replace (mitral and aortic being the most common); bioprosthetic porcine or bovine tissue valve replacements not easily visualized.
Intra-aortic counterpulsation balloon device (IACB or IABP)	Consists of an inflatable balloon about 25 cm long, the tip of which generally can be visualized just distal to the left subclavian artery in the descending thoracic aorta, about 2 cm from the aortic arch.

Table 2-23 Radiographic Findings: Croup Versus Epiglottitis

View	Condition	
	Croup	**Epiglottitis**
Chest film (antero-posterior [AP])	"Steeple sign" (i.e., narrowed and tapering airway below larynx due to subglottic edema); tracheal dilation possibly present if the film was taken during expiration	Usually appears normal (little or no evidence of subglottic involvement)
Lateral neck film	May appear normal (little or no evidence of supraglottic involvement)	"Thumb sign" due to prominent shadow caused by a swollen epiglottis

objects are readily visualized on x-ray. Some plastic objects or food matter may be more difficult to identify and often require laryngoscopy or bronchoscopy to confirm and resolve.

In terms of serious upper airway infections in pediatric patients, croup and epiglottitis are the most commonly encountered diseases. **Table 2-23** compares the typical radiographic findings in these two conditions.

T⁴—TOP TEST-TAKING TIPS

You can improve your score on this section of the NBRC exam by reviewing these tips:

- Only alert patients ("oriented × 3") can fully cooperate and participate in their care.
- A Glasgow Coma Scale (GCS) score of ≤ 8 indicates coma.
- A patient's pain/interference rating of > 4 requires intervention.
- Use/recommend the Borg Scale to assess a patient's shortness of breath/dyspnea or degree of exertion; values ≥ 5 indicate severe shortness of breath/dyspnea with strong exertion.
- Tachypnea, thoracic–abdominal dyssynchrony, and the use of accessory muscles always indicate increased work of breathing.
- Sputum production > 30 mL/day indicates the need for airway clearance.
- Job *and* home factors must be included in an environmental assessment.
- Health literacy is associated with low educational levels and manifests as a lack of knowledge regarding care or difficulty following a care plan.
- Use teach-back (knowledge) or return demonstration (skills) to evaluate patient learning.
- Peripheral cyanosis (acrocyanosis), coolness of the extremities, and slow capillary refills indicate circulatory failure.
- When assessing a patient, especially one who has been bedridden, the skin integrity should be examined for signs of breakdown and, when detected, should be documented and treated.
- A short/thick neck, large tongue, and limited visibility of pharyngeal structures (Mallampati classification) predict difficult intubation.
- Pink, watery, frothy secretions suggest pulmonary edema.
- An infant with an Apgar score (**A**ppearance, **P**ulse, **G**rimace, **A**ctivity, **R**espirations) of < 4 should be resuscitated.
- Fetal maturity is indicated by a lecithin/sphingomyelin (L/S) ratio of > 2 and the presence of phosphatidylglycerol (PG).
- A pulse deficit usually indicates a cardiac arrhythmia, such as atrial fibrillation or flutter, PVCs, or heart block.
- A pulse that varies with the breathing cycle (pulsus paradoxus) indicates severe airway obstruction (e.g., status asthmaticus) or cardiac tamponade.
- The trachea tends to shift *toward areas of collapse/atelectasis* and *away from space-occupying lesions,* such as pneumothoraces and pleural effusions.
- Rhonchial fremitus is associated with excess secretions in the large airways.
- Especially in patients receiving positive-pressure ventilation, neck/upper chest crepitus suggests a pneumothorax.

- Increased percussion resonance indicates hyperinflation, whereas a dull/flat note suggests increased tissue density (e.g., pneumonia, atelectasis).
- "All that wheezes is not asthma"—consider CHF/pulmonary edema in adults and foreign-body obstruction in toddlers/children.
- Stridor indicates tracheal/laryngeal/upper airway obstruction (e.g., croup, epiglottitis, post-extubation edema).
- A chest x-ray is aligned correctly if the thoracic spine lines up under the center of the sternum and equally between the medial ends of each clavicle.
- A patient with a condition affecting the phrenic nerve, such as quadriplegia, often shows signs of an *elevated* diaphragm.
- A properly functioning diaphragm may have a *flattened* appearance due to hyperinflation associated with a chronic condition such as severe emphysema or an acute one such as asthma or pneumothorax.
- A blunted costophrenic angle on x-ray suggests a pleural effusion.
- Pulmonary artery engorgement and enlargement due to pulmonary emboli or other conditions may manifest themselves on a chest x-ray and often warrant further testing.
- On an AP x-ray, croup may show narrowing and tapering of the trachea below the larynx ("steeple sign"); epiglottitis may appear on lateral neck films as a prominent shadow in the laryngopharynx ("thumb sign").

POST-TEST

To confirm your mastery of each chapter's topical content, you should create a content post-test, available online via the Navigate Premier Access for Comprehensive Respiratory Therapy Exam Preparation Guide, which contains Navigate TestPrep (access code provided with every new text). You can create multiple topical content post-tests varying in length from 10 to 20 questions, with each attempt presenting a different set of items. You can select questions from all three major NBRC TMC sections: Patient Data, Troubleshooting and Quality Control of Devices and Infection Control, and Initiation and Modification of Interventions. A score of at least 70–80% indicates that you are adequately prepared for this section of the NBRC TMC exam. If you score below 70%, you should first carefully assess your test answers (particularly your wrong answers) and the correct answer explanations. Then return to the chapter to re-review the applicable content. Only then should you reattempt a new post-test. Repeat this process of identifying your shortcomings and reviewing the pertinent content until your test results demonstrate mastery.

Perform Procedures to Gather Clinical Information (Section I-C)

CHAPTER 3

Albert J. Heuer

Although the title "respiratory therapist" (RT) emphasizes *therapy*, to be effective, your clinical interventions must be based on pertinent *clinical information*. Thus, a competent RT must be able to determine which data are relevant to each patient's care and—in many cases—perform the procedures needed to obtain the data. To assess this general competency, the NBRC exams include a heavy emphasis on questions or scenarios that test your knowledge of common diagnostic and monitoring procedures. To succeed on these exams, you must demonstrate a high level of proficiency on this critical topic.

OBJECTIVES

In preparing for this section of the NBRC exams (TMC/CSE), you should demonstrate the knowledge needed to perform the following procedures:

1. 12-lead ECG
2. Noninvasive monitoring (pulse oximetry, transcutaneous P_{O_2}/P_{CO_2}, capnography)
3. Bedside measures of ventilation (V_T, f, $\dot{V}e$, VC, MIP, MEP)
4. Pulmonary function tests (peak flow, screening spirometry, full lab-based PFT exam)
5. Blood gas sample collection
6. Blood gas collection and analysis, including hemoximetry
7. Exercise-related tests (6-minute walk test [6MWT], O_2 titration with exercise, cardiopulmonary stress test)
8. Cardiopulmonary calculations
9. Hemodynamic monitoring
10. Airway pressures, compliance, and resistance during mechanical ventilation
11. Auto-PEEP detection and measurement
12. Spontaneous breathing trials (SBT)
13. Apnea monitoring
14. Sleep-related studies (overnight pulse oximetry, CPAP/BPAP titration)
15. Tracheal airway cuff management
16. Therapeutic bronchoscopy

WHAT TO EXPECT ON THIS CATEGORY OF THE NBRC EXAMS

TMC exam: 12 questions; 4 recall, 7 application, 1 analysis
CSE exam: indeterminate number of questions; however, section I-C knowledge is a prerequisite to succeed on the CSE, especially on Information Gathering sections.

WHAT YOU NEED TO KNOW: ESSENTIAL CONTENT

12-Lead ECG

The 12-lead electrocardiogram (ECG) is used to assess rhythm disturbances, determine the heart's electrical axis, and identify the site and extent of myocardial damage. Here we focus on the basic procedure, as outlined in the accompanying box (**Box 3-1**). Chapter 4 provides details on ECG interpretation.

Box 3-1 Basic 12-Lead ECG Procedure

1. Turn on the machine (plug it into an outlet if AC-powered); run the self-test/calibration process.
2. Place the patient appropriately in supine or semi-Fowler's position.
3. Have the patient remove all jewelry or metal and relax completely.
4. Apply limb electrodes to muscular areas of the arms and legs.
5. Place chest leads in the proper locations (see Figure 3-1).
6. Ensure patient comfort, and respect patient privacy and modesty.
7. Run the 12-lead ECG to obtain a good recording (stable isoelectric baseline, no extraneous noise/electrical interference).

Figure 3-1 shows the proper lead placement for obtaining a 12-lead ECG. Note that there are only 10 actual leads to place, not 12. One (the right leg) does not count because it is just a ground lead. The difference is the three augmented limb leads (aVR, aVL, and aVF), which use the right arm (RA), left arm (LA), and left leg (LL) electrodes to obtain their data.

Most units automatically detect common problems and will not begin recording until a good signal is obtained. The two most common problems are absent or "noisy" signals. Failure to obtain a signal usually is due to a loose, missing, or defective lead or the patient's hair preventing the lead from making proper skin contact. A noisy ECG signal may be caused by a poor electrical connection,

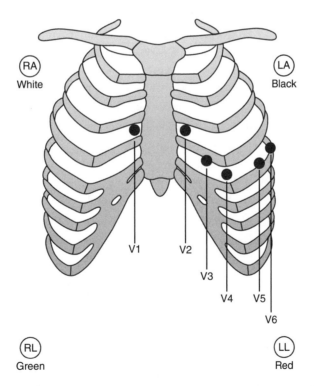

Figure 3-1 Diagnostic ECG Lead Placement. Place the RL/green lead on the right leg, the LL/red lead on the left leg, the RA/white lead on the right arm, and the LA/black lead on the left arm. Then place the six chest leads as follows: V1—fourth intercostal space, right sternal border; V2—fourth intercostal space, left sternal border; V3—between V2 and V4; V4—fifth intercostal space, midclavicular line; V5—fifth intercostal space, anterior axillary line; and V6—fifth intercostal space, midaxillary line.

motion artifact, or improper filtering of extraneous electrical activity. In either case, you should follow these steps:

- Verify that the ECG snaps and connectors are clean and corrosion free.
- Verify that the lead electrodes are connected properly to the patient.
- Verify that the electrode gel is not dry; replace any suspect electrodes.
- Check the ECG main cable for continuity; replace it if damaged.
- Confirm that the patient is motionless; if necessary, support the patient's limbs.
- Verify that the device's filter settings (if available) are appropriately set.

Noninvasive Monitoring

Pulse Oximetry

You use a pulse oximeter to spot check, monitor, or obtain trend data on a patient's pulse oxygen saturation (SpO_2). **Table 3-1** outlines the basic steps, including key considerations for obtaining good saturation data.

Table 3-1 Key Considerations in the Setup of Pulse Oximeters

Setup Steps	Key Considerations
1. If AC powered, connect the power cord to an appropriate power source.	• Most oximeters use a battery to provide power if an AC outlet is unavailable.
2. Connect the appropriate probe to the oximeter.	• There are special probes for infants and children. • Proper probe size is essential for accurate readings.
3. Turn the power on.	• Most oximeters perform a power-on-self-test (POST) before reading the SpO_2. • Always verify that the unit has passed the POST.
4. Select a site for probe application	• Check for adequate perfusion. • If applied on a finger, remove any nail polish. • Clean the site with an alcohol prep pad.
5. Attach the probe to the patient.	• For continuous monitoring, use a disposable probe attached with adhesive or Velcro strips. • For spot checks, a nondisposable, multiuse probe is satisfactory. • Always disinfect a multiuse probe with alcohol before use. • Overly tight oximeter probes may cause venous pooling and inaccurate readings or skin damage.
6. Verify a good signal.	• If displayed, observe the waveform to verify a good pulse signal. • Alternatively, use the oximeter's LED display to verify a good signal. • Always validate the oximeter's rate against an electrocardiogram (ECG) monitor or palpated pulse.
7. For continuous monitoring, set the alarm limits.	• Set the low alarm according to institutional protocol, typically 90–94% for adults and 85–88% for infants.
8. For overnight oximetry, set the devices for trend recording.	• Select the planned period (e.g., 8 hours, 12 hours). • Adjust the capture rate/response time to the fastest allowable value (usually 2–6 seconds). • Confirm sufficient memory is available to record for the specified period/capture rate. • If needed or appropriate, turn alarms off.

Capnography

Capnography involves the measurement and display of exhaled CO_2 levels during breathing. The key procedural steps in monitoring exhaled CO_2 are as follows:

1. Obtain a calibrated capnograph or calibrate the device as per the manufacturer's instructions.
2. Select, obtain, and connect sensor or sampling system/filter appropriate for the situation (e.g., intubated/invasive ventilation, noninvasive ventilation, patient breathing spontaneously via intact airway).
3. Connect capnograph to a power source (check battery charge), turn on, and confirm completion of the power-on-self-test (some units will perform a one-point/low calibration at start-up).
4. Connect sensor or sampling system to the patient and confirm a good inspiratory baseline ($Petco_2$ = 0 torr) and expiratory waveform on the display.
5. Compare the monitor $Petco_2$ reading with the patient's current arterial Pco_2 ($Petco_2$ typically runs 1–5 torr less than the $Paco_2$, more with high deadspace ventilation).
6. Set alarms (example settings only; follow institutional protocol):
   - $Petco_2$: High 50–55 torr; low 25–30 torr
   - Respiratory rate: appropriate for age/condition (7–35/min for adults)
   - Apnea alarm: 20–30 seconds

Transcutaneous Po_2/Pco_2

Transcutaneous blood gas monitoring provides continuous, noninvasive estimates of arterial Po_2 and Pco_2 via a sensor placed on the skin (some units combine a Pco_2 sensor with a pulse oximeter probe instead of an O_2 sensor). These pressures are referred to as transcutaneous (tc) partial pressures, abbreviated as $Ptco_2$ and $Ptcco_2$.

Common indications for transcutaneous blood gas monitoring are listed in Chapter 5.

Transcutaneous monitoring also may be used in children or adults to continuously assess the adequacy of ventilation (via $Ptcco_2$) when capnography is not available or technically difficult, such as during noninvasive ventilation or high-frequency ventilation.

You should avoid using a transcutaneous monitor on patients with poor skin integrity or those with an adhesive allergy. Because accurate $Ptco_2$ and $Ptcco_2$ values generally require good perfusion, you should not use these devices on patients in shock or with poor peripheral circulation. Lengthy setup and stabilization time (5–20 minutes) also make transcutaneous monitoring a poor choice in emergencies.

Key elements of the transcutaneous blood gas monitoring procedure include the following:

- Membrane the sensor and calibrate the device as per the manufacturer's instructions.
- Ensure proper temperature setting (usually 44°C if monitoring $Ptco_2$ and $Ptcco_2$, with temperatures as low as 37°C adequate if monitoring only $Ptcco_2$).
- Choose a site that has good superficial circulation (e.g., the side of the chest, below the clavicles, the abdomen, inner thigh), and clean it with alcohol.
- Apply the adhesive fixation ring to the sensor (some protocols apply the ring to the skin first).
- Apply the contact gel to the sensor face and inside the fixation ring; avoid air bubbles.
- Apply the sensor to the selected site; make sure the edges are sealed, with the sensor lying flat on the skin.
- Allow sufficient time for the reading to stabilize (5–20 minutes).
- Set the high/low $Ptco_2$ and $Ptcco_2$ alarms (varies by patient/protocol; high $Ptco_2$ for infants typically set to 80 torr).
- To avoid burns/skin damage, change the sensor site frequently (every 2–6 hours, depending on the sensor temperature, infant size, and manufacturer's recommendation).

Peak Flow

A patient's peak expiratory flow rate (PEFR) is the maximum flow generated on forced expiration and is a simple measure used to assess for airway obstruction. However, because the PEFR is highly effort-dependent, it is not used for diagnosis but instead is considered a monitoring tool. For this reason, the PEFR is mainly used for the following purposes:

- Monitoring the effect of bronchodilator therapy (using pre- and post-test measures)
- Assessing the severity of asthma symptoms
- Detecting early changes in asthma control that require adjustments in treatment

Often, the patient makes these measurements at home and records them in a log. Inspection of this log can help RTs assess the pattern of a patient's symptoms and response to therapy.

Typically, you measure a patient's PEFR with a mechanical peak-flow meter or electronic spirometer and report the value in liters per second (L/sec) or liters per minute (L/min) body at temperature pressure, saturated (BTPS). *To convert L/sec to L/min, multiply by 60; to convert L/min to L/sec, divide by 60.*

To make this measurement, the patient must be able to follow simple instructions and coordinate breathing with the use of the measurement device. Data needed for interpretation (see Chapter 4) include the patient's gender, age, and height. Also, you should determine the patient's smoking history and current medications, including bronchodilators and steroids. Key points needed to ensure valid measurement include the following:

- If using a mechanical meter, it must be set to zero and properly positioned (some devices must be held level).
- Ideally, the patient should sit or stand up straight and inhale fully to total lung capacity (TLC).
- The mouthpiece should be inserted above the tongue, with the patient making a tight lip seal.
- The patient should exhale in a sharp burst with maximum force (complete exhalation is not needed).
- The measurement should be repeated until three values are obtained that vary by less than 10%; record the highest of the three values.
- If assessing bronchodilator therapy:
  ○ Allow the drug to reach its full effect before the post-test (usually 10–30 min).
  ○ Compute the percent change from pre-test to post-test (see Chapter 4).

Mechanics of Spontaneous Ventilation

Bedside assessment of spontaneous ventilation involves measurement of a patient's tidal volume (V_T), rate of breathing (f), minute ventilation ($\dot{V}E$), vital capacity (VC), and maximum inspiratory pressure (MIP). Here we discuss the basic procedures for obtaining these measures. Chapter 4 covers their interpretation.

You should recommend measuring these parameters when there is a need to do either of the following:

- Assess the progress of diseases affecting respiratory muscle strength (e.g., neuromuscular disorders)
- Evaluate a patient's potential need for mechanical ventilation

These measures can also be used to assess whether a patient is ready to be weaned from mechanical ventilation. However, new evidence-based guidelines have established different criteria to evaluate a patient's readiness to wean.

You typically measure V_T, f, and $\dot{V}E$ on spontaneously breathing patients using a respirometer attached to a one-way valve, as described in Chapter 6. Over a 1-minute interval, you measure the accumulated exhaled volume and count the frequency of breaths. To compute the tidal volume, you divide the minute ventilation by the frequency (i.e., $V_T = \dot{V}E \div f$). For example, the tidal volume of a patient breathing at a rate of 38/min with a minute ventilation of 11.4 L/min would be computed as follows:

$$V_T = 11.4 \text{ L/min} \div 38 \text{ breaths/min} = 0.3 \text{ L or } 300 \text{ mL}$$

A different and more useful measure called the *rapid shallow breathing index* (RSBI) can be computed using the same data. You compute the RSBI by dividing the patient's rate of breathing by the average tidal volume in liters: $RSBI = f \div V_T$ (L). For example, the RSBI for a patient breathing spontaneously at a rate of 38/min with an average tidal volume of 300 mL would be computed as follows:

$$RSBI = f \div V_T \text{ (L)}$$
$$RSBI = 38 \div 0.3$$
$$RSBI \approx 127$$

Fast and shallow breathing as in the previous example increases deadspace ventilation, which is evident in the formula for alveolar minute ventilation—**a point commonly tested on the NBRC exams**. Alveolar minute ventilation ($\dot{V}_A$) is the volume of "fresh" gas reaching the alveoli per minute. To compute $\dot{V}_A$, you multiply a patient's breathing frequency (f) by the *difference* between the tidal volume (V_T) and the physiologic deadspace per breath (V_D):

$$\dot{V}_A = f \times (V_T - V_D)$$

Unless otherwise indicated, *you should assume a deadspace of approximately 1 mL per pound of predicted body weight*. Using the above formula and assuming a 125-lb patient (57 kg) breathing at a rate of 15/min with a tidal volume of 400 mL, you would compute this patient's alveolar minute volume as follows:

$$\dot{V}_A = f \times (V_T - V_D)$$
$$\dot{V}_A = 15 \times (400 - 125) = 4125 \text{ mL/min}$$

In this case, approximately 70% of the patient's ventilation per minute is "fresh" gas ($\dot{V}_A \div \dot{V}_E = 4125 \div 6000 = 0.69 = 69\%$), with the remaining 30% being deadspace ventilation. Thirty percent of deadspace ventilation is considered roughly normal.

The VC indicates how well the entire ventilatory "pump" is working, including both lung/chest wall interaction and respiratory muscle function. For this reason, along with the pressure measures discussed subsequently, the VC is a good indicator of the progress of diseases affecting respiratory muscle strength, such as neuromuscular disorders. In these cases, you typically use either a mechanical respirometer or an electronic spirometer to measure the *slow* vital capacity (SVC). To obtain the SVC, have the patient inhale as deeply as possible (*deeper, deeper, deeper,...*) and then exhale slowly and completely for as long as possible (*more, more, more,...*) or until no volume change occurs for at least 2 seconds. This procedure should be performed at least three times to ensure maximum effort and repeatability; the best result is recorded. The SVC can be obtained only with alert and cooperative patients.

The MIP assesses the patient's inspiratory muscle strength. You measure MIP (aka negative inspiratory force [NIF]) using a manometer attached to a one-way valve configured to allow exhalation but not inspiration. With this setup, the patient "bucks down" toward residual volume (RV) on each successive breath, at which point a maximum effort is ensured (the patient need not be conscious). Given that this process can cause anxiety in alert patients, you should provide a careful and reassuring explanation before performing the procedure.

Blood Gas Sample Collection

Indications for blood gas and hemoximetry sampling and analysis are detailed in Chapter 5. Chapter 4 covers the interpretation of arterial blood gas (ABG) and hemoximetry data, and Chapter 8 reviews sample analysis and related quality-control procedures. Here we focus on the key elements involved in obtaining samples via arterial puncture, indwelling vascular lines, or capillary "stick."

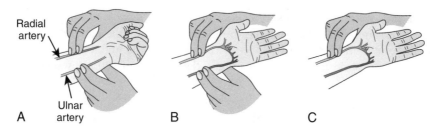

Figure 3-2 Modified Allen's Test. (A) Patient's hand is clenched while you obstruct flow to both the radial and ulnar arteries for about 5 seconds. **(B)** The patient opens his or her hand while you maintain pressure; the hand should appear blanched. **(C)** Upon the release of pressure on the ulnar artery, the palmar surface should flush within 5–10 seconds and color should be restored. Prolonged delay before flushing indicates decreased ulnar artery flow.

Hess, Dean. *Respiratory Care: Principles and Practice, Third Edition*. Burlington, MA: Jones & Bartlett Learning, 2016. Data from Dudley HAF, Eckersely JRT, Paterson-Brown S. *A Guide to Practical Procedures in Medicine and Surgery*. Butterworth-Heinemann; 1989.

Arterial Sampling by Puncture

The radial artery is the preferred site for obtaining arterial blood because (1) it is located near the skin surface and not close to any large veins, and (2) the ulnar artery provides collateral circulation. Other potential sites for sampling include the brachial, femoral, and dorsalis pedis arteries. These sites carry greater risk and should be used only by those with the proper training.

Key points in performing a radial arterial puncture for ABG analysis include the following:

- Review the patient's prothrombin time (PT), partial thromboplastin time (PTT), or International Normalized Ratio (INR) to anticipate longer bleeding time.
- Choose the nondominant wrist first.
- Assess collateral circulation by performing the modified Allen's test (**Figure 3-2**).
  - If collateral circulation is not present on the initial side, assess the other wrist.
  - If both sides lack collateral circulation, use the brachial artery.
- After needle withdrawal, compress the site until the bleeding stops (patients with a prolonged PT, PTT, or INR may require longer compression times).
- After hemostasis is ensured, apply a sterile bandage over the puncture site; recheck the site after 20 minutes, and document the procedure.
- Apply the methods outlined in Chapter 8 to avoid preanalysis errors by performing quality control procedures.

Sampling Blood from Vascular Lines

If you need to obtain repeated arterial samples over several days or need to monitor blood pressure continually, you should recommend placement of an indwelling arterial catheter, or "A-line." In the NBRC hospital, RTs may be responsible for the insertion and care of arterial lines. The accompanying box (**Box 3-2**) outlines the key elements involved in inserting an arterial line. Chapter 7 provides details on infection control procedures for indwelling catheters.

Either direct cannulation or the guidewire (Seldinger) technique are used to insert the catheter. With direct cannulation, you puncture the artery with a needle sheathed in a catheter. Once blood is observed "flashing" at the needle hub, the catheter sheath is advanced over the needle into the artery, and the needle is removed. With the Seldinger technique, you puncture the artery with a needle, then thread a small guidewire through the needle into the vessel. Next, you remove the needle, leaving the guidewire in place. Finally, you advance the catheter over the guidewire into the artery and remove the guidewire.

Figure 3-3 shows the basic equipment used to maintain an indwelling arterial catheter. Once inserted, this catheter is connected to a continuous flush device. The flush device keeps the line open via a continuous low flow of fluid through the system. To maintain continuous flow, the IV bag

Box 3-2 Key Elements Involved in Arterial Line Insertion

- Ensure that a "time-out" is performed before the procedure.

- Ensure that the monitoring system is set up and calibrated, with lines properly flushed.

- Scrub the insertion site with chlorhexidine, and cover area with a sterile drape.

- Puncture skin at the point of pulsation at 30-degree angle, with needle bevel and hub arrow up.

- Advance catheter into position, connect to transducer tubing and flush the line.

- Confirm proper arterial waveform on the monitor; reposition catheter if needed.

- Secure line to prevent traction on the catheter.

- Cover line insertion point with a clear sterile dressing.

- Recheck for the adequacy of distal blood flow and patient comfort.

- Instruct patient on line use and safety considerations

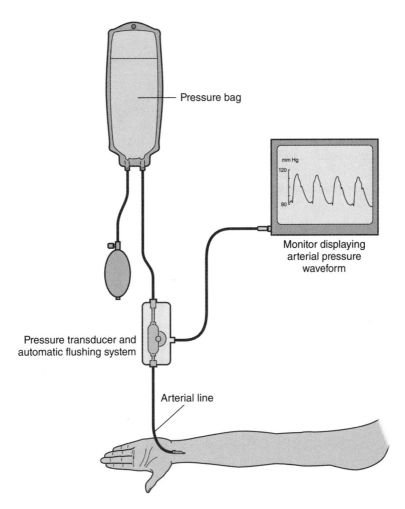

Figure 3-3 Indwelling Arterial Catheter System.

Modified from Kacmarek RM, Stoller JK, and Heuer AJ, eds. *Egan's Fundamentals of Respiratory Care* (11th ed.). St. Louis, MO: Mosby; 2017. Courtesy of Elsevier Ltd.

must be pressurized at least to 300 mm Hg, usually by a hand bulb pump. A pressure transducer, connected to the flush device, provides an electrical signal to a monitor, which displays the arterial pressure waveform. A sampling port (not shown in Figure 3-3) typically is included to allow intermittent blood withdrawal.

Table 3-2 Procedures for Obtaining Blood Samples from an Arterial Line (Adult Patient)

Three-Way Stopcock Sampling	In-Line Closed-Reservoir Sampling
• Swab sample port with chlorhexidine, povidone-iodine, or alcohol.	• Slowly draw blood into the reservoir to the needed fill volume.
• Attach waste syringe and turn the stopcock off to flush solution/bag.	• Close the reservoir shut-off valve.
• Aspirate 5–6 mL blood (at least 6 times the "dead" volume).	• Swab sample port with chlorhexidine, povidone-iodine, or alcohol.
• Turn stopcock off to the port.	• Attach the blunt/needleless sampling syringe to the valved sampling port.
• Remove waste syringe; properly discard it.	• Aspirate the needed volume of blood.
• Secure heparinized syringe to port, reopen stopcock, and collect the sample.	• Open the reservoir shut-off valve.
• Turn stopcock off to the port; remove syringe.	• Slowly depress reservoir plunger to reinfuse blood into the patient.
• Flush line until clear.	• Reswab sample port; flush line until clear.
• Turn stopcock off to patient, briefly flush sampling port, and swab sample port.	• Confirm restoration of arterial pulse pressure waveform.
• Turn stopcock off to the port; confirm restoration of arterial pulse pressure waveform.	

Two different procedures are used to obtain blood samples from vascular lines: the three-way stopcock method and the in-line closed reservoir method (**Table 3-2**). The closed-reservoir sampling method is becoming the standard approach in many ICUs since it minimizes blood waste, reduces the potential for contamination, and better protects against exposure to bloodborne pathogens than the stopcock method.

When obtaining a blood sample from a pulmonary artery (PA) or Swan-Ganz catheter (mixed venous blood), the following points must be considered:

- To avoid contamination with arterialized blood and falsely high O_2 levels, the sample must be drawn *slowly* from the catheter's distal port with the balloon *deflated*.
- Attention must be paid to the IV infusion rate through the catheter to prevent sample dilution.
- When obtaining arterial and mixed venous samples to calculate cardiac output (using the Fick equation), both samples must be drawn *at the same time*.

Obtaining a Capillary Blood Sample

Capillary blood gas (CBG) sampling is used in infants and toddlers when a blood sample is needed to assess ventilation and acid-base status, but arterial access is not available. Capillary sampling is less invasive, quicker, and easier to perform than an arterial puncture. This sampling technique is contraindicated when accurate analysis of oxygenation is needed and in neonates less than 24 hours old.

Obtain a capillary blood sample as follows:

- Gather the needed equipment: lancet, alcohol pad, sterile gauze, adhesive bandage, and pre-heparinized capillary tube with tube caps.
- Select the site (e.g., heel, great toe, earlobe). Avoid inflamed, swollen, or edematous tissue and cyanotic or poorly perfused areas. For heel sticks, avoid the posterior curvature, and puncture the lateral side only (see **Figure 3-4**).
- Use a warm cloth or warming pack to warm the site for 3–5 minutes to no higher than 42–45°C.
- Puncture the skin with the lancet and wipe away the first drop of blood.
- Allowing the free flow of blood, collect the sample from the middle of the blood drop (do not squeeze the site).
- Fill the tube, cap its ends, label it, and send it for analysis.

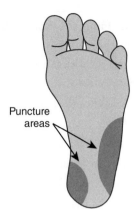

Puncture
areas

Figure 3-4 Capillary Blood Sampling Sites.

Blood Gas Analysis/Hemoximetry

Indications for blood gas and hemoximetry sampling and analysis are detailed in Chapter 5. Chapter 4 covers the interpretation of ABG and hemoximetry data, and Chapter 8 reviews quality-control procedures for these tests. Here we focus on the key elements involved in the actual procedure for analyzing blood samples, both in the laboratory and at the point of care.

Current regulations require that laboratory tests must be performed by individuals who meet the competency requirements for the procedure, as documented at least annually. Testing also must follow the protocol recommended by the instrument manufacturer. If you are responsible for performing the analysis in a blood gas lab, you always must take the following key steps:

- Confirm that the specimen was labeled correctly and stored before analysis.
- Assess the sample for obvious preanalytical errors, such as air bubbles or clots (see Chapter 8).
- Confirm that the analyzer was properly calibrated before running the sample (see Chapter 8).
- Ensure that analysis occurs within an acceptable time period, as follows:
  - < 30 minutes if sample at room temperature in a plastic syringe
  - < 5 minutes if sample used for a shunt study
  - Immediately if sampled from a patient with an elevated leukocyte or platelet count.
  - If kept for > 30 min, the sample should be in a glass syringe chilled to 0–4°C.
- Mix the sample thoroughly, and then discard a drop or two of blood from the syringe.
- Confirm that the sample is properly aspirated/injected into the analyzer.

Outside the ABG lab, point-of-care testing (POCT) may be conducted on patients in urgent need of assessment. Most POCT instruments measure blood samples using disposable cartridges specifically designed for each desired set of tests. The most common POCT tests done by RTs are for ABGs, alone or in combination with measurement of other parameters used in managing critically ill patients, such as electrolytes, hemoglobin, glucose, lactate, and blood urea nitrogen (BUN).

If POCT is ordered for ABG analysis, in addition to the analyzer, you will need an ABG kit and the appropriate analysis cartridge. Key elements in using a common POCT unit (Abbott Laboratories I-STAT) for blood analysis are outlined in the accompanying box (**Box 3-3**). Other devices may employ slightly different procedures.

Whenever you report the results of any test you conduct, you should also provide a brief statement addressing test quality, including any problems encountered with the specimen or its measurement.

Box 3-3 Key Procedural Elements in Using the Abbott Laboratories I-STAT POCT Instrument

- Select the appropriate test cartridge (as per physician order).
- Turn the analyzer on, and confirm its power-on-self-test (POST).
- From the menu provided, specify the cartridge type/test panel to be performed.
- Scan or enter the operator and patient IDs.
- Carefully remove the cartridge from its pouch; avoid touching any contact pads.
- Obtain the sample as usual and analyze it within 3 minutes (do *not* place it in ice).
- Mix the sample thoroughly, and then dispense it into the cartridge well to the fill mark.
- Close the sample well cover, insert the cartridge into its port, and confirm placement.
- Enter any requested information—for example, type of sample, Fi_{O_2}, patient temperature.
- View the results shown on the analyzer's display screen.
- Remove the cartridge when indicated by the analyzer.
- Turn analyzer off, and place in the downloader/recharger.

Oxygen Titration with Exercise

According to the American Association for Respiratory Care (AARC), O_2 titration with exercise is indicated for the following purposes:

- Assessing arterial oxygenation during exercise in patients suspected of desaturation, especially those with pulmonary disease who complain of dyspnea on exertion or have a decreased DLco and low Pa_{O_2} at rest
- Optimizing the level of O_2 therapy for patients with documented exertion-related desaturation

Contraindications and patient preparation are the same as for cardiopulmonary stress testing (discussed subsequently), with additional cautions against performing this test on patients with a resting Sp_{O_2} less than 85% on room air.

This test is often performed during exercise capacity testing and requires the same basic equipment, except for the metabolic cart. If a treadmill is not available, a step test or the 6MWT can be substituted. A cycle ergometer is not recommended because patients' O_2 needs during exercise must be established while carrying the portable system they use or that is planned for use. Heart rate monitoring via pulse oximeter is mandatory; ECG monitoring should be used if possible.

Cardiopulmonary Calculations

Where it is essential for an explanation, we include selected cardiopulmonary calculations in this chapter. Appendix C (see Navigate 2 Premier companion website) provides a complete summary of all calculations that might appear on the NBRC exams.

Hemodynamic Monitoring

Hemodynamic monitoring involves bedside measurement of pressures and flows in the cardiovascular system. **Table 3-3** outlines the key information that hemodynamic monitoring provides by sampling location.

General considerations that apply to the proper use of indwelling catheters for hemodynamic monitoring include the following:

- For accurate pressure measurements, you need to ensure that the transducer is at the same level as the pressure it measures; for central venous pressure (CVP) and PA pressures, this is the patient's *phlebostatic axis* (intersection of the fourth intercostal space and midaxillary line).

Table 3-3 Hemodynamic Monitoring Information by Sampling Location

Location	Pressure(s)	Reflects
Systemic artery	Systemic arterial pressure	• LV afterload • Vascular tone • Blood volume
Central vein (cv)	Central venous pressure (CVP)	• Fluid volume • Vascular tone • RV preload
Pulmonary artery (PA)	Pulmonary artery pressure (PAP)	• RV afterload • Vascular tone • Blood volume
	Pulmonary artery wedge pressure (PAWP), balloon inflated	• LV preload
LV, left ventricular; RV, right ventricular.		

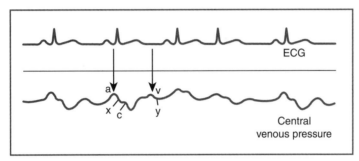

Figure 3-5 Monitor Display of CVP Waveform and ECG. The "a" wave reflects a contraction in the atrial systole and follows the "p" wave in the ECG. The "x" descent reflects fall in right atrial pressure following atrial systole. The "c" wave, often small, represents the closure of the tricuspid valve. The "v" wave represents ventricular systole, as well as passive atrial diastolic filling, and follows the "t" wave of the ECG. The "y" descent represents the fall in the right atrial pressure following the opening of the tricuspid valve and the initiation of passive filling of the right ventricle.

- Both CVP and PA wedge pressure (PAWP) are affected by changes in intrathoracic pressure during spontaneous and positive-pressure breathing; to minimize this effect, make your measurements at end-expiration.
- Do not remove patients from positive end-expiratory pressure (PEEP) or continuous positive airway pressure (CPAP) to measure CVP or PAWP. If PEEP is less than or equal to 10 cm H_2O, simply obtain the end-expiratory reading; if PEEP is greater than 10 cm H_2O, use the following correction formula:

$$\text{Corrected pressure} = \text{measured pressure} - [0.5 \times (\text{PEEP}/1.36)]$$

In critical care settings, vascular pressures are often measured and displayed continuously on a monitor at the bedside. **Figure 3-5** provides an example of a display of CVP and the ECG, as well as annotations depicting the key events.

Common problems you may encounter when obtaining hemodynamic pressure measurements, as well as their solutions, are outlined in **Table 3-4**.

As noted in Table 3-4, any partial obstruction in the measurement system, such as that caused by air bubbles or small clots, can "dampen" the pressure signal (i.e., reduce its amplitude).

Table 3-4 Common Problems with Hemodynamic Pressure Measurement and Their Solutions

Problem/Causes	Solution
Unexpectedly High or Low Venous/Pulmonary Artery (PA) Pressure Readings	
Change in transducer reference level	Position transducer at the phlebostatic axis (midchest)
Damped Pressure Waveform	
Catheter tip against the vessel wall	Pull back, rotate, or reposition catheter while observing pressure waveform.
Partial occlusion of catheter tip by a clot	Aspirate clot with syringe and flush with heparinized saline.
A clot in stopcock or transducer	Disconnect and flush stopcock and transducer; if no improvement, change stopcock and transducer.
Air bubbles in transducer or connector tubing	Disconnect transducer and flush out air bubbles.
Absent Waveform/No Pressure Reading	
Catheter occluded	Aspirate blood from the line.
Catheter out of the vessel	Notify the doctor, and prepare to replace the line.
Stopcock off to the patient	Position stopcock correctly.
Loose connection	Tighten loose connection.
Transducer not connected to monitor	Check and tighten the cable connection.
Monitor set to zero, calibrate, or off	Make sure monitor set to proper function/display.
Incorrect scale selection	Select appropriate scale (arterial = high; venous = low).
Signal Artifacts	
Patient movement	Wait until the patient is quiet before taking a reading.
Electrical interference	Make sure electrical equipment is connected and grounded correctly.
Catheter fling	Notify physician to reposition catheter.

Airway Pressures and Pulmonary Mechanics

During mechanical ventilation, you typically monitor the peak inspiratory pressure (PIP), the baseline or PEEP level, and the difference between the two (PIP – PEEP), referred to as the *driving pressure* or ΔP. Depending on the patient and mode of ventilation, you also may monitor (1) the plateau pressure (P_{plat}), (2) the difference between PIP and P_{plat}, (3) the difference between P_{plat} and PEEP, (4) the auto-PEEP pressure, and (5) the mean airway pressure (P_{mean} or MAP). **Figure 3-6** depicts these pressures as an idealized graphic of single-breath pressure versus time during volume-control ventilation.

Auto-PEEP Detection and Measurement

Auto-PEEP represents the abnormal and often undetected residual pressure above baseline remaining in the alveoli at end-exhalation due to air-trapping. Auto-PEEP is also referred to as occult PEEP, intrinsic PEEP, and dynamic hyperinflation. Patients at greatest risk for developing auto-PEEP are those with high airway resistance and high compliance who are being supported by ventilator modes that limit expiratory time.

As indicated in **Table 3-5**, auto-PEEP is not visible on a normal pressure-versus-time graphic. Instead, to detect auto-PEEP, you need to inspect either the ventilator's flow-versus-time waveform (Figure 3-6) or the flow–volume loop.

Figure 3-6 also demonstrates what occurs when an end-expiratory pause is implemented on a patient with auto-PEEP. Once flow ceases, the airway pressure will equilibrate with the *higher* alveolar pressure, causing a momentary rise in the pressure baseline. This rise in baseline pressure corresponds to the level of residual pressure (and volume) "trapped" in the alveoli that does not fully

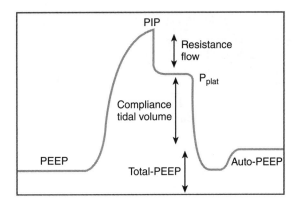

Figure 3-6 Airway Pressure Waveform During Volume Control Ventilation. An end-inspiratory and end-expiratory breath hold are applied to measure P_{plat} and auto-PEEP, respectively. The PIP-P_{plat} difference is a function of the flow setting and the ventilator and airway resistance. The P_{plat}-PEEP difference is determined by the set VT and the total level of PEEP (including auto-PEEP).

Table 3-5 Pressures Commonly Monitored During Mechanical Ventilation

Pressure	Definition	Key Points
Peak inspiratory pressure (PIP)	Peak airway pressure at the end of the breath	• During volume-control (Vc) ventilation PIP varies with patient mechanics (C_{rs} and Raw) and ventilator settings. • During pressure-control (PC) ventilation PIP is set/held constant. • During noninvasive positive-pressure ventilation (NPPV) PIP is equivalent to IPAP.
Positive end-expiratory pressure (PEEP)	Baseline pressure throughout inspiration and exhalation	• Set during all ventilator modes. • Active throughout the entire respiratory cycle (inspiration and exhalation) • Depending on the mode, also may be referred to as CPAP or EPAP
Driving pressure (ΔP)	Difference between PIP and PEEP	• Pressure applied to overcome total impedance to inflation (equation of motion*) • Equivalent to IPAP – EPAP during NPPV
Plateau pressure (P_{plat})	Airway pressure at the end of breath after cessation of inspiratory flow ($\dot{V}I$)	• During volume-control ventilation, requires an end-inspiratory pause or hold (0.5–2.0 sec) • During PC ventilation, equals set PIP only if $\dot{V}I$ has completely ceased
PIP – P_{plat}	Drop in pressure from PIP during an inspiratory pause (volume-control ventilation only)	• Represents the component of ΔP due to inspiratory Raw • Inspiratory Raw calculated as (PIP – P_{plat}) ÷ $\dot{V}I$ (L/sec)

Pressure	Definition	Key Points
P_{plat} – PEEP	Difference between the airway pressure at the end of breath (during a breath-hold maneuver) and the baseline pressure	• Represents the component of ΔP due to C_{rs} • C_{rs} computed as VT ÷ (P_{plat} – PEEP)
Auto-PEEP	Residual pressure (above set PEEP) in alveoli due to air-trapping	• Not visible on normal pressure-versus- time graphic (and thus also called "occult" PEEP) • Requires an end-expiratory pause for measurement
Mean airway pressure ($\bar{P}_{AW}$)	Average pressure over several breathing cycles	• Function of PIP, I:E ratio, and PEEP • A key determinant of functional residual capacity (FRC) and oxygenation • Used in the computation of oxygenation index (OI)

*Simplified equation of motion: $\Delta P = (V_T/C_{rs}) + (Raw \times \dot{V}_I)$.

C_{rs}, compliance of the respiratory system; CPAP, continuous positive airway pressure; EPAP, expiratory positive airway pressure; IPAP, inspiratory positive airway pressure; Raw, airway resistance.

escape during exhalation. Chapter 4 covers the management of auto-PEEP. Table 3-5 defines these pressures and provides key points regarding their application at the bedside.

Plateau Pressure

It is particularly noteworthy that plateau pressures (P_{plat}) are useful in many respects. As described above, it is a key component of determining static compliance. Also, it can be quite useful as a guideline in minimizing lung injury caused by mechanical ventilation. P_{plat} can be determined by performing an inspiratory pause maneuver (while employing a square inspiratory flow pattern) during volume-targeted ventilation. In general, plateau pressures should be kept below 30 cm H_2O during mechanical ventilation to reduce the likelihood of ventilator-induced lung injury.

Pulmonary Compliance and Airway Resistance

The simplified equation of motion noted in Table 3-5 tells us that the driving pressure during mechanical ventilation consists of two components: (1) the pressure needed to overcome the elastic recoil of the lungs and thorax (V_T/C_{rs}) and (2) the pressure due to airway resistance (Raw $\times \dot{V}_I$). During volume-control ventilation, an end-inspiratory pause or hold allows us to separate or "partition" out these two components of ΔP and thus compute both C_{rs} and Raw. Specifically, because compliance equals volume ÷ pressure, we can compute C_{rs} using the following equation:

$$C_{rs} = \frac{V_T}{P_{plat} - PEEP}$$

Because this measure is obtained under conditions of zero flow, many clinicians and the NBRC refer to it as the *static* compliance.

With resistance equaling pressure ÷ by inspiratory flow, we can also use the pressures obtained during an inspiratory pause to compute Raw as follows:

$$R_{aw} = \frac{(PIP - P_{plat})}{\dot{V}_i}$$

Note that the NBRC also may assess your understanding of a measure called *dynamic compliance* (C_{dyn}). Dynamic compliance is a measure of the total impedance to inflation during volume-control ventilation, reflecting *both* C_{rs} and Raw. As such, you perform a computation similar to that for static compliance, but instead, use the driving pressure ($\Delta P = PIP - PEEP$) in the equation:

$$C_{dyn} = \frac{V_T}{(PIP - PEEP)}$$

Because ($PIP - PEEP$) always will be greater than ($P_{plat} - PEEP$) during volume-control ventilation, C_{dyn} *always will be less than* C_{rs}, with the difference between the two ($C_{rs} - C_{dyn}$) due to airway resistance. *Specifically, the greater the difference between C_{rs} and C_{dyn}, the greater the contribution of airway resistance to the driving pressure.*

The accompanying box provides an example of these computations for an adult patient receiving volume-control ventilation. Note that you usually need to convert the ventilator flow from L/min to L/sec to compute airway resistance (L/min $\div$ 60 = L/sec).

Example of Compliance and Resistance Computations

Scenario

An adult patient receiving volume-control (Vc), assist-control (AC) ventilation exhibits the following parameters:

Parameter	Value
V_T (mL, corrected)	500
Inspiratory flow (L/min)	40
PIP (cm H_2O)	50
P_{plat} (cm H_2O)	30
PEEP (cm H_2O)	5

Calculating Static Compliance:

$$C_{rs} = V_T \div (P_{plat} - PEEP) = 500 \div (30 - 5) = 500 \div 25 = 20 \text{ mL/cm } H_2O$$

Calculating Dynamic Compliance:

$$C_{dyn} = V_T \div (PIP - PEEP) = 500 \div (50 - 5) = 500 \div 45 = 11 \text{ mL/cm } H_2O$$

Calculating Airway Resistance:
  First convert L/min to L/sec:

$$\text{L/min} \div 60 \text{ sec/min} = \text{L/sec}$$

$$40 \div 60 = 0.67 \text{ L/sec}$$

Then compute the airway resistance:

$$\text{Raw} = (PIP - P_{plat}) \div \dot{V}I$$

$$= (50 - 30) \div 0.67 = 20 \div 0.67 = 29.9 \text{ cm } H_2O/\text{L/sec}$$

Today, many ventilators automate computation of these parameters. However, the NBRC expects candidates to be able to perform these computations manually and interpret their results, as discussed in Chapter 4.

Spontaneous Breathing Trials

Patients receiving mechanical ventilation for respiratory failure should undergo a weaning assessment whenever the following criteria are met:

- Evidence for some reversal of the underlying cause of respiratory failure
- Adequate oxygenation (e.g., P/F ≥ 150–200, PEEP ≤ 5–8 cm H_2O, Fio_2 ≤ 0.4–0.5)
- pH ≥ 7.25
- Hemodynamic stability (no myocardial ischemia or significant hypotension)
- Capability to initiate an inspiratory effort

Daily *spontaneous breathing trials* (SBTs) provide the quickest route for discontinuing mechanical ventilation in patients who meet these criteria. Tracking measures such as vital capacity and MIP/NIF while the patient is receiving ventilatory support can provide useful insights into weaning potential. However, a carefully monitored SBT provides the most valid information for deciding whether a patient can stay off the ventilator.

Spontaneous breathing modes used in SBT weaning protocols include (1) straight T-tube breathing, (2) CPAP, (3) pressure support, and (4) pressure support plus CPAP (bi-level ventilation). Based on current evidence, no one approach appears better than the others. However, CPAP can help improve breath-triggering in patients who experience auto-PEEP.

Figure 3-7 provides a decision-making algorithm for a typical SBT protocol. All such protocols involve an initial "readiness" assessment of the patient, using criteria such as those delineated previously. The next step is typically the application of a brief supervised period (2–5 minutes) of carefully monitored spontaneous breathing. During this "screening" phase, you assess the patient's breathing pattern, vital signs, and comfort level. If the patient tolerates the screening phase, you continue the SBT for at least 30 minutes but no more than 120 minutes. If after this time interval ABGs are acceptable and the patient remains stable, mechanical ventilation can be discontinued.

Conversely, if the patient fails the SBT, you should restore the patient to the prior level of ventilatory support and work with the physician to determine why the trial failed. Chapter 4 provides additional details on the criteria you should use to determine SBT success or failure.

Apnea Monitoring

Apnea monitoring warns caregivers of life-threatening cardiorespiratory events, particularly in neonates being treated for recurrent apnea accompanied by bradycardia or O_2 desaturation. At-risk babies also may be discharged from the hospital with a prescription for home apnea monitoring, as will some older children and adults with conditions affecting the control of breathing.

Most apnea monitors use two sensors placed on the chest wall to detect respiratory movements via changes in electrical impedance. Typically, hospital monitors display a continuous waveform representing the cycle of chest motion, with the respiratory and heart rates also provided. *Although these systems can warn of adverse events, you should always confirm a patient's status by visual inspection.* Moreover, because impedance changes measure only chest wall movement and not airflow, simple apnea monitoring cannot be used to detect obstructive sleep apnea. Patients suspected of obstructive sleep apnea should undergo polysomnography.

Key points in performing apnea monitoring include the following:

- Set the low/high heart rate alarm limits (typically 80–210 for neonates; lower limits for older babies).
- Set the apnea time alarm limit (typically 15–20 seconds).
- For event recording:
  - Clear memory, and set the desired option for waveform recording.
  - Set the event log limits for low/high heart rate and apnea time.
  - Secure the sensors on the right and left sides of the chest, midway between the nipple line and the midaxillary line where the greatest chest motion is occurring (a sensor "belt" facilitates placement).
  - Connect the patient cable, turn the monitor on, and confirm a successful system check.
  - Confirm that the monitor signals match the patient's heart and respiratory rate.

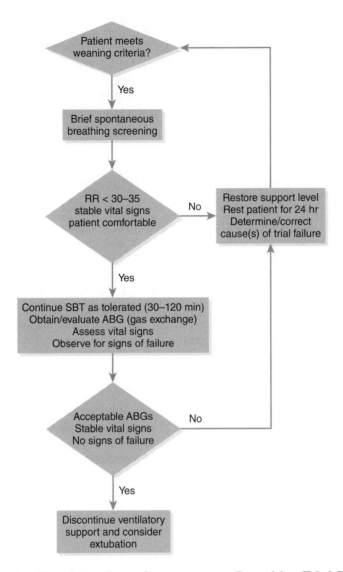

Figure 3-7 Example Algorithm for a Spontaneous Breathing Trial Protocol.

Apnea Test

The apnea test is one of three major components of the neurologic evaluation for brain death. This test assesses whether or not high levels of blood/brain CO_2 ($Paco_2 \geq 60$ torr) stimulate breathing. Complementing the apnea test in the neurologic evaluation for brain death is an assessment of the level of coma and for the presence/absence of brainstem reflexes, including pharyngeal and tracheal reflexes.

Prerequisites

- Evidence of an acute central nervous system (CNS) lesion consistent with a diagnosis of brain death
- Absence of severe acid-base, electrolyte, or endocrine abnormalities
- Absence of CNS depressants or neuromuscular blocking/paralytic agents
- Core temperature $\geq 36°C/96.8°F$ (may be supported artificially)
- Stable systolic blood pressure ≥ 100 mm Hg (may be supported with vasopressors)
- Normal $Paco_2$ (35–45 torr)*
- P/F ratio > 200

If any of the prerequisites cannot be met, and there are any other contraindications to safely performing the apnea test, an ancillary study of should be performed. Ancillary tests supporting the diagnosis of brain death include electroencephalography, conventional cerebral angiography, single-photon emission computed tomography (SPECT) radioisotope brain scan, and transcranial Doppler ultrasonography.

*If evidence of chronic CO_2 retention (e.g., chronic obstructive pulmonary disease [COPD], severe obesity), the patient's baseline Pa_{CO_2} should be considered the normal value.

Procedure

1. Preoxygenate the patient for at least 10 minutes with 100% O_2 and PEEP = 5 cm H_2O.
2. Obtain a baseline ABG and confirm a "normal" Pa_{CO_2} and a $Pa_{O_2} > 200$ torr.
3. Remove the patient from the ventilator.
4. Provide O_2 via a catheter at 6–10 L/min inserted through ET tube to the level of the carina.*
5. Monitor oxygen saturation and blood pressure.
6. Watch closely for any respiratory movements (i.e., abdominal or chest excursions).
7. Terminate the test if spontaneous respiratory effort occurs, a serious ectopic heart rhythm arises, the Sp_{O_2} falls below 85% for more than 30 seconds, or the systolic blood pressure decreases to less than 90 mm Hg.
8. Draw repeat ABGs at 10 minutes.
9. Place the patient back on the ventilator and restore all original settings (while awaiting further tests or decisions).

*As an alternative, you can oxygenate the patient using continuous-flow continuous positive airway pressure (CPAP) at 10 cm H_2O and 100% O_2.

Note that spontaneous body movements may be observed during the test even when cerebral blood flow is absent. These movements are spinal in origin and can occur with physical stimulation. To avoid the misinterpretation that might occur with such movements, you must avoid any physical stimulation of the patient during the test. See Chapter 4 for results interpretation.

Sleep-Related Studies

Sleep-related studies that the NBRC expects candidates to be familiar with include overnight oximetry and CPAP and bilevel positive airway pressure (BPAP) titration. Here we focus on the actual test procedures. Chapter 4 covers the interpretation of their results.

Overnight Pulse Oximetry

Overnight or *nocturnal* oximetry uses a recording pulse oximeter to log changes in Sp_{O_2} and heart rate while the patient is sleeping. Overnight oximetry can help identify patients with sleep apnea-hypopnea syndrome (SAHS) and assess their response to therapy. Also, overnight oximetry can determine whether serious desaturation occurs in certain COPD patients during sleep.

Key points in performing overnight oximetry include the following:

- Set up and verify equipment operation:
  - Set the device to trend monitoring and select the period (e.g., 8 hours).
  - If settable, adjust the capture rate to the shortest allowable (usually 2–6 seconds).
  - Confirm that there is sufficient memory to capture the data for the planned period.
  - If needed, turn the low alarm off and begin trend monitoring.
  - Instruct and prepare the patient (remove artificial fingernails and nail polish).
  - Attach the sensors and begin recording.
  - Return in the morning to gather the data.

If overnight oximetry is conducted in the home:

- Provide simple, step-by-step, written instructions for the patient and family.
- Demonstrate proper setup and operation of the equipment on the patient.
- Require a return demonstration to verify its proper use.
- Provide a phone number where the patient can get help.

Upon completion of the procedure, you transfer the data to a computer for storage and analysis using the applicable data-acquisition software.

CPAP/ NIPPV Titration

Once a patient is diagnosed with SAHS, most physicians will order a CPAP/BPAP titration study to assess the effectiveness of this therapy and tailor it to patient needs. Titration studies can be conducted via laboratory polysomnography or using an unattended auto-CPAP system.

Polysomnography CPAP/NIPPV Titration

All patients undergoing CPAP/NIPPV titration (via polysomnography or auto-CPAP) should first receive appropriate instructions (with demonstration), be carefully fitted with a comfortable mask, and be given the time needed to get used to the device. Once this is accomplished, the titration procedure commences as follows:

- Start CPAP at 4 cm H_2O (use a higher pressure if the patient complains of "not getting enough air" or cannot fall asleep).
- Maintain each CPAP pressure level for an observation interval of at least 5 minutes.
- If *any* of the following events occur during the interval, increase the CPAP level by at least 1 cm H_2O:
  - Two or more obstructive apneas
  - Three or more hypopneas
  - Five or more respiratory effort–related arousals (RERAs)
  - Three or more minutes of loud snoring
  - Continue increasing the CPAP level until the obstructive events are abolished or controlled or until you reach a maximum CPAP level of 20 cm H_2O.
- If the patient cannot tolerate high CPAP pressures, *or* obstructive respiratory events continue at higher levels of CPAP (> 15 cm H_2O), *or* the patient exhibits periods of central sleep apnea during titration, consider a trial of BPAP:
  - Starting EPAP = 4 cm H_2O and IPAP = 8 cm H_2O.
  - Recommended min/max IPAP – EPAP differential = 4/10 cm H_2O.
  - Recommended maximum IPAP = 30 cm H_2O.
  - Raise EPAP to abolish obstructive events.
  - Raise IPAP to abolish hypopnea and snoring.
  - If events persist at the maximum tolerated IPAP, increase EPAP in increments of 1 cm H_2O.

Auto-CPAP Titration

Many modern CPAP units incorporate a mode in which pressure levels are automatically optimized to abolish or control obstructive events. Typically, these units use sensors to monitor pressure, flow, and system leaks (see Chapter 6). Using these input data, a computer algorithm identifies the event and adjusts the pressure accordingly. For example, if the device detects a defined number of apnea events, the algorithm will begin a programmed step-up in CPAP pressure until the problem resolves or the maximum preset pressure is reached. **Figure 3-8** provides a trend graph of CPAP pressure and obstructive events over 7 hours that demonstrates how auto-CPAP functions.

Tracheal Airway Cuff Management

Monitoring tracheal airway cuff pressures is a standard of care for respiratory therapy and a mandatory part of the routine patient–ventilator system checks. Cuff pressures over 25–30 cm H_2O can obstruct tissue blood flow (ischemia), causing ulceration and necrosis. Conversely, if cuff pressures are too low, leakage-type aspiration can occur, which may lead to ventilator-associated pneumonia (VAP). Thus, the goal is to avoid tracheal mucosal damage without increasing the risk of VAP.

Cuff pressures should be monitored and adjusted regularly (e.g., once per shift) and more often if the tube is changed, if its position changes, if the air is added to or removed from the cuff, or if a leak occurs. To measure and adjust cuff pressures, you need a calibrated manometer, a three-way stopcock, and a 10- or 20-mL syringe. Many institutions use a commercially available bulb device that

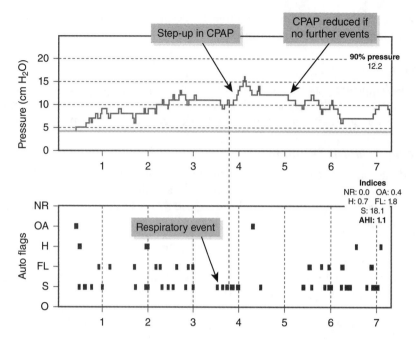

Figure 3-8 Trend Graph of Auto-CPAP (REMstar Auto). The occurrence of a respiratory event (snoring) 4 hours into sleep triggers a programmed step-up in CPAP pressure until the problem resolves, at which point the pressure is incrementally reduced if no additional events occur.

AHI, apnea/hypopnea index (sum of OA + H); FL, flow limitation; H, hypopnea; NR, nonresponsive apnea/hypopnea; OA, obstructive apnea; S, snore.

Courtesy of Philips Respironics, Murrysville, Pennsylvania.

combines the functions of these components. Newer electronic devices to measure and manage the cuff pressures are also available.

If using the three-way stopcock system:

1. Attach the syringe and manometer to the stopcock set so that all three ports are open.
2. Attach the third stopcock port to the cuff's pilot tube valve, being sure that the connection is leak free.
3. With the stopcock open to the syringe, manometer, and cuff, add or remove air while observing the pressure changes on the manometer.
4. If the patient is receiving positive-pressure ventilation, adjust the pressure to eliminate gurgling sounds at the cuff throughout inspiration (indicating a leak-free seal) but at a pressure no higher than 30 cm H_2O.

Additional fine points in the procedure that may appear on NBRC exams include the following:

- Most hospitals (including the NBRC "hospital") set 25 cm H_2O as the high-pressure limit.
- Attaching a manometer and syringe to a pilot tube line causes volume loss and lowers cuff pressure; for this reason, you must always adjust the pressure—never just measure it.
- Any change in ventilator settings that alters peak pressures may require pressure readjustment.
- Cuff pressure and the method used to obtain it should be recorded as part of the airway management or ventilator documentation.
- Obtaining a leak-free seal at acceptable cuff pressures during mechanical ventilation may be difficult when (1) high peak pressures are required or (2) the tracheal tube is too small for the patient's airway. In these cases, it is best to keep pressures below 25–30 cm H_2O but recommend exchanging the airway either for a larger one or one that provides continuous aspiration of subglottic secretions (see Chapter 9).

- Even at pressures of 20–30 cm H_2O, low-pressure cuffs may still allow some leakage. Again, the solution is using a tube that provides continuous aspiration of secretions above the cuff.

Some clinicians recommend recording and tracking cuff inflation *volume* in addition to pressure. *Increases in inflation volume over time likely indicate tracheal dilation*, which can lead to permanent damage such as tracheomalacia. However, because this technique requires emptying the cuff, it can increase the likelihood of aspiration. Given that this hazard outweighs the potential benefits of this procedure, it is not recommended.

Two unique cuff designs can help avoid tracheal trauma: the Lanz tube and the Bivona Fome-Cuf (also called the Kamen-Wilkinson tube). The Lanz tube incorporates an external regulating valve and control reservoir that automatically maintains cuff pressure at about 30 cm H_2O. Bivona Fome-Cuf tubes have a foam cuff that seals the trachea at atmospheric pressure. With the Bivona Fome-Cuf tube:

- Before insertion, you deflate the cuff with a syringe and close off the pilot tube.
- Once the tube is positioned properly in the trachea, you open the pilot tube to the atmosphere and allow the foam to expand against the tracheal wall.

Sputum Induction

Sputum induction is used to gather specimens of lower airway secretions and cellular matter in patients who cannot spontaneously produce an adequate sample for analysis. The procedure involves having the patient inhale a hypertonic saline aerosol, which promotes coughing and facilitates sputum collection. Specimens obtained via sputum induction can be used to assist in the following:

- Diagnosing respiratory tract infections (microbiological analysis)
- Confirming the presence of lung cancer (cytological analysis)
- Assessing the immunological status of the lungs (cytological and immunological analysis)

Sputum induction is a simple, noninvasive, and relatively safe procedure that, if successful, can eliminate the need for a bronchoscopy. The key "need-to-know" points regarding sputum induction, synthesized from various published protocols, are as follows:

- If being performed to diagnose respiratory tract infections, the procedure should be performed in a negative-pressure room or booth with the therapist using airborne respiratory precautions, including donning of an N-95 mask.
- To minimize contamination of specimens with saliva and oropharyngeal debris, before induction, the patient should rinse out the mouth and gargle with water until the returned fluid is clear (requires emesis basin).
- Because hypertonic saline can cause bronchospasm, patients with reactive airway disease (e.g., asthma, COPD) should receive pretreatment with a fast-acting beta agonist such as albuterol. Measure the patient's FEV_1 10–15 minutes after bronchodilator treatment for use as the baseline for in-treatment comparison. Patients taking a long-acting controller such as Advair (fluticasone and salmeterol) may not need pretreatment with an inhaled fast-acting bronchodilator.
- Although most protocols specify using an ultrasonic nebulizer (due to its higher aerosol density), a jet nebulizer is satisfactory if it can continuously deliver aerosol over the 15- to 20-minute induction session (may require refilling).
- Regardless of the type of nebulizer used, when collecting a specimen for microbiological analysis, you should use a valved breathing circuit with an expiratory HEPA filter.
- Depending on the protocol, 3%, 5%, 7%, or 10% sterile saline solution may be used; some procedures increase the concentration 1–2 times if the lower strength fails to produce a specimen.
- Every 5 minutes (or whenever the patient wants to), encourage coughing and expectoration of sputum into the sterile collection cup. In patients with reactive airway disease, measure the FEV_1 at the end of each induction attempt; and terminate the procedure if the FEV_1 falls by 20% or more from the initial post-bronchodilator value or symptoms of respiratory distress occur (wheezing/complaints of dyspnea or chest tightness).
- Specimen collection in pediatric patients may require the application of airway clearance therapy followed by nasotracheal or oropharyngeal suction.

- Terminate the procedure if unsuccessful after 15–20 minutes or if the patient is showing signs of respiratory distress or is lightheaded or feels nauseous.
- An adequate sample should be between 2 and 5 mL in volume (4–5 mL is needed for reliable acid-fast bacilli [AFB] analysis); the presence of plugs or mucous strands (visible when the specimen is held up to the light) is a good indicator that the sputum is from the lower airway.
- Label/contain the specimen and ensure proper transport in accordance with the College of American Pathologists (CAP)/Joint Commission/Occupational Safety and Health Administration (OSHA) guidelines and your laboratory protocols.
- To ensure reproducible results for immunological assessment additional induction, attempts should be spaced at least 24 hours apart.

Exercise-Related Diagnostic Procedures

In addition to oxygen titration with exercise described earlier in this chapter, the NBRC expects candidates to be familiar with two other exercise-related assessments: the cardiopulmonary stress test and the 6-minute walk test, and O_2 titration with exercise. Refer to Chapter 4 for discussion of test interpretation.

Cardiopulmonary Exercise Testing

Cardiopulmonary exercise testing involves measurement of heart and lung function during progressive increases in workload, usually performed on a treadmill. The standard work unit used for exercise testing is the metabolic equivalent of task (MET): 1 MET = 3.5 mL O_2 consumption/kg of body weight, about equal to normal resting O_2 consumption per minute. MET levels are varied during exercise by altering treadmill speeds and inclinations. Most protocols increase exercise intensity by 1–2 METs at each step-up in workload.

Exercise testing is conducted under direct physician supervision in a cardiac, pulmonary, or exercise physiology lab. A fully stocked crash cart with a defibrillator, O_2, suction, and airway equipment must be on hand, and all involved staff should be ACLS certified. General contraindications against exercise testing include acute MI, uncontrolled heart failure, unstable angina, significant cardiac dysrhythmias, acute pulmonary disorders, and severe hypertension.

Two types of exercise tests are commonly performed: the cardiac stress test and the comprehensive exercise capacity assessment. The classic cardiac "stress test" assesses the patient's 12-lead ECG, heart rate, and blood pressure and may include radionuclide imaging of coronary perfusion. The classic stress test is indicated as follows:

- To diagnose coronary artery disease (CAD)
- To evaluate risk and prognosis in patients with a history of CAD
- To assess prognosis after MI
- To provide the basis for the rehabilitation prescription
- To evaluate the impact of medical treatment for heart disease

Data are continuously gathered at each increment in workload, and patient symptoms are monitored. ST-segment depression or elevation indicates myocardial ischemia and constitutes a positive test result. Imaging information enhances diagnostic precision by identifying the location and extent of ischemia.

The more comprehensive exercise capacity test employs a metabolic cart to measure ventilation parameters (tidal volume, respiratory rate) and gas exchange (O_2 consumption and CO_2 production) during the test protocol. This approach is used for the following purposes:

- Differentiating between cardiac and pulmonary limitations to exercise capacity
- Evaluating responses to treatments intended to increased exercise tolerance
- Determining appropriate exercise levels in rehabilitation programs
- Detecting exercise-induced bronchospasm
- Evaluating exercise capacity in heart transplant candidates
- Evaluating claims for cardiopulmonary disability

Box 3-4 Basic Comprehensive Exercise Capacity Test Procedure (Treadmill)

Procedure

1. Obtain the appropriate medical and medication history and pulmonary function test (PFT) results; measure the patient's height and weight.
2. Place and secure the electrocardiogram (ECG) leads, pulse oximetry probe, and blood pressure cuff.
3. Obtain a baseline resting 12-lead ECG, SpO_2, and blood pressure (BP).
4. If ordered, obtain a baseline arterial blood sample (ABG/lactate level).
5. Instruct the patient in the operation of the treadmill.
6. Confirm leak-free fit of the breathing interface; have the patient breathe through the system for 2–3 minutes, until stable.
7. Provide 2–3 minutes of unloaded warm-up activity (e.g., 1–2 mph, 0% grade).
8. Apply the prescribed protocol to increment the patient workload.
9. Measure BP, heart rate (HR), SpO_2, Borg exertion rating, and symptoms (if any) toward the end of each graded interval.
10. End the test as follows:
    a. When $\dot{V}O_{2max}$ or the maximum steady-state heart rate is achieved (stop at the end of that stage)
    b. When the patient cannot continue due to exhaustion
    c. If an abnormal or hazardous response occurs (e.g., a cardiac arrhythmia)
11. If ordered, obtain an arterial sample immediately following test cessation.
12. Provide 2–3 minutes of unloaded cool-down activity (e.g., 1–2 mph, 0% grade).
13. Have the patient stop activity.
14. Continue to monitor BP and HR until they return to baseline.
15. If assessing for exercise-induced bronchospasm, immediately obtain PFT measures.

The accompanying box (**Box 3-4**) outlines the elements commonly included in the comprehensive exercise capacity test procedure. In most cases, patients scheduled for an exercise test should be told to take their regular medications and avoid strenuous activity on the day of the test. Also, you should instruct patients to avoid caffeine and to not smoke or eat for at least 2 hours before the test and to wear loose, comfortable clothing and nonslip footwear suitable for walking, such as sneakers.

Abnormal or hazardous responses that justify ending the test include wide swings in blood pressure; development of severe angina, dyspnea, or a serious arrhythmia; or the patient becoming dizzy, confused, or cyanotic.

6-Minute Walk Test

The 6-minute walk test (6MWT) measures the distance a patient can walk on a flat surface in 6 minutes. It evaluates how well the body responds to exertion and is used to determine the overall functional capacity or changes in capacity due to therapy in patients with moderate to severe heart or lung disease. **Table 3-6** summarizes the indications for the 6MWT.

The 6MWT does not measure O_2 uptake nor does it help identify either the cause of dyspnea or the factors limiting exercise tolerance. *If such information is needed, you should recommend a comprehensive cardiopulmonary exercise test.*

The 6MWT should *not* be performed on patients who have either had a myocardial infarction (MI) or experienced unstable angina during the month before the test. Relative contraindications include a resting heart rate > 120 beats/min, a systolic blood pressure > 180 mm Hg, or a diastolic blood pressure > 100 mm Hg.

The American Thoracic Society (ATS) has developed a standardized protocol for the 6MWT. The first consideration is the walking course itself, which must be 30 meters in length, with a clear set starting line and turnaround point, and with the distance marked in 3-meter increments. In terms of equipment, you will need a stopwatch, a movable chair, and a recording worksheet. **Figure 3-9** provides a 6MWT worksheet like that recommended by the ATS.

Table 3-6 Indications for the 6-Minute Walk Test

Functional Status (Single Measurement)	Pre-/Post-Treatment Comparisons
Chronic obstructive pulmonary disease (COPD)	Lung transplantation
Cystic fibrosis	Lung resection
Heart failure	Lung volume reduction surgery
Peripheral vascular disease	Pulmonary rehabilitation
Fibromyalgia	COPD
Effects of aging	Pulmonary hypertension
	Heart failure

6-Minute Walk Test		Walk #:	Date:	
Patient Name:		Patient ID:		Gender: M F
Race/ Ethnicity:		Height (cm):	Weight (kg):	Blood Pressure:
Medications taken before the test (dose and time):				
Supplemental O_2 during the test?	No	Yes	Flow L/min:	Device:

Lap counter	1	2	3	4	5	6	7	8	9	10	11	12	13	14	15

	Start/baseline	End of test
Time		
Heart rate		
SpO_2		
Dyspnea (Borg scale)		
Fatigue (Borg scale)		

Stopped or paused before 6 minutes?	Yes	No	Reason:
Other symptoms at end of exercise:	☐ Angina ☐ Dizziness	☐ Hip or leg pain ☐ Diaphoresis	☐ Ashen appearance ☐ Other:
Number of laps:	x 60 m/lap	+ partial lap of m =	Total distance (6MWD)
Predicted 6MWD:	m	% Predicted (actual/predicted)	%
Comments:			
Interpretation:			
Test administrator (name):		Signature:	

Figure 3-9 American Thoracic Society Recommended Documentation Form for the 6-Minute Walk Test.

Modified from ATS statement: Guidelines for the six-minute walk test. *Am J Respir Crit Care Med.* 2002;166:111–117.

You will also need a sphygmomanometer to measure blood pressure, as well as a visual Borg Scale to assess the patient's dyspnea and level of exertion. If used, a pulse oximeter must be lightweight and not have to be held by the patient while walking. Last, for potential emergencies, you must have immediate access to a source of oxygen, an automated electronic defibrillator (AED), and a telephone.

To prepare for the 6MWT, patients should wear comfortable clothing and walking shoes/sneakers, bring their usual walking aid (e.g., cane, walker), follow their usual medical regimen, and avoid vigorous exercise for 2 hours before testing. If a recent ECG is available, the results should be reviewed by a physician before testing. For patients with a history of stable angina on exercise, direct them to take their angina medication before the test and have rescue nitrates available. For patients on supplemental O_2, oxygen should be provided at the prescribed flow using the same portable system normally used.

The ATS-recommended 6MWT protocol is outlined in the accompanying box (**Box 3-5**). You should immediately stop the test if the patient develops chest pain, severe dyspnea, leg cramps, staggering, diaphoresis, or a pale or ashen appearance. In these cases, seat the patient in a chair, retake

---

Box 3-5 ATS 6-Minute Walk Protocol

1. With the patient sitting at rest for at least 10 minutes, gather all needed data and measure/record vital signs.
2. Assemble all equipment (lap counter, stopwatch, colored tape, Borg Scale, recording worksheet).
3. If SpO_2 is to be monitored, record the baseline value.
4. Have the patient stand and rate his or her baseline dyspnea and exertion levels using the Borg Scale.
5. Move to the starting point and set the stopwatch to zero.
6. Position the patient at the starting line and provide the requisite ATS-mandated demonstration and instructions.
7. Start the timer as soon as the patient starts to walk.
8. Remain at the starting line while you watch the patient and tally the completed "laps."
9. After each lap, make sure the patient sees you tallying the lap.
10. At the end of each minute, encourage the patient and specify the remaining time.
11. After exactly 6 minutes, firmly say "Stop," mark the stop point on the floor with tape, and have the patient sit down.
12. Repeat the Borg Scale assessment, being sure to remind the patient of the prior ratings. Also, ask, "What, if anything, kept you from walking farther?"
13. If using a pulse oximeter, record the end-of-walk SpO_2 and pulse rate.
14. Record the number of laps, additional distance covered in any partial lap, and the total distance walked (rounded to the nearest meter).
15. Congratulate the patient on a good effort.

Modified from the American Thoracic Society. ATS statement: Guidelines for the six-minute walk test. *Am J Respir Crit Care Med.* 2002;166:111–117.

---

the vital signs, administer O_2 as appropriate, and arrange for a physician assessment. Once you are sure the patient is stable, record the time stopped, distance walked, and the reason the patient could not continue.

Pulmonary Function Tests

In addition to measuring peak expiratory flow rates (PEFR) discussed earlier in this chapter, the NBRC expects candidates to be able to measure conduct screening spirometry; and perform laboratory testing of forced vital capacity (FVC), static lung volumes, and diffusing capacity (DLco).

Spirometry Outside and Inside a Pulmonary Function Testing Laboratory

Screening spirometry involves the measurement of the FVC and related measures (e.g., PEFR, FEV_t, FEF_{25-75}) at the point of care using a portable electronic spirometer. Chapter 6 provides details on the selection, use, and troubleshooting of bedside spirometers, and Chapter 4 describes the interpretation of spirometry results. Here we focus on performing spirometry.

As with peak flow, FEV measurements depend on proper patient performance, as instructed and coached by the RT. The accompanying box (**Box 3-6**) outlines a basic procedure designed to help ensure accurate and reproducible results.

Pulmonary Function Laboratory Studies

Pulmonary function laboratory studies include the same FVC measurements assessed at the bedside, plus static lung volumes (TLC, functional residual capacity [FRC], vital capacity [VC], inspiratory capacity [IC], expiratory reserve volume [ERV], and residual volume [RV]) and sometimes the diffusing capacity.

Static Lung Volumes

The key static lung volume from which the others are derived is the FRC. If the FRC is known, both the RV and TLC are computed as follows:

$$RV = FRC - ERV$$
$$TLC = FRC + IC$$

Box 3-6 Screening Spirometry Procedure

1. Turn the spirometer on and connect a new mouthpiece or sensor (some sensors require inputting individual calibration data).
2. Input all requested patient data accurately (e.g., age, sex, height, ethnicity).
3. Remove candy, gum, or dentures from the patient's mouth; loosen any tight clothing.
4. Have the patient sit or stand, but be consistent, and record the patient's position.
5. Demonstrate the procedure using your own mouthpiece/sensor, being sure to emphasize the following points:
   a. How to hold the sensor steady and avoid jerky motions (can cause flow or start-of-test errors)
   b. How deeply to inhale
   c. How to correctly place the mouthpiece on top of the tongue
   d. How fast and long to exhale (at least 6 seconds)
6. Use nose clips to prevent patient leaks.
7. Have the patient perform the maneuver while you carefully observe test performance:
   a. Ensure that the patient breathes in as deeply as possible (to full TLC).
   b. Coach the patient to forcibly blast the breath out, *as fast and as long as possible* (at least 6 seconds; patients with severe chronic obstructive pulmonary disease [COPD] may take up to 15 seconds to fully exhale).
   c. Carefully observe the patient for poor technique and correct as needed.
8. Repeat the procedure until you have three acceptable maneuvers.
9. Print and review the results.

Table 3-7 describes the three methods most commonly used to measure FRC in pulmonary function laboratories. Note that whereas the helium dilution and nitrogen washout methods both measure actual FRC (lung volume communicating with the airways), body plethysmography measures total thoracic gas volume (TGV). Normally, the FRC and TGV are equal. *A TGV that exceeds FRC indicates the presence of "trapped" gas that is not in communication with the airways, as seen in bullous emphysema and air-trapping.*

Diffusing Capacity

The diffusing capacity of the lung (DLco) is assessed by measuring the transfer of carbon monoxide (CO) from the lungs into the pulmonary capillaries. The *single-breath test* is the most common procedure, the key elements of which include the following:

- The patient exhales completely to RV
- The patient inspires from RV to TLC, inhaling a mixture of 21% O_2, 10% He, and 0.3% CO.
- The patient performs a 10-second breath-hold.
- The first portion of the patient's exhalation (anatomic deadspace) is discarded.
- After that, a sample of 0.5–1.0 L of expired gas is collected and analyzed for % He and % CO.
- The test is repeated after at least a 4-minute wait until results are within 5% or 3 mL/min/mm Hg.
- Reported measures include the DLco in mL/min/mm Hg (Hb and HbCO corrected), the alveolar volume (VA, an estimate of TLC), the ratio of DLco to VA, and the inspiratory VC.

Tests of Respiratory Muscle Strength

As described earlier in this chapter, MIP assesses the patient's inspiratory muscle strength. Also, maximal expiratory pressure (MEP) measures a patient's expiratory muscle strength. Like MIP, MEP measurements also are obtained with a manometer. However, unlike MIP measurements, MEP does not require a one-way valve and can only be measured on an alert and cooperative patient.

Therapeutic Bronchoscopy

Bronchoscopy is a procedure which involves the insertion of a fiber optic or occasionally rigid catheter through the upper airway and vocal cords into the trachea and bronchi. It can be done for diagnostic

Table 3-7 Comparison of Methods Used to Measure Functional Residual Capacity

Method/Description	Key Points
Helium (He) Dilution (Closed-Circuit Method)	
• At the end of a normal exhalation (FRC), the patient is connected to a spirometer containing 5–10% He, and then the patient breathes normally. • CO_2 is chemically absorbed by soda lime, and O_2 is added to keep a constant end-expiratory level (about 0.25 L/min). • The test continues until equilibration is reached (% He is constant for 2 minutes). • FRC is calculated based on initial and final % He, the volume of He and O_2 added to the system and system deadspace.	• The spirometer must be leak free and the He analyzer properly calibrated. • After the FRC is obtained, VC, IC, ERV, and IRV should be measured. • FRC may be underestimated in individuals with air trapping. • Hypercapnia or hypoxemia may occur if CO_2 is not removed or O_2 not added. • Test results should be repeatable ($\pm$500 mL in adults). • Test validity depends on the proper starting point (at FRC) and an absence of leaks (e.g., poor mouth seal, perforated eardrums, tracheostomies).
Nitrogen (N_2) Washout (Open-Circuit Method)	
• At the end of a normal exhalation (FRC), the patient is connected to a 100% O_2 reservoir. • Expired N_2 and expired volume are measured continuously. • The test continues for 7 minutes or until % N_2 falls below 1.0% (more time may be needed for patients with air trapping). • FRC is computed based on total expired volume and final % N_2.	• The system must be leak-free and the N_2 analyzer properly calibrated. • Some patients cannot maintain a good mouth seal or cooperate adequately. • The ventilatory drive may be depressed in some patients who breathe 100% O_2. • An initial alveolar % N_2 of 80% is assumed if the patient has been breathing room air for at least 15 minutes. • After the FRC is obtained, VC, IC, ERV, and IRV should be measured. • A minimum of 15 minutes should elapse before the test is repeated. • Test results should be repeatable ($\pm$500 mL in adults). • Test validity depends on starting at FRC and an absence of leaks (increased % N_2 in the middle of the test indicates a leak).
Body Box (Body Plethysmography)	
• Transducers measure chamber + mouth pressure and flow. • A mouthpiece shutter occludes the airway at end-expiration. • The patient "pants" against the closed shutter (compressing and expanding gas in the thorax and the chamber). • Changes in chamber pressure are proportional to changes in alveolar gas volume. • The volume of gas in the thorax is computed according to Boyle's law: $P_1V_1 = P_2V_2$.	• Careful calibration of multiple transducers is required. • The test measures total thoracic gas volume (TGV), which may be greater than He dilution or N_2 washout FRC (due to "trapped gas" in cysts or bullae, as can occur in emphysema). • Plethysmographic TGV is usually measured together with airway resistance/conductance. • Claustrophobic patients may not tolerate the procedure. • Test validity requires proper panting (as evidenced by "closed" P-V loops) at about 1 cycle/sec with hands against the patient's cheeks to avoid "bowing." • TGV should be averaged from a minimum of three to five acceptable panting maneuvers. • After the FRC is obtained, VC, IC, ERV, and IRV should be measured.

ERV, expiratory reserve volume; FRC, functional residual capacity; IC, inspiratory capacity; IRV, inspiratory reserve volume; VC, vital capacity.

and therapeutic reasons. Chapter 5 of this text describes the diagnostic and therapeutic indications as well as the major contraindications for this procedure. In addition, Chapter 16 details the procedure, required equipment, and the role of the respiratory therapist in performing a bronchoscopy.

T⁴—TOP TEST-TAKING TIPS

You can improve your score on this section of the NBRC exam by reviewing these tips:

- Know your ECG chest lead placements: V1—fourth intercostal space (ic), R sternal border; V2—fourth intercostal space, L sternal border; V3—between V2 and V4; V4—fifth intercostal space, midclavicular; V5—fifth intercostal space, anterior axillary line; V6—fifth intercostal space, midaxillary line.
- Validate an oximeter's signal by comparing its pulse rate against an ECG monitor or palpated pulse; the typical alarm setting is 90–94% for adults and 85–88% for infants.
- Change the transcutaneous monitor sensor site frequently (every 2–6 hours).
- Set capnograph alarms to $Petco_2$ 50–55 torr (high)/25–30 torr (low).
- The rapid shallow breathing index (RSBI) = f ÷ V_T (L).
- Unless otherwise indicated, assume a deadspace of approximately 1 mL per pound of predicted body weight (PBW).
- Use peak expiratory flow rate (PEFR) to monitor airway obstruction, not diagnose it.
- To convert L/sec to L/min, multiply by 60; to convert L/min to L/sec, divide by 60.
- Always get three repeatable/acceptable measures for any PEFR or $FE\dot{V}$
- Age, sex, height, and ethnicity are required to compute a patient's predicted normal spirometry values.
- Ideally, an FEV breath maneuver should last at least 6 seconds.
- Helium dilution FRC measurement must begin at the end of a normal exhalation.
- The FRC is required to compute both the RV and TLC.
- The radial artery is the preferred site for obtaining arterial blood; always check for collateral circulation (modified Allen's test) and clotting measures (PT, PTT, INR).
- When obtaining a mixed venous blood sample from a PA catheter, the sample must be drawn slowly from the catheter's distal port with the balloon deflated.
- For heel sticks/capillary samples, puncture the lateral side of the heel, not the posterior curvature; capillary samples are only useful for assessing Pco_2 and pH, not oxygenation.
- Analyze ABG samples in plastic syringes within 30 min; if kept for > 30 min, the sample should be in a glass syringe chilled to 0–4°C (in ice slush).
- The 6-minute walk test (6MWT) measures overall functional capacity; it does not measure O_2 uptake or identify either the cause of dyspnea or the factors limiting exercise tolerance.
- The standard work unit for exercise testing is the metabolic equivalent of task or MET; 1 MET = 3.5 mL O_2 consumption/kg of body weight, about equal to normal resting $\dot{V}o_2$.
- Terminate an O_2 titration with exercise if the Sao_2 drops below 85%.
- Arterial blood pressure reflects LV afterload, vascular tone, and blood volume; central venous pressure (CVP) reflects the fluid volume and RV preload, and pulmonary artery wedge pressure (PAWP or PCWP) indicates LV preload.
- On an arterial pressure waveform, the dicrotic notch corresponds to aortic valve closure.
- Pulse pressure is the difference between systolic and diastolic pressures, normally about 40 mm Hg.
- For accurate CVP/PA pressure measurements, (1) the transducer should be level with the intersection of the fourth intercostal space and midaxillary line, (2) measurements should be made at end-expiration, and (3) the patient should not be removed from PEEP/CPAP.
- Damped vascular pressure waveforms indicate partial occlusion by a clot or air bubbles in the system.
- To measure respiratory system compliance (C_{rs}) and airway resistance (Raw) during volume-control ventilation, you institute an end-inspiratory pause or hold, which creates a static or "no-flow" pressure plateau (P_{plat}); computations are as follows:
  - Raw = (PIP – P_{plat}) ÷ inspiratory flow (L/sec)
  - C_{rs} (aka "static compliance") = V_T ÷ (P_{plat} – PEEP)

- A *combined* measure of compliance and resistance called *dynamic compliance* (C_{dyn}) may appear on the NBRC exams: $C_{dyn} = V_T \div (PIP - PEEP)$.
- C_{dyn} always will be less than C_{rs}, with the difference between the two ($C_{rs} - C_{dyn}$) due to airway resistance; the greater the difference between C_{rs} and C_{dyn}, the greater the contribution of airway resistance to the driving pressure.
- To detect auto-PEEP, look for a failure of expiratory flow to return to baseline before the next mechanical breath (flow scalar or flow–volume loop).
- To measure auto-PEEP, institute an end-*expiratory* pause; auto-PEEP = end-expiratory pause pressure – PEEP.
- Assess a patient for weaning from mechanical ventilation who (1) is hemodynamically stable and can initiate an inspiratory effort, (2) has adequate oxygenation (P/F ≥ 150–200, PEEP ≤ 5–8 cm H_2O, Fio_2 ≤ 0.4–0.5), and (3) has a pH ≥ 7.25.
- Daily spontaneous breathing trials provide the quickest route for weaning from mechanical ventilation.
- For neonates, set the low/high heart rate alarm limits on an apnea monitor to 80–210 (lower limits for older babies) and the apnea time alarm limit to 15–20 seconds.
- For polysomnography CPAP/BPAP titration, begin at 4 cm H_2O and increment in a stepwise manner by at least 1 cm H_2O when frequent apneas, hypopneas, or prolonged snoring occurs; continue if needed to a maximum of 20 cm H_2O.
- If the patient cannot tolerate high CPAP pressures, *or* obstructive events continue at CPAP > 15 cm H_2O, *or* if the patient exhibits periods of central sleep apnea during titration, consider a trial of BPAP.
- Maintain tracheal tube cuff pressure on mechanically ventilated patients in the range of 20–30 cm H_2O *without inspiratory gurgling* to prevent mucosal damage and leakage-type aspiration.
- If leakage-type aspiration cannot be prevented at a cuff pressure of 30 cm H_2O, recommend exchanging the airway for one that provides continuous aspiration of subglottic secretions.
- For diagnosing respiratory tract infections, perform sputum induction in a negative-pressure room or booth, use a filtered/valved breathing circuit, and wear an N-95 mask.
- Pre-administer a beta agonist, and monitor the FEV_1 before, during, and after hypertonic sputum induction in patients with reactive airway disease.
- Bronchoscopy involves the insertion of a fiber optic or occasionally rigid catheter through the upper airway and vocal cords into the trachea and bronchi and can be done for both diagnostic and therapeutic reasons.

POST-TEST

To confirm your mastery of each chapter's topical content, you should create a content post-test, available online via the Navigate Premier Access for Comprehensive Respiratory Therapy Exam Preparation Guide, which contains Navigate TestPrep (access code provided with every new text). You can create multiple topical content post-tests varying in length from 10 to 20 questions, with each attempt presenting a different set of items. You can select questions from all three major NBRC TMC sections: Patient Data, Troubleshooting and Quality Control of Devices and Infection Control, and Initiation and Modification of Interventions. A score of at least 70–80% indicates that you are adequately prepared for this section of the NBRC TMC exam. If you score below 70%, you should first carefully assess your test answers (particularly your wrong answers) and the correct answer explanations. Then return to the chapter to re-review the applicable content. Only then should you reattempt a new post-test. Repeat this process of identifying your shortcomings and reviewing the pertinent content until your test results demonstrate mastery.

Evaluate Procedure Results (Section I-D)

Narciso E. Rodriguez

Respiratory therapists (RTs) must be proficient in the assessment of a patients' response to a procedure and therapies. The ability to evaluate pertinent clinical information helps RTs determine the patient's condition, develop good treatment plans, and evaluate responses to therapy. For this reason, the NBRC exams include numerous questions requiring interpretation of data obtained from common diagnostic and monitoring procedures. Your success on these exams depends heavily on your knowledge in this area.

OBJECTIVES

In preparing for this section of the NBRC exams (TMC/CSE), you should demonstrate the knowledge needed to interpret the information obtained from the following procedures:

1. 12-lead ECG
2. Noninvasive monitoring (pulse oximetry, transcutaneous P_{O_2}/P_{CO_2}, capnography)
3. Bedside measures of ventilation (V_T, f, $\dot{V}e$, Vc, MIP, MEP)
4. Blood gas analysis and hemoximetry
5. O_2 titration with exercise
6. Cardiopulmonary calculations
7. Hemodynamic monitoring
8. Pulmonary Compliance and resistance during mechanical ventilation
9. Plateau pressure (P_{plat}) and auto-PEEP determination
10. Spontaneous breathing trials
11. Apnea monitoring
12. Apnea test (brain death determination)
13. Overnight pulse oximetry and CPAP/BPAP titration during sleep
14. Tracheal tube cuff pressure measurement and management
15. Cardiopulmonary stress testing and the 6-minute walk test (6MWT)
16. Pulmonary function tests (peak flow, screening spirometry, full lab-based PFT exam)

WHAT TO EXPECT ON THIS CATEGORY OF THE NBRC EXAMS

TMC exam: 10 questions; 2 recall, 4 application, 4 analysis
CSE exam: indeterminate number of questions; however, section I-D knowledge is a prerequisite to succeed on the CSE, especially on Information Gathering sections.

WHAT YOU NEED TO KNOW: ESSENTIAL CONTENT

Interpreting a 12-Lead ECG

The NBRC expects all candidates to be proficient in identifying common abnormalities from an electrocardiogram (ECG) rhythm strip. To do so, you systematically assess the rate, rhythm, P waves, PR interval, QRS complex, QT interval, ST segment, and T waves. The easiest way to estimate heart rate is to use the "rule of 300," as depicted in **Figure 4-1**. At the standard recording speed of 25 mm/sec, each little 1-mm box represents 0.04 sec, with each large box representing 5 × 0.04 or 0.20 sec. Therefore, if a QRS complex were to occur with *each large box*, then the R-R interval would be

0.20 sec, and the rate would be 5 beats/sec × 60 sec/min or 300 beats/min. As long as the rhythm is regular, dividing 300 by the number of big boxes spanned by the R-R interval provides a good estimate for any cardiac rate. For example, if the R-R interval spans three large boxes, the rate would be about 300 ÷ 3 = 100/min. **Table 4-1** summarizes key findings defining major abnormalities in rhythm, P waves, PR interval, QRS complex, QT interval, ST segment, and T waves, as well as their most common causes.

In addition to rhythm assessment, the NBRC expects *basic* knowledge of 12-lead ECG interpretation, including the ability to recognize axis deviation, confirm hypertrophy, and identify the

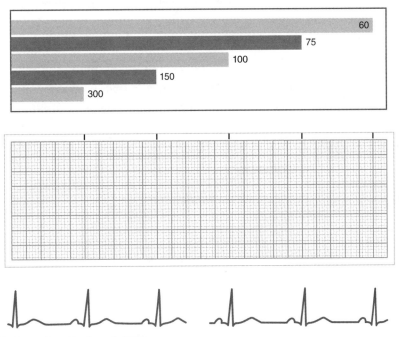

Figure 4-1 Using the Rule of 300.

Table 4-1 Major ECG Rhythm Abnormalities and Their Common Causes

Abnormal ECG Findings	Common Causes
P waves—*abnormal*	Left or right atrial hypertrophy, premature atrial contractions (PACs)
P waves—*absent*	Atrial fibrillation, junctional rhythms
P-P interval—*variable*	Sinus arrhythmia, atrial fibrillation
PR interval—*prolonged* (> 0.20 sec)	First-degree or Mobitz-type I atrioventricular (AV) block
QRS complex—*widened* (> 0.12 sec)	Premature ventricular contractions (PVCs), right (R) or left (L) bundle branch block, ventricular tachycardia, hyperkalemia
QT interval—*prolonged* (> 0.45 sec)	Myocardial ischemia/infarction, electrolyte imbalance, antiarrhythmics, tricyclic antidepressants
QT interval—*shortened* (< 0.30 sec)	Electrolyte imbalance, digoxin
R-R interval—*shortened* (< 0.60 sec)	Tachycardia (R-R < 0.60 sec or rate > 100/min)
R-R interval—*prolonged* (> 1.00 sec)	Bradycardia (R-R > 1.00 sec or rate < 60/min)
R-R interval—*variable* (> 0.12 sec or > 10% variation)	Sinus arrhythmia; atrial fibrillation; second-degree heart block (type I)
ST segment—*depressed* (chest leads)	Non-ST-elevation myocardial ischemia/infarction (NSTEMI), ventricular hypertrophy, conduction disturbances, hyperventilation, hypokalemia, digoxin

Abnormal ECG Findings	Common Causes
ST segment—*elevated* (chest leads)	ST elevation myocardial ischemia/infarction (STEMI), left bundle branch block, ventricular hypertrophy, hyperkalemia, digoxin
T wave—*tall*	Hyperkalemia, acute myocardial infarction, conduction disturbances, ventricular hypertrophy
T wave—*small, flattened, or inverted*	Myocardial ischemia, hyperventilation, anxiety, left ventricular hypertrophy, digoxin, pericarditis, pulmonary embolism, conduction disturbances, electrolyte imbalances
U wave—*prominent*	Hypokalemia, hypomagnesemia, ischemia

Table 4-2 Common 12-Lead ECG Findings

Abnormality	12-Lead ECG Findings
Axis Deviation (normally QRS is positive in leads I and aVF)	
Left axis deviation	QRS is positive (upward) in lead I but negative in lead aVF.*
Right axis deviation	QRS is negative (downward) in lead I but positive in lead aVF.
Extreme right axis deviation	QRS is negative in leads I and aVF.
Hypertrophy	
Left ventricular hypertrophy (Sokolow-Lyon index)	Left axis deviation (up to –30 degrees is normal)
	Lead V1 S wave + lead V5 or V6 R wave ≥ 35 mm
	Lead aVL R wave ≥ 11 mm
Right ventricular hypertrophy	Right axis deviation (> 100 degrees)
	Increase in voltage in V1, V5, and V6
	R waves in lead V1 > 7 mm
	R waves > S waves in lead V1 or R waves < S waves in lead V5 or V6
Myocardial Ischemia/Infarction*	
Ischemia/NSTEMI	ST-segment depression (horizontal or downsloping ≥ 0.5 mm)
	T-wave flattening or inversion ≥ 1 mm
Acute STEMI	ST-segment elevation ≥ 2 mm (men) or ≥ 1.5 mm (women) in two contiguous precordial leads
	Pathologic (deep/prolonged) Q waves
	Prominent R waves in V1–V2

STEMI, ST-segment elevation myocardial infarction; NSTEMI, non-ST-segment elevation myocardial infarction.
*Electrical events occurring in the leads "facing" the damage; may vary according to time since insult.

presence of myocardial ischemia or myocardial infarction (MI). **Table 4-2** summarizes the common 12-lead ECG findings associated with these problems. *The most common pattern in patients with chronic lung disease is right axis deviation/right ventricular hypertrophy.* Also important is your understanding that the 12-lead ECG alone cannot diagnose an MI. Other clinical data, including patient presentation and cardiac biomarkers, are needed to establish this diagnosis. Moreover, the distinction between ST-segment elevation MI (STEMI) and non-ST-segment elevation MI (NSTEMI) is essential because the treatment of the two conditions differs substantially. Patients with STEMI typically undergo thrombolytic therapy and angioplasty, whereas those with NSTEMI usually receive antiplatelet drugs and anticoagulants.

Interpreting Noninvasive Monitoring Data

The NBRC expects candidates to be proficient in interpreting SpO_2, $PtcCO_2$, $PtcO_2$, and $PetCO_2$ data and using this information to enhance patient care.

Interpreting Spo₂

Chapter 3 outlines the procedure for obtaining accurate SpO_2 data. Chapter 5 lists the indications for monitoring of SpO_2, and Chapter 6 describes the setup, use, and troubleshooting of oximeters.

The emphasis here is on interpreting SpO_2 data, based on the following key points:

- Pulse oximeters provide relatively accurate ($\pm$2–4%) estimates of oxyhemoglobin saturation when there is good perfusion.
- As measured by standard two-wavelength pulse oximeters, the SpO_2 *overestimates* oxyhemoglobin saturation when abnormal hemoglobins such as carboxyhemoglobin (HbCO) are present (e.g., smoke inhalation).
- The SpO_2 is typically greater than 93–95% when breathing room air.
- Assuming an accurate reading, a SpO_2 < 90% (on any FiO_2) indicates the need for supplemental O_2.
- To relate SpO_2 to the approximate PaO_2, use the "40–50–60/70–80–90" rule of thumb: PaO_2s of 40, 50, and 60 torr are about equal to SpO_2s of 70%, 80%, and 90%, respectively.
- Always assess the SpO_2 together with the hemoglobin (Hb) content/hematocrit—a patient with severe anemia may have a normal SpO_2 but still be suffering from hypoxemia due to low oxygen content (CaO_2).
- *Dual* pulse oximetry (pre-/postductal) is used to screen for critical congenital heart defects (CCHDs) in neonates; a CCHD may be present if both right hand (pre-) and foot (post-) SpO_2 are < 95% *or* the difference between them is $\geq$ 3%.
- Significant declines in SpO_2 (> 4–5%) during exercise or sleep are abnormal.

The most common source of errors and false alarms with pulse oximetry is motion artifact. To minimize this problem, consider relocating the sensor to an alternative site. **Table 4-3** outlines other factors that can cause erroneous SpO_2 readings and the expected direction of the error. Note also that pulse oximeters provide few useful data when the PaO_2 rises above 100 torr (hyperoxia).

Interpreting Transcutaneous Po₂ and Pco₂

Chapter 5 lists the indications for transcutaneous monitoring of arterial PO_2 and PCO_2, and Chapter 6 describes the setup and assembly, use, and troubleshooting of these devices. Here the focus is on the interpretation of transcutaneous monitoring data.

Regarding $PtcCO_2$, research indicates that it closely approximates $PaCO_2$ under most clinical conditions. The close correlation between $PtcCO_2$ and $PaCO_2$ makes this measure useful in assessing real-time changes in ventilation during mechanical ventilation. Conversely, $PtcO_2$ is equivalent to PaO_2 only in well-perfused patients, and when PaO_2 is less than 100 torr. The $PtcO_2$ underestimates the PaO_2 in perfusion states causing vasoconstriction (e.g., low cardiac output, shock, and dehydration) and when the PaO_2 is higher than 100 torr. $PtcO_2$ also underestimates PaO_2 in children and adults (due to their thicker skin) and when the sensor is underheated, when the sensor is placed on a bony surface, or when too much pressure or contact gel is applied.

Table 4-3 Factors Causing Erroneous Spo₂ Readings

Factor	Potential Error
Presence of HbCO (e.g., smoke inhalation)	Falsely high % HbO_2*
Presence of high levels of metHb	Falsely low % HbO_2 if SaO_2 > 85%
	Falsely high % HbO_2 if SaO_2 < 85%
Vascular dyes (e.g., methylene blue)	Falsely low % HbO_2
Dark skin pigmentation and nail polish	Falsely high % HbO_2 (3–5%)
Ambient light	Varies (e.g., falsely high % HbO_2 in sunlight); may also cause falsely high pulse reading
Poor perfusion and vasoconstriction	Inadequate signal; unpredictable results

*Multiple-wavelength pulse oximeters can detect HbCO.

Modified from Gentile MA, Heuer AJ, Kallet RH. Analysis and monitoring of gas exchange. In Kacmarek RM, Stoller JK, Heuer AJ, eds. *Egan's Fundamentals of Respiratory Care* (11th ed.). St. Louis, MO: Mosby; 2017.

Due to the many factors affecting the correlation between $Ptco_2$ and Pao_2, most clinicians recommend that continuous measurement of this parameter be used primarily for trend monitoring, *with the $Ptco_2$ maintained in the range of 50–80 torr in neonates.* If more precision is needed, the $Ptco_2$ must be "calibrated" against a simultaneous Pao_2 measurement. If the Pao_2 value is substantially higher than the $Ptco_2$ values, poor peripheral circulation is the likely cause.

As with pulse oximetry, dual-sensor $Ptco_2$ measurements can be used to screen for CCHD in newborns. Using this method, CCHD may be present if the *preductal* $Ptco_2$ (measured on the right upper chest) is at least 15 torr higher than the *postductal* Po_2 (measured on the lower abdomen or thigh).

The transcutaneous Po_2 also can be used to assess wound healing. In general, wound tissue $Ptco_2$ values > 30–40 torr indicate that perfusion is adequate to promote healing.

Interpreting Capnography Data

Chapter 3 outlines the procedure for obtaining accurate $Petco_2$ data. Chapter 5 describes the indications for capnography (waveform display) and capnometry (numeric value only). Chapter 6 provides details on the setup and calibration of capnographs. Here we address the interpretation of basic capnography data.

In healthy individuals, $Petco_2$ averages 2–5 torr less than arterial CO_2. **Table 4-4** differentiates between the causes of sudden and gradual changes in $Petco_2$ readings.

Most capnographs provide a continuous breath-by-breath display of inspired and exhaled CO_2 concentrations. **Figure 4-2** depicts the components of the normal CO_2 waveform for one full breathing cycle. Note that in patients with chronic obstructive pulmonary disease (COPD), congestive heart failure (CHF), auto-positive end-expiratory pressure (auto-PEEP), ventilation-perfusion (V/Q) mismatch, and pulmonary emboli, a clear alveolar plateau phase may never occur. **Table 4-5** describes the most common scenarios found during capnography.

Interpreting Bedside Ventilation Measures (VT, f, Ve, VC, MIP, MEP)

Table 4-6 defines the common measures used at the bedside to assess a patient's ventilation and provides both the approximate adult normal and critical values for each.

Interpretation of Blood Gas and Hemoximetry Data

When assessing blood gas results, we recommend that you *first* determine acid-base status and then separately evaluate oxygenation.

Table 4-4 Conditions Associated with Changes in $Petco_2$

	Rise in $Petco_2$	Fall in $Petco_2$
Sudden change	• A sudden increase in cardiac output (e.g., return of spontaneous circulation [ROSC] during cardiopulmonary resuscitation [CPR]) • Sudden release of a tourniquet • Injection of sodium bicarbonate	• Sudden hyperventilation • A sudden drop in cardiac output/cardiac arrest* • Massive pulmonary/air embolism • Circuit leak/disconnection* • Esophageal intubation* • Endotracheal (ET)/tracheostomy tube obstruction or dislodgement*
Gradual change	• Hypoventilation • Increased metabolism/CO_2 production • Rapid rise in temperature (malignant hyperthermia)	• Hyperventilation • Decreased metabolism/CO_2 production • Decreased pulmonary perfusion • Decrease in body temperature

*Can result in a $Petco_2$ of 0 torr.

Modified from Gentile MA, Heuer AJ, Kallet RH. Analysis and monitoring of gas exchange. In Kacmarek RM, Stoller JK, Heuer AJ, eds. *Egan's Fundamentals of Respiratory Care* (11th ed.). St. Louis, MO: Mosby; 2017.

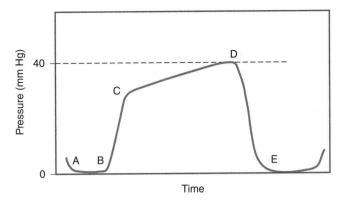

Figure 4-2 Normal End-Tidal CO$_2$ Waveform. A to B: Exhalation of pure deadspace gas. No exhaled CO$_2$ is present. B to C: Combination of deadspace and alveolar gas. Exhaled CO$_2$ begins to rise. C to D: Alveolar plateau, exhalation of alveolar CO$_2$. Petco$_2$ is typically measured at the end of the alveolar plateau. D to E: Inhalation of fresh gas (% CO$_2$ drops to zero).

Table 4-5 Common Petco$_2$ Waveform Descriptions

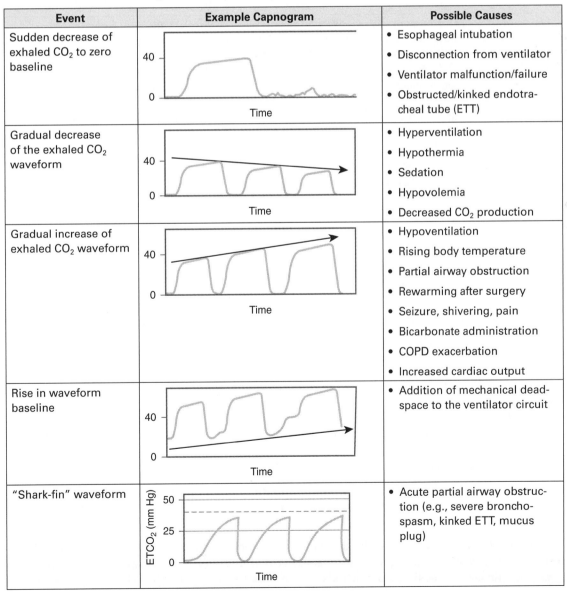

Event	Example Capnogram	Possible Causes
Sudden decrease of exhaled CO$_2$ to zero baseline		• Esophageal intubation • Disconnection from ventilator • Ventilator malfunction/failure • Obstructed/kinked endotracheal tube (ETT)
Gradual decrease of the exhaled CO$_2$ waveform		• Hyperventilation • Hypothermia • Sedation • Hypovolemia • Decreased CO$_2$ production
Gradual increase of exhaled CO$_2$ waveform		• Hypoventilation • Rising body temperature • Partial airway obstruction • Rewarming after surgery • Seizure, shivering, pain • Bicarbonate administration • COPD exacerbation • Increased cardiac output
Rise in waveform baseline		• Addition of mechanical deadspace to the ventilator circuit
"Shark-fin" waveform		• Acute partial airway obstruction (e.g., severe bronchospasm, kinked ETT, mucus plug)

Table 4-6 Bedside Ventilation Parameters

Measure (Abbreviation)	Definition	Approximate Adult Normal	Critical Adult Value*
Tidal volume (V_T)	Volume inhaled *or* exhaled on each breath	5–7 mL/kg PBW	< 4–5 mL/kg or < 300 mL
Rate (f)	Number of breaths inhaled *and* exhaled in 1 min	12–20/min	< 5/min > 30–35/min
Rapid shallow breathing index (RSBI)	Frequency of breathing divided by tidal volume in liters; RSBI = f ÷ V_T (L)	< 50	> 105[†]
Minute ventilation (Ve)	Total volume exhaled per minute; equals rate times tidal volume (f × V_T)	5–10 L/min (depends on body size/ metabolic rate)	< 4 L/min or > 10 L/min
Deadspace fraction	Ratio of physiologic deadspace to tidal volume (V_D/V_T)	0.25–0.35	> 0.60–0.70
Slow vital capacity (SVC)	Maximum volume exhaled after a maximum inhalation measured during a slow exhalation	70 mL/kg PBW	< 10–15 mL/kg
Maximum inspiratory pressure (MIP, NIF)	Maximum pressure generated against airway occlusion at or near residual volume (RV) after successive inspiratory efforts for 15–25 sec	−80 to −120 cm H_2O	0 to −20 or −25 cm H_2O

*Critical values represent the threshold above or below which patients likely cannot maintain adequate spontaneous ventilation.

[†] The RSBI is used primarily to predict *failure* to wean from mechanical ventilation, as indicated by values > *105 early in a spontaneous breathing trial.*

PBW, predicted body weight.

PBW males (kg) = 50 + 2.3 (height (in.) − 60)

PBW females (kg) = 45.5 + 2.3 (height (in.) − 60)

Acid-Base Status

Follow these steps to assess the acid-base components of an arterial blood gas accurately:

1. Categorize the pH (increased, decreased, or normal).
2. Determine the respiratory involvement ($Paco_2$ increased, decreased, or normal).
3. Determine metabolic involvement (HCO_3^- increased, decreased, or normal).
4. Assess for compensation.

Chapter 1 reviews normal arterial blood gas (ABG) parameters and describes how to identify the four *primary* acid-base disturbances using just the pH and $Paco_2$. Here we focus on assessing *compensation* for these primary disturbances and identifying combined acid-base problems.

Blood pH is determined by the ratio of the blood buffer/base bicarbonate (HCO_3^-) to the dissolved CO_2 in the blood:

$$pH \propto \frac{HCO_3^-}{Paco_2}$$

Compensation occurs when the system *not* affected by the primary disturbance attempts to restore the pH to normal. Using respiratory acidosis as an example, if the lungs retain CO_2, the $Paco_2$ rises (the primary event). Based on the balance between the base (HCO_3^-) and acid (dissolved CO_2), an increase in the $Paco_2$ will lower the blood pH (respiratory acidosis). To compensate, the system *not affected* (the kidneys) tries to restore the pH by increasing blood levels of HCO_3^- (the compensatory response). As HCO_3^- levels rise, the pH is restored toward normal. **Table 4-7** summarizes both the primary events and compensatory responses, as well as the expected changes in base excess (BE).

As shown in **Table 4-8**, by combining assessment of the $Paco_2$ and BE, you can quickly identify whether compensation is occurring, and which disturbance is primary. *Compensation is occurring if both the $Paco_2$ and BE are abnormally high or low.* Once that is established, you look at the blood pH. If the blood pH is less than 7.40, the primary problem is the one causing acidosis. If the blood pH is above 7.40, the primary problem is the one causing alkalosis.

You can also use the pH to determine whether compensation is full or partial. Compensation is "full" if the pH is in the normal range (7.35–7.45); otherwise, compensation is termed "partial." In general, renal/metabolic compensation for primary respiratory disorders is slow (hours to days), whereas respiratory compensation for primary renal/metabolic disorders is fast (minutes). Indeed, *a failure of the lungs to quickly compensate for a primary renal/metabolic acid-base disturbance indicates impaired pulmonary function.*

When the $Paco_2$ and BE diverge in opposite directions (one abnormally high and the other abnormally low), *a combined acid-base disturbance exists.* A high $Paco_2$ and low BE define a combined respiratory *and* metabolic acidosis, whereas a low $Paco_2$ and high BE define a combined respiratory *and* metabolic alkalosis.

Table 4-7 Primary Acid-Base Disorders and Compensatory Responses

Acid-Base Disorder	Primary Event	Compensatory Response	Base Excess
Respiratory acidosis	$\downarrow pH = \dfrac{HCO_3^-}{\uparrow Paco_2}$ hypoventilation	$\leftrightarrow pH = \dfrac{\uparrow\uparrow HCO_3^-}{\uparrow Paco_2}$ kidneys retain HCO_3^-	> +2 mEq/L
Respiratory alkalosis	$\uparrow pH = \dfrac{HCO_3^-}{\downarrow Paco_2}$ hyperventilation	$\leftrightarrow pH = \dfrac{\downarrow\downarrow HCO_3^-}{\downarrow Paco_2}$ kidneys excrete HCO_3^-	< −2 mEq/L
Metabolic acidosis	$\downarrow pH = \dfrac{\downarrow HCO_3^-}{Paco_2}$ loss of base/gain of acid	$\leftrightarrow pH = \dfrac{\downarrow HCO_3^-}{\downarrow\downarrow Paco_2}$ Hyperventilation	< −2 mEq/L
Metabolic alkalosis	$\uparrow pH = \dfrac{\uparrow HCO_3^-}{Paco_2}$ gain of base/loss of acid	$\leftrightarrow pH = \dfrac{\uparrow HCO_3^-}{\uparrow\uparrow Paco_2}$ hypoventilation	> +2 mEq/L

$\uparrow$, primary increase; $\downarrow$, primary decrease; $\uparrow\uparrow$, compensatory increase; $\downarrow\downarrow$, compensatory decrease; $\leftrightarrow$, restoration.

Table 4-8 Using Base Excess (BE) to Assess for Compensation

$Paco_2$	BE	pH	Acid-Base Disturbance
> 45 torr	> +2 mEq/L	Between 7.40 and 7.45	Compensated metabolic alkalosis
		Between 7.35 and 7.40	Compensated respiratory acidosis
< 35 torr	< −2 mEq/L	Between 7.40 and 7.45	Compensated respiratory alkalosis
		Between 7.35 and 7.40	Compensated metabolic acidosis

The accompanying box (**Box 4-1**) provides some common examples of acid-base reports similar to those commonly appearing on the NBRC exams, along with their interpretation.

Oxygenation

Given that the PaO_2 represents only dissolved oxygen, getting the "full picture" requires that you also consider both the Hb content and its saturation. Also, a full assessment needs to account for age, FiO_2, and sometimes altitude. Last, the NBRC exams will often assess your ability to interpret mixed venous oxygenation data.

Box 4-1 Example Acid-Base Blood Gas Sets with Interpretations

Example Report	Interpretation
pH = 7.22 PCO_2 = 65 torr HCO_3^- = 26 mEq/L BE = −1 mEq/L	Abnormal report. pH < 7.35 (acidemia) and PCO_2 > 45 torr; therefore, primary problem is respiratory acidosis. HCO_3^- and BE are within normal limits; therefore, there is no compensation. *Conclusion*: acute (uncompensated) respiratory acidosis
pH = 7.35 PCO_2 = 62 torr HCO_3^- = 33 mEq/L BE = +7 mEq/L	Abnormal report. pH normal (in the acidic side), PCO_2 > 45 torr, HCO_3^- > 26 mEq/L, BE > +2 mEq/L. Because PCO_2 and BE have both risen together, compensation is occurring. With the pH (7.35) on the acid side *but within normal limits*, the primary problem is respiratory acidosis, and the compensation is complete. *Conclusion*: fully compensated respiratory acidosis
pH = 7.57 PCO_2 = 25 torr HCO_3^- = 22 mEq/L BE = 0	Abnormal report. pH > 7.45 (alkalemia) and PCO_2 < 35 torr; therefore, the primary problem is respiratory alkalosis. HCO_3^- and BE are within normal limits; therefore, there is no compensation. *Conclusion*: acute (uncompensated) respiratory alkalosis
pH = 7.32 PCO_2 = 24 torr HCO_3^- = 12 mEq/L BE = −13 mEq/L	Abnormal report. pH < 7.35 (acidemia), PCO_2 < 45 torr; therefore, the primary problem is metabolic acidosis. Because PCO_2 and BE have both fallen together, compensation is occurring. However, because the pH is below the normal limit, compensation is only partial. *Conclusion*: partially compensated metabolic acidosis
pH = 6.90 PCO_2 = 100 torr HCO_3^- = 19 mEq/L BE = −12 mEq/L	Abnormal report. The PCO_2 and BE are diverging in opposite directions. The PCO_2 is abnormally high (would by itself cause respiratory acidosis), and the BE is abnormally low (would by itself cause metabolic acidosis). Together they are driving the pH down to a lethally low level. *Conclusion*: combined respiratory and metabolic acidosis

---

Normal Arterial Oxygenation

Table 4-9 specifies the normal ranges for these measures for a healthy young adult breathing room air at sea level.

Normal PaO_2 and SaO_2 values are affected by age, FiO_2, and altitude. As one gets older, the PaO_2 declines in a predictable way. For the NBRC exams, we recommend using the following simplified equation to estimate the PaO_2 based on age:

$$\text{Normal } PaO_2 \text{ (breathing room air) based on age} = 100 - \text{age}/3$$

For example, this simple estimation rule would be applied to a 70-year-old as follows:

$$\text{Normal } PaO_2 \text{ for 70-year-old} = 100 - 70/3 = 100 - 23 = 77 \text{ torr}$$

Table 4-9 Normal Reference Ranges for Arterial Oxygenation Measures

Parameter	Normal Range
Pao_2	80–100 torr
Sao_2 (Hb saturation)	95–98%
Hemoglobin (Hb)	M: 13.5–16.5 g/dL
	F: 12.0–15 g/dL
Cao_2 (O_2 content)*	16–22 mL/dL
*Cao_2 = (total Hb $\times$ 1.36 $\times$ Sao_2) + (0.003 $\times$ Pao_2). F, female; M, male	

Note that recent research indicates that the age-associated declines in Pao_2 level off at around 70–75 years of age. Thus, 75–80 torr is the lower limit of a normal Pao_2 for essentially all age groups breathing air at sea level.

Supplemental O_2 increases the alveolar and arterial PO_2. Again, assuming normal lung function, increasing the Fio_2 has a predictable effect on blood oxygenation, as dictated by the alveolar air equation (see Appendix B in Navigate 2 companion website). However, for rapid assessment at the bedside, we recommend the following rule of thumb:

Assuming normal lung function, the Pao_2 should be at least 5 times the O_2% delivered.

Applying this simple rule to clinical practice, if a subject with normal lung function is receiving 50% O_2, we would expect an arterial PO_2 of at least 5 $\times$ 50 or about 250 torr. Of course, the "flip side" of this rule is that any a patient with a Pao_2 significantly lower than this estimate would have abnormal oxygenation.

Although the concentration of oxygen remains at a near constant 21% regardless of altitude, its partial pressure falls as the barometric pressure decreases. Given that the barometric pressure drops by about 5 torr per 1000 ft (up to 10,000 ft), the effect of altitude on "normal" Pao_2 is also predictable, as stated in this additional rule of thumb:

Assuming normal lung function, the Pao_2 declines by ~5 torr per every 1000 ft altitude

Applying this rule, if we were working in Denver, Colorado, at an altitude of 5000 ft, we would estimate a "normal" Pao_2 when breathing room air as being about 100 – (5 $\times$ 5) = 100 – 25 = 75 torr. If we were transporting a patient in an unpressurized aircraft at an altitude of 10,000 ft, we could predict that the Pao_2 would be about 50 torr lower than at sea level.

Abnormal Arterial Oxygenation (Hypoxemia)

To judge the severity of hypoxemia, you must consider the Fio_2. The four most common measures used to judge the severity of hypoxemia—any of which can appear on the NBRC exams—are the A-a gradient or $P(A\text{-}a)o_2$, a/A ratio (Pao_2/Pao_2), P/F ratio (Pao_2/Fio_2), and oxygenation index (OI). Example computation of these parameters is covered in Appendix B in the Navigate 2 companion website. **Table 4-10** summarizes their interpretation.

As indicated in Table 4-10, the most severe forms of hypoxemia are due to physiologic shunting in the lungs (areas of perfusion without ventilation). The NBRC expects candidates to be able to *estimate* the percentage of shunting occurring in critically ill patients. The accompanying box (**Box 4-2**) provides a useful rule of thumb for making this estimate and an example computation.

Mixed Venous Oxygenation

Mixed venous blood samples are obtained from the distal port of a pulmonary artery (PA) catheter with the balloon *deflated*. For patients not having a PA catheter in place, samples obtained from a central venous pressure (CVP) line may be considered as an alternative.

Table 4-10 Interpretation of Measures Used to Assess the Severity of Hypoxemia

Measure	Formula	Interpretation

P/F ratio	Pao_2/Fio_2	• Normal P/F > 350–380
		• Abnormal P/F ratios*:
		  ○ 200–300: V/Q mismatch/mild ARDS
		  ○ 100–200: some shunting/moderate ARDS
		  ○ < 100: refractory hypoxemia, severe shunting/ARDS

A-a gradient	$P(A-a)o_2$	• Abnormal oxygenation:
		  ○ $P(A-a)o_2$ on room air > 5–10 torr
		  ○ $P(A-a)o_2$ on 100% O_2 > 25–65 torr
		  ○ $P(A-a)o_2$ on 100% > 300 torr: severe shunting

a/A ratio	Pao_2/PAo_2	• Normal a/A ratio > 0.75
		• Abnormal a/A ratios:
		  ○ 0.35–0.75: hypoxemia; likely due to V/Q mismatch
		  ○ < 0.35: hypoxemia due to shunting

Oxygenation index (OI)	$\dfrac{Fio_2 \times MAP \times 100}{Pao_2}$	• Used during MV (includes MAP)
		• Normal < 5–8
		• Abnormal:
		  ○ 8: P/F ratio < 200 (moderate/severe RDS)
		  ○ 20: severe hypoxemia; may justify HFOV (neonates)
		  ○ > 40: high mortality; indication for ECMO (neonates)

ARDS, acute respiratory distress syndrome; ECMO, extracorporeal membrane oxygenation; HFOV, high-frequency oscillatory ventilation; MAP, mean airway pressure; MV, mechanical ventilation; RDS, respiratory distress syndrome; V/Q, ventilation/perfusion ratio.

*In addition to P/F ratio, diagnosis of ARDS requires acute onset and bilateral opacities consistent with pulmonary edema on computed tomography (CT) or chest x-ray that are not fully explained by cardiac failure or fluid overload.

Box 4-2 Estimating the Percent Shunt [Assuming Pao_2 > 100 torr and $C(a-\bar{V})o_2$ = 5 mL/dL]

Rule of Thumb: When breathing 100% oxygen, every 100 torr $P(A-a)o_2$ difference equals about a 5% shunt.

Example: A patient breathing 100% O_2 has a $P(A-a)o_2$ of 300 torr. What is her approximate percent shunt?

Solution: 300/100 = 3

Approximate % shunt = 3 × 5 = 15%

Mixed venous blood is useful for assessing tissue oxygenation. When obtained at the same time, arterial and mixed venous samples can be used to compute cardiac output and physiologic shunt. **Table 4-11** provides the commonly cited reference ranges for mixed venous oxygen parameters obtained via a PA catheter (values obtained from a CVP catheter typically are slightly lower).

In general, with a normal Hb level; *if the $S\dot{V}o_2$ is less than 50% or the $P\bar{V}o_2$ is less than 27 torr, the patient has impaired tissue oxygenation.* A $S\dot{V}o_2$ less than 30% (corresponding to a $P\bar{V}o_2$ of about 20 torr) can lead to unconsciousness and permanent organ damage.

Full interpretation of mixed venous oxygenation requires an understanding that these parameters vary *directly* with O_2 delivery to the tissues (CO × Cao_2) and *inversely* with tissue O_2 consumption. Thus, mixed venous O_2 will fall if either O_2 delivery decreases or if O_2 consumption increases (all else being equal). In contrast, mixed venous O_2 will rise if either O_2 delivery increases or if O_2 consumption decreases. **Table 4-12** demonstrates these relationships and summarizes the common clinical conditions associated with changes in mixed venous O_2 content.

Table 4-11 Normal Reference Ranges for Mixed Venous Oxygen Measures

Parameter	Normal Range
$P\bar{v}O_2$	38–42 torr
$S\bar{v}O_2$ (Hb saturation)	68–77%
$C\bar{v}O_2$ (O_2 content)*	14–16 mL/dL
* $C\bar{v}O_2$ = (total Hb × 1.36 × $S\bar{v}O_2$) + (0.003 × $P\bar{v}O_2$)	

Table 4-12 Conditions Associated with Changes in Mixed Venous O_2 Content ($C\bar{v}O_2$)

Low $C\bar{v}O_2$	
Decreased Oxygen Delivery*	**Increased Oxygen Demand**
↓ Hb (e.g., anemia, hemorrhage)	Hyperthermia
↓ PaO_2, SaO_2 (e.g., hypoxemia, suctioning)	Trauma/burns
↓ CO (e.g., hypovolemia, shock, arrhythmias)	Shivering
	Seizures
High $C\bar{v}O_2$	
Increased Oxygen Delivery	**Decreased Oxygen Demand**
↑ CO	Hypothermia
Hyperoxemia (e.g., ↑ FiO_2, polycythemia)	Anesthesia
	Pharmacologic paralysis
	Cyanide poisoning†
	Sepsis†
*Oxygen delivery = CO × CaO_2; oxygen demand = whole-body $\dot{V}O_2$.	
† In both cyanide poisoning and sepsis, $C\bar{v}O_2$ can be higher than normal, even if tissue hypoxia is present. For this reason, in patients with pathologic conditions that decrease O_2 demand, mixed venous lactate may be a better indicator of tissue oxygenation.	

Instead of assessing your knowledge of mixed venous O_2 parameters by themselves, the NBRC may evaluate your understanding of the difference between the arterial and mixed venous oxygen content or $C(a-\bar{V})O_2$. Normally, $C(a-\bar{V})O_2$ is less than 7.0 mL/dL. $C(a-\bar{V})O_2$ will increase if O_2 consumption increases or cardiac output decreases. In contrast, $C(a-\bar{V})O_2$ decreases when oxygen consumption falls or cardiac output increases.

Interpreting Exercise-Related Test Results

The NBRC expects you to be familiar with three exercise-related assessments: the 6MWT, the cardiopulmonary stress test, and O_2 titration with exercise. Here we focus on test interpretation. Chapter 3 discusses the key elements involved in each procedure.

6-Minute Walk Test (6MWT)

The outcome measure for the 6MWT is the 6-minute walk distance (6MWD). Prediction equations for the 6MWD exist, but they are not very useful in assessing those with cardiopulmonary disease. In general, *a 6MWD less than 500–600 meters can be used to screen for abnormal functional capacity*. However, because the test is not diagnostic of any specific condition, patients who exhibit a low 6MWD should undergo further pulmonary and cardiac function testing. *If you are using the 6MWT to assess treatment, you should expect at least a 10–20% improvement in the 6MWD to consider it effective.*

Cardiopulmonary Stress Testing

Depending on their condition or suspected diagnosis, patients may undergo either a cardiac stress test or a comprehensive exercise capacity assessment.

Table 4-13 Measurements Made During Comprehensive Exercise Capacity Testing

Measurement	Definition	Typical Values at Peak Exercise Capacity
Vo_{2max}	Maximum uptake of O_2 per minute at peak exercise capacity	Men: 35–90 mL/kg/min Women: 25–75 mL/kg/min
Anaerobic threshold	Exercise intensity beyond which progressive increases in blood lactate occur	> 40% Vo_{2max}
HR_{max}	Maximum heart rate at peak exercise capacity	220 – age
Breathing reserve	The proportion of MVV that is unused after reaching maximum minute ventilation at peak exercise capacity	> 30%
Spo_2	O_2 saturation (pulse oximetry)	> 88%
O_2 pulse	Oxygen consumption per heartbeat at peak exercise capacity	Men: > 12 mL/beat Women: > 8 mL/beat

HR, heart rate; MVV, maximum voluntary ventilation; Vo_2, oxygen consumption.

A positive cardiac stress test occurs when either ST-segment depression or elevation occurs at elevated workloads, indicating myocardial ischemia. If radionuclide imaging is included in the procedure, comparison of the resting and exercise "pictures" can help reveal the location and extent of any ischemia. On a color scan, areas of good blood flow will appear as bright orange or red, whereas ischemic areas appear dark blue or violet.

Interpreting the results of a comprehensive exercise capacity test is a bit more complicated. **Table 4-13** provides the common parameters measured during exercise capacity testing, including their typical values at peak capacity.

General guidelines for interpretation are as follows:

- Normal result if the patient can do the following:
  - Attain predicted Vo_{2max} and HR_{max} at peak exercise
  - Increase ventilation in response to increased work intensity
  - Maintain normal Spo_2 levels at all levels of exercise
- Exercise capacity is reduced with the following results:
  - Vo_{2max} < 15 mL/kg/min or a peak exercise level *or*
  - Exercise level ≥ 5 metabolic equivalents of task (MET; 1 MET = 3.5 mL O_2/kg body weight) cannot be attained
- Causes of reduced exercise capacity/↓ Vo_{2max} and typical findings include the following:
  - Poor physical conditioning (normal anaerobic threshold, high ↓ HR_{max})
  - Pulmonary disorder (breathing reserve < 30%, desaturation common)
  - Cardiovascular disorder (↓ anaerobic threshold, ↓ O_2 pulse, ↓ HR_{max})

If the test is being done to detect exercise-induced bronchospasm, look for at least a 20% drop in FEV_1 post-exercise. If the test is being conducted to justify participation in a pulmonary rehabilitation program, the patient's Vo_{2max} should be less than 75% of predicted, with a breathing reserve of less than 30%.

Oxygen Titration with Exercise

Interpretation of the results of O_2 titration during exercise is built into the procedure. Evaluation is based on using a Spo_2 of 88% or a Pao_2 of 55 torr as the decision point. Applying this point to a patient at peak activity level results in the following:

- Spo_2 ≥ 88% (Pao_2 ≥ 55 torr): the patient does not need additional O_2/terminate test.
- If ↓ Spo_2 ≥ 2% *or* Spo_2 < 88% (Pao_2 < 55 torr), ↑ O_2 by 1 L/min until Spo_2 ≥ 88%.

Note that to *provide an extra margin of safety, the American Association for Respiratory Care (AARC) recommends setting the target Spo₂ during titration to 93%.* The resulting liter flow should be the value prescribed by the ordering physician for use during applicable activities.

Interpreting Hemodynamic Monitoring Data

The NBRC expects that candidates know the common reference ranges of vascular pressures and the causes of abnormal values, as outlined in **Table 4-14**. In general, pressures rise above normal due to increased cardiac activity (increased contractility and rate), hypervolemia, distal vasoconstriction, or flow obstruction. Pressures fall below normal due to decreased cardiac activity, hypovolemia, or distal vasodilation.

Table 4-14 Vascular Pressures: Reference Ranges and Causes of Abnormalities

Reference Ranges	Increased	Decreased
Systemic Arterial Pressure (SAP)		
Systolic: 90–120 mm Hg Diastolic: 60–80 mm Hg Mean: 70–105 mm Hg	• Increased LV contractility (e.g., inotropes) • Vasoconstriction (e.g., alpha agonist) • Hypertension • Increased cardiac rate • Arteriosclerosis • Essential hypertension • Sympathetic stimulation	• LV failure (e.g., MI, CHF) • Vasodilation (e.g., alpha blockers) • Hypovolemia • Decreased cardiac rate • Arrhythmias • Shock • Systemic hypotension
Central Venous/Right Atrial Pressure (CVP)		
2–6 mm Hg	• Increased venous return/hypervolemia • RV failure (e.g., cor pulmonale) • LV failure/cardiogenic shock • Tricuspid or pulmonary valve stenosis • Pulmonary hypertension • Hypoxemia (e.g., COPD) • Pulmonary embolism • Cardiac tamponade/constrictive pericarditis • Positive-pressure ventilation/PEEP • Pneumothorax	• Vasodilation • Hypovolemia • Shock • Spontaneous inspiration
Pulmonary Artery Pressure (PAP)		
Systolic: 15–30 mm Hg Diastolic: 8–15 mm Hg Mean: 9–18 mm Hg	• Increased RV contractility • Hypervolemia • Pulmonary hypertension • Hypoxemia (e.g., ARDS, COPD) • Pulmonary embolism • Left ventricular failure • Cardiac tamponade • Mitral stenosis • Vasoconstriction (e.g., vasopressors)	• RV failure • Vasodilation (e.g., INO, sildenafil) • Hypovolemia

Reference Ranges	Increased	Decreased
Pulmonary Arterial Wedge Pressure (PAWP or PCWP)		
6–12 mm Hg	• LV failure/cardiogenic shock • Hypervolemia • Cardiac tamponade/constrictive pericarditis • Mitral stenosis • Positive-pressure ventilation/PEEP • Pneumothorax	• Shock other than cardiogenic • Hypovolemia • Spontaneous inspiration

ARDS, acute respiratory distress syndrome; CHF, congestive heart failure; COPD, chronic obstructive pulmonary disease; INO, inhaled nitric oxide; LV, left ventricular; MI, myocardial infarction; PEEP, positive end-expiratory pressure; RV, right ventricular.

Table 4-15 Commonly Measured Hemodynamic Parameters

Parameter	Formula	Normal Range (70-kg patient)
Cardiac output (CO)	Fick equation or thermal dilution value	4–8 L/min
Cardiac index (CI)	CI = CO (L/min) ÷ BSA	2.5–4.0 L/min/m^2
Stroke volume (SV)	SV = CO (mL/min) ÷ HR	60–130 mL/beat
Stroke Index (SI)	SI = CI ÷ HR or SV/BSA	30–50 mL/m^2
Systemic vascular resistance (SVR)	SVR = [(MAP – CVP) ÷ CO] × 80*	900–1400 dynes-sec/cm^5 (15–20 Wood units)
Pulmonary vascular resistance (PVR)	PVR = [(MPAP – PAWP) ÷ CO] × 80*	110–250 dynes-sec/cm^{5*}

BSA, body surface area (m^2); CVP, central venous pressure (mm Hg); HR, heart rate (beats/min); MAP, mean arterial pressure (mm Hg); MPAP, mean pulmonary artery pressure (mm Hg); PAWP, arterial wedge pressure (mm Hg).

*To convert dynes-sec/cm^5 to Wood units (mm Hg/L/min), divide by 80.

Although most hemodynamic monitors compute mean vascular pressures, the NBRC exams can test your ability to estimate these measures. You can estimate both the systemic and pulmonary arterial mean pressures using the following formula:

$$\text{Estimated mean pressure} = \text{diastolic} + 1/3(\text{systolic} - \text{diastolic})$$

For example, the mean arterial pressure (MAP) of a patient with a systolic value of 110 mm Hg and a diastolic value of 70 mm Hg would be calculated as follows:

$$\text{Estimated mean pressure} = 70 + 1/3(110 - 70)$$
$$= 70 + (40 \div 3) = 70 + 13.3$$
$$\approx 83 \text{ mm Hg}$$

Interpreting Blood Flows and Resistances

Knowledge of cardiac output (CO), heart rate, CVP, mean arterial and pulmonary arterial pressures, and pulmonary arterial wedge pressure (PAWP) allows computation of several other hemodynamic parameters, as defined in **Table 4-15**.

The NBRC expects that you know the normal ranges for adult CO, cardiac index (CI), and stroke volume (SV) and—given the necessary data—compute a patient's CI and SV. In addition, you should be able to interpret all of the values in Table 4-15. See the accompanying box (**Box 4-3**) for a simple example.

As with resistance to gas flow through a tube, vascular resistance represents a change in pressure (ΔP) per unit flow. In terms of vascular resistance, the "tubes" are the systemic and pulmonary circulations, and the flow equals the CO. For the systemic circulation, ΔP = mean arterial pressure – CVP, and for the pulmonary circulation, ΔP = mean PA pressure – left ventricular end-diastolic pressure (LVEDP), which is equivalent to the PAWP.

The causes of increased vascular resistance are complex. Except those conditions causing hypervolemia or affecting cardiac contractility, virtually all the factors specified in Table 4-14 as increasing pressures in the systemic and pulmonary circulations are caused by increased vascular resistance—for example, hypertension (systemic or pulmonary), arteriosclerosis, hypoxemia (pulmonary circulation only), and vasopressor drugs. In addition, one of the body's responses to cardiogenic and hypovolemic shock (which both *decrease* systemic and pulmonary vascular pressures) is to increase vascular resistance by vasoconstriction.

Finally, the NBRC may ask a question or two that require you to integrate your knowledge of pressure, flow, and resistance parameters as related to common clinical conditions. **Table 4-16**

Box 4-3 Hemodynamic Computations and Interpretation

Problem

Given a patient with a cardiac output of 4.0 L/min, a heart rate of 100/min, and a body surface area of 2.0 m^2 compute this patient's stroke volume and cardiac index.

Solution

Stroke volume (SV)

SV (mL) = CO (mL/min) ÷ HR

SV = 4000 ÷ 100 = 40 mL

Cardiac index (CI)

CI (L/min/m^2) = CO ÷ BSA

CI = 4.0 ÷ 2 = 2.0 L/min/m^2

Interpretation

The patient's stroke volume and cardiac index are both below normal. Decreased stroke volume is associated with decreased cardiac contractility (e.g., a myocardial infarction) or increased afterload (e.g., vasoconstriction).

Table 4-16 Hemodynamic Changes in Common Clinical Conditions

Condition	BP	CVP	CO	PAP	PAWP
Dehydration/hypovolemic shock	↓	↓	↓	↓	↓
LV failure/cardiogenic shock	↓	N or ↑	↓	↑	↑
RV failure/cardiogenic shock	↓	↑	↓	↓	↓
Septic shock (early)	↓	↓	↑	↓	↓
Neurogenic shock	↓	↓	↓	↓	↓
Pulmonary hypertension	N	↑	N or ↓	↑	N
Pulmonary embolism	↓	↑	↓	↑	N or ↓

↑, increased; ↓, decreased; BP, arterial blood pressure; CVP, central venous pressure; CO, cardiac output; LV, left ventricular; N, normal; PAP, pulmonary artery pressure; PAWP, pulmonary artery wedge pressure; RV, right ventricular.

Box 4-4 Example of a Hemodynamic Interpretation

Problem

Measurements taken via a pulmonary artery (PA) catheter on a patient with a decreased cardiac output and low arterial blood pressure indicate the following:

- Increased central venous pressure (CVP)
- Increased pulmonary artery pressure (PAP)
- Increased pulmonary artery wedge pressure (PAWP)

Interpretation

The increased CVP and PAP could be due to left ventricular (LV) failure/cardiogenic shock, pulmonary hypertension, or pulmonary embolism. However, the elevated PAWP is most consistent with LV failure/cardiogenic shock. The actual impact on cardiac output could be determined using the thermal dilution method via the PA catheter.

---

outlines the typical hemodynamic changes you will see in selected critically ill patients. The accompanying box (**Box 4-4**) provides an example of interpretation.

Pulmonary Compliance and Airway Resistance During Mechanical Ventilation

Key points in evaluating patient compliance during positive-pressure ventilation (PPV) are as follows:

- "Normal" C_{rs} for intubated adult patients ranges between 40 and 80 mL/cm H_2O.
- C_{rs} values below 25–30 mL/cm H_2O are associated with increased work of breathing (WOB) and potential weaning difficulties.
- If C_{rs} decreases during volume-control ventilation (Raw unchanged), you will observe the following:
  - Increased peak inspiratory pressure (PIP)
  - Increased P_{plat}
  - *No change* in PIP – P_{plat}
  - Decreased C_{dyn}
- C_{rs} – C_{dyn} unchanged (both decrease proportionately)
- Decreased slope of the pressure-volume loop
- If C_{rs} decreases during pressure-control (PC) ventilation (Raw unchanged), you will observe the following:
  - Decreased V_T
  - Decreased slope of the pressure-volume loop
- Increases/improvements in C_{rs} will produce changes opposite to those just described above.
- Common causes of acute decreases in C_{rs} include the following:
  - Atelectasis
  - Pulmonary edema/CHF
  - Acute respiratory distress syndrome (ARDS)
  - Tension pneumothorax
  - Pleural effusion
  - Overdistention/hyperinflation
  - Endotracheal (ET) tube slippage into mainstem bronchi
  - Bronchial obstruction by a mucus plug
  - Ascites/abdominal distention

Key points in evaluating patient airway resistance (Raw) during PPV are as follows:

- "Normal" Raw for intubated adults ranges between 5 and 12 cm H_2O/L/sec
- If Raw increases during volume-control ventilation (C_{rs} unchanged), you will observe the following:
  - Increased PIP
  - Increased PIP – P_{plat} difference

- *No change* in P_{plat}
- Decreased C_{dyn}
- Increased $C_{rs} - C_{dyn}$ (C_{rs} unchanged; C_{dyn} decreases)
- Increased width of the pressure-volume loop
- If Raw increases during PC ventilation (C_{rs} unchanged), you will observe the following:
  - Decreased V_T—*but only if the flow continues to the end of breath* (V_T will remain unchanged if flow ceases before the end of the breath)
  - Increased width of the pressure-volume loop
  - Decreases/improvements in Raw will produce changes opposite to those just described above.
- Common causes of acute increases in Raw are as follows:
  - Bronchospasm
  - Excessive secretions
  - Peribronchial/airway edema and swelling
  - Partial artificial airway occlusion (mucus plug, kinking/biting)

Other than computing compliance or resistance, you will likely see NBRC exam questions on evaluation trends/changes in these parameters over time. The accompanying box (**Box 4-5**) provides an example scenario like those commonly appearing on the TMC and CSE exams.

Evaluating and Correcting Auto-PEEP

Due to its deleterious effects, once you confirm the presence of auto-PEEP, you need to determine its cause and apply the appropriate corrective strategy. Chapter 3 describes how to detect and measure auto-PEEP.

As outlined in **Table 4-17**, equipment and patient-related factors can cause auto-PEEP.

Once the source of the problem is identified, you need to implement or recommend a corrective strategy. If the cause is high ventilator rate, short expiratory time, or high I:E ratio, you can lower or eliminate auto-PEEP by taking the following actions:

- Decreasing the rate (volume control or PC)
- Increasing the inspiratory flow (volume control)

Box 4-5 Example Compliance and Resistance Interpretation

Scenario

An adult patient receiving volume-control AC ventilation exhibits the following parameters over time:

Parameter	7:00 AM	8:00 AM	9:00 AM	10:00 AM
V_T (mL)	500	500	500	500
Inspiratory flow (L/min)	40	40	40	40
PIP (cm H_2O)	50	55	60	65
P_{plat} (cm H_2O)	30	30	30	30
PEEP (cm H_2O)	5	5	5	5

Potential Questions

1. What major change in this patient's lung mechanics is occurring over these 4 hours?
2. What are the potential causes of this change/problems to look for?

Solutions

1. Identify the major change in this patient's lung mechanics over these 4 hours:
   - P_{plat} – PEEP remains constant, so C_{rs} remains unchanged (at 20 mL/cm H_2O).
   - PIP – P_{plat} increases from 20 cm H_2O to 35 cm H_2O, so Raw is increasing.
2. Possible causes include bronchospasm, excessive secretions, airway edema, and partial artificial airway occlusion (mucus plug, kinking/biting).

Table 4-17 Causes of Auto-PEEP

Equipment-Related Factors	Patient-Related Factors
High ventilator rate	Bronchospasm
Short expiratory time/high I:E ratio	Small airway collapse
High minute ventilation	Increased secretions
Partially obstructed ETT or heat and moisture exchanger (HME)	Mucus plug ("one-way valve" effect)
Wet expiratory filters	Patient-ventilator asynchrony
Malfunctioning exhalation valve ("sticky valve")	Decreased elastic recoil/high compliance

- Decreasing the tidal volume (volume control)
- Decreasing the inspiratory time (PC)

If the problem is high minute ventilation, decrease the rate and tidal volume, and be willing to accept a rise in $Paco_2$ if the pH can be maintained above 7.25 (permissive hypercapnia). If the cause is a partially obstructed ETT, heat and moisture exchanger (HME) or expiratory filter, suction or un-kink the tube or replace the HME and filter. For malfunctioning exhalation valves, you may have to change the ventilator unit as some expiratory valves are housed inside the unit.

For patient-related problems such as bronchospasm or increased secretions, implement or recommend the appropriate therapy (e.g., a bronchodilator or airway clearance). If auto-PEEP is due to small airway collapse or decreased elastic recoil/high compliance, recommend the incremental application of external PEEP up to 50–80% of the measured auto-PEEP level.

Evaluating Spontaneous Breathing Trials (SBTs)

Chapter 3 outlines the methods and basic procedure for conducting a spontaneous breathing trial (SBT).

An SBT is considered successful if, after at least 30 minutes, the following goals are achieved:

- Acceptable gas exchange
- $Spo_2 \geq 85$–90% or $Pao_2 \geq 50$–60 torr
- pH ≥ 7.30
- Increase in $Paco_2 \leq 10$ torr
- Stable hemodynamics
- Heart rate < 120–140/min; change < 20% from baseline
- Systolic blood pressure < 180–200 mm Hg and > 90 mm Hg; change < 20% from baseline
- No vasopressors required
- Stable ventilatory pattern
- Respiratory rate ≤ 30–35/min
- Change in respiratory rate < 50% from baseline

If the patient can maintain acceptable physiologic parameters and can tolerate the SBT for its full duration (30–120 min), you can consider extubation. The decision of whether to proceed with extubation should be a separate consideration, based on an assessment of the patient's airway patency and protective reflexes. Chapter 9 provides details on when and how to extubate a patient.

If these goals are not met, you should return the patient to a sufficient level of ventilatory support to maintain adequate oxygenation and ventilation and prevent muscle fatigue. Even when the patient meets these physiologic measures, you may need to discontinue the SBT if you note one or more of the following subjective indicators of intolerance or failure:

- Change in mental status (e.g., somnolence, coma, agitation, anxiety)
- Onset or worsening of discomfort
- Diaphoresis

- Signs of increased work of breathing:
  - Use of accessory respiratory muscles
  - Thoracoabdominal paradox

If a patient fails an SBT, you should work with the physician to determine the cause(s). Once these factors are identified and corrected, you should resume performing an SBT every 24 hours.

Assessing Apnea Monitor Data and Alarms

In terms of evaluating apnea monitor data, the device's event recording (chest motion, heart rate trend) can be used to identify the following conditions:

- *Apnea*: the cessation of respiratory effort. Short periods (less than 10 seconds) of central apnea can be normal for all ages.
- *Pathologic apnea*: apnea occurring for longer than 20 seconds or associated with cyanosis, abrupt marked pallor, hypotonia, or bradycardia (< 80–100 beats/min in neonates).
- *Periodic breathing*: a breathing pattern characterized by three or more respiratory pauses of more than 3 seconds' duration with less than 20 seconds of respiration between pauses. *Periodic breathing is not associated with cyanosis or changes in heart rate and can be a normal event.*

To differentiate the various causes of altered respiratory rate, you compare the apnea monitor's respirations to the heart rate, as summarized in **Table 4-18**. Note that apnea monitoring cannot identify the cause of apnea (central versus obstructive) or by itself identify related symptoms (e.g., cyanosis, pallor, hypotonia, choking).

Evaluating Sleep-Related Studies

Chapter 3 outlines the procedures involved in conducting sleep-related studies and covers the management of sleep disorders.

Here we focus on assessing overnight oximetry and continuous positive airway pressure (CPAP)/bilevel positive airway pressure (BPAP) titration results.

Evaluating Overnight Pulse Oximetry Data

Figure 4-3 provides a 5-hour segment of a typical overnight oximetry trend graph for a patient being assessed for sleep apnea. The graph includes both the SpO_2 and the pulse rate, as well as marks indicating potential periods of motion artifact (to help eliminate false-positive results). This graph shows several major desaturation periods, visible as "valleys" in the SpO_2 trend, associated with increases in heart rate. *A desaturation event occurs when the SpO_2 drops by 4% or more.* The average number of desaturation events per hour of sleep is the oxygen desaturation index (ODI). Oximetry software typically reports the total number of desaturation events and the ODI, along with the percentage of time that the SpO_2 was below a given level, most commonly 90%.

In general, an ODI of 15 or more indicates the presence of sleep apnea-hypopnea syndrome (SAHS). In these cases, a follow-up polysomnography exam is not needed to confirm the diagnosis or begin therapy, except as may be required to titrate CPAP treatment (described subsequently). Patients suspected of sleep-disordered breathing who exhibit fewer than 15 desaturation events per hour should undergo full polysomnography to diagnose SAHS and help determine its cause.

In COPD patients, decreases in arterial O_2 saturation may occur in the absence of apnea, hypopnea, or snoring. For this reason, the ODI is not as useful in assessing COPD patients' nocturnal

Table 4-18 Interpretation of Apnea Monitor Signals

Respirations	Heart Rate	Likely Significance
Absent	Decreased	Pathologic apnea
Decreased	Increased	Hypoxemia*
Decreased/irregular	Unchanged	Periodic breathing
Increased	Increased	Motion/activity artifact
*Confirmed via simultaneous pulse oximetry.		

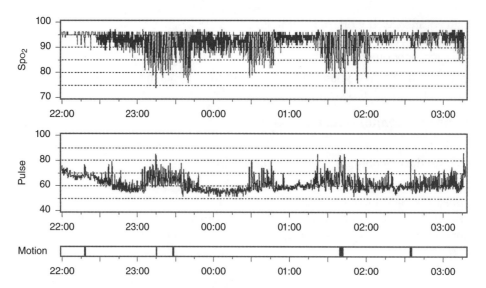

Figure 4-3 Overnight Oximetry Trend Graph.

Courtesy of Sleep Solutions, Inc., Pasadena, Maryland.

desaturation. Instead, Medicare allows reimbursement for nocturnal O_2 therapy in the following circumstances:

- Nocturnal oximetry demonstrates a greater than 5% drop in SpO_2 or a SpO_2 of less than 88%.
- The patient has signs or symptoms of hypoxemia (e.g., impaired cognitive process, insomnia).

These criteria are the same as for continuous long-term O_2 therapy (LTOT) in COPD ($SaO_2 \leq$ 88% or $PaO_2 \leq 55$ torr on room air). When nocturnal desaturation is associated with pulmonary hypertension, daytime somnolence, or cardiac arrhythmias, continuous (as opposed to just nighttime) O_2 therapy is indicated. For those patients already certified for continuous LTOT who also exhibit nocturnal desaturation, the liter flow can be titrated upward in increments of 1 L/min until the nighttime SpO_2 consistently exceeds 88% and desaturation events cease.

Evaluating CPAP/BPAP Titration Results

The goal of CPAP/BPAP titration is to determine the level of control afforded by the therapy at selected pressure settings. You quantify the control level using the respiratory disturbance index or RDI during an observation interval of at least 15 minutes that includes a period of rapid eye movement (REM) sleep. Control is classified as follows:

- *Optimal*: the titrated CPAP level reduces the RDI to **less than 5**, and REM sleep is not continually interrupted by arousals.
- *Good*: the titrated CPAP level reduces the RDI to **10 or less** (or by 50% if the baseline RDI was less than 15), and REM sleep is not continually interrupted by arousals.
- *Adequate*: at the titrated CPAP level, the RDI remains **above 10 but is reduced 75% from baseline, and REM sleep is not continually interrupted by arousals**.

If the control level is less than adequate during the requisite observation period, pressure levels are incrementally increased until at least adequate control is achieved.

Assessing Tracheal Tube Cuff Status

Assessment of airway integrity should be performed on a routine basis according to institutional protocols. Cuff pressures (in cuffed airways) should be part of this assessment, and it should be done at least per shift in an 8-hour period or whenever needed after airway manipulation has occurred.

Key points in assessing tracheal tube cuff pressure include the following:

- For patients receiving positive-pressure ventilation, the desired outcome is a leak-free seal (no gurgling at peak inspiration) at cuff pressures between 20 and 30 cm H_2O (the "minimal leak" technique is no longer recommended).

- After intubation, if cuff pressures > 30 cm H_2O are needed to avoid leakage, the tube is likely too small for the patient's airway; evaluate and recommend exchange for a proper size tube if required.
- If progressively higher and higher cuff pressures are needed to avoid leakage over time, the likely problem is either tracheal dilation/tracheomalacia (often visible on anterior-posterior [AP] x-ray) or cuff/pilot balloon malfunctioning.
- To keep pressures below 30 cm H_2O and help avoid leakage aspiration, recommend that the tube be exchanged for one that provides continuous aspiration of subglottic secretions.

Apnea Test Interpretation (Brain Death Determination)

Apnea test indications and procedure are discussed in Chapter 3. Here we'll discuss the final interpretation of its results.

At the end of an apnea study if respiratory movements are absent and the final arterial blood gas shows a $Paco_2$ of at least 60 torr (> 20 torr increase from baseline for CO_2 retainers) after 10 minutes, then apnea has been demonstrated, which supports a diagnosis of brain death. If the $Paco_2$ does not equal or exceed 60 torr, and the patient was stable and did not develop hypoxemia, the test may be repeated with the time extended to 12–15 minutes if necessary.

Spirometry Outside or Inside a Pulmonary Function Laboratory

The NBRC expects candidates to be able to interpret peak-flow measurements, screening spirometry results, and data obtained via a full laboratory PFT evaluation.

Interpreting Peak Expiratory Flow Rate (PEFR)

Table 4-19 lists the commonly cited peak expiratory flow rate (PEFR) reference ranges by patient age and sex. When using an electronic spirometer to measure PEFR, the patient's gender and height must be entered to determine the predicted value from which the percent predicted is then computed.

As with all pulmonary function tests, a patient's percent predicted value is calculated as follows:

$$\% \text{ predicted} = \frac{\text{actual}}{\text{predicted}} \times 100$$

In asthma management, we often substitute the patient's *personal best* value for the predicted value in computing the percent predicted measure. A patient's personal best PEFR is the highest value achieved over a 2-week asymptomatic period.

As indicated in **Table 4-20**, when a patient presents to the emergency department with a history of asthma and corresponding symptoms, the percent predicted PEFR can help determine the severity of the exacerbation and the proper course of therapy.

For example, in an adult male with a predicted PEFR of 10 L/sec, if his actual PEFR was 7 L/sec, his % predicted would be 7 ÷ 10 = 0.70 = 70%. In general, *PEFR values < 80% of predicted indicate expiratory flow obstruction.* However, because the test is so dependent on patient effort and starting lung volume, you should always consider the possibility of either poor effort or poor technique whenever the PEFR is significantly below normal.

Table 4-19 Reference Ranges for Peak Expiratory Flow Rate (PEFR)

Patient Category	Common Reference Ranges	
	L/min	L/sec
Adult males	450–750	8–12
Adult females	350–530	6–9
Children (depends on height)	150–450	3–8

Table 4-20 Peak Expiratory Flow Rate (PEFR), Asthma Severity, and Recommended Therapy

% Predicted or % Personal Best	Severity (Including Symptoms)	Recommended Therapy
> 80%	Mild	Short-acting beta agonist (SABA) bronchodilator
50–80	Moderate	O_2 to keep saturation > 90% SABA Consider anticholinergic + oral steroids
< 50	Severe	Admit to hospital O_2 to keep saturation > 90% SABA + anticholinergic + oral steroids Consider epinephrine or magnesium sulfate Frequent vital sign monitoring

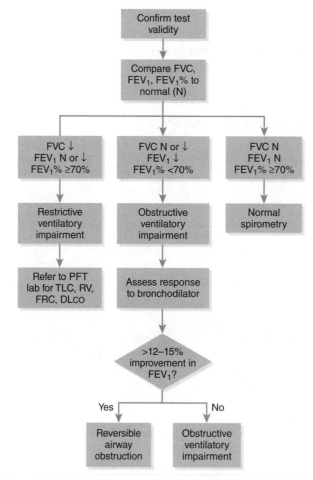

Figure 4-4 Basic Procedure for Interpreting the Bedside or Ambulatory Spirometry.

Data from Barreiro TJ, Perillo I. An approach to interpreting spirometry. *Am Fam Phys.* 2004;69:1107–1114.

Interpreting Screening Spirometry

Figure 4-4 outlines the basic process for interpreting spirometry results. Because the results require proper patient performance, the first step is always to assess test validity. Assuming valid test results,

Table 4-21 Bedside Spirometry Categorization of Pulmonary Function Impairment

Parameter	Normal	Obstructive	Restrictive	Mixed
FVC (% predicted)	N	↓ or N	↓	↓
FEV$_1$ (% predicted)	N	↓	↓ or N	↓
FEV$_1$% (N ≥ 70%)	N	↓	↑ or N	↓

N, normal; ↓, decreased; ↑, increased. For obstructive impairments, judge severity by FEV$_1$% predicted as follows: > 79% normal; 70–79% mild; 50–69% moderate; < 50% severe.

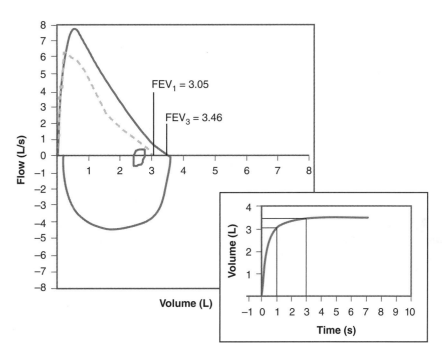

Figure 4-5 A flow volume loop and volume-time curve from a patient with normal pulmonary function. Normal subjects can forcibly exhale 80–90% of the vital capacity (FVC) in about 3 seconds.

you first compare the patient's forced vital capacity (FVC), FEV$_1$, and FEV$_1$% to the patient's computed reference ranges. In general, the FVC and FEV$_1$ are considered normal if the patient's values are at least 80% of those predicted. *A normal FEV$_1$% (FEV$_1$/FVC × 100) is 70% or more for all patients.* As indicated in **Table 4-21**, by comparing these three values, you can immediately categorize the type of impairment present.

Graphic analysis should always supplement numeric assessment. Depending on the spirometer used, the FVC graph may be volume versus time or flow versus volume. **Figure 4-5** shows a healthy patient with normal results. **Figure 4-6** shows the typical results of a patient with severe airflow obstruction showing the concave downward slope of the flow-volume loop representing dynamic airway collapse due to the airway obstruction and the reduced expiratory flows. **Figure 4-7** shows the results of a patient with a severe restrictive disorder showing the high flows and the rapid empty-ing of the vital capacity together with a significant reduction on lung volumes.

If the analysis indicates an obstructive impairment, you should recommend assessing the pa-tient's response to bronchodilator therapy, with repeat spirometry timed to correspond to the peak response time of the drug, usually after 15–30 minutes. You then compute the % change as follows:

$$\% \ change = \frac{post - pre}{pre} \times 100$$

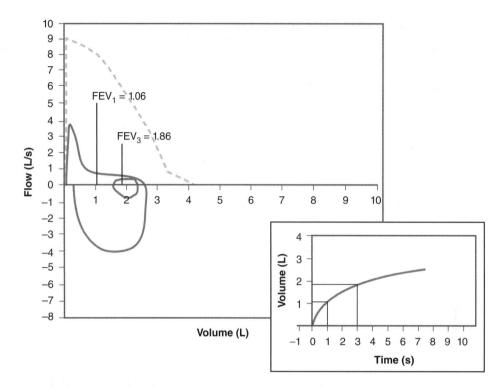

Figure 4-6 A flow volume loop and volume-time curve from a patient with severe emphysema (obstruction). Note the concave downward slope of the flow-volume loop representing dynamic airway collapse due to the airway obstruction and the reduced expiratory flows.

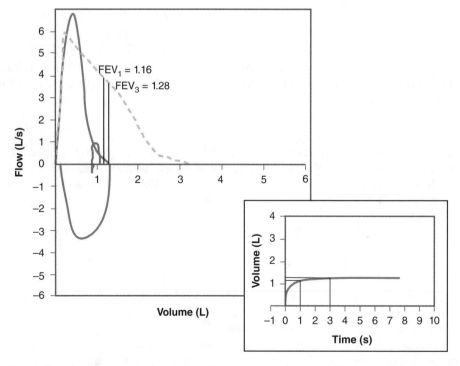

Figure 4-7 A flow volume loop and volume-time curve from a patient with severe pulmonary fibrosis (restriction). Note the high flows and the rapid emptying of the vital capacity together with a significant reduction on lung volumes.

Where "post" is the patient's FEV₁ after bronchodilator, and "pre" is the FEV₁ before bronchodilator. For example, if a patient's FEV₁ before bronchodilator was 3.0 liters and after bronchodilator was 3.3, you would compute the % change as [(3.3 − 3.0) ÷ 3.0] × 100% = [0.3 ÷ 3.0] × 100% = 0.10 × 100% = 10%.

If the patient's FEV₁ improves by at least 12–15% (or by 200 mL or more in adults during PFTs), then the obstruction is classified as reversible, as in asthma. Lesser improvement indicates that the obstruction is not reversible, as in most forms of COPD.

If analysis indicates a restrictive or mixed impairment, you should recommend that the patient undergo a full evaluation in the pulmonary laboratory, to include measurement of static lung volumes and diffusing capacity. In combination, these tests will help differentiate among the various causes of restriction.

Evaluating Pulmonary Function Laboratory Studies

In addition to basic spirometry, the typical PFT lab tests will include measurement of static lung volumes (especially the FRC, residual volume [RV], and total lung capacity [TLC]), as well as the single-breath diffusing capacity or D𝐿co. As with all PFT measurements, assessment of lung volumes requires a comparison of the patient's values to the patient's normal values or reference ranges based on gender, height, age, and ethnicity. Approximate average values for the key static lung volumes for a healthy, young 70-kg male and the likely disease pattern indicated by abnormal findings are summarized in **Table 4-22**.

In terms of the DLCO, the severity of impairment in diffusion capacity is judged against the patient's predicted normal value (based on age, gender, height, and weight), with the "typical" normal ranging between 25 and 30 mL/min/mm Hg. The DLCO is low in conditions that impair alveolar-capillary diffusion (as in pulmonary fibrosis) or decrease surface area (as in emphysema). The DLCO also is low when Hb levels, pulmonary capillary blood flow, or alveolar volumes are reduced. Values in the 65–80% range represent mild impairment, between 50% and 65% represent moderate abnormality, and less than 50% of normal indicates a severe problem. Note that the DLCO may be higher than usual in patients with increased Hb (as in secondary polycythemia). High DLCO values also occur with increases in pulmonary blood flow, such as during exercise.

Once the results of the FVC, static lung volume, *and* diffusing capacity tests are known, the nature of the impairment can be determined. **Figure 4-8** provides an algorithm for interpreting pulmonary lab test results based on the FEV₁%, slow vital capacity (SVC), TLC, and DLCO. You assess the FEV₁% first, followed by the VC, TLC, and then (if needed) the DLCO.

An FEV₁% < 70% indicates either an obstructive disorder or a mixed obstructive and restrictive disorder. For obstructive diseases, the DLCO helps to differentiate between emphysema (low DLCO) and other forms of airway obstruction—such as asthma or chronic bronchitis—in which the DLCO is normal. To differentiate asthma from chronic bronchitis, you should recommend a pre-/post-bronchodilator assessment or (in advanced labs) a methacholine challenge.

If the FEV₁% is ≥ 70%, the patient has either normal pulmonary function or a restrictive disorder. The disorder is restrictive if the TLC is low. Again, the DLCO helps differentiate the two most common types of restrictive disorders, with a normal or high value suggesting a chest wall or neuromuscular problem and a low value consistent with interstitial lung diseases that limit diffusing capacity, such as pulmonary fibrosis.

Table 4-22 Normal Static Lung Volumes and Their Obstructive/Restrictive Patterns

Measure	Normal (Mean)*	Obstructive Pattern†	Restrictive Pattern
RV	1200 mL	↑	↓
FRC	2400 mL	↑	↓
TLC	6000 mL	N or ↑	↓

*Healthy young 70-kg male.
†Requires spirometry (e.g., FEV₁, FEV₁%) to confirm.
N, normal; ↓, decreased (< 80% predicted); ↑, increased (> 120% predicted).

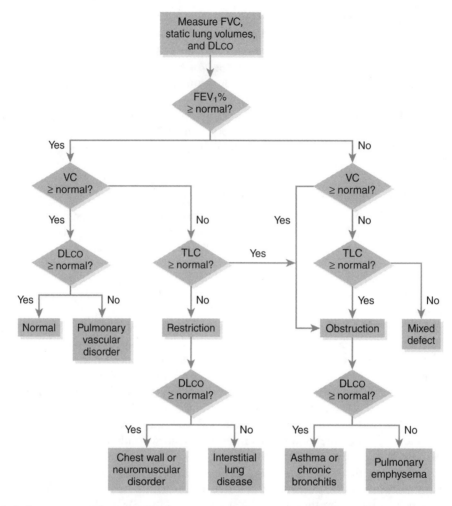

Figure 4-8 Interpretation of Pulmonary Laboratory Test Results. Less than normal is < 70% for the FEV_1% and < 80% predicted for the VC, TLC, and DLCO.

Data from Pellegrino R, Viegi G, Brusasco V, et al. Interpretative strategies for lung function tests. *Eur Respir J.* 2005;26:948–968.

Cardiopulmonary Calculations

Where essential for an explanation, we include selected cardiopulmonary calculations in this chapter. Appendix B, found in the Navigate 2 companion website, provides a complete summary of all calculations that might appear on the NBRC exams.

T⁴—TOP TEST-TAKING TIPS

You can improve your score on this section of the NBRC exam by reviewing these tips:

- Key ECG tips: (1) absent P waves indicate atrial fibrillation or a junctional rhythm; (2) widened QRS complexes denote a PVC, bundle branch block, ventricular tachycardia, or hyperkalemia; (3) a variable R-R interval suggests sinus arrhythmia, atrial fibrillation, or second-degree heart block; (4) ST elevation or depression signals myocardial ischemia, K^+ imbalances, or digoxin effects.
- The most common 12-lead ECG pattern in patients with chronic lung disease is right axis deviation/right ventricular hypertrophy.
- To relate SpO_2 to the approximate PaO_2, use the "40–50–60/70–80–90" rule of thumb: PaO_2s of 40, 50, and 60 torr are about equal to SpO_2s of 70%, 80%, and 90%.

- When using dual oximetry (pre-/postductal), critical congenital heart defects (CCHDs) may be present if both right hand (pre-) and foot (post-) SpO_2 are < 95% *or* the difference between them is ≥ 3%.
- When using a standard pulse oximeter, abnormal hemoglobins (e.g., HbCO, metHb), dark skin pigmentation, nail polish, and ambient light interference will cause erroneous SpO_2 readings. Always use hemoximetry when accurate measurement of SaO_2 is essential.
- The $PtcO_2$ accurately reflects the PaO_2 only in well-perfused patients and when PaO_2 is less than 100 torr; if in doubt, calibrate the $PtcO_2$ against a simultaneous PaO_2 measurement.
- Lack of a clear alveolar plateau phase in the expired CO_2 waveform can occur in patients with COPD, CHF, auto-PEEP, V/Q mismatch, and pulmonary emboli.
- A rise in the expired CO_2 waveform baseline indicates an increase in mechanical deadspace.
- MIP/NIF values less negative than −20 to −25 cm H_2O indicate that muscle strength likely is insufficient to support spontaneous ventilation.
- A rapid shallow breathing index (RSBI) > 105 predicts weaning failure.
- You detect a compensation process in ABG data if the $PaCO_2$ and BE *both* are abnormally high or low; in such cases, if the pH is < 7.40, the primary problem is the one causing acidosis; if the pH is > 7.40, the primary problem is the one causing alkalosis.
- If the $PaCO_2$ and BE diverge in opposite directions (one abnormally high and the other abnormally low), a *combined* acid-base disturbance exists. A high $PaCO_2$ with a low BE define a combined respiratory and metabolic acidosis, and a low $PaCO_2$ with a high BE define a combined respiratory and metabolic alkalosis.
- Assuming normal lung function, the PaO_2 should be at least 5 times the O_2% a patient is receiving.
- Breathing 100% O_2, every 100 torr $P(A-a)O_2$ difference equals about a 5% shunt.
- A P/F ratio < 100 (e.g., a PaO_2 < 60 torr on > 60% O_2) indicates refractory hypoxemia and severe shunting/ARDS.
- An oxygenation index (OI) > 8 corresponds to a P/F ratio < 200 (moderate/severe RDS); values > 20 may justify high-frequency ventilation in neonates.
- A low mixed venous O_2 content or abnormally high $C(a-\dot{V})O_2$ indicates (1) reduced O_2 delivery (decreased CaO_2 or CO) and/or (2) increased tissue O_2 consumption (e.g., hyperthermia, burns, shivering).
- A 6MWD < 500–600 meters indicates abnormal functional capacity; used as a treatment measure, a pre-/post-treatment gain of at least 10–20% is needed to confirm effectiveness.
- ST-segment depression or elevation during a cardiac stress test indicates myocardial ischemia; accompanying imaging data can identify the location and extent of ischemia.
- A patient has a normal exercise capacity if the patient can attain the predicted VO_{2max} and HR_{max} (220 − age) at peak exercise, increase ventilation in response to increased work, and maintain a normal SpO_2; a low VO_{2max} (< 15 mL/kg/min) indicates reduced capacity.
- Patients with a pulmonary disorder affecting exercise capacity will exhibit a low VO_{2max}, limited breathing reserve, and (usually) O_2 desaturation.
- The goal of O_2 titration with exercise is to find the O_2 flow at which the patient's SpO_2 equals or exceeds 88%.
- The normal mean arterial pressure is 70–105 mm Hg; values < 60–70 mm Hg indicate hypotension, most commonly due to LV failure, vasodilation, hypovolemia, or shock.
- Positive-pressure ventilation and PEEP typically increase the CVP above its normal 2–6 mm Hg.
- Normal systolic pulmonary artery pressure (PAP) is 15–30 mm Hg, with a normal mean of 9–18 mm Hg; pulmonary hypertension, hypoxemia (e.g., ARDS, COPD), pulmonary embolism, and left ventricular failure all increase PAP.
- LV failure increases the pulmonary arterial wedge pressure (PAWP or PCWP) above its normal 6–12 mm Hg.
- Compute any vascular mean pressure as diastolic + 1/3 (systolic − diastolic).
- Compute cardiac output (CO) as stroke volume (SV) × heart rate (SV = CO ÷ HR).
- Compute the normal cardiac index (CI) as CO (L/min) ÷ BSA; adult normal is 2.5–4.0 L/min/m².
- To differentiate hypovolemic shock from LV failure/cardiogenic shock, look at the CVP and pulmonary artery pressures—they are low in hypovolemic shock, high in LV failure.

- If C_{rs}/static compliance decreases during volume-control ventilation (Raw unchanged), you will observe ↑ PIP, ↑ P_{plat}, no change in PIP – P_{plat}, ↓ C_{dyn}, C_{rs} – C_{dyn} unchanged (both decrease proportionately), and ↓ slope of the pressure-volume loop.
- If C_{rs}/static compliance decreases during PC ventilation (Raw unchanged), you will observe decreased V_T and decreased the slope of the pressure-volume loop.
- If Raw increases during volume-control ventilation (C_{rs} unchanged) you will observe ↑ PIP, ↑ PIP – P_{plat}, no change in P_{plat}, ↓ C_{dyn}, ↑ C_{rs} – C_{dyn} (C_{rs} unchanged; C_{dyn} decreases), and ↑ width of the pressure-volume loop.
- If the cause of auto-PEEP is high ventilator rate, short expiratory time, or high I:E ratio, you can decrease or eliminate auto-PEEP by decreasing the rate (volume control or PC), increasing the inspiratory flow (volume control), decreasing the tidal volume (volume control), or decreasing the inspiratory time (PC).
- If auto-PEEP is due to small airway collapse or decreased elastic recoil/high compliance, recommend the incremental application of external PEEP.
- A spontaneous breathing trial (SBT) is considered successful if after at least 30 minutes, the patient has (1) acceptable gas exchange (SpO_2 ≥ 85–90%, pH ≥ 7.30, $PaCO_2$ increase ≤ 10 torr); (2) stable hemodynamics (heart rate < 120–140/min; change < 20%, systolic blood pressure < 180–200 mm Hg and > 90 mm Hg); and (3) a stable ventilatory pattern (< 50% increase in rate, rate ≤ 30–35/min).
- Based on apnea-monitored parameters, an absence of respirations and a decreased heart rate for > 15–20 sec indicates pathologic apnea; decreased respirations and a decreased heart rate signal hypoxemia.
- As measured by overnight oximetry, an oxygen desaturation index (ODI) ≥ 15 indicates the presence of sleep apnea-hypopnea syndrome.
- During CPAP titration, optimum control for sleep apnea is indicated if the respiratory disturbance index (RDI) is < 5 and REM sleep is not continually interrupted by arousals.
- If increases in tracheal tube cuff inflation pressure or volume are needed over time to prevent leakage, the likely problem is tracheal dilation or a malfunctioning ETT.
- A peak expiratory flow rate (PEFR) < 50% of personal best in a patient with asthma indicates severe obstruction and the need for immediate acute care.
- An FEV_1% (FEV_1/FVC × 100) < 70% confirms a diagnosis of airway obstruction, usually accompanied by an increase in FRC and RV (hyperinflation).
- A decreased FVC with a normal or increased FEV_1% suggests a restrictive pulmonary condition, confirmed by an overall reduction in static lung volumes (RV, FRC, and TLC).
- An increase in FEV_1 of at least 12–15% (or by 200 mL or more in adults) after bronchodilator indicates reversible airway obstruction.
- Normal DL_{CO} is 25–30 mL/min/mm Hg; low values occur in pulmonary fibrosis (reduced diffusion), emphysema (decreased surface area), and when Hb levels, pulmonary capillary blood flow, or alveolar volumes are reduced; the DL_{CO} may be higher than normal in patients with secondary polycythemia.

POST-TEST

To confirm your mastery of each chapter's topical content, you should create a content post-test, available online via the Navigate Premier Access for Comprehensive Respiratory Therapy Exam Preparation Guide, which contains Navigate TestPrep (access code provided with every new text). You can create multiple topical content post-tests varying in length from 10 to 20 questions, with each attempt presenting a different set of items. You can select questions from all three major NBRC TMC sections: Patient Data, Troubleshooting and Quality Control of Devices and Infection Control, and Initiation and Modification of Interventions. A score of at least 70–80% indicates that you are adequately prepared for this section of the NBRC TMC exam. If you score below 70%, you should first carefully assess your test answers (particularly your wrong answers) and the correct answer explanations. Then return to the chapter to re-review the applicable content. Only then should you reattempt a new post-test. Repeat this process of identifying your shortcomings and reviewing the pertinent content until your test results demonstrate mastery.

Recommend Diagnostic Procedures (Section I-E)

Narciso E. Rodriguez

Aside from providing therapy, your role as a respiratory therapist (RT) often involves making recommendations to others to improve patient care. This includes making recommendations related to enhancing therapeutic outcomes. However, the NBRC also assesses your ability to recommend needed *diagnostic procedures* for your patients.

OBJECTIVES

In preparing for the shared NBRC exam content (TMC/CSE), you should demonstrate the knowledge needed to recommend:

1. Testing for tuberculosis
2. Laboratory tests
3. Imaging studies
4. Bronchoscopy (diagnostic and therapeutic)
5. Bronchoalveolar lavage (BAL)
6. Pulmonary function testing
7. Noninvasive monitoring
8. Blood gas and/or hemoximetry (CO-oximetry)
9. Electrocardiography (ECG)
10. Exhaled gas analysis
11. Hemodynamic monitoring
12. Sleep studies
13. Thoracentesis

WHAT TO EXPECT ON THIS CATEGORY OF THE NBRC EXAMS

TMC exam: 8 questions; 2 recall, 4 application, 2 analysis.
CSE exam: indeterminate number of sections; however, section I-E knowledge is a prerequisite to succeed on both CSE Information Gathering and Decision-Making sections.

WHAT YOU NEED TO KNOW: ESSENTIAL CONTENT

Testing for Tuberculosis (TB)

You should recommend a tuberculin skin test for the diagnosis of a *latent* TB infection. However, a serial sputum specimen collection (for acid-fast bacilli [AFB] stain) is recommended to detect an *active* TB infection. Concurrently, you can recommend additional tests, such as chest x-ray and interferon-gamma release assays that will help to confirm the diagnosis of active TB or previous exposure to *Mycobacterium tuberculosis (M. tuberculosis)*.

Tuberculin Skin Test (Mantoux Test)

The Mantoux tuberculin skin test measures an individual's response to exposure to *M. tuberculosis*. You should recommend the tuberculin skin test for people at high risk for TB infection, including the following:

- Those who have symptoms of TB (fever, night sweats, cough, and weight loss)
- Those who have been exposed to someone who has TB
- Those from a country where TB is prevalent (most countries in Latin America, the Caribbean, Africa, Asia, Eastern Europe, and Russia)
- Those who live or work somewhere in the United States where TB is common (e.g., homeless shelters, prison or jails, some nursing homes)
- Those with HIV infection or other medical problems that weaken the immune system
- Those who use illegal drugs

Interferon-Gamma Release Assay (IGRA)

IGRA is as sensitive as the Mantoux test for detecting latent TB and more sensitive for detecting active TB. This is a blood test that measures how the immune system reacts to exposure to *M. tuberculosis*.

Skin Testing for Allergies

You should recommend allergy skin testing for patients with symptoms consistent with an immunoglobulin E (IgE)–mediated hypersensitivity reaction to an environmental, food, or drug allergen. Allergy symptoms may include skin itching, dizziness, diaphoresis, wheezing (from bronchoconstriction), nausea, vomiting, and diarrhea.

Disorders for which skin testing can support a diagnosis include allergic asthma, rhinitis, and conjunctivitis; food allergies; drug allergies (primarily penicillin); venom allergies (e.g., bee/wasp venom); and latex allergy. Skin testing should not be performed routinely on patients at high risk for an anaphylactic reaction (such as poorly controlled asthma) or those taking medications that interfere with the IgE immune response (e.g., antihistamines), steroids, and anti-IgE antibodies such as omalizumab (Xolair; use to treat asthma).

Laboratory Tests

Blood test results can provide valuable information regarding a patient's status. **Table 5-1** lists some of the most common lab tests you should recommend based on selected patient scenarios commonly seen on the NBRC exams. Table 1-4 (Chapter 1) lists common lab reference ranges for adult patients for the tests likely to appear on NBRC exams as well as the significance of their results.

Imaging Studies

Table 5-2 outlines the primary imaging studies used in patients with respiratory disorders and reasons for recommending them.

You also should be able to recommend proper x-ray positions according to the patient scenario. Posteroanterior (PA) films are recommended for ambulatory patients, who stand upright and take a deep breath. The anteroposterior (AP) projection is most commonly used for intensive care unit (ICU) portable films. Lateral views (in combination with AP or PA films) help assess for pleural effusions.

Bronchoscopy

You should recommend a *diagnostic* bronchoscopy in the following circumstances:

- Assessing lesions of unknown etiology that appear on a chest x-ray
- Evaluating recurrent atelectasis or pulmonary infiltrates
- Assessing the patency of the upper airway
- Investigating the source of hemoptysis
- Evaluating unexplained cough, localized/unilateral wheeze, or stridor
- Following up on suspicious or positive sputum cytology results
- Obtaining lower respiratory tract secretions, cell washings, or biopsies for cytological or microbiological assessment
- Determining the location and extent of injury from toxic inhalation or aspiration
- Evaluating problems associated with artificial airways—for example, tube placement or tracheal damage

CHAPTER 5   Recommend Diagnostic Procedures (Section I-E)

Table 5-1 Recommending Blood Tests

Patient Scenario	Recommended Test(s)
Patients with evidence of tissue hypoxia but normal PaO_2 and SpO_2	• Hemoglobin (Hb) and hematocrit (Hct) to determine O_2-carrying capacity • Hemoximetry to assess for actual SaO_2 and abnormal saturation (e.g., HbCO, metHb) • Lactic acid to assess for tissue hypoxia/anaerobic metabolism
Postoperative patients with a low-grade fever	• White blood cell count (WBC) with differential to rule out possible bacterial pneumonia • Blood culture and sensitivities (for sepsis)
Postoperative patients with sudden dyspnea, hemoptysis, chest pain, or tachycardia (signs of pulmonary embolism)	• d-Dimer test • Ischemia-modified albumin • Arterial blood gases to assess the degree of hypoxemia
Patients with fluid-balance disturbances	• Electrolytes to assess possible causes of fluid imbalance • Hemoglobin and hematocrit to assess for hemodilution or concentration
Patients with decreased (< 25 mL/h) or absent urine output (oliguria) over time	• Urinalysis for specific gravity and pH • Electrolytes • Blood urea nitrogen (BUN) and creatinine to assess for possible renal disease/failure • Glomerular filtration rate (GFR)
Patients with chest pain likely due to myocardial infarction (MI) or ischemia	• Cardiac biomarkers (CK, CK-MB, troponin I) to assess for cardiac muscle damage • Electrolytes
Patients with suspected hepatitis, history of alcohol or drug abuse	• Liver enzymes (ALT, AST, ALP) to assess liver function • Selected drug-screening panels
Patients with acid-base disturbances	• Arterial blood gas (ABG) • Electrolytes • Albumin and total protein • Bilirubin
Patients with unexplained muscle weakness	• Electrolytes to assess for low potassium, calcium, and magnesium • Glucose to assess for hypoglycemia • Thyroid-stimulating hormone to assess for hypothyroidism
Patients with premature ventricular contractions (PVCs) or cardiac dysrhythmias without previous history of cardiac disease	• Electrolytes (especially potassium and calcium) • Thyroid-stimulating hormone to assess for hypo-/hyperthyroidism (thyrotoxicosis)
Patients on anticoagulation therapy or with uncontrolled bleeding	• Platelet count to assess for clotting ability • Coagulation measures (prothrombin time [PT], International Normalized Ratio [INR], activated partial thromboplastin time [APTT]) to assess for clotting problems • Hb/Hct, red blood cell (RBC) measures to assess for bleeding/blood loss
Patient with shock-like symptoms	• Cardiac biomarkers to assess for cardiogenic shock • Renal function tests to assess for hypovolemia • Blood culture to assess for sepsis/septic shock • Hb/Hct to assess for bleeding/blood loss • Lactic acid to assess for tissue hypoxia/anaerobic metabolism

Table 5-2 Recommending Imaging Studies

Recommend to	Comments
Chest X-Ray	
• Evaluate signs and symptoms of respiratory and cardiovascular disorders • Follow known chest disease processes to assess progression • Monitor patients receiving ventilatory support • Monitor patients after thoracic surgery • Assess surgical risk in patients with cardiac or respiratory symptoms • Confirm proper placement of endotracheal tubes (ETTs), CVP and PA catheters, and NG/OG and chest tubes • Comply with government requirements for chest radiography, as in occupational lung disease	Although performing a chest x-ray after thoracentesis is common practice, the American College of Radiology recommends it only if a pneumothorax is suspected (e.g., if air rather than fluid is aspirated) Perform a chest x-ray only when indicated. Routine daily chest x-ray is no longer recommended to monitor mechanically ventilated patients
Neck X-Ray	
• Help diagnose causes of stridor and respiratory distress • Detect the presence of radiopaque aspirated foreign bodies (e.g., coins) • Detect retropharyngeal abscesses and hematomas	AP versus lateral neck films are taken to differentiate croup from epiglottitis; however, the classic AP-view "steeple sign" described for croup is not specific to that disorder and may be absent.
Thoracic Computed Tomography (CT) Scan	
• Evaluate abnormalities identified by chest x-ray (e.g., interstitial lung disease, pleural effusions, and pulmonary nodules) • Stage lung cancer • Detect tumor metastases to the lung • Detect mediastinal masses/nodes and other abnormalities • Detect pulmonary embolism (spiral CT and CT angiography) • Detect and evaluate aortic aneurysm • Assess trauma to thoracic organs and structures	The patient must remain motionless. Spiral CT and CT angiography are replacing V/Q scans for diagnosing pulmonary embolism (PE).
Thoracic Magnetic Resonance Imaging (MRI)	
• Evaluate the heart, major vessels, and lungs for pathologic abnormalities • Assess the chest wall and surrounding soft tissues for abnormalities • Evaluate posterior mediastinal masses • Detect and evaluate aortic aneurysm • Detect/assess mediastinal, vascular, and chest-wall metastasis of lung cancer • Stage lung cancer in patients who are allergic to radiographic contrast media	Patients must remain motionless. It is contraindicated in patients with pacemakers, metallic surgical clips or heart valves, or infusion or chemotherapy pumps. Ventilatory support must be provided by a manual all plastic resuscitator or via a ventilator certified for MRI use. MRI is less accurate than CT for assessing lung parenchymal disease.
Positron Emission Tomography (PET) Scan	
• Differentiate malignant versus benign masses • Assess tumor metastases/response to therapy • Determine tumor biopsy site(s) • Detect and localize impaired blood flow to the myocardium	Often combined with CT scanning to enhance diagnostic accuracy. Most common use in pulmonary medicine is to diagnose, stage, and evaluate treatment of non–small-cell lung cancer.

Recommend to	Comments
Pulmonary Angiography	
• Evaluate the pulmonary arteries for pulmonary embolism, stenosis, AV malformation, or aneurysm	Contraindicated in patients with bleeding abnormalities, extremely high blood pressure, or shock.
	It is being replaced by CT angiography.
Ventilation/Perfusion (V/Q) Scan	
• Detect and quantify the size of a pulmonary embolism • Assess regional pulmonary blood flow in patients undergoing lung resection surgery	Patients must be able to breathe through a mouthpiece, hold the breath for 10 seconds or more, and remain still during the procedure.
Transthoracic Ultrasound	
• Detect free fluid in the thorax (e.g., pleural or pericardial effusion, hemithorax) • Detect pneumothorax • Detect mediastinal masses • Detect pulmonary atelectasis or consolidation • Assess the pleural surfaces for pleuritis or granulomatous processes • Assess thoracic wall lesions and rib masses • Assess trauma to the diaphragm, heart, and large thoracic vessels, as well as bone fractures • Guide thoracentesis and percutaneous needle biopsies	Generally ineffective in imaging tissues or organs through aerated lung tissue or pneumothorax.
AP, anteroposterior; AV, arteriovenous; CVP, central venous pressure; ET, endotracheal; NG, nasogastric; OG, orogastric; PA, pulmonary artery.	

You should recommend a *therapeutic* bronchoscopy in the following circumstances:

- Facilitating ETT insertion during difficult intubations
- Achieving selective intubation of a main stem bronchus
- Locating and clearing mucus plugs causing lobar or segmental atelectasis
- Removing abnormal endobronchial tissue or foreign bodies
- The need to place and assess airway stent function
- The need for airway balloon dilatation in the treatment of tracheobronchial stenosis

According to the American Association for Respiratory Care (AARC), you should recommend *against* bronchoscopy in patients with the following criteria:

- Cannot be adequately oxygenated during the procedure
- Have a bleeding disorder that cannot be corrected
- Have severe obstructive airway disease
- Have severe refractory hypoxemia
- Are hemodynamically unstable

Bronchoalveolar Lavage (BAL)

Bronchoalveolar lavage (BAL) involves the instillation and removal of sterile saline solution into a lung segment via the suction channel of a fiberoptic bronchoscope. The withdrawn fluid then undergoes chemical, cytological, and microbiological assessment. According to the American Thoracic Society (ATS), BAL is indicated in patients with nonresolving pneumonia, unexplained lung infiltrates (interstitial or alveolar), or suspected alveolar hemorrhage and in patients with interstitial lung disease (ILD). BAL is a key tool for diagnosing bacterial ventilator-associated pneumonia (VAP) and helps confirm a diagnosis of various lung cancers. Moreover, BAL can also be used for pulmonary toilet in certain conditions such as pulmonary alveolar proteinosis by removing the abnormal surfactant material that accumulates in the alveolar space with this disease. The only major contraindication to BAL is a predisposition for bleeding.

Pulmonary Function Tests

Table 5-3 outlines the primary reasons why you would recommend specific pulmonary function tests for your patients.

Table 5-3 Recommending Pulmonary Function Tests

Specific Test	Recommend to
Peak expiratory flow rate (PEFR)	• Monitor airway tone of patients with asthma over time (via diary) • Assess changes in airway tone in response to bronchodilator therapy (forced expiratory volume [FEV] spirometry is preferred). • A post-bronchodilator improvement of 12% or more is considered significant.
Screening/bedside spirometry	• Screen for lung dysfunction suggested by history and physical indicators or other abnormal diagnostic tests • Assess changes in lung function in response to treatment • Assess the risk for surgical procedures known to affect lung function • Monitor disease progression
Pre-/post-bronchodilator spirometry (bedside or lab)	• Confirm the need for bronchodilator therapy • Individualize the patient's medication dose • Determine patient status during acute and long-term drug therapy • Determine if a change in dose, frequency, or medication is needed
Laboratory spirometry (forced vital capacity [FVC] volumes and flows)	• Quantify the severity and prognosis associated with lung disease • Follow up on bedside spirometry results that are not definitive (e.g., restrictive conditions) • Assess the potential pulmonary effects of environmental or occupational exposures • Monitor for adverse reactions to drugs with known pulmonary toxicity • Assess the degree of pulmonary impairment for rehabilitation or disability claims
Maximum voluntary ventilation (MVV)	• Assess the integrated function of the airways, lungs, thoracic cage, and respiratory muscles • Evaluate preoperative pulmonary function • Predict breathing reserve for exercise testing • Evaluate respiratory disability
Functional residual capacity (FRC) and total lung capacity (TLC)	• Evaluate the degree of hyperinflation in obstructive abnormalities • Determine the volume of gas trapped in cysts or bullae (by comparing it to body box thoracic gas volume [TGV]) • Assess the presence and severity of restrictive abnormalities

Specific Test	Recommend to
Carbon monoxide diffusing capacity (DLCO)	• Evaluate/follow the course of interstitial lung diseases such as pulmonary fibrosis and pneumoconiosis
	• Evaluate/follow the course of emphysema and cystic fibrosis
	• Differentiate among chronic bronchitis, emphysema, and asthma in patients with obstructive patterns
	• Quantify the degree of pulmonary impairment for disability claims
	• Evaluate cardiovascular disorders affecting diffusion or pulmonary blood flow
	• Evaluate the pulmonary effects of systemic diseases such as rheumatoid arthritis and lupus
	• Evaluate the effects of drugs known to cause pulmonary damage, such as amiodarone and bleomycin
	• Help predict arterial desaturation during exercise in patients with lung disease
Bronchial provocation (e.g., methacholine challenge test)	• Assess the presence of/severity of airway hyperreactivity
	• Evaluate occupational asthma
	• Determine the relative risk of developing asthma
	• Assess response to therapeutic interventions
Airway resistance (body plethysmography)	• Evaluate airway responsiveness to provocation
	• Identify the specific type and severity of obstructive lung disease
	• Localize the primary site of flow limitation

Noninvasive Monitoring, Blood Gas Analysis, and Hemoximetry (CO-oximetry)

Respiratory care often requires monitoring of patient oxygenation, ventilation, and acid-base balance. You can assess arterial oxygenation by arterial blood gas (ABG) analysis, hemoximetry, pulse oximetry, or transcutaneous Po_2 monitoring. You can evaluate ventilation by ABG analysis, transcutaneous monitoring of Pco_2, or capnography (discussed here in a separate section). A full assessment of acid-base status requires an ABG. **Table 5-4** outlines the key indications for these various measurements.

Some additional key points regarding recommending these assessments are mentioned below.

ABG Analysis

- If the goal is the *most accurate* evaluation of oxygenation, ventilation, and acid-base status, always recommend ABG analysis.
- Standard ABG analysis does not measure actual Hb content, Hb saturation, or abnormal hemoglobins, such as carboxyhemoglobin (HbCO) or methemoglobin (metHb).

Hemoximetry (CO-oximetry)

- If you need accurate measures of any Hb parameters, use or recommend hemoximetry (CO-oximetry).
- The most common patient scenario in which you should recommend hemoximetry is smoke inhalation/CO poisoning. Hemoximetry is also recommended during inhaled nitric oxide therapy to monitor metHb concentrations.
- You also should recommend hemoximetry when you need to calibrate a pulse oximetry reading (Spo_2) against the actual arterial saturation.

Table 5-4 Indications for Various Invasive and Noninvasive Blood Measurements

Method	Indications
Invasive	
Blood gas analysis (ABG)	• Evaluate ventilation ($Paco_2$), acid-base (pH, $Paco_2$, and HCO_3^-), and oxygenation (Pao_2, Sao_2) status • Assess the patient's response to therapy or diagnostic tests (e.g., O_2 therapy, exercise testing) • Monitor severity and progression of a documented disease process
Hemoximetry (CO-oximetry)	• Determine actual blood oxyhemoglobin saturation (%HbO_2) • Measure abnormal Hb levels (HbCO, metHb, and sulfhemoglobin)
Noninvasive	
Pulse oximetry (Spo_2)	• Monitor the adequacy of Spo_2 • Quantify the response of Spo_2 to therapeutic or diagnostic interventions • Screen for critical congenital heart disease in neonates ("dual" oximetry) • Comply with regulations or recommendations by authoritative groups (e.g., anesthesia monitoring)
Transcutaneous monitoring ($Ptco_2$, $Ptcco_2$)	• Continuously monitor the adequacy of arterial oxygenation and ventilation • Continuously monitor for excessive arterial oxygenation (hyperoxemia) • Quantify real-time changes in ventilation and oxygenation during diagnostic or therapeutic interventions • Screen for functional shunts in babies with congenital heart disease ("dual" $Ptco_2$)
Invasive and Noninvasive	
Capnography & capnometry	• Confirm proper placement of an ETT during intubation (invasive) • Monitoring patients receiving moderate sedation or opioid analgesia for suppression of ventilation (noninvasive) • Continuous monitoring of ventilation during mechanical ventilation (invasive) • Monitor the effectiveness of compressions during CPR (capnometry only, invasive) • Assess the metabolic rate (noninvasive and invasive)

Pulse Oximetry

- Pulse oximetry should not replace ABG analysis or hemoximetry when the clinical situation demands accurate assessment of oxygenation.
- Recommend against pulse oximetry in patients with poor peripheral perfusion and when there is a need to monitor for hyperoxemia (higher-than-normal PO_2s).

Transcutaneous Monitoring ($Ptco_2$, $Ptcco_2$)

- $Ptco_2$ monitoring is most accurate in infants, less so in children and adults.
- Infant $Ptco_2$ monitoring is the best way to assess for hyperoxemia and help prevent retinopathy of prematurity (ROP).
- $Ptcco_2$ can be measured reliably in hemodynamically stable adults, making it an excellent choice for monitoring ventilation when capnography is difficult (e.g., during noninvasive positive-pressure ventilation [NPPV]).
- Due to lengthy setup times, do not recommend transcutaneous monitoring in emergencies.

Capnography

You should recommend capnography for the following situations:

- Monitoring the adequacy of ventilation in patients receiving mechanical ventilation (required during transport of mechanically ventilated patients)
- Providing graphic data to help evaluate the ventilator–patient interface
- Monitoring the adequacy of ventilation in unstable patients, those undergoing moderate sedation, or those receiving opioid analgesia
- Monitoring the severity of pulmonary disease and assessing the response to therapies intended to lower physiologic deadspace and better match ventilation to pulmonary perfusion (V/Q)
- Confirming and monitoring ETT placement in the lungs after intubation
- Optimizing chest compressions and detecting the return of spontaneous circulation (ROSC) during cardiopulmonary resuscitation (CPR)
- Measuring CO_2 production (to assess metabolic rate)

The utility of capnography during CPR is based on the fact that $Petco_2$ correlates well with cardiac output. With poor or absent blood flow to the lungs, $Petco_2$ levels remain low (< 10 torr). With good blood flow to the lungs—either due to effective chest compressions or due to the restoration of cardiac function—$Petco_2$ levels rise.

In terms of assessing ventilation-perfusion relationships (V/Q), deadspace, and CO_2 production, you will need to recommend *volumetric* capnography. Volumetric capnography simultaneously measures expired CO_2 levels and tidal volumes, thereby allowing computation of deadspace and CO_2 production. Interestingly, there is some evidence that deadspace and CO_2 production measurements also can be used to titrate positive end-expiratory pressure (PEEP) levels in patients receiving mechanical ventilation.

Regarding graphic evaluation of the ventilator–patient interface, end-tidal CO_2 trend analysis can indicate potential hyperventilation/hypoventilation, which should be confirmed by ABG analysis. Analysis of the shape of the capnogram also can help identify conditions such as circuit rebreathing, disconnection, and airway obstruction.

Electrocardiography

You should recommend obtaining a 12-lead electrocardiogram (ECG) to meet the following needs:

- Screening for heart disease (e.g., coronary artery disease [CAD], left ventricular hypertrophy)
- Ruling out heart disease in surgical patients
- Evaluating patients with chest pain
- Following the progression of patients with CAD
- Evaluating heart rhythm disorders (using rhythm strips)

A 12-lead ECG also can be used to assess the effect of metabolic disorders associated with electrolyte disturbances—in particular, calcium and potassium imbalances.

Exhaled Gas Analysis

Exhaled gases commonly analyzed for diagnostic purposes include carbon dioxide (CO_2), carbon monoxide (CO), and nitric oxide (NO). The need for exhaled CO_2 analysis was previously covered in this chapter's section on capnography.

Exhaled CO Analysis

You should recommend exhaled CO analysis to monitor patients' smoking status. Exhaled CO levels are associated with the number of cigarettes consumed daily. Readings below 6–8 ppm signify a nonsmoking status, with values below 3–4 ppm typically confirming true smoking abstinence. Readings above 6–8 ppm indicate that smoking has likely occurred within the past 12–24 hours. A higher cutoff (10–11 ppm) should be applied to patients with inflammatory lung diseases such as asthma or chronic obstructive pulmonary disease (COPD) because inflammation boosts endogenous CO production.

You also can recommend exhaled CO analysis to assess for moderate levels of CO poisoning in conscious and cooperative patients. Divide the CO concentration in ppm by 6 to estimate the HbCO%. For example, an exhaled CO reading of 48 ppm would indicate a HbCO saturation of about 8%.

Fractional Exhaled Nitric Oxide (FeNO) Analysis

Nitric oxide (NO) is a chemical mediator produced primarily by endothelial cells in the lung, as well as by epithelial cells, macrophages, eosinophils, and neurons. Because it is a gas, NO appears in the exhaled breath, with its concentration increasing in the presence of airway inflammation—particularly in patients with asthma. In patients with asthma symptoms, exhaled NO analysis can help establish the correct diagnosis. In those with a confirmed asthma diagnosis, you can recommend exhaled NO analysis to do the following:

- Predict the response to corticosteroids
- Titrate anti-inflammatory medication
- Monitor the level of asthma control
- Predict impending exacerbation
- Monitor medication adherence

Table 5-5 outlines the normal and abnormal ranges of NO for adult and pediatric patients and related key management points, as recommended by the American Thoracic Society (ATS).

Table 5-5 Exhaled NO Levels and Key Patient Management Points

	Exhaled NO Levels (in parts per billion)		
	Low	**Intermediate**	**High**
Adult	< 25 ppb	25–50 ppb	> 50 ppb
Children (< 12 years)	< 20 ppb	20–35 ppb	> 35 ppb
Eosinophilic Inflammation?	Unlikely	Likely	Present
Management Points			
Symptomatic	• Unlikely to respond to ICS • Consider alternative diagnosis including chronic cough, vocal cord dysfunction, non-allergic asthma, GERD, ciliary dyskinesia, cystic fibrosis, chronic lung disease of prematurity	• Be cautious but consider asthma. • Consider increasing ICS dose and possible ICS resistance • If no asthma history, consider other causes (e.g., gastroesophageal reflux, sinusitis, cardiac disease, persistent allergen exposure)	• Generally, confirms asthma diagnosis in patients with respiratory symptoms who are not taking ICS • If asthma Dx confirmed, assess for medication compliance, proper dose, and proper inhaler technique • If asthma Dx confirmed and patient complying with treatment, consider increasing ICS dose or adding a beta-agonist
Asymptomatic	• Adequate ICS dose, taper steroids	• Adequate ICS dose and adherence • Continue to monitor	• Continue with present treatment • Assess exposure to aeroallergens

ICS, inhaled corticosteroid; ppb, parts per billion.

Modified from Dweik, R. A., Boggs, P. B., Erzurum, S. C., Irvin, C. G., Leigh, M. W., . . . Lundberg, J. O. (2011). An Official ATS Clinical Practice Guideline: Interpretation of Exhaled Nitric Oxide Levels (FeNO) for Clinical Applications. *American Journal of Respiratory and Critical Care Medicine*, 184(5), 602–615. doi:10.1164/rccm.9120-11st.

Hemodynamic Monitoring

Noninvasive Blood Pressure Measurement

As a component of the vital signs, blood pressure should be measured noninvasively and regularly for all patients. The frequency of measurement varies according to the patient's cardiovascular stability. Automated noninvasive bedside systems allow measurement intervals as short as every 5 minutes.

Invasive Hemodynamic Monitoring

Although the decision to insert an indwelling catheter is a medical one, you need to be aware of the circumstances in which your patients could benefit from hemodynamic monitoring. Likewise, given the many complications associated with indwelling lines and catheters, you must be familiar with the contraindications. **Table 5-6** summarizes the key indications and contraindications for indwelling catheters by type and location.

Sleep Studies

Sleep studies that RTs might recommend include overnight pulse oximetry and polysomnography.

Overnight Oximetry

You should recommend overnight oximetry for the following purposes:

- Helping identify patients with sleep apnea-hypopnea syndrome (SAHS)
- Helping assess the response of patients with sleep apnea to therapy, such as continuous positive airway pressure (CPAP)
- Identifying whether serious desaturation occurs in patients with COPD during sleep

For in-home assessment of sleep disorders, "limited" polysomnography (PSG) has mostly replaced overnight oximetry. Limited PSG monitors up to seven key parameters, including Spo_2, airflow, and respiratory effort. Although it does not assess sleep stages, you can recommend limited PSG for individuals who have a high likelihood of obstructive sleep apnea (OSA). You also can recommend limited PSG testing as to follow-up on the effectiveness of treatment for those already diagnosed with OSA.

Regarding screening individuals with COPD, it is well known that some of these patients experience large drops in O_2 saturation during sleep. This nocturnal desaturation generally can be predicted from daytime saturation levels and is probably due to hypoventilation occurring during rapid eye movement (REM) sleep. When screening COPD patients for nocturnal desaturation, the focus should be on those with hypercapnia, erythrocytosis, or evidence of pulmonary hypertension.

Laboratory Polysomnography

Laboratory PSG is the gold standard for diagnosing sleep apnea. You should recommend lab PSG for patients who exhibit signs or symptoms associated with sleep-disordered breathing, such as daytime somnolence and fatigue, morning headaches, pulmonary hypertension, and polycythemia. According to the AARC, lab PSG is specifically indicated in patients with the following conditions:

- COPD with awake $Pao_2 > 55$ torr and whose condition includes pulmonary hypertension, right heart failure, polycythemia, or excessive daytime sleepiness
- Chest wall or restrictive neuromuscular disorders and whose condition includes chronic hypoventilation, polycythemia, pulmonary hypertension, disturbed sleep, morning headaches, daytime somnolence, or fatigue
- Disorders of respiratory control with chronic hypoventilation (daytime $Paco_2 > 45$ torr) or whose illness is complicated by pulmonary hypertension, polycythemia, disturbed sleep, morning headaches, daytime somnolence, or fatigue
- Excessive daytime sleepiness or sleep maintenance insomnia
- Snoring associated with observed apneas and excessive daytime sleepiness

Laboratory PSG also is indicated to help diagnose certain neurologic and movement disorders, such as restless legs syndrome and nocturnal seizures, as well as parasomnias such as sleepwalking. Also, lab PSG is used to assess the adequacy of sleep-related interventions, including titrating CPAP/

Table 5-6 Indications and Contraindications for Indwelling Catheters

Indications	Contraindications
Systemic Arterial Monitoring (A-Line)	
• To continuously monitor arterial pressure in unstable/hypotensive patients or those receiving vasoactive drugs • To obtain frequent ABGs/labs for patients in respiratory failure, receiving mechanical ventilation, or with severe metabolic disturbances.	• Inadequate collateral arterial circulation (as confirmed by Allen's test [radial site only]) • Evidence of infection or peripheral vascular disease in the selected limb • Severe bleeding disorder • Presence of a surgical/dialysis shunt in the selected arm (consider the opposite arm)
Central Venous Pressure (CVP) Monitoring	
• To monitor CVP/right ventricular function in unstable or hypotensive patients • To provide and monitor volume resuscitation • To infuse drugs that can cause peripheral phlebitis (certain vasopressors and chemotherapeutic agents) • To sample blood for P_VO_2 or S_VO_2 (a surrogate for mixed venous measures) • To provide a route for total parenteral nutrition • To perform plasmapheresis or hemodialysis • To introduce transvenous pacing wires • To provide venous access in patients with poor peripheral veins	• Evidence of infection at the insertion site • Abnormalities at the insertion site (vascular injury, prior surgery, rib/clavicle fractures, chest wall deformity) • Suspected injury to the superior vena cava • Severe bleeding disorder (Note: The subclavian vein cannot be compressed to stop bleeding.) • Presence of an intravascular pacemaker or vena cava filter • Severe obesity (a technical difficulty) • Bullous lung disease (high risk of pneumothorax)
Pulmonary Artery (PA) Monitoring	
• To identify the cause of various shock states • To identify the cause of pulmonary edema • To diagnose pulmonary hypertension • To diagnose valvular disease, intracardiac shunts, cardiac tamponade, and pulmonary embolus • To monitor and manage complicated MI • To assess the hemodynamic response to therapies • To manage multiple organ failure • To manage hemodynamic instability after cardiac surgery • To optimize fluid and inotropic therapy • To measure tissue oxygenation and cardiac output • To perform atrial and ventricular pacing	• Certain dysrhythmias (Wolff-Parkinson-White syndrome, LBBB) • Tricuspid or pulmonary valve endocarditis, stenosis, or mechanical prosthesis • Right heart mass (thrombus and/or tumor) • Infection at the insertion site • The presence of an RV assist device, transvenous pacemaker, or defibrillator • Severe bleeding disorder
ABG, arterial blood gas; CVP, central venous pressure; LBBB, left bundle branch block; MI, myocardial infarction; RV, right ventricular.	

bilevel positive airway pressure (BPAP) in patients with sleep apnea and determining BPAP levels for respiratory insufficiency due to chronic neuromuscular disorders, such as amyotrophic lateral sclerosis. When nocturnal seizures are considered as part of the differential diagnosis of abnormal movements or behaviors during sleep, extended electroencephalogram (EEG) monitoring is typically performed during the PSG.

Thoracentesis

Thoracentesis is a physician-performed procedure involving the withdrawal of fluid from the pleural space for either diagnostic or therapeutic purposes. You would recommend a *diagnostic* thoracentesis to help determine the cause of the accumulated fluids in the pleural space (e.g., transudative versus exudative) or to obtain cell samples to assess for certain malignancies. You would recommend a *therapeutic* thoracentesis for any patient with a pleural effusion large enough to cause respiratory distress. Contraindications to thoracentesis include insufficient pleural fluid, skin infection or wound at the needle insertion site, and severe bleeding disorder.

T⁴—TOP TEST-TAKING TIPS

You can improve your score on this section of the NBRC exam by reviewing these tips:

- Recommend the tuberculin skin test for people at high risk for TB infection (i.e., those with HIV infection or other medical problems that weaken the immune system).
- Recommend a serial sputum specimen collection (for AFB stain) to detect an active TB infection.
- You should recommend additional tests, such as chest x-ray and interferon-gamma release assays, that will help to confirm the diagnosis of active TB or previous exposure to *M. tuberculosis.*
- Recommend hemoximetry to assess for actual HbO_2 and abnormal Hb saturation (e.g., HbCO, metHb).
- Recommend lactic acid (lactate) blood test to assess for tissue hypoxia/anaerobic metabolism in patients with shock-like symptoms or those with normal arterial oxygenation but signs and symptoms of tissue hypoxia.
- Recommend a white blood cell count (WBC) with differential to rule out possible bacterial pneumonia.
- Recommend blood urea nitrogen (BUN) and creatinine to assess for possible renal disease/failure.
- Recommend liver enzymes (ALT, AST, ALP) to assess liver function.
- Recommend coagulation measures (prothrombin [PT], International Normalized Ratio [INR], activated partial thromboplastin time [APTT]) to assess for clotting problems.
- Recommend AP and lateral neck x-rays to (1) help diagnose causes of stridor and respiratory distress, (2) detect radiopaque aspirated foreign bodies, and (3) detect retropharyngeal abscesses and hematomas.
- Recommend transthoracic ultrasound to (1) detect pleural or pericardial effusions; (2) assess trauma to the diaphragm, heart, and large thoracic vessels; and (3) guide thoracentesis and percutaneous needle biopsies.
- Recommend diagnostic bronchoscopy to evaluate unexplained cough, localized/unilateral wheeze, or stridor (usually associated with foreign-body aspiration).
- Recommend a V/Q scan to detect and quantify the effects of a pulmonary embolism and to assess regional pulmonary blood flow in patients undergoing lung resection surgery.
- Recommend bronchoalveolar lavage (BAL) in patients with nonresolving pneumonia; unexplained lung infiltrates and suspected VAP.
- Recommend a posteroanterior (PA) film for ambulatory patients who can stand upright and take a deep breath.
- Recommend a portable anteroposterior (AP) chest x-ray for ICU patients who are bedridden.
- Recommend lateral views (in combination with AP or PA films) to help assess for pleural effusions.
- Recommend pre-/post-bronchodilator spirometry to confirm the need for bronchodilator therapy (reversible obstruction) and to individualize the patient's medication dose. A 12% improvement is considered significant.
- Recommend FRC/TLC measurement to assess the presence and severity of restrictive abnormalities.
- Recommend Dʟᴄᴏ testing to quantify the degree of pulmonary impairment for disability claims.

- Recommend CO-oximetry for patients suffering from smoke inhalation (to measure HbCO) and for those suspected of having abnormal Hb (e.g., metHb, sulfhemoglobin).
- If the goal is the most accurate evaluation of oxygenation, ventilation, and acid-base status, always recommend an ABG analysis.
- Standard ABG analysis does not measure actual Hb content, Hb saturation, or abnormal hemoglobins, such as carboxyhemoglobin (HbCO) or methemoglobin (metHb).
- Recommend dual pulse oximetry to screen for critical congenital heart disease in neonates.
- Recommend waveform capnography to confirm ETT placement in the lungs and detect the return of spontaneous circulation during CPR.
- Recommend a 12-lead ECG to screen for heart disease (e.g., CAD, left ventricular hypertrophy) and evaluating patients with chest pain.
- Recommend exhaled CO analysis to monitor a patient's smoking status.
- Recommend exhaled nitric oxide measurement to titrate corticosteroids dosing in patients with asthma.
- Recommend a CVP catheter to monitor fluid volume and right heart function in unstable or hypotensive patients.
- Recommend a pulmonary artery catheter when patient management requires frequent assessment of cardiac output.
- Recommend overnight oximetry to identify whether serious desaturation occurs in patients with COPD during sleep.
- Recommend laboratory polysomnography for patients with snoring associated with observed apneas and excessive daytime sleepiness.
- Recommend diagnostic thoracentesis to determine the cause of accumulated fluids in the pleural space and therapeutic thoracentesis for any patient with a pleural effusion large enough to cause respiratory distress.

POST-TEST

To confirm your mastery of each chapter's topical content, you should create a content post-test, available online via the Navigate Premier Access for Comprehensive Respiratory Therapy Exam Preparation Guide, which contains Navigate TestPrep (access code provided with every new text). You can create multiple topical content post-tests varying in length from 10 to 20 questions, with each attempt presenting a different set of items. You can select questions from all three major NBRC TMC sections: Patient Data, Troubleshooting and Quality Control of Devices and Infection Control, and Initiation and Modification of Interventions. A score of at least 70–80% indicates that you are adequately prepared for this section of the NBRC TMC exam. If you score below 70%, you should first carefully assess your test answers (particularly your wrong answers) and the correct answer explanations. Then return to the chapter to re-review the applicable content. Only then should you reattempt a new post-test. Repeat this process of identifying your shortcomings and reviewing the pertinent content until your test results demonstrate mastery.

CHAPTER 6 — Assemble and Troubleshoot Devices (Section II-A)

Michael J. Chaney

The Assemble and Troubleshoot Devices section is the second-largest topic on the NBRC TMC exam and is also one of the most difficult for candidates. We recommend that you spend a significant portion of your time reviewing this section before attempting the TMC exam.

OBJECTIVES

In preparing for the NBRC exams (TMC/CSE), you should demonstrate the knowledge needed to assemble and troubleshoot the following devices:

1. Medical gas delivery interfaces
2. Long-term oxygen therapy
3. Medical gas delivery, metering, and clinical analyzing devices
4. CPAP/NPPV with patient interfaces
5. Humidifiers
6. Nebulizers
7. Metered-dose inhalers, spacers, and valved holding chambers
8. Dry-powder inhalers (DPI)
9. Resuscitation equipment
10. Mechanical ventilators
11. Intubation equipment
12. Artificial airways
13. Suctioning equipment
14. Blood analyzers
15. Patient breathing circuits
16. Hyperinflation devices
17. Secretion clearance devices
18. Heliox delivery device
19. Portable spirometer
20. Testing equipment in a pulmonary function laboratory
21. Pleural drainage
22. Noninvasive monitoring
23. Bronchoscopes and light sources
24. Hemodynamic monitoring

WHAT TO EXPECT ON THIS CATEGORY OF THE NBRC EXAMS

TMC exam: 15 questions; 4 recall, 8 application, and 3 analysis
CSE exam: indeterminate number of sections; however, section II-A knowledge can appear in both the CSE Information Gathering and Decision-Making sections.

WHAT YOU NEED TO KNOW: ESSENTIAL CONTENT

Medical Gas Delivery Devices and Interfaces

You will select or recommend O_2 therapy for patients with documented hypoxemia ($Pao_2 < 60$ torr or $Sao_2 < 90\%$ on room air) or signs of hypoxemia (e.g., dyspnea, tachypnea, tachycardia, cyanosis, confusion). O_2 therapy may also be indicated for patients suffering from severe shock, trauma, or acute myocardial infarction (MI) and those undergoing procedures likely to cause hypoxemia, such as bronchoscopy, or during/following surgery.

Most equipment used for O_2 delivery are disposable, single-patient devices categorized as either low- or high-flow systems. These classifications are based on the device ability or inability to deliver a fixed oxygen concentration independently of a patient's inspiratory needs.

Table 6-1 summarizes common oxygen devices, their flow settings, Fio_2 ranges, advantages, disadvantages, and their best use.

Low-Flow Devices/Systems

These devices deliver O_2 at flows at less than the patient's inspiratory flow, so the O_2 is always variable and diluted with some inspired room air (see Table 6-1). Masks overcome some of this

Table 6-1 Common Oxygen Administration Devices

Device	Flow/Fio_2	Advantages	Disadvantages	Best Use
Nasal cannula	• For adults, each L/min of O_2 raises the Fio_2 by approximately 4% above room air. • Air-entrainment causes Fio_2 dilution (see **Table 6-2**) • 1-6 L/min (adult range) • 22–45%	• Can be used on adults, children, and infants • Easy to apply • Disposable • Low cost • Generally, well-tolerated at flows ≤ 6 L/min	• Unstable, easily dislodged • Fio_2 varies with rate, depth of breathing, and inspiratory flows • Flows > 6 L/min can be uncomfortable • Can cause dryness/bleeding • Polyps or a deviated septum may block the flow	• Stable patient needing low Fio_2 • Home care patient requiring long-term O_2 therapy
Simple mask	• 5–10 L/min • 35–50%	• Can be used on adults, children, and infants • Quick, easy to apply • Disposable • Low cost	• Uncomfortable, claustrophobia • Must be removed for eating or taking oral meds • Prevents radiant heat loss • Blocks vomitus in unconscious patients	• Emergencies • Short-term therapy requiring moderate Fio_2
Partial rebreathing mask	• 6–10 L/min (to prevent the bag from collapsing) • 40–70%	• Same as for simple mask • Moderate to high Fio_2s	• Same as for simple mask • Potential suffocation hazard	• Emergencies • Short-term therapy requiring moderate to high Fio_2s
Nonrebreathing mask	• Minimum 10 L/min (to prevent the bag from collapsing) • 60–80%	• Same as for simple mask • High Fio_2s	• Same as for simple mask • Potential suffocation hazard	• Emergencies • Short-term therapy requiring high Fio_2s • Heliox therapy

Table 6-2 Factors Affecting the Fio₂ of Low-Flow Oxygen Systems

Less Air Dilution/Higher Fio₂	More Air Dilution/Lower Fio₂
Device-Related	
Higher O₂ flow input	Lower O₂ flow input
Reservoir present (masks)	Reservoir absent (cannula)
Leak absent (masks)	Leak present (masks)
Valves present (masks)	Valves absent (masks)
Patient-Related	
Lower inspiratory flow	Higher inspiratory flow
Lower tidal volume	Higher tidal volume
Slower rate of breathing	Faster rate of breathing
Lower minute ventilation	Higher minute ventilation

air dilution by providing an external O₂ reservoir. Most low-flow devices are reported in L/min because Fio₂ varies with breathing pattern, rate, depth, and inspiratory flow. Therefore, Fio₂ ranges are estimates only.

Because the Fio₂ delivered by a low-flow system varies, you should always evaluate the patient's response to therapy to determine the proper flow setting, as described in Chapter 11. Table 6-2 summarizes factors affecting the amount of air dilution and the Fio₂ in low-flow systems.

Table 6-3 summarizes the most common problems with low-flow O₂ therapy devices, along with their causes and potential solutions.

High-Flow Devices/Systems

These devices deliver O₂ at flows exceeding the patient's inspiratory flow. For this reason, they are reported in Fio₂, rather than liters of flow. The Fio₂ remains precise regardless of changes in breathing pattern, rate, depth, and inspiratory flow.

Table 6-4 describes the two major categories of high-flow systems: (1) air-entrainment devices and (2) manual or mechanical blending systems. Although technically a reservoir system, the infant oxyhood meets the definition of a high-flow device when used at the recommended flow of 6–8 L/min.

Air-Entrainment Systems

Air-entrainment systems mix air and O₂ at specific ratios, which vary by jet and port size. Bigger ports and smaller jets cause more air dilution, lower Fio₂s, and higher total flows, whereas smaller ports and bigger jets cause less air dilution and higher Fio₂s but lower total flows. Note that obstructing an entrainment device's entrainment port *decreases* air entrainment, resulting in a higher *delivered* O₂ concentration but a lower overall flow, with an unpredictable effect on the actual *inspired* O₂ concentration delivered to the patient.

It is also essential to note that high-flow devices must be titrated by changing Fio₂, not the flow. If the flow is reduced on a high-flow device, the Fio₂ remains unchanged, but flow reduction may result in insufficient flow to meet the patient's inspiratory demand and therefore, the delivered O₂ becomes variable. If using a reservoir system, flow reductions can also *cause CO₂ rebreathing and suffocation.*

Table 6-5 lists air-to-O₂ ratios, and total output flows of air-entrainment systems. This table shows that *the lower the Fio₂, the higher the total output of the device, and vice versa.* For example, at 0.8 Fio₂, for every L/min setting on the O₂ flowmeter, the output is 1.3 L/min. For 0.24 Fio₂, for every 1 L/min setting on the flowmeter, there is 26 L/min of output. *Therefore, the higher the Fio₂, the higher the input flow (flowmeter setting) required to meet the patient's inspiratory demand.*

For this reason, in general, the best way to ensure a stable Fio₂ is to provide a total flow of at least 40 L/min. As indicated in Table 6-5, for an input flow of 10 L/min, this occurs only at or below the 40% O₂ settings. Total output flow can be increased somewhat by increasing the O₂ input flow, although this flow is limited by the backpressure created at the device jet, typically to 12–15 L/min.

Table 6-3 Troubleshooting Common Problems with Low-Flow O₂ Devices

Problem/Clue	Cause(s)	Solution
Nasal Cannulas		
No gas flow can be felt coming from the cannula	Flowmeter not on	Adjust flowmeter as needed
	System leak	Check all connections
	Humidifier down tube is obstructed	Repair or replace the device
Humidifier pop-off sounding	Obstruction distal to the humidifier	Find and correct obstruction
	Flow set too high	Lower flow
	Obstructed naris	Use alternative O₂ appliance
The patient complains of soreness over lips or ears	Irritation/inflammation due to appliance straps/loops	• Loosen straps • Use skin-protecting pads or dressing at pressure points • Use an alternative device
Signs of airway dryness	Delivered medical gas is not humidified	Use a simple bubble humidifier for low-flow systems set to deliver ≥ 4 L/min.
Masks		
The patient constantly removes the mask	Claustrophobia	Use an alternative device
	Confusion	• Restrain or sedate the patient • Consider alternative device
No gas flow detected	Flowmeter is not on	Adjust flowmeter as needed
	System leak	Check connections
Reservoir bag collapses when the patient inhales	• Inadequate flow • Increased minute ventilation	Increase flow
Reservoir bag remains fully inflated during inhalation	Too much flow	Decrease flow until bag slightly deflates during inspiration
	Large mask leak	Correct leak
	Inspiratory valve jammed/reversed	Repair or replace the mask
The patient develops erythema over the face or the ears	Irritation/inflammation due to appliance or straps	• Reposition mask/straps • Use skin-protecting pads or dressing over the ear pressure points • Provide skin care

An alternative is to combine two air-entrainment nebulizers, which will double the provided flow to generate enough output that the mist does not disappear on inspiration.

Blending Systems

A better way to provide *very precise* high FIO₂s (> 0.60) at high flows (> 40 L/min) is to use a mechanical or manual blending system capable of unrestricted flow delivery. All blenders require a 50-psi air and oxygen source. Most blenders output 50 psi at the set O₂%, which can be applied directly to power respiratory equipment or to control the flow going to the patient by using a flowmeter.

To set up a standard O₂ blender:

1. Connect the air and O₂ 50-psi hoses to the respective gas sources.
2. If only one gas hose is connected, the blender will sound a loud, high-pitched alarm. This is normal until the other gas hose is connected. This alarm will also sound if one of the gas sources fails during use.
3. Verify the prescribed O₂% using an O₂ analyzer.

Table 6-4 Common High-Flow Oxygen Administration Devices

Device	Flow/FIO₂	Advantages	Disadvantages	Best Use
Air-entrainment nebulizer	• 10–15 L/min input • The output should be ≥ 60 L/min to ensure stable FIO₂ • 28–100%	• Provides temperature control and extra humidity	• FIO₂ < 28% or ≥ 0.35 not ensured • FIO₂ varies with back-pressure (e.g., condensation in the tubing) • Infection risk	• Patients with artificial airways requiring low to moderate FIO₂s (T-piece or tracheal mask) • Post-extubation or post-upper airway surgery (cool aerosol mask)
Air-entrainment mask (Venturi mask)	• 4–12 L/min input • The output should be ≥ 60 L/min to ensure stable FIO₂ • 24–50%	• Inexpensive • Easy to apply	• Because total flow output decreases with increasing FIO₂, the FIO₂ becomes less precise at FIO₂ ≥ 0.35 • Varies with back pressure and entrainment port size • Not appropriate for use if vomiting or claustrophobic • Must be removed for oral meds and eating	• When a precise, stable low to moderate FIO₂ delivery is needed (e.g., unstable COPD needing low FIO₂)
High-flow nasal cannula (HFNC)	• 1–40 L/min adults† • 1–20 L/min children • 1–8 L/min neonates/infants • 24–100%	• Easy to apply • Stable, precise FIO₂s • Provides gas at BTPS without condensation • Meets/exceeds the nonrebreather performance • Decreases anatomic deadspace (CO₂ washout from the upper airway)	• Requires special (proprietary) cannulas and humidification system • Can create CPAP (may be an advantage if desired) • Potential electrical risks • Some units associated with contamination/infection • Higher risk of barotrauma in infants and children due to inadvertent CPAP	• An alternative to a nonrebreather for those needing high FIO₂ or patients with claustrophobia, facial burns, or hypothermia • Provides humidified O₂ therapy • Alternative to nasal CPAP
Oxyhood*	• 6–8 L/min • 21–100%	• Full range of FIO₂s	• Difficult to clean, disinfect • Excessive noise • Difficult to maintain stable FIO₂s at higher concentration due to leaks and frequent opening	• For neonates/infants requiring supplemental oxygen

BTPS, body temperature pressure, saturated (37°C and 100% relative humidity); CPAP, continuous positive airway pressure.

*Oxyhood technically an enclosure that provides enough O₂ flow to meet infant inspiratory needs and ensure CO₂ removal.

†Some units may deliver up to 80 to 100 L/min.

Modified from Kacmarek RM, Stoller JK, Heuer AJ, eds. *Egan's Fundamentals of Respiratory Care* (11th ed.). St. Louis, MO: Mosby; 2017.

Table 6-5 Air-to-O$_2$ Ratios and Total Flow Output of Air-Entrainment Devices

O$_2$%	Air-to-O$_2$ Ratio	Total Ratio Parts (Air + O$_2$)	Total Flow at 10 L/min O$_2$ Input*
80	0.3:1	1.3	13
70	0.6:1	1.6	16
60	1:1	2	20
50	1.7:1	2.7	27
40	3:1	4	40
35	5:1	6	60
31	7:1	8	80
28	10:1	11	110
24	25:1	26	260
*Total flow (air + oxygen) = O$_2$ input flow (L/min) × total ratio parts.			

If a blender pressure alarm sounds after both gas sources are attached, or if you observe a large discrepancy between the blender setting and the measured O$_2$%:

1. Verify that both gas sources are at the required inlet pressures (usually $\geq$ 35 psig).
2. Check for leaks between the gas source and the blender.
3. If these check out, replace the blender.

F$_{IO_2}$s vary according to the blender setting and to a small degree flow. Higher flow rates minimize or eliminate air dilution, so in general, you should set the desired O$_2$ concentration on the blender and use the higher end of the patient flow range to guarantee the F$_{IO_2}$, with little to no additional room air added to the patient's inspiratory flow stream.

High-Flow Nasal Cannula

One commonly used system that uses a blender is a heated high-flow nasal cannula (HFNC). This system includes a blender to mix air and O$_2$, a flowmeter (high-flow flowmeter for adults [0–80 L/min]), a heated humidification system, an O$_2$ analyzer, a heated delivery system to prevent tubing condensation and gas cooling, and a proprietary nasal cannula. By providing warm, humidified gas to the airway, an HFNC overcomes the discomfort patients experience with standard nasal cannulas at high flows.

HFNC flow settings depend on the age/size of the patient but generally fall within the following ranges:

- Adults: 1–40 L/min or higher
- Children: 1–20 L/min
- Infants: 1–8 L/min

High flows can also produce continuous positive airway pressure (CPAP), which may provide an added benefit, especially for neonates and infants with hypoxemic respiratory failure. For patients with hypercapnia, a high-flow nasal cannula can decrease ventilatory demand by "washing out" CO$_2$ from upper airway deadspace.

Table 6-6 summarizes the most common problems with high-flow O$_2$ therapy devices, along with their causes and potential solutions. If a problem cannot be corrected and no replacement is available, select an O$_2$ system that closely matches the HFNC's F$_{IO_2}$—for example, a nonrebreathing mask if delivering a high F$_{IO_2}$.

O$_2$ Device Selection

In general, sicker patients require higher and more stable F$_{IO_2}$s, whereas less acutely ill patients usually can be managed with lower, less precise F$_{IO_2}$s. **Table 6-7** provides guidance in selecting an O$_2$ delivery system based on these factors.

Table 6-6 Troubleshooting Common Problems with High-Flow O₂ Therapy Devices

Problem/Clue	Cause(s)	Solution(s)
Air-Entrainment Masks		
Patient's SaO₂ lower than expected	Inadequate total flow	• Increase input flow • Check for/correct any flow obstructions or leaks
	Inadequate O₂ concentration	• Increase the FIO₂ or switch to a device capable of higher FIO₂
	Displacement of device	• Reposition device
The patient complains of dryness	Inadequate water vapor content	• Use aerosol collar plus an air-driven nebulizer to increase humidification
Air-Entrainment Nebulizers		
Patient's SaO₂ lower than expected	Inadequate total flow (only for high O₂% settings, such as > 35–40%)	• Maximize input flow • Add open reservoir to the expiratory side of T-tube • Connect multiple nebulizers in parallel • Provide inspiratory reservoir with a one-way expiratory valve • Set nebulizer to low O₂% and bleed in extra O₂
	Aerosol tubing is *entirely* blocked by condensate buildup (tubing filled with water and no gurgling sound)	• Drain tubing condensate • Add a water trap
Delivered O₂% higher than set or expected	Obstruction to flow in circuit creating back pressure	• Drain tubing condensate • Add a water trap • Check/correct kinking or other outlet obstructions
Blender Systems		
Blender alarm sounds (continuous high-pitched sound)	• One of the gas sources is leaking, disconnected, or the pressure is inadequate	• Ensure that both the air and O₂ hoses are securely connected • Verify that both gas sources are at the required inlet pressures (usually ≥ 35 psig) • Check for leaks between the gas source and the blender • If these check out, replace the blender

Table 6-7 Selecting an O₂ Administration Device Based on Desired FIO₂ and Stability

Desired O₂%	Needed Stability in Delivered O₂%	
	Stable/Fixed	**Variable**
Low (< 35%)	• Air-entrainment mask • Air-entrainment nebulizer • Heated high-flow cannula	• Standard nasal cannula • Isolette (infant)
Moderate (35–60%)	• Air-entrainment nebulizer • Heated high-flow cannula	• Simple mask • Isolette (infant)
High (> 60%)	• 2+ air-entrainment nebulizers in parallel • Heated high-flow nasal cannula • Oxyhood (infant)	• Partial rebreathing mask • Nonrebreathing mask

Modified from Kacmarek RM, Stoller JK, Heuer AJ, eds. *Egan's Fundamentals of Respiratory Care* (11th ed.). St. Louis, MO: Mosby; 2017.

Table 6-8 Example O$_2$ Device Selection Scenarios

Patient Scenario	Recommended O$_2$ Delivery System
A stable adult patient needing a low to moderate F$_{IO_2}$	Nasal cannula, 1–6 L/min
A patient admitted to the emergency department with chest pain and a suspected MI	Nonrebreathing mask, > 10 L/min or high-flow nasal cannula ($\geq$ 20 L/min @ 100%)
A patient just extubated from ventilatory support on 30% O$_2$	Air-entrainment nebulizer and aerosol mask
An unstable COPD patient requiring a precise low F$_{IO_2}$	Air-entrainment mask at 24 or 28%
A postoperative patient with an ETT requiring a moderate F$_{IO_2}$	Air-entrainment nebulizer (40–50% O$_2$) and T-tube with an open reservoir
A stable postoperative patient with a tracheostomy tube needing low F$_{IO_2}$	Air-entrainment nebulizer, 30–35%, and tracheostomy collar
An ICU patient with a high minute volume needing high, precise F$_{IO_2}$ (intact upper airway)	Two air-entrainment nebulizers in parallel with an aerosol mask. A high-flow nasal cannula ($\geq$ 30-40 L/min)
A stable 2-year-old child needing a low F$_{IO_2}$	Nasal cannula ¼–2 L/min with a calibrated low-flow flowmeter
An infant requiring short-term supplemental moderate O$_2$	Simple O$_2$ mask
An infant requiring high F$_{IO_2}$ and temperature control	Oxyhood at 6-8 L/min with servo-controlled heated humidification system or high-flow nasal cannula (1–8 L/min)

COPD, chronic obstructive pulmonary disease; ETT, endotracheal tube; ICU, intensive care unit; MI, myocardial infarction.

Table 6-8 applies these concepts to the selection of specific O$_2$ systems in a variety of common clinical scenarios you are likely to see on the NBRC exams.

Gas Delivery, Metering, and Clinical Analyzing Devices

There are several types of gas delivery systems available. Concentrators and liquid oxygen (LOX) systems are covered in the long-term oxygen therapy (LTOT) section of this chapter. Which gas delivery system to use depends on its application and where it is being used. In hospitals, O$_2$ and air are supplied to the bedside via piped-in wall gas at the standard working pressure of 50 psi to use with respiratory equipment, such as ventilators and O$_2$ blenders, or to connect to flowmeters to deliver specific flow rates.

High-pressure gas cylinders are used in a hospital setting in areas that lack piped wall gas or during patient ambulation or transport. Oxygen tanks are also used in other settings such as a back-up at home for oxygen concentrators. If specialized gas delivery is needed (He, NO, CO, and CO$_2$), they are only available in gas cylinders. Air compressors can be used in those same areas for specific applications. **Table 6-9** provides guidelines for selecting gas delivery equipment.

Gaseous Oxygen Cylinders

If portability is the first consideration, select either a small cylinder (A through E, or M), a portable liquid O$_2$ system, or a portable O$_2$ concentrator (covered in the LTOT section of this chapter).

H cylinders in the home are used primarily as a backup system in case the concentrator fails or there is a power outage. H systems can also be used for infants who require very little flow, or if flows higher than concentrator capabilities are required. This is not very practical, though, as often H tanks need to be tied together and replaced frequently.

Table 6-9 Guidelines for Selecting Gas Delivery Equipment

Purpose	Setting	Needed Equipment
To provide 50-psi unrestricted flow to ventilators or blenders	Piped source available (most hospital units)	None; connect directly to the piped gas source at 50 psi using a DISS connection
	Piped source not available	• Large gas cylinder (H or K) with a preset (50-psi) pressure-reducing valve • For air, piston air compressor with reservoir
To deliver a controlled flow of gas to a patient or equipment	Piped source available (most hospital units)	Connect calibrated Thorpe tube flowmeter to piped gas source at 50 psi
	Piped source not available	• Gas cylinder with reducing valve and flowmeter—cylinder size selected based on portability needs and planned duration of usage • For air, portable diaphragm compressor (limited flow/pressure)

When using cylinders for transport, use a flowmeter that is unaffected by gravity—either a Bourdon gauge or an integrated regulator/variable orifice flow controller like the Praxair Grab 'n Go™ or Western Medica's Oxytote™. If the patient is being transported for a magnetic resonance imaging (MRI) study, you must use iron-free equipment (e.g., aluminum cylinders and carts and brass and aluminum regulators). If there is no need for portability or the duration of use is expected to be lengthy, you should select a large cylinder (G, H, or K).

Once you have selected the appropriate cylinder and attachments, apply the following guidelines for proper and safe use:

1. Check the tank by checking the label to ensure it contains the proper gas.
2. Ensure you have enough gas for the duration of planned use.
3. Transport large cylinders chained to a wheeled cart; place small cylinders in the gurney/wheelchair holder.
4. If you hear the tank leaking (hissing sound), check for a loose connection or missing/damaged washers (PISS regulators).
5. Slowly open the cylinder valve all the way and then turn back half a turn to prevent valve "freezing" when fully open.
6. Record pressure, and compute flow duration (**Table 6-10**).
7. Before disconnecting equipment, close the cylinder valve and release pressure from any attached devices.

Duration of flow = [gauge pressure (psi) × cylinder factor] ÷ flow (L/min).

It assumes a full cylinder is at 2200 psi. Cylinder filling pressures may vary—always check before computation.

Air Compressors

Although medical-quality air can be provided via cylinders, air compressors are the preferred source. Small portable compressors generally are limited to powering devices such as small-volume nebulizers. If a portable compressor fails to operate when the switch is turned on, check the electrical outlet for power and the unit's fuse or circuit breaker. If an operating compressor's output appears inadequate:

1. Check the inlet filter for obstruction.
2. Check the tubing and connected equipment for obstruction.
3. Check the tubing and connections for leaks.

Table 6-10 Cylinder Factor and Duration of Flow @ 1 L/min for Full O_2 Cylinders

	M-6/B	M-9/C	D	E	G	H/K
Cylinder factor	0.07	0.11	0.16	0.28	2.14	3.14
Hours flow @ 1 L/min	2.6	4.0	5.9	10.3	78.5	115.1

O_2, He, CO, and Specialty Gas Analyzers

Most respiratory therapists (RTs) are skilled in monitoring Fio_2s using portable O_2 analyzers. Details on the use and troubleshooting of these devices are provided in Chapter 8. However, the NBRC also expects RTs to be familiar with other specialty gas analyzers. **Table 6-11** outlines the method employed, use, performance standards, and calibration considerations for all gas analyzers that you may encounter in practice.

As noted in Table 6-11, essentially all gas analyzers should undergo a two-point calibration before each use.

Long-Term Oxygen Therapy (LTOT)

Special consideration is required for patients receiving continuous low-flow O_2 therapy outside the hospital. Bulk oxygen systems with wall outlets is not an option within the home, so a system that is safe and compatible within the home environment must be used. Portability is also a consideration as these patients are often active and, in some cases, go to work or school with oxygen. Home systems can include one or a combination of oxygen cylinders, a concentrator, LOX, or a conserving device.

Oxygen Concentrators

An O_2 concentrator is an electrically powered device that physically separates the O_2 found in room air from nitrogen. Most concentrators use sodium-aluminum silicate pellets to absorb nitrogen, CO_2, and water vapor and produce about 90–95% O_2 at flows up to 10 L/min. O_2 concentrators are the most cost-efficient supply method for patients in alternative settings who need continuous low-flow O_2.

Portable O_2 concentrators (POCs) are smaller versions of standard home concentrators, powered by household AC, 12-volt DC (available in cars, RVs, and motor homes), or batteries. The typical battery life is 1 to 4 h, with some models having optional battery packs that can extend use time to more than 6 h.

Most POCs deliver O_2 only in the pulse-dose mode, which is enough for those with low O_2 needs (30% or less O_2). Some units also can operate in a continuous-flow mode. In general, only continuous-flow units can provide more than 30% O_2, which is needed to provide adequate Fio_2 at high altitudes (e.g., in airliner cabins). Unfortunately, most continuous-flow POCs are bigger and heavier than pulse-dose-only units and, therefore, are less portable.

The basic procedure for start-up and operation of a POC is as follows:

1. Before operation, make sure the air intake filter is clean and positioned correctly.
2. Locate and position the unit in a well-ventilated area with the air inlets and outlets unobstructed; in a small room or car, keep a window open.
3. Connect the unit to the best available power source (AC first, auto-DC next, battery last).
4. Connect a pulse dose nasal cannula to the O_2 outlet.
5. Turn the unit on, confirm power-up status, and set the prescribed flow.
6. Confirm that the unit is sensing inhalation (flashing indicator with pulse sound).
7. After start-up, the unit should reach its maximum O_2 output in approximately 1–2 minutes.

Liquid Oxygen (LOX) Systems

With the availability of portable concentrator oxygen, LOX systems are less commonly used than in the past. However, since 1 L of liquid O_2 vaporizes into 860 L of gaseous O_2, LOX systems are an efficient way to store supplemental O_2.

Table 6-11 Therapy and Diagnostic Gas Analysis

Gas	Analysis Method(s)	Usage	Performance Standards and Calibration Considerations

O_2	• Paramagnetic
	• Electrochemical:
	  ○ Galvanic cell
	  ○ Polarographic
	• ZRO_2
		• Bedside Fio_2 monitoring
		• Metabolic analysis ($\dot{V}o_2$)
			• For bedside monitoring (primarily Galvanic cell or polarographic sensors):
			  ○ Accuracy: $\pm$ 2% for bedside monitoring
			• For metabolic analysis (primarily ZRO_2 sensors):
			  ○ Accuracy: 1.0%
			  ○ Precision: 0.01%
			• Two-point calibration (21% and 100%) should be done just before each test according to manufacturer's specification.

N_2	• Emission spectroscopy • Mass spectrometry	Functional residual capacity (FRC) determination (nitrogen washout)	• For real-time (breath) analysis: ○ Accuracy: $\pm$ 0.2% over the entire range N_2% (0–80%) • Two-point calibration should be done just before each test • Linearity should be checked every 6 months with a 40% N_2 calibration gas mixture
He	• Thermal conductivity	• FRC determination (helium dilution) • Single-breath DLco (as tracer gas)	• For FRC or DLco: ○ Measurement range: 0–10% • Two-point calibration (zero and full scale) should be done just before each test • CO_2 and water must be removed before the sample is analyzed.
CO	• Infrared absorption • Electrochemical	• Single-breath DLco • Assessment of smoking status	• Accuracy is less important than linearity and stability (DLco is based on relative changes in CO%) • Two-point calibration (zero and full scale) should be done just before each test

NO, NO_2	• Chemiluminescence
	• Electrochemical
		• Nitric oxide therapy
		• Monitoring airway inflammation (expired NO)
			• For nitric oxide:
			  ○ Resolution: 1 ppm
			  ○ Accuracy between 1 and 20 ppm: $\pm$ (0.5 ppm + 20% actual concentration)
			  ○ Accuracy above 20 ppm: $\pm$ (0.5 ppm + 10% actual concentration)
			• For NO_2:
			  ○ Accuracy: $\pm$ 20% of the actual %, or 0.5 ppm, whichever is greater
			  ○ Daily one-point automated "zero" calibration (room air) while on the patient
			  ○ Monthly two-point high range using 45 ppm NO/10 ppm NO_2 calibrating gases

Depending on the model, a stationary home storage cylinder (the "base" unit) holds between 45 and 100 pounds of LOX. To calculate the duration of flow, first convert the LOX weight in pounds to the equivalent volume of gaseous O_2 in liters. At normal operating pressures, 1 pound of LOX equals approximately 344 L of gaseous O_2. To determine how long the contents will last in minutes, divide the total available gaseous O_2 by the prescribed flow (L/min).

Table 6-12 Troubleshooting Concentrators or LOX Systems

Problem/Clue	Cause(s)	Solution
No oxygen is delivered	Kinks in delivery tubing	Check all tubing to ensure there are no kinks, bends, obstructions, or objects putting pressure on the tube
	The oxygen source is off (concentrator) or empty (liquid oxygen [LOX] reservoir or gas cylinder)	Turn concentrator on, fill/refill LOX reservoir, replace gas cylinder
Concentrator alarm	Intake filters are blocked or dirty	• Clean intake filters • Ensure filters are the proper distance from the wall or curtains
	Low F_{IO_2} output	• Be sure the flow is turned on • Unit needs maintenance (call provider for service or maintenance)

Portable LOX systems are used in conjunction with a stationary base unit, from which they are filled as needed. When full, the typical portable unit holds about 1 L of LOX and weighs less than 6 pounds. When used with a demand-flow delivery device (described subsequently), these systems can provide 8 hours or more of supplemental O_2.

Table 6-12 summarizes the most common problems with concentrators and LOX systems, along with their causes and potential solutions.

Oxygen-Conserving or Demand-Flow Devices

Oxygen cylinders and LOX systems can last longer if an *oxygen-conserving device* is used. The following points are important regarding O_2-conserving devices:

- All O_2-conserving devices minimize O_2 waste that occurs during exhalation with standard nasal cannulas.
- O_2-conserving devices can reduce O_2 usage by 50–75%, doubling or tripling duration of flow from bulk sources.
- There are two types of O_2-conserving devices:
  - Simple reservoir cannulas
    - Store O_2 in a small reservoir during exhalation and release it during inhalation
    - Bulky appearance not well tolerated by patients
  - Pulse-dose/demand-flow systems
    - These systems use sensors to trigger a valve that delivers O_2 only during inspiration
    - Systems differ, so flow must be individually adjusted to achieve the desired Sp_{O_2}
    - If the device fails, the patient must switch to continuous O_2 source at 2–3 times the conserving device flow

Table 6-13 summarizes the most common problems with demand-flow devices, along with their causes and potential solutions.

CPAP/NPPV Devices

Continuous positive airway pressure (CPAP) is the application of positive pressure to the airway throughout the spontaneous breathing cycle. In adults, CPAP is used to treat obstructive sleep apnea, acute cardiogenic pulmonary edema, and postoperative atelectasis. In infants, CPAP most commonly is used to treat respiratory distress syndrome and apnea of prematurity.

In both adults and infants, CPAP also may facilitate weaning from invasive mechanical ventilation. During CPAP application the source gas is provided via either high-pressure air/O_2 (blender or ventilator) or an air blower (typical source for home CPAP). At a minimum, a CPAP system also should provide a way to monitor and limit airway pressures. Ideally, hospital-based systems also should incorporate an O_2 analyzer.

Table 6-13 Troubleshooting Common Problems with Demand-Flow Systems

Problem/Clue	Cause(s)	Solution
Sensor alarm	No inspiration is sensed	• Turn unit off, then back on to reset the alarm • Check cannula and tube connections to ensure they are tight and not kinked/obstructed • Adjust the cannula to ensure a comfortable fit, then initiate inspiration
	Leaks in the delivery system	• Check cannula and tubing connections to ensure they are tight
No oxygen is delivered	Kinks in delivery tubing	• Check all tubing to ensure there are no kinks, bends, obstructions, or objects putting pressure on the tube
	The oxygen source is off or empty	• Turn concentrator on, fill/refill LOX reservoir, replace gas cylinder
Oxygen is delivered continuously	Unit is in bypass mode due to failure to sense inspiration, and/or selector knob is set to continuous flow mode	• Turn the unit off, then back on to reset the alarm • Check cannula and tube connections to ensure they are tight and not kinked or otherwise obstructed • Adjust the cannula to ensure a comfortable fit, then initiate inspiration • Check the selector to ensure it is set to pulse

Assembly and Application

Assembly of CPAP systems generally involves connecting and confirming proper operation of the gas source, humidifier, and patient circuit, then selecting and applying the patient interface. Ventilator, blender, and humidifier setup, as well as the typical patient circuits used on servo-controlled ventilators (dual-limb) and CPAP machines (single limb with leakage valve), are described later in this chapter. Fluidic control CPAP circuits include the fluidic valve system and are specific to each manufacturer's device.

Adult CPAP interfaces include nasal and oronasal masks (most common) or nasal pillows. For infants, short nasal prongs and nasal masks are used. Infant airway interfaces include a head cap with fasteners for securing the system to the infant. A proper fit is essential for pressure maintenance and patient tolerance. Prongs that are too small can cause difficulty in maintaining the prescribed pressure, whereas prongs that are too large can cause tissue erosion.

Additional points related to equipment setup of CPAP systems include the following:

- Adult CPAP application
  - If using a full oronasal mask, be sure that it is equipped with a safety inlet valve.
  - Make sure that the circuit is long enough and free to move with the patient during sleep.
  - Always position the exhaust port so that the vented air is directed away from the patient.
  - Make sure that nothing blocks the unit's air inlet filter or the circuit exhaust port.
  - If supplemental O_2 is required, it is bled in from a concentrator or liquid O_2 system.
  - Use a skin-protecting pad, dressing, or lining to prevent irritation and skin breakdown on pressure areas if necessary.
  - For cardiogenic pulmonary edema, select/use a CPAP or a noninvasive positive pressure ventilation (NPPV) device capable of providing 100% O_2.
- Infant CPAP application
  - Recommend insertion of an orogastric tube to prevent gastric distention.
  - For bubble systems, use sterile H_2O (add 0.25% acetic acid for infection control).
  - Set the flow to 5–10 L/min (continuous flow systems, e.g., bubble CPAP).
  - Start therapy at 4–6 cm H_2O, 40–50% O_2.
  - Switch to ventilatory support if $Pao_2 < 50$ torr on CPAP > 7 cm H_2O and $Fio_2 > 0.60$ or hypercapnic respiratory failure develops.

Troubleshooting

To troubleshoot a CPAP system, you first must identify the likely component problem. Blender and humidifier troubleshooting are covered separately in this chapter. Common problems for infants and adults, possible causes, and solutions for circuit, interface, and pressure control are outlined in **Table 6-14**.

Chapter 17 covers the common problems with home use of CPAP for obstructive sleep apnea and their solutions.

Table 6-14 Adult and Infant Troubleshooting of CPAP Circuit, Interface, and Pressure Control Problems

Problem	Likely Cause(s)	Solution
Excessive airway pressure (≥2 cm H_2O above set level)	Flow too high (continuous flow systems)	Reduce flow
	Occlusion of the expiratory limb	Find and remove obstruction/drain condensate
	Blocked silencer/bacteria filter	Check/replace if needed
	Excess water in water seal (bubble CPAP)	Raise submersed expiratory limb or lower water level to prescribed CPAP pressure
	Nasal or oropharyngeal obstruction	Check nasal passages, suction if needed; reposition head/neck (slight extension)
Low airway pressure (≤2 cm H_2O below set level)	Flow too low (continuous flow systems)	Increase flow
	Circuit leak/disconnect	Check/correct leaks
	Insufficient water/evaporation in water seal (bubble CPAP)	Lower submersed expiratory limb or increase the water level to prescribed CPAP pressure
	Airway interface not snug, mask leak	• Check for the proper fit/position; select a larger size if needed • Use mask spacers and adjusters • Ensure nasal prongs are not too small
	Mouth open	Use chin strap
Skin irritation/ breakdown	Mask too tight or not sized properly Nasal prongs not sized properly	• Check proper size (infant nasal prongs that are too large can cause erosion/nasal septum damage) • Loosen/straighten mask • Use a skin-protecting pad, dressing, or lining to prevent irritation and skin breakdown on pressure areas (Duoderm or Tegaderm)
Pressure setting not tolerated	Prescribed pressure too high	• Use ramp function if available • Switch to NPPV
Hypercapnia develops	Prescribed pressure too low	• Recommend increase in pressure • Switch to NPPV
Condensate draining into the airway	Improper positioning of the unit	• Place unit lower than the airway interface
Gastric distention (especially infants)	Usually from pressure settings > 20 cm H_2O	• Insert orogastric tube
Pneumothorax	Always a possibility when applying positive pressure to the airway of small infants. More likely to occur at CPAP pressure > 6 cm H_2O	• Confirm via chest x-ray or a transilluminator (neonates) • If small and no distress present, continue to monitor • If a tension pneumothorax is present, insert a thoracotomy tube to evacuate the gas

Humidifiers

A *humidifier* adds or retains molecular water to gas via evaporation from a water surface. There are three types of humidifiers: bubble humidifiers, passover humidifiers, and heat and moisture exchangers (HMEs).

With any humidifier set up, be sure that all connections are properly placed, tight, and not cross-threaded. If setting up a bubble humidifier, confirm that the pressure pop-off is functional by crimping the end of the cannula so that the bubbler whistles. When using a heated passover system, make sure you select the appropriate mode setting (invasive or noninvasive). If using an HME, be sure you place it between the "wye" and the airway interface (endotracheal or "trach" tube [ETT]) and no contraindications are present.

An HME does not add humidity to the system; it merely retains and redelivers the patient's exhaled humidity. Because of this, HMEs should not be used if the patient is dehydrated, has a high minute volume, is hypothermic or a large exhalation leak is present as these conditions will decrease the amount of exhaled humidity. An HME should also be avoided if there are excessively thick or bloody secretions being coughed out of the airway as this may block the airflow through the HME and increase circuit resistance.

To avoid humidification or temperature-regulation problems in mechanically ventilated patients with artificial airways, you must ensure that gas delivered to the patient's airway is carrying *at least* 30 mg/L of water vapor content. Most HMEs meet this standard if the minute ventilation is not excessive and there are no expiratory leaks. Heated humidifiers also meet and exceed this requirement, typically delivering gas saturated with water vapor (100% relative humidity) to the airway at temperatures between 34°C and 41°C.

In heated humidification systems that do not use heated wires, the condensate resulting from cooling gas is a potential source of nosocomial infection. Methods that can help minimize nosocomial infections associated with ventilator circuits include the following:

- Using HMEs or heated-wire circuits to eliminate condensate (not applicable to all patients)
- Changing circuits only when visibly soiled or malfunctioning
- Avoiding unnecessary disconnections—for example, for suctioning (consider an in-line/closed-suction system)
- Preventing excessive condensate in the circuit and accidental drainage into the patient's airway
- Avoiding contamination during circuit disconnection or disposal of condensate
- Using a drainage system in the circuit to avoid disconnection

Table 6-15 summarizes problems commonly encountered with humidification devices, along with their causes and potential solutions.

Table 6-15 Troubleshooting Common Problems with Humidifiers

Problem/Clue	Cause(s)	Solution
Bubble Humidifier		
No gas flow coming from the cannula	Flowmeter not on	Adjust flowmeter
	System leak*	Check connections
Humidifier pop-off sounding	Obstruction distal to the humidifier	Find/correct obstruction
	Flow is set too high	Use an alternative device
	Obstructed naris	Use an alternative device
Heated Passover Humidifier		
Intermittent flow or "bubbling" in tubing circuit	Water vapor condensation	• Drain condensate (away from the patient) • Place water traps in the circuit • Use a heated-wire circuit

(continues)

Table 6-15 Troubleshooting Common Problems with Humidifiers (*continued*)

Heated Passover Humidifier		
Airway temperature too high	Temperature set too high	• Reset to 34–41°C
	An abrupt decrease in flow	• Ensure proper flow (change sensitivity to flow instead of pressure)
	Temperature probe not in circuit	Insert temperature probe in the circuit
	Unit warmed up without flow through the circuit	Let temperature equilibrate with the flow before application
	Unit failure	Replace unit
Airway temperature too low	Temperature set too low	Reset to 34–41°C
	Cool water added to the reservoir	System will readjust
	An abrupt increase in flow	System will readjust
	Reservoir low or empty	Refill/replenish the reservoir
	External fan or A/C vent blowing on temp probe	Redirect fan / Cover temp probe with cloth
Heat and Moisture Exchanger (HME)		
Increased PIP (volume control) or decreased V_T (pressure control) during invasive mechanical ventilation	Device partially obstructed with secretions	Replace device
Copious, thick secretions	Inadequate humidification	Assure good systemic hydration / Switch to heated (active) humidification
Need to administer aerosolized medications	Failure to deliver medication due to the filtering effect of HME. Potential to obstruct HME with aerosolized medication	Switch to heated (active) humidification

PIP, peak inspiratory pressure; V_T, tidal volume.

*Check via folding the delivery tubing

Nebulizers

A *nebulizer* generates and disperses small particles of liquid into a carrier gas as an aerosol. There are several different types of nebulizers, each with a specific use. Nebulizer types include large-volume (air-entrainment) nebulizers, small-volume nebulizers (SVNs), ultrasonic nebulizers, or vibrating-mesh nebulizers. **Table 6-16** compares these devices in terms of operating principles and best use.

Devices used to generate bland aerosols include large-volume jet nebulizers and ultrasonic nebulizers. **Table 6-17** summarizes problems commonly encountered with common aerosol delivery systems, along with their causes and potential solutions.

Table 6-18 outlines the problems commonly encountered with nondisposable mesh nebulizers, including their causes and potential solutions.

Metered-Dose Inhalers, Spacers, Valved Holding Chambers, and DPIs

In the previous section we covered nebulizers, which included the ones that deliver medications. In this section, we will continue with medication delivery devices to include MDIs and DPIs and their accessories.

Table 6-16 Nebulizer Types, Characteristics, and Best Uses

Type	Characteristics	Best Use(s)
Large-volume air-entrainment nebulizer (LVN)	• Large volume, high output of aerosol • Can be heated for higher humidity output • Interfaces include t-piece (Briggs adapter), trach mask, aerosol mask, or face tent • If the liquid is water or normal saline, it is called bland aerosol therapy • If connected to an O_2 source, supplemental oxygen can be given (see O_2 delivery section)	• To provide humidification (and O_2) for a bypassed upper airway • To reduce inflammation (cool aerosol) for patients with upper airway edema (e.g., croup, post-extubation) • To help thin secretions • Sputum induction
Small-volume nebulizer (SVN)	• Comes in several types to include a standard jet nebulizer, a breath-actuated nebulizer (BAN), or continuous nebulizer • Delivers small volumes (2.5–4 mL) of respirable aerosol (1–5 microns) • Perfect for medication delivery • Input gas flow 6–8 L/min for optimal particle size	• Deliver aerosolized medications
Ultrasonic nebulizer	• High-volume and high-density output compared to jet nebulizers • Can come in higher volume models to be used with water or normal saline to deliver bland aerosol therapy • Can come in small-volume models for medication delivery • Needs inspiratory flow or circuit flow to deliver, so these can be used in-line to deliver meds without adding additional flow to the system	• Small volume model to deliver inhaled medications • Large volume model to help thin secretions or for sputum induction
Vibrating-mesh nebulizer	• Agitation created by vibrations creates aerosol droplets • Needs inspiratory flow or circuit flow to deliver	• Deliver inhaled medications • Prefer with mechanically ventilated patients because no additional flow or volume introduced into the circuit

Table 6-17 Troubleshooting Common Problems with Common Aerosol Delivery Systems

Problem/Clue	Cause(s)	Solution
Large-Volume Jet Nebulizer		
Inadequate mist output	Inadequate input flow	Increase input flow
	Corrugated tube obstruction	Drain condensate
	Jet orifice misalignment	Repair or replace unit
	Low water level	Refill the unit
Aerosol mist disappears during inspiration (T-tube or mask)	Inadequate flow Increased patient's inspiratory flow demands	• Maximize input flow • Add open reservoir to the expiratory side of T-tube • Connect multiple nebulizers in parallel • Use gas injection nebulizer

(continues)

Table 6-17 Troubleshooting Common Problems with Common Aerosol Delivery Systems (*continued*)

Small Volume Jet Nebulizer (SVN)		
Inadequate or no output	• Missing cone • Clogged jet orifice • Flow setting too low • Med cup not tight • Insufficient fill volume • Nebulizer positioned incorrectly	• Replace nebulizer • Adjust flow to 6–8 L/min • Tighten the med cup • Ensure there is adequate volume in the nebulizer • Position vertically
Ultrasonic		
No mist is seen in the nebulizer chamber	Unit not "on" or connected to the power	Connect the unit to power and turn on
	Inadequate fluid level	Ensure adequate fluid level
Misting in the chamber but no aerosol delivered	Inadequate flow through the chamber	Increase flow through the chamber

Table 6-18 Troubleshooting Electronic Nondisposable Mesh Nebulizers

Problem	Cause	Solution
No visible aerosol when using batteries	Batteries inserted incorrectly or low in charge	• Insert batteries properly • Replace/recharge batteries or use AC power
	Cable from power unit to nebulizer not properly connected or damage	Make sure that the cable is properly connected; replace the cable if needed
	Mesh plate clogged with residual drug	Clean or replace the device as per the manufacturer's protocol
No visible aerosol when using AC power	AC power unit not correctly plugged into a working outlet	Insert the plug into a working outlet and verify that the power light is lit
	Cable from power unit to nebulizer not properly connected	Make sure that the cable is properly connected
	Mesh plate clogged with residual drug	Clean or replace the device as per the manufacturer's protocol
No visible aerosol when the power source is properly functioning	No solution in the medication reservoir	Fill the reservoir with the prescribed solution
	Mesh plate clogged with residual drug	Clean or replace the device as per the manufacturer's protocol
Weak nebulization/longer than the expected treatment time	Mesh plate clogged with residual drug	Clean or replace the device as per the manufacturer's protocol
	Batteries low in charge (power warning)	Replace/recharge batteries or use AC power
Medication left in unit after treatment	Batteries low in charge (power warning)	Replace/recharge batteries or use AC power
	Mesh plate clogged with residual drug	Clean or replace the device as per the manufacturer's protocol

Table 6-19 summarizes some considerations and the problems you are likely to encounter with pMDI and DPI medication delivery devices and their solutions.

Spacers and Valved Holding Chambers

One of the common problems with pMDI technique is with timing or coordinating the actuation of an MDI with inspiration. Actuating the MDI too late after inspiration has begun results in the

Table 6-19 Considerations for pMDI and DPI Medication Delivery and Troubleshooting

Metered-Dose Inhaler	Dry-Powder Inhaler
• Shake the canister and "prime" it (i.e., waste a dose into the air) if it is a new MDI or has not been used for a few days	• Poor patient response: check and correct patient technique
• A cold canister should be warmed in the hands to function properly	• Higher inspiratory flows are needed (>60 L/min) compared to an MDI
• Wait ~1 minute between puffs	• Timing and coordination are not needed because the drug only moves with the inspiratory flow (no propellant)
• Have patient hold breath for 10 seconds to allow maximum drug deposition	• Breath-hold is encouraged but not required
• Open-mouth technique: MDI is positioned 4 cm (2 finger widths) away from the open mouth. Keep the tongue down	• If no powder is felt, medication is not loaded on the chamber
• Closed-mouth technique: place MDI between the lips with tongue down	• Powder residue in the outlet (may indicate patient exhaling back into the device): clean with a dry cloth or small brush; advise patient on proper technique; make sure device stored with cap on in dry place
• Timing/coordination or oral deposition problems may be solved by using a spacer or valved holding chamber	

medication not being inhaled as deeply. Actuating it too soon before inspiration has begun results in oral deposition. Problems with timing and coordination can be alleviated by using a spacer or valved holding chamber.

Spacers and chambers create space between the MDI and the mouth, allowing the propellant to dry and larger particles to be removed from the stream. A valved holding chamber provides a bit more deposition compared to a spacer because it reduces the effect of a patient exhaling into the chamber, so it is a better choice between the two, although cost and availability may be an issue for some patients.

A key consideration when using these devices has to do with cleaning them, specifically the plastic ones. Manually drying them may cause an electrostatic charge to generate in their surface that draws medication to the insides of the chamber or spacer. Most manufacturers recommend periodic cleaning with soap and water and letting them air dry.

Resuscitation Devices

Manual Resuscitators

Resuscitation devices provide ventilation and oxygenation in emergencies and during patient transport. Resuscitation devices include self-inflating manual resuscitators (aka bag-valve-mask [BVM] systems), flow-inflating resuscitators, gas-powered resuscitators, and mouth-to-valve mask resuscitators (typically used outside of the hospital setting). **Table 6-20** summarizes the selection and troubleshooting of these devices.

Assembly and Use

Most BVMs are disposable and need minimal assembly. Key considerations in their use include the following:

- Use an O_2 reservoir with a volume at least equal to the bag stroke volume.
- If needed, attach a PEEP valve to the expiratory port and adjust it to the desired level.
- Always test the device for proper function before application (see the discussion of troubleshooting).
- To ensure the highest possible F_{IO_2}, (1) manually provide for slow refilling of the bag (if time permits), (2) make sure a reservoir is connected to the BVM device, and (3) provide for adequate input flow.

Table 6-20 Selection and Troubleshooting of Resuscitation Devices

Best Use	Characteristics/ Advantages	Disadvantages	Troubleshooting
Self-Inflating BVM			
First choice in most resuscitation and transport situations	• Can ventilate without a gas source • Easy to use and reliable • Can add a PEEP valve • If reservoir tube or bag is attached, it can deliver high FIO_2 • Has a pressure pop-off to limit excessive pressure delivery (usually set at 40 cm H_2O pressure)	• Does not provide "blow-by" oxygen (requires squeezing to operate) • It will deliver room air if not connected to an O_2 source • Unable to ventilate if pop-off valve is activated due to increased airway resistance/decreased compliance.	• Most are disposable so malfunctioning BVMs should be replaced • Ensure reservoir tube is attached for high FIO_2 • Set flow high enough so that the reservoir bag does not collapse when the bag is released to fill • Secretions or vomit can clog valves; replace the bag • Deactivate pop-off valve if needing pressures > 40 cm H_2O • If there is no resistance or chest rise when the bag is squeezed, valves may be faulty. May occlude with hand and check before use or during troubleshooting.
Flow-Inflating Resuscitator			
• Most often used for infant resuscitation, delivery, or NICU • Often used in the OR	• Can easily deliver high FIO_2 • Can control PEEP by adjusting the exhalation port (usually a screw-type adjustment) • Can deliver "blow-by" oxygen	• Must have a good mask seal to operate • Cannot operate without a gas source • Difficult to determine PEEP level being delivered	• If the bag does not inflate fast enough, increase input flow or decrease exhalation port size. Ensure a good mask seal. • If the bag is overinflated, turn down the input flow or open the exhalation port
Gas-Powered Resuscitator			
Connects directly to a 50-psi gas source	• Can deliver high minute volumes with 100% FIO_2 • Good for OR or code situations	• Needs a 50-psi gas source	• Ensure connections are tight from the gas source
Mouth-to-Valve Mask Resuscitators			
Out of hospital resuscitation	• Inexpensive, small and portable (some can fit on a keychain) • Does not need a gas source • One-way valve protects the rescuer from the victim's exhaled gas	• Delivers the FIO_2 of exhaled gas (~ 17%) • Tiring to use for prolonged periods	• Ensure one-way valve is in place and there is a good seal
BVM, bag-valve-mask; NICU, neonatal intensive care unit; OR, operating room; PEEP, positive end-expiratory pressure.			

Troubleshooting

Before applying a resuscitator to a patient, check it for proper function. For BVMs, follow these two simple steps:

1. Occlude the patient connector, and then squeeze the bag. If the bag has a pressure relief valve, it should pop off. If the bag does not have a relief valve, it should not be possible to compress the bag.
2. Squeeze the bag, and then occlude the patient connection. The bag should reinflate via the inlet valve, and any attached O_2 reservoir bag should deflate (if applicable).

Failure of the first test indicates that either the nonrebreathing valve or the bag inlet valve is missing or leaking. Failure of the second test indicates that the bag inlet valve is jammed or positioned incorrectly. *If the BVM fails either test, replace it.*

Automated External Defibrillators (AEDs)

AEDs are used to provide early defibrillation in pulseless patients with pulseless ventricular tachycardia or ventricular fibrillation, as this *has been shown to improve survival rates in those who need defibrillation*. These units are typically found outside of the hospital and are easily accessible and easily operated by the general public.

Key points for the setup and use of an AED includes:

- Once a pulseless victim is identified and an AED is available, turn the unit on, then apply the pads to the victim's bare chest and connect the cables to the unit.
- Clear the victim so the unit can identify a shockable rhythm.
- If the unit prompts that a shock is needed, clear the victim again and push the shock button after it charges.
- If the unit says that no shock is needed, resume CPR (remember that your patient is pulseless). Pulseless, nonshockable situations would include asystole or pulseless electrical activity.
- Repeat analyzing and the steps that follow every 2 minutes (approximately five CPR cycles). Remember to switch rescuer positions at that time as well.

Additional considerations:

- Use a child AED and child pads on those younger than 8 years old.
- Place one pad on the upper right chest below the collarbone. The other goes on the left side a few inches below the armpit. An alternate anterior-posterior placement option is to place one pad on the left side of the chest between the left side of the breastbone and below the left nipple. The other pad goes on the left side of the victim's back at the same level as the one in the front.
- Hairy chest: If good contact cannot be made, either shave the chest or if you have an extra set of pads, apply and quickly pull off to remove the hair.
- Wet situations: If the victim is wet, lying in a puddle or snow, or is in the water, dry the chest before using the AED.
- Implanted defibrillators/pacemakers: Do not place pads directly over these devices or on top of transdermal medication patches; remove the medication patch and wipe the area.

Mechanical Ventilators and Breathing Circuits

Selection

Four key questions dictate the choice of a ventilator device:

1. Which patient variables apply?
2. Where will the device be used, and for how long?
3. How will the device be used?
4. Which added capabilities are needed or desired?

Table 6-21 provides common answers to these key questions and guidance on recommending the type of ventilator you should select for each circumstance.

Ventilator Assembly (Breathing Circuits)

Most ventilators require little or no assembly. However, before applying a ventilator to a patient, you need to select and assemble the appropriate breathing circuit *and* confirm its operation. Here we focus on the breathing circuit. Ventilator and operational verification procedures are described in Chapter 8.

Most adult and pediatric ventilators and CPAP circuits use large-bore corrugated tubing. Two general types of breathing circuits are used: (1) the dual-limb or "wye" circuit and (2) the single-limb circuit. Single-limb circuits may include a true expiratory "mushroom" valve or a leakage-type exhaust port. **Table 6-22** summarizes the appropriate use of these different breathing circuits.

Dual-Limb Circuits

Figure 6-1 shows a typical dual limb "wye" circuit (middle), the type most commonly used with critical care ventilators. It includes three basic components that together resemble the letter "Y": (1) an inspiratory limb that delivers fresh gas from the ventilator to the patient, (2) a standard 15-mm patient connector/swivel adapter, and (3) an expiratory limb that directs expired gas to the ventilator's expiratory valve or PEEP/CPAP valve. Additional components may include plug connectors for the heated wires, a pressure-sensing line, and ports for temperature probes.

Table 6-21 Selecting a Ventilator

Question	Answer	Recommended Device
Which patient variables apply?	The patient is an infant or small child	Ventilator certified for use on specific age group
	The patient has or needs an artificial tracheal airway	Standard multipurpose ICU ventilator; if artificial tracheal airway not needed, select a noninvasive positive-pressure ventilator
	The patient has hypoxemic respiratory failure only, adequate ventilation	Ventilator capable of high levels of oxygen and PEEP or airway pressure release ventilation (APRV)
	The patient is a candidate for weaning	Ventilator capable of SIMV, CPAP, pressure support, bilevel ventilation with the capability to monitor spontaneous breathing parameters
Where will the device be used and for how long?	In the acute care setting	Standard multipurpose pneumatically powered microprocessor-controlled ICU ventilator capable of volume control or pressure control (PC)
	Home or long-term care setting	Electrically powered ventilator with volume control, assist control (A/C) and volume control, SIMV
	For short-term transport	BVM or simple pneumatically powered transport ventilator (for long-term transport, consider an electrically powered ventilator capable of running on 12-volt DC)
	During MRI procedures	Ventilator certified for MRI use
How will the device be used?	On critically ill/unstable patients	Standard multipurpose microprocessor-controlled ICU ventilator with graphics display
	On stable home or long-term care patients	A ventilator with vent-inoperative, high-pressure, and disconnect alarms
Which additional capabilities are needed or desired?	Advanced alarm and monitoring functions	Standard multipurpose microprocessor-controlled ICU ventilator with graphics display
	Data analysis/storage and programmability	Standard multipurpose microprocessor-controlled ICU ventilator with graphics display

BVM, bag-valve-mask; CPAP, continuous positive airway pressure; ICU, intensive care unit; MRI, magnetic resonance imaging; PEEP, positive end-expiratory pressure; SIMV, synchronized intermittent mandatory ventilation.

The mechanical deadspace or rebreathed volume in dual-limb circuits is found between the ventilator circuit wye and the patient's airway. *Any tubing or device (such as an HME, MDI, and end-tidal CO_2 adaptor) added between these connections will increase mechanical deadspace.*

Single-Limb Circuits

As shown in Figure 6-1, there are two types of single-limb circuits: (1) those with built-in expiratory valves and (2) those with leakage-type exhaust ports. Those with the expiratory valve (Figure 6-1,

Table 6-22 Appropriate Use of Common Ventilator/Continuous Positive Airway Pressure (CPAP) Circuits

Circuit Type	Appropriate Use
Dual limb "wye" circuit	Most critical care ventilators
	Continuous-flow CPAP circuit
Single-limb circuit with an expiratory valve	Transport and home care ventilators
Single-limb circuit with leakage-type exhaust port	Noninvasive positive-pressure ventilators

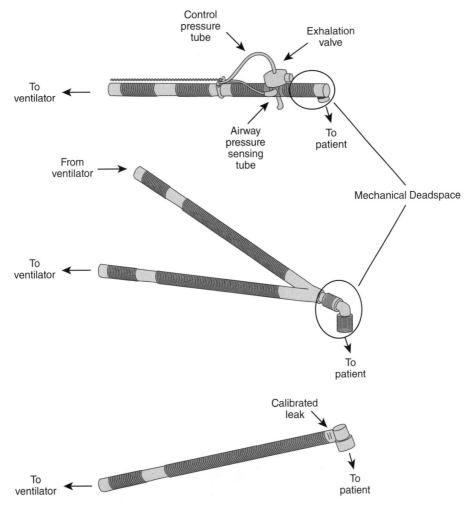

Figure 6-1 Type of Patient Breathing Circuits. Top: Single-limb circuit with exhalation valve used in home- care or transport ventilators. **Middle:** Double-limb circuit used on intensive care ventilators. **Bottom:** Single-limb circuit *without* exhalation valve used in noninvasive ventilators.

top) have a separate pneumatic line running from the ventilator to the expiratory valve. When pressurized, the expiratory valve blocks gas outflow during inspiration. At the beginning of expiration, this valve depressurizes and allows expired gases to escape. By maintaining a set level of pressure throughout expiration, the expiratory valve also can provide CPAP/PEEP. *The mechanical deadspace in these circuits is that between the built-in expiratory valve and the patient's airway.*

Figure 6-1 (bottom) also shows a single-limb circuit with a leakage-type exhaust port, as used with most NPPV ventilators. The continuous flow that noninvasive ventilators provide forces expired gas out this exhaust port during exhalation. Combined with the leakage common to all NPPV interfaces, this simple setup prevents rebreathing of most expired gas, thereby minimizing mechanical deadspace. When provided, PEEP/CPAP is created by the continuous regulation of pressure and system flow/leakage via the ventilator's demand valve.

Special Considerations

Figure 6-2 depicts the three most common NPPV interfaces: the oronasal or full-face mask, the nasal mask, and nasal pillows. The lower leakage associated with full face masks may make them the best choice for short-term treatment of hypoxemic and hypercapnic respiratory failure in the acute care setting, although they should be avoided if the patient has a high risk of vomiting or aspiration.

For patients with hypercapnic respiratory failure, nasal appliances are preferred due to their lesser deadspace. Oral devices have proved successful in managing patients with chronic hypercapnic respiratory failure in need of intermittent support, such as those with progressive neuromuscular diseases. Whichever device is selected, it must be positioned and secured well enough to prevent major leakage yet remain loose enough to avoid discomfort or pressure sores. To prevent tissue damage during long-term usage, you may need to consider special cushioning materials or alternative interfaces.

Circuit Assembly

Proper circuit assembly involves connecting all components to the proper ventilator outlets and inlets and checking to confirm that all connections are tight and leak-free. Generally, you connect the inspiratory limb to either a high-efficiency particulate air (HEPA) filter at the ventilator's gas outlet or to the outlet side of a heated humidifier.

All patients needing ventilatory support via a tracheal airway require properly humidified gas, provided via either an active heated humidifier or a passive HME. Water traps can be placed at low points in the circuit to prevent condensate generated by heated humidifiers from obstructing flow. If a heated-wire circuit is used, the connector(s) must be plugged into the low-voltage outlets on the humidifier. If an HME is used, it must be placed to ensure bidirectional flow, where it will always add some deadspace.

Circuit Testing/Calibration

After connection to a ventilator, all standard circuits should be tested for leaks. On a conventional microprocessor-controlled ventilator, the leak test typically is conducted during the device's pre-use check. Never use a "cheater hose" for the pre-use check. Use the actual circuit so that it can be checked for leaks, measured and compensated for compressible volume, and ensure that the circuit can withstand the flow and pressure applied to it during the pre-use check.

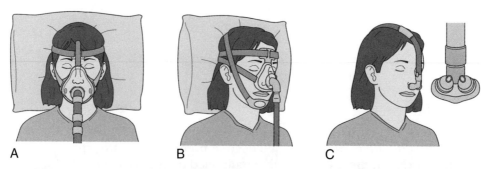

Figure 6-2 Common Noninvasive Positive-Pressure Ventilation (NPPV) Patient Interfaces. (A) Oronasal mask. **(B)** Nasal mask. **(C)** Nasal pillows.

Troubleshooting Ventilator Circuits and Interfaces

Problems that occur during mechanical ventilation can be due to the ventilator, its circuit, or the patient. **Important**: *because you must always attend to patient needs first, when any major problem is suspected, immediately remove the patient from the ventilator and provide appropriate support using a manual resuscitator with a PEEP valve connected to an O_2 source.* If this action resolves the problem, you know that the ventilator or circuit was the cause and can have others troubleshoot the system while you continue to support the patient manually.

Chapter 11 describes how you should respond to alarms and changes in the status of patients receiving mechanical ventilation. Here we focus on troubleshooting the ventilator circuit and related equipment.

The most common problems encountered with ventilator circuits include leaks, obstructions, expiratory/PEEP valve problems, humidification and temperature regulation problems, and infection/cross-contamination (**Table 6-23**). Specific to NPPV are problems with the patient interface.

In addition to airway cuff or pilot tube problems, circuit leaks are among the most common problems causing loss of ventilator volume and pressure. To distinguish a circuit leak from a ventilator malfunction, run a circuit leak test. If the leak test fails, then the ventilator may not be delivering the preset volume.

Circuit obstructions always are associated with low-volume and high-pressure alarms. Expiratory obstruction is the more serious of the two conditions, as it can result in rebreathing, asphyxia, or barotrauma. The most dangerous type of expiratory obstruction occurs when the exhalation port on single-limb circuits becomes obstructed. To avoid this problem, you must prevent patients from grasping the circuit, and make sure that nothing obstructs the exhalation port, such as bedding.

NPPV patient interfaces are the last major area of ventilator circuit troubleshooting. **Table 6-24** summarizes the most common problems with these interfaces and their potential solutions.

Intubation Equipment

Equipment need for routine intubation includes the following:

- Personal protective equipment (e.g., gloves, gowns, masks, eyewear)
- Towels (for positioning)
- BVM resuscitator with O_2 flowmeter and connecting tubing

Table 6-23 Troubleshooting Common Ventilator Circuit Problems

Problem	Clue	Solution
Leaks	Low-volume + low-pressure alarms	• Check/correct loose circuit connections
Inspiratory obstructions (e.g., kinks, condensate, excessive secretions, HME blockage, artificial airway blockage)	Low-volume + high-pressure alarms	• Find/correct obstruction • Drain condensate • Replace HME • Suction patient
Expiratory obstructions (e.g., kinks, condensate, blocked exhalation port [patient, bedding])	Low-volume + high-pressure alarm	• Find/correct obstruction • Drain condensate • Prevent expiratory port blockage

Expiratory/PEEP valve malfunction	• Open or leaking:
	  ○ Low-volume alarm
	  ○ Low PEEP/CPAP alarm
	• Obstructed/sticking:
	  ○ High-pressure alarm
	  ○ High PEEP/CPAP
	• Expiratory flow impeded
		• Single-limb circuits:
		  ○ Check expiratory valve line
		  ○ Replace circuit
		• Double-limb circuit with internal expiratory valve:
		  ○ Replace ventilator

Table 6-24 Common Problems with NPPV Patient Interfaces

Interface	Problems	Remedy
Nasal masks	Mouth leakage	Use chin strap
	Discomfort	Refit, adjust strap tension, change mask type
	Nasal bridge redness, pressure sores	Reduce strap tension, use forehead spacer, use nasal pillows, use artificial skin or a nose pad
Oronasal (full face) masks	Rebreathing	Use nonrebreathing (plateau) exhalation valve
	Impedes speech/eating	Permit periodic removal if tolerated
	Claustrophobia	Choose a clear mask with minimal bulk
	Aspiration risk	Exclude patients who cannot protect their airway or are at high risk of aspiration; use nasogastric (NG) tube for abdominal distention
Nasal pillows	Mouth leakage	Use chin strap
	Discomfort	Ensure proper fit, adjust strap tension, change mask type
	External nares redness, pressure sores	Clean/replace or use different-size pillows; reduce strap tension; temporarily use a nasal mask
Oral devices	Dry mouth, throat, lips	Provide supplemental humidification; apply oral lubricant/saliva replacement
	Numb lips	Extend the distance between lips and flange
	Gum discomfort	Try a smaller seal
	The device falls out at night	Tighten the holder/use a flanged mouthpiece
	Nasal leak	Consider nose clips/plugs
	Sore jaw	Discourage biting down on appliance; the device should "float" in mouth
	Excessive salivation	Usually temporary/resolves after initial use

- Oropharyngeal airways
- Suction apparatus (vacuum source, flexible suction catheters, Yankauer tip)
- Water-soluble lubricating jelly
- Laryngoscope handles (two) with assorted blades, batteries, and bulbs
- Video laryngoscope (if available)
- ETTs (at least three different age-appropriate sizes)
- Stylet
- Magill forceps (if nasal intubation)
- Syringe
- CO_2 detector (good), waveform capnograph (best)
- Tube securing device

When a difficult airway is present or expected, accessory equipment should be available to assist a skilled clinician—usually a pulmonologist or anesthesiologist—in performing the procedure. Typically, this equipment may include the following:

- Tracheal tube introducer (aka "bougie")
- Lighted stylet
- Intubating laryngeal mask airway ("Fastrach")
- Optical/video-assisted laryngoscope
- Fiberoptic bronchoscope
- Supraglottic airways (e.g., LMA, King)

Table 6-25 provides more detail on the accessory equipment needed for intubation, including its selection, use, and troubleshooting.

Table 6-25 Accessory Intubation Equipment

Description	Selection and Use	Troubleshooting
Laryngoscope and blades	May choose Macintosh or Miller depending on preference	If the bulb does not light: • Check handle/blade connection • Check/replace the batteries • Check/replace the bulb
Stylet	• Adds rigidity and maintains the shape of an ETT during insertion • Used only for oral intubation • Some video laryngoscopes use a special proprietary stylet	To prevent trauma, make sure stylet tip does not extend beyond the ETT tip and bend stylet at a right angle at the ETT adaptor if no flange is provided
Tracheal Tube Introducer (Bougie)	• A bendable plastic stylet with a small "hockey-stick" angle at the distal tip inserted directly into the trachea and used as a guide over which the ETT can be passed. • Some types have a central channel for ventilation/oxygenation	• Bougie is stiff enough to cause damage to pharynx/vocal cords or perforation of the trachea, bronchi, and potentially the esophagus • For intubation, not tube exchange (used standard tube exchanger instead)
Light Wand	• A flexible stylet with a lighted bulb at the tip passed with the ETT. Characteristic glow ("jack-o'-lantern" effect) under the skin indicates tracheal placement • No glow if the tube is in the esophagus	Does not confirm proper tracheal position; always check breath sounds and confirm with x-ray
Magill Forceps	• Used to manipulate the ETT during nasal intubation by direct visualization • Once the tip of the ETT is in the oropharynx, insert the laryngoscope, and visualize the glottis. Then use the forceps to grasp the tube just above the cuff and direct it between the cords	To prevent trauma, never use forceps without direct visualization and avoid forceful movements
Colorimetric CO_2 Detector	• Disposable CO_2 indicator used to confirm ETT placement in airway • Select correct type based on patient size/weight • Place between ETT and bag-valve resuscitator • Tube position in lungs indicated when the color changes from purple to tan/yellow as the patient is ventilated (at least six breaths)	• Failure to change color can occur even with the proper position during cardiac arrest (false negative). If CPR, must resume compressions and ventilate for an accurate reading. • The color change can occur with improper placement in mainstem bronchus (false positive)
Capnograph monitor (if available)	• Provides numerical $Petco_2$ display as well as capnography waveform • Confirms placement (accuracy secondary only to direct bronchoscopic visualization)	• Condensation or secretions on the sensor site can affect accuracy. Replace sensor if that happens. • Consider a different confirmation device if secretions are excessive • Ensure the sensor is placed on the ETT. Placing further away can affect accuracy.
Bite Block/Tube Holder	• Stabilizes oral ETT, prevents biting on the tube, minimizes movement/accidental extubation • Options include oral airway taped to ETT or flanged tube holder with straps	• Gagging response may require sedation • Can make oral care difficult

Artificial Airways

An artificial airway is required when the patient's natural airway can no longer perform its proper functions. Conditions requiring these devices include airway compromise, respiratory failure/need for ventilatory support, and the need to protect the lower airway.

Table 6-26 outlines the basic indications, key factors in selection and use, and troubleshooting considerations associated with the airways you will encounter most frequently.

In addition to these devices, you may encounter four other specialized tracheal airway devices: (1) fenestrated tracheostomy tubes, (2) "speaking" tracheostomy tubes, (3) speaking valves, and (4) tracheostomy buttons. **Table 6-27** outlines the basic indications, key factors in selection and use, and troubleshooting considerations associated with these devices.

Suctioning Equipment

Airway suctioning is indicated to remove retained pulmonary secretions, to obtain a sputum specimen, maintain a patent airway, or stimulate a cough in patients who are unable to cough effectively.

All suction equipment includes three components: (1) a negative-pressure or vacuum source, (2) a collection system, and (3) a suction device for removing secretions or other fluids. Suction devices in a hospital usually consist of a quick connector or a DISS connection to a wall system of piped vacuum. Where wall vacuum is unavailable, as in some ambulatory clinics, patient transport, or in the home, a portable battery system can be used. Less common are the hand-powered portable suction pump or (believe it or not) a mouth-powered one.

Table 6-28 outlines the key considerations in selecting suction equipment and specifies the appropriate device given the circumstances.

Suction systems incorporate either a trap or float valve in the collection bottle/canister to prevent aspiration of fluids into the suction pump or regulator. Before suctioning, always confirm that the canister is not full and that the valve is not closed. Also, you should ensure that all tubing connections are tight because any leaks reduce vacuum and therefore secretion removal. Fold/occlude the connecting suction tubing coming from the canister to set the suction level and adjust the vacuum control while you observe and set the negative-pressure gauge.

Table 6-29 provides guidelines for setting the initial negative pressure levels for suctioning adults, children, and infants using portable and wall suction systems. Note that the portable (in. Hg) versus wall regulator pressures (mm Hg) are not equal. This is because it is the *flow* that ultimately determines suction device performance. Because wall regulators provide higher flows for a given pressure, less vacuum pressure is required.

After adjusting the vacuum pressure, connect the selected suction device to the system, and implement the procedure. Chapter 10 provides details on procedures used to remove bronchopulmonary secretions, including suctioning.

Now that you have chosen and set up your system, there are a few other considerations listed in **Table 6-30** that you need to consider. Further troubleshooting of this procedure is described in **Table 6-31.**

Blood Analyzers

Blood analyzers that RTs use include benchtop/lab arterial blood gas (ABG) analyzers and hemoximeters (CO-oximeters), as well as portable point-of-care testing (POCT) systems. Benchtop/lab analyzers are highly automated devices for which the NBRC expects only key knowledge of measurement procedures and quality control methods.

POCT Analyzers

POCT analyzers are highly reliable devices. Because calibration occurs with each cartridge test, minimal user intervention is needed. **Table 6-32** summarizes the few problems that you may encounter in using a POCT analyzer, along with their causes and potential solutions.

Note that you may obtain POCT results outside the device's critical range, such as a pH less than 7.20 or greater than 7.60. Such readings are *not* the same as flagged or outside-reportable-range results and should be treated as potentially valid data. To validate measures falling outside a device's

Table 6-26 Indications, Selection, Use, and Troubleshooting of Selected Artificial Airways

Indications	Selection and Use	Troubleshooting
Oropharyngeal Airways (OPA)		

• To prevent the tongue from obstructing the upper airway during bag-mask ventilation
• For comatose patients who develop upper airway occlusion
• As a "bite block" in intubated patients
• For patients having seizures
• Generally, not indicated in conscious patients
	• Proper sizing: measure from the corner of the mouth to the angle of the jaw. Size 9 fits medium size adults.
	• If too large, may occlude trachea and cause gastric insufflation
	• If too small, is not effective or may push the tongue back and occlude the airway
	• Proper positioning: airway should curve over and extend past the base of the tongue
		• If airway obstruction due to the tongue is not relieved:
		  ○ Remove the airway, reinsert
		  ○ Recheck the size of the airway
		• If patient gags or retches, remove the device and maintain the airway by positioning the head/neck; consider a nasopharyngeal airway as an alternative

Nasopharyngeal Airways (NPA)		

• To prevent airway obstruction
• For patients having seizures that prevent opening the mouth
• To minimize the trauma associated with repetitive suctioning via the nasal route
• Avoid in patients with nasal or nasopharyngeal trauma or blockage (e.g., polyps, adenoid hypertrophy in children)
	• Proper sizing: for an average-size female, select a #6 (24-Fr); for an average-size male, select a #7 (28-Fr)
	• When lubricated, the airway should fit through the inferior meatus without force
	• If too large, it can cause mucosal trauma, gagging, vomiting, and gastric distention. Never cut an NPA as the cut edge is sharp.
	• Always insert with the beveled side pointed toward the nasal septum (patient's midline)
	• To prevent slippage into the nasal cavity, always use a flanged or "trumpet" type of airway
		• If you cannot pass the airway:
		  ○ Be sure the NPA is lubricated
		  ○ Try the other naris
		  ○ Try a smaller airway
		• If a suction catheter will not pass:
		  ○ Lubricate the catheter
		  ○ Consider a larger airway or smaller suction catheter

(continues)

Table 6-26 Indications, Selection, Use, and Troubleshooting of Selected Artificial Airways (*continued*)

Endotracheal Tubes (ETT)		
• To establish and protect the airway against aspiration in emergencies or with unconscious patients • To bypass an upper airway obstruction (may require tracheotomy) • To provide short-term positive-pressure ventilation	• Proper sizing is critical • Inflate cuff to confirm integrity before intubating; deflate fully and lubricate before insertion • Typical adult insertion length from tip to incisors: 19–21 cm for females and 21–23 cm for males • Always check tracheal insertion by breath sounds + CO_2 analysis; confirm the proper position with x-ray • See Chapter 9 for intubation procedure and Chapter 16 for assisting with intubation	• Tube position (breath sounds): o If breath sounds are not equal bilaterally, deflate the cuff, withdraw tube 1–2 cm (adults), reinflate cuff, recheck o If breath sounds are not heard, or the stomach distends, remove the tube, oxygenate, and reintubate • Leaks: o If large leak occurs, reinflate cuff, recheck for leaks o If the leak persists, check pilot balloon, inflation line, and valve for leaks (bypass by inserting a small-gauge needle with three-way stopcock into the pilot line) o If the inflation line system is leak-free, the cuff is likely blown; reintubate o Obstruction—follow the obstruction algorithm provided in Chapter 15
• Subglottic suction ETT (e.g., high-low evac)	• To evacuate subglottic secretions and reduce the likelihood of ventilator-associated pneumonia (VAP)	• Connected to low-level suction (–20 to –30 cm H_2O) pressure) • Should be flushed with air periodically to maintain patency

Laryngeal Mask Airways (LMAs)		
• Alternative to ETT intubation for emergency ventilatory support and airway control • To provide ventilatory support and airway control for patients who are difficult to intubate • Contraindicated if high risk of aspiration (intubate or use Combitube) • Contraindicated in patients who are conscious/have intact gag reflexes and those with trauma or obstructive lesions in the mouth or pharynx	• Proper sizing is critical (infant/small child, 1–1.5; child, 2–3; adolescent/small adult, 3–4; adult, 4–6) • Before insertion, fully deflate mask cuff and lubricate mask rim and posterior surface • After proper positioning, inflate mask and confirm effective ventilation; do not exceed maximum cuff volume	• If you need maximum inflation volume to seal, consider a larger mask • Malposition of the airway can cause obstruction or leaks—reposition the patient's head, readjust tube position, or adjust cuff inflation volume • A fiberoptic scope can confirm proper placement

Esophageal–Tracheal Combination Tubes	
• As an alternative to ET intubation for emergency ventilatory support and airway control in or out of the hospital • To provide ventilatory support and airway control for patients who are difficult to intubate due to trauma, bleeding, vomiting, or other factors obscuring the vocal cords • Available only for adults and large children • Contraindicated in conscious patients or those with intact gag reflexes • Contraindicated in patients with esophageal disease	• Proper sizing: 41-Fr for patients more than 5 ft tall; 37-Fr for smaller patients • Leak-test cuffs and then deflate before insertion • Insert until two black marks at the proximal end of the tube are between upper incisors • Inflate blue cuff (100 mL) and white cuff (15 mL) • Ventilate first through the longer blue pharyngeal tube connector; good breath sounds confirm normal esophageal placement with ventilation via the tube's pharyngeal holes • If gurgling is heard over the epigastrium and breath sounds are absent, the tube is in the trachea; inflate white cuff (15 mL) and ventilate through the white tracheal connector	• If you cannot ventilate through either connector, the tube may be inserted too far (pharyngeal cuff can obstruct glottis); to rectify, withdraw 2–3 cm at a time while ventilating until breath sounds are heard over lungs • Confirm tube placement via capnography

Tracheostomy Tubes	
• To provide long-term positive-pressure ventilation • To bypass upper airway obstruction (when oral or nasal intubation is not feasible due to trauma or obstructive airway) • For patients needing a permanent artificial airway	• Proper sizing is critical (see Chapter 9) • Inflate cuff to confirm integrity before intubating; deflate fully and lubricate before insertion • Always check position by breath sounds + CO_2 analysis; confirm with x-ray • Be sure to secure neckplate/flange to avoid extubation; change disposable ties as needed for comfort and cleanliness • Make sure that a correctly sized spare inner cannula is kept at the bedside • See Chapters 9 and 16 for guidance on changing tracheostomy tubes and providing tracheostomy care	Leaks • If a large leak occurs, reinflate cuff, recheck for leaks • If the leak persists, check pilot balloon, inflation line, and valve for leaks (bypass by inserting a small-gauge needle with three-way stopcock into the pilot line) • If the inflation line system is leak-free, the cuff likely is blown; reintubate Obstruction: follow the obstruction algorithm provided in Chapter 15

Table 6-27 Indications, Selection, Use, and Troubleshooting of Specialty Tracheal Airway Devices

Indications	Selection and Use	Troubleshooting
Fenestrated Tracheostomy Tubes		
• To facilitate weaning from a tracheostomy tube • To support patients needing intermittent (e.g., nocturnal) ventilatory support • To facilitate speech	• Sized the same as regular tracheostomy tubes • Outer cannula has fenestration (opening) above cuff • Removal of inner cannula opens the fenestration • Plugging tube *after* cuff deflation allows normal upper airway function • Remove the plug to suction • To provide positive pressure or protect the lower airway, reinsert inner cannula and reinflate cuff	• *Never* plug tube with the cuff inflated (attach a warning tag to the plug) • If respiratory distress occurs when the tube is plugged, make sure cuff is fully deflated • If a deflation of cuff does not relieve distress, the tube may be improperly positioned; carefully reposition
"Speaking" Tracheostomy Tubes		
• To allow patients with a tracheostomy tube to vocalize, even when receiving mechanical ventilation • For patients not needing a cuff for airway protection, consider a speaking valve instead	• Sized the same as tracheostomy tubes • Include a separate small line that adds gas flow (4–6 L/min) to an outlet above the cuff, allowing patient vocalization • A "wye" connector controls when the flow is applied • Cuff must be inflated for vocalization	• Leaks and obstructions are managed the same as a regular tracheostomy tube • Separately label gas supply and cuff lines to avoid mix-up (connecting cuff line to a flowmeter will burst cuff)
Tracheostomy Buttons		
• To maintain an open stoma after tracheostomy tube removal • To facilitate weaning from a tracheostomy tube • To provide long-term access for suctioning of the lower airway	• Consists of a short cannula flanged at both ends • Exact insertion length controlled using spacers • A cap seals the button and forces the patient to use upper airway • Some buttons provide an adaptor for positive-pressure ventilation	• Regularly pass a suction catheter through a button to ensure patency • If respiratory distress occurs, the tube may be protruding too far into the trachea; reposition by changing the number of spacers
Speaking Valves		
• To allow patients with tracheostomy tubes/buttons and good protective reflexes to vocalize, swallow, and cough normally • Contraindicated for unconscious patients or with HMEs	• The one-way valve allows inspiration through the tube but blocks expiration • When used with tracheostomy tubes, it is critical that the cuff must be *fully* deflated. Failure to do so can cause suffocation or very high airway pressures that could cause trauma or may launch the PMV forcefully from the trach tube • Always suction through the tube and above cuff before attaching • To provide O_2, use a tracheostomy collar or an O_2 adaptor • If used with ventilator, select time- or volume-cycled mode and adjust alarms (expiration will not occur through breathing circuit)	• If patient experiences distress with valve and cuff deflated, likely causes are upper airway obstruction, secretion problems, or too-large tracheostomy tube; remove the valve immediately. Downsize trach, use fenestrated trach, switch to low-profile cuff trach. Ensure all air has been removed from the cuff. • The valve should be cleaned daily in soapy water, rinsed, and air-dried to prevent sticking due to dried secretions. • Should not be worn during sleep because the valve could become clogged and cause obstruction

Table 6-28 Selection of Suctioning Devices and Catheters

Selection	Considerations	Recommendations
Suction scenario	Oral cavity/nasal passages (newborn)	Choose bulb suction
	Oropharynx	Choose Yankauer tip (oropharyngeal)
	Trachea	Select standard suction catheter
	Bronchus (right or left)	Use a Coude directional tip catheter
	Nasal route (frequent)	Select a standard suction catheter with an NPA
	Meconium aspiration	Use meconium aspirator connected to ETT
	Ventilator/PEEP	Use in-line/closed suction system
	Tracheal cuff leakage-type aspiration	Consider continuous supraglottic aspiration system
	Sputum collection	Use sputum collection (Lukens) trap
Catheter size	• The external diameter of suction catheters should be less than half the diameter of the airway lumen in children and adults. • Use this formula: ETT or trach ID size × 2; then choose the next smallest catheter size (adult size catheters come in even numbers)	

Table 6-29 Guidelines for Initial Negative Pressure Levels

Patient Group	Portable Suction Pump	Wall Regulator
Adults	−12 to −15 in. Hg	−100 to −150 mm Hg
Children/Infants	−7 to −12 in. Hg	−100 to −120 mm Hg
Infants	−5 to −7 in. Hg	−80 to −100 mm Hg

Table 6-30 Additional Troubleshooting Considerations

Goal/Objective	Recommendations
Catheter depth	• The catheter should be inserted only to just beyond the tip of the tracheal airway (shallow suctioning), a distance equal to the tube plus adapter length.
Reduce hypoxemia, VAP risk, and lung derecruitment in mechanically ventilated patients	• Use an in-line/closed-suction system. • Oxygenate for 30 to 60 seconds pre- and post-procedure (neonates increase F_{IO_2} by 10% only). Use oximeter to monitor high-risk patients. • Limit vacuum application time to 15 seconds. • Use the least vacuum pressure needed to remove secretions.
Minimize trauma	• Use the least vacuum pressure needed to remove secretions. • Use an NPA for frequent nasotracheal (NT) suction.
Reduce VAP risk from secretions leaking around the cuff	• Provide routine mouth care. • Ensure proper cuff pressure. • Consider a continuous subglottic aspiration system (Hi-Lo Evac Tube).
To collect a sputum sample	• Use the sputum collection (Lukens) trap.

Table 6-31 Suction Troubleshooting

Problem(s)	Solution(s)
No vacuum pressure	• Make sure that the vacuum source is turned on and set to the continuous suction mode. • For a portable electrical pump, confirm that it has electrical power and that it is switched on (if the pump still does not run, check the fuse/circuit breaker). • Ensure the canister is not full, which will block the system from operating.
Inadequate vacuum	• Check vacuum setting. • Check system for leaks/disconnects. Start at the wall and work your way back to the patient, disconnecting, and checking each part of the system as you go. • Check the canister—ensure the lid is tight and does not have a hairline crack. Check that plugs and caps are on securely. • Tubing: make sure all suction tubing is tightly secured. • Be sure you occlude the thumb port while suctioning. • Check for obstructions or restrictions. Check for dried secretions that were not adequately rinsed from the line. • Check for kinks or crimped lines.
The patient becomes hypoxemic or bradycardic during the procedure	• Stop, oxygenate, and monitor

Table 6-32 Troubleshooting Common Problems with Point-of-Care Testing (POCT) Analyzers

Problem/Clue	Cause	Solution
The analyzer does not turn on	Batteries discharged or dead	Confirm that the batteries are properly charged; if you cannot properly charge the batteries, replace them.
Analyzer turns on but fails to display proper start-up information	Software start-up/boot error	Reboot the analyzer (turn it off, wait for 10–20 seconds, turn it on); replace the device if the second start-up fails.
Calibration error message	A problem with the sample, calibrating solutions, sensors, or device's electrical or mechanical functions	Follow the error message guidance and report findings (maybe a numeric error code referenced in the user's manual); repeat the analysis using a fresh sample and new cartridge.
Flagged results	Results outside the analyzer's reportable ranges	Send the sample to the ABG lab for analysis.
Results rejected based on quality control criteria	A problem with the sample, calibrating solutions, sensors, or device's electrical or mechanical functions	Repeat the analysis using a fresh sample and new cartridge. If sample integrity is not in question, results that are not rejected should be reported as usual. If results are rejected twice, send the sample to the central lab.

critical range, repeat the analysis using a fresh sample and new cartridge. Some protocols require that out-of-range results be repeated in the central lab. *Either way, never wait for repeat results if the findings are life-threatening or coincide with a deteriorating clinical picture.* For example, if the POCT result indicates a PO_2 of less than 40 torr, and the patient exhibits signs of severe hypoxemia, increase the FIO_2 while awaiting the repeat test results.

Hyperinflation Devices

These devices include incentive spirometers, IPPB units, CPAP devices (when used for lung expansion), or any of the proprietary devices like EzPAP® or AccuPAP™. They are designed to provide lung expansion therapy, which is discussed in further detail in Chapter 10.

Secretion Clearance Devices

Several mechanical devices are used to aid patients in secretions clearance. These units include mechanical percussors and vibrators, oscillators, and positive expiratory pressure (PEP) devices. Because these devices all are used to aid airway clearance, they are covered in Chapter 10.

He/O$_2$ Delivery Systems

Due to their reduced density, mixtures of helium with oxygen (heliox) can help decrease the work of breathing, especially in patients with large airway obstruction or severe asthma. Most centers use heliox cylinders that are available in one of three common combinations of He%/O$_2$%: 80/20, 70/30, or 60/40. *To ensure patient safety, NEVER use 100% He to mix with O$_2$ to achieve the desired ratio. ALWAYS use premixed heliox combined with at least 20% O$_2$.*

   If the gas mixture is delivered by a flowmeter, you must either use a device calibrated for the specified He% or use an oxygen flowmeter and apply a correction factor of 1.8 for 80/20 mixtures, 1.6 for 70/30 mixtures, and 1.4 for 60/40 mixtures. For example, for every 10 L/min of indicated flow on an O$_2$ flowmeter delivering an 80/20 mixture, the actual heliox flow is 18 L/min (10 L/min × 1.8 = 18 L/min).

   For spontaneously breathing patients, heliox generally is delivered via a tight-fitting nonrebreathing mask at a flow enough to meet the patient's inspiratory demands. Alternatively, you can deliver heliox using a high-flow cannula delivery system. Heliox mixtures also can be delivered to mechanically ventilated patients—both those with cuffed artificial airways and via the noninvasive route. Heliox, however, can alter ventilator performance. For this reason, only ventilators approved by the FDA for delivering heliox should be used. Even with approved ventilators, you may need to add special modules or use conversion factors to adjust settings.

   Irrespective of the delivery method, all patients receiving helium-oxygen mixtures should be closely monitored, and an O$_2$ analyzer with active alarms should always be used to continuously measure the F$_{IO_2}$ of the mixture provided to the patient. Details on providing/modifying heliox therapy are provided in Chapter 12.

Portable Spirometers

Portable spirometers are useful for bedside measurement of directly measurable lung volumes and capacities, as well as basic measurements of flow (electronic spirometers). They can also be used to obtain a flow/volume loop or perform basic pre- and post-bronchodilator studies.

   Devices used to measure pulmonary function at the bedside include mechanical "vane-type" respirometers and portable electronic spirometers. Use a mechanical "vane-type" respirometer to measure tidal volume, minute volume, inspiratory capacity, slow vital capacity, or to measure or confirm exhaled V$_T$ on a ventilator. Use a portable electronic spirometer to obtain measures of forced expiratory volumes/flows (FVC maneuver).

Mechanical "Vane Type" Respirometers

Mechanical respirometers, such as the Wright or Haloscale, measure gas volume via a rotating vane, with a gear mechanism translating these rotations into the movement of indicator hands on a watch-like dial. An *on/off* switch unlocks and locks the gear mechanism, and a reset button resets the indicator hands to zero.

   Mechanical respirometers generally are accurate to within 2% of their recommended flow range. Like any turbine system, however, these devices tend to overread at high flows and under read at low flows. Moreover, these devices are easily damaged by flows outside their recommended range. For this reason, they should never be used to measure forced flows or volumes. In other words, never use them for an FVC maneuver.

Before each use, you should check the respirometer for proper function:

1. Inspect the device's inlet and outlet to make sure they are clean and dry.
2. Check the foil vane—if it is bent or damaged, send the device for repair.
3. Check for proper function by resetting the indicators to zero, turning the unit on, and then performing these steps:
   a. Cup the device in the palm of your hand, with the inlet unobstructed.
   b. Gently blow toward the device's inlet (the indicators should rotate smoothly).
4. Check the on/off control while the indicators are rotating.
5. Press the reset button to return the indicators to zero.

Once you confirm proper function, you should set up the device for expired volume measurements, as depicted in **Figure 6-3**. As assembled, this setup can be attached directly to an ET or tracheostomy tube, a mask, or a mouthpiece (use nose clips with a mouthpiece).

To use a respirometer to obtain expired volume measurements, follow these steps:

1. Attach the device to the *exhalation side of the one-way valve*.
2. Instruct the patient in the desired maneuver (slow vital capacity, minute volume).
3. Connect the patient to the one-way valve breathing port.
4. Move the on/off switch to the *on* position during patient *inhalation*.
5. Have the patient perform the desired maneuver (timed for minute volume).
6. When the maneuver is completed, move the on/off switch to the *off* position (avoid resetting to "0" before reading).
7. Record the desired measures (for minute volume, compute $V_T = \dot{V}_E \div f$).
8. For multiple measures on the same patient, store the valve/filter assembly in a clean bag at the bedside.

If a properly functioning device fails to operate, you should recheck the position of the on/off switch and make sure the respirometer is appropriately positioned concerning the valve assembly (Figure 6-3).

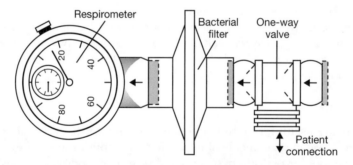

Figure 6-3 Basic Equipment Setup of Wright Respirometer for Bedside Volume Measures. A one-way breathing valve separates the patient's inspiratory and expiratory volumes. A HEPA filter protects the patient and respirometer from contamination. Replacement of the valve and filter allows the respirometer to be used on multiple patients (if the respirometer becomes contaminated, gas sterilize and properly aerate it). Here the respirometer is positioned to measure expiratory volumes (its normal use), with its inlet attached to the expiratory side of the breathing valve. To measure inspiratory volumes, you would reverse this positioning by connecting the filter and the respirometer's *outlet* to the inspiratory side of the valve.

Modified from Kacmarek RM, Foley K, Cheever P, Romagnoli D. Determination of ventilatory reserve in mechanically ventilated patients: a comparison of techniques. *Respir Care.* 1991;36:1085–1092.

Portable Electronic Spirometers

Portable electronic spirometers combine a flow sensor with a computer module. The computer module converts the flow signal into volume and outputs data via a screen and printer. The flow sensor may either sense flow directly (e.g., using a hot wire or Doppler technology) or by measuring the "back pressure" created as gas flows through a restriction. **Figure 6-4** depicts a spirometer pneumotachometer that quantifies flow by measuring pressure differences across a resistive element.

Proper use of portable spirometers involves (1) regular calibration and (2) a procedure that provides valid results. Calibration of pulmonary function test (PFT) equipment is covered in Chapter 8. Here we focus on the proper application of the procedure.

Unlike many physiologic measurements, forced expiratory measures are very dependent on the patient correctly performing the procedure. Key procedural elements required to ensure accurate and reproducible results when performing bedside spirometry are outlined in Chapter 3. The most common technique-related problems include the following:

- Incomplete inhalation (less than inspiratory capacity)
- Inadequate expiratory force
- Breathing during maneuver
- Leakage (poor lip seal/exhalation through the nose)
- Too slow a start to forced exhalation
- Stopping exhalation before all gas is expelled
- Coughing during the maneuver

Devices that incorporate automated validity checks can detect many of these errors. To detect and correct these problems, the National Lung Health Education Program (NLHEP) recommends several validity checks and corrective prompts, as specified in **Table 6-33**. If the spirometer does not provide automated checks, you will need to detect these errors by carefully observing the patient during the maneuver and examining the graphic results. Chapter 8 provides details on how to detect patient-related errors affecting the validity of spirometry measurements.

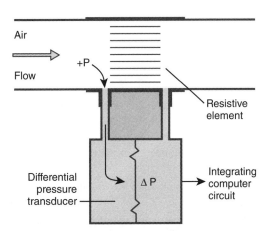

Figure 6-4 Differential Pressure (Fleisch) Pneumotachometer. Air flowing through a resistive element (parallel tubes) creates a pressure difference across the element, directly proportional to flow. These pressure changes are measured by a pressure transducer that sends its output signal to a computerized circuit, which converts the flow signal to volume via electronic integration. For continuous use, the pneumotachometer typically is heated to maintain a constant temperature and prevent condensation.

Modified from Sullivan WJ, Peters GM, Enright PL. Pneumotachography: Theory and clinical application. *Respir Care.* 1984;29:736–749.

When used and maintained according to the manufacturer's instructions, portable spirometers are generally trouble-free. As outlined in **Table 6-34**, malfunctions that do occur usually involve power source problems, computer software or hardware errors, incorrect calibration or assembly, or damage to the sensor.

Table 6-33 Validity Checks and Corrective Prompts for Portable Spirometers

Problem Observed on Validity Check	Corrective Prompts
Back-extrapolated volume > 150 mL	"Don't hesitate."
Time to peak expiratory flow > 120 ms*	"Blast out faster."
Forced expiratory time < 6.0 sec and end-of-test volume† > 100 mL	"Blow out longer."
Repeat FEV_6 values do not match within 150 mL	"Take a deeper breath."

*More than 160 ms for school-age children and adolescents.

†End-of-test volume = change in exhaled volume during the last 0.5 sec of the maneuver.

Table 6-34 Troubleshooting Common Problems with Portable Spirometers

Problem/Clue	Cause(s)	Solution(s)
The device does not turn on	The device lacks electrical power	• If AC powered, confirm connection to working line power outlet • If battery-powered, check/replace batteries
The device turns on, but does not complete or fails the power-on-self-test (POST)	Failure of boot/start-up program or central processing unit (CPU) failure	• Record error message • Turn the device off, wait 20 seconds, then turn it back on • Replace device if continued boot failure
The sensor will not zero	The sensor is moving during zeroing	• Place sensor on tabletop and repeat
Device fails volume calibration (± 3%)	Incorrect temperature or pressure/altitude input	• Recalibrate device, being sure to enter proper temperature and pressure/altitude
	Loose connections or leaks in the spirometer system	• Tighten connections and correct leaks
	Flow sensor assembled incorrectly or damaged	• Reassemble or replace flow sensor
	Flow sensor obstructed with foreign matter	• Clean or replace the flow sensor
The test begins/volume accumulates before patient exhales	Sensor and tubing are not stationary at the start of the test	• Have the patient hold the sensor assembly steady until prompted to begin
Flow measures appear to be reversed (differential pressure sensors only)	Flow sensor inlet and outlet pressure tubing connections reversed	• Check/correct and confirm proper tubing connections
The device does not sense the beginning of exhalation	Sensor pressure tubing not connected	• Check/correct and confirm proper tubing connections
	Flow sensor assembled incorrectly or damaged	• Reassemble or replace flow sensor

Problem/Clue	Cause(s)	Solution(s)
Falsely high or low volume or flow readings suspected	Device out of calibration	• Recalibrate device, being sure to enter the proper temperature and pressure/altitude
	Incorrect temperature or pressure/altitude input	• Recalibrate device, being sure to enter proper temperature and pressure/altitude
	Flow sensor assembled incorrectly or damaged	• Reassemble or replace flow sensor
	Leaks in the patient or spirometer system (low readings only)	• Correct leaks • Use nose clips • Ensure proper lip seal
	Teeth, lips, or tongue obstructing mouthpiece (low readings only)	• Correct patient technique
Falsely high or low percent normal computations suspected	Incorrect patient data entry (e.g., age, height, gender)	• Verify/re-enter correct patient data

Testing Equipment in a Pulmonary Function Laboratory

Previously discussed portable spirometers have their use for basic bedside measurements. If, however, more complex pulmonary function testing is needed, then it needs to be conducted in a pulmonary function lab. Like a portable electronic spirometer, testing in a PFT lab includes an FVC maneuver, pre- and post-bronchodilator studies, a flow/volume loop, a volume/time curve, and basic volumes and capacities measurements. Additional testing in a PFT lab includes measurement of lung volumes and capacities that cannot be directly measured by spirometry (RV, FRC, TLC), more in-depth testing of flows and volumes, airway resistance, maximum voluntary ventilation (MVV), diffusing capacity (DLco), closing volumes, distribution of ventilation, and bronchoprovocation studies.

PFT lab testing and equipment can be quite extensive, and because there are separate NBRC CPFT and RPFT credentialing exams that cover this information in detail, here we will cover some basics as they relate to equipment found in the PFT lab.

The American Thoracic Society (ATS) provides standards for PFT lab testing equipment that must be followed to obtain accurate and reproducible results so that proper evaluation and reporting can be done. **Table 6-35** lists the most common tests and the ATS recommendations for obtaining accurate and reproducible test results.

"Indirect spirometry" techniques are used to measure lung volumes and capacities that cannot be exhaled and therefore cannot be directly measured. This includes RV, FRC, and TLC. **Table 6-36** describes these techniques and their advantages and disadvantages.

Pleural Drainage Systems

Pleural drainage systems remove air or fluid from the pleural space via a tube properly positioned inside the chest cavity. As depicted in **Figure 6-5**, all standard pleural drainage systems have three key components:

1. A one-way seal to prevent air from returning to the pleural space
2. A suction control for adjusting the negative pressure applied to the chest tube
3. A collection chamber for gathering fluid aspirated through the chest tube

Traditional pleural drainage systems like that shown in Figure 6-5 use a "wet" seal and a water column for suction control. Some newer units employ a dry seal and a "dry" suction control mechanism. Here we focus on the use of the traditional "wet" systems.

Table 6-35 ATS Guidelines for Obtaining Accurate and Reproducible Results

Issue/Troubleshooting	Recommendation
FVC Maneuver	
Indications	• To obtain VC and other volumes as well as flows to help determine the presence and the severity of obstructive and restrictive disease processes
Back extrapolation volume	• Must be < 5% of the FVC or 150 mL
Beginning of the maneuver	• Must be notably distinguished
Graphics produced from the FVC maneuver	• Must be smooth
Length of FVC	• Minimum of 6 seconds with a 1-second plateau unless coughing or dizziness occurs
Reproducibility	• Three acceptable maneuvers, with a max of eight attempts. • If three acceptable maneuvers cannot be obtained, do not report the results • The two largest FVC and FEV_1 measurements must be within 200 mL or 5% of each other
Reporting	• The two largest FVC and FEV_1 values are reported, even if they do not come from the same attempt • The best flows are reported • The maneuver with the biggest sum of the FVC and FEV_1 is the best overall test
Maximum Voluntary Ventilation [MVV]	
Indications	• Calculates how much gas the patient can move in a minute. • Helps quantify the degree of impairment from obstructive and restrictive disease processes.
Procedure	• The patient breathes deep and rapid for 12 to 15 seconds. • Data are extrapolated, calculated, and reported as an L/min value
Reliability	• Extremely effort dependent, so suboptimal effort could be interpreted as impairment
Diffusion Test [DLco]	
Indications	• To measure the amount of carbon monoxide (CO) that crosses the alveolar-capillary membrane in units of mL per minute per unit of pressure (mL/min/torr). • Helps to quantify the diffusing capacity of the lungs. • CO is used because it is naturally in negligible amounts in the body, and it is highly attracted to Hb.
Procedure	• Single inhalation of gas that includes a small amount of CO and He (trace gas) with a 10-second breath-hold to allow for diffusion. Exhaled concentrations are then measured to determine diffusing capacity.
Disadvantage	• Patients incapable of a breath-hold may not be able to perform the test.

To assemble a pleural drainage system for evacuation of pleural air or fluid:

1. Aseptically open the package, being sure not to touch any tube connectors or internal surfaces.
2. Position the system *below the patient's chest level*, usually by hanging it on the bed frame.
3. Fill the *water seal* chamber with sterile water to the desired level, usually 2 cm.
4. Fill the *suction control chamber* with sterile water to the desired level, usually to obtain a negative pressure of −20 cm of H_2O; make sure the chamber vent is unobstructed.
5. Connect the *collection chamber* tubing to the chest tube, avoiding kinks or loops.

Table 6-36 Indirect Spirometry Equipment

Description	Advantages/Disadvantages
He Dilution	
• The patient breathes into a "closed circuit" system for up to 7 minutes with a known concentration of He • At the end of the test, the final He concentration can be used to calculate the previously unknown volumes/capacities (RV, FRC, TLC) • The lower the final He concentration, the larger the volumes/capacities	• *Advantage*: easy to do as only tidal breathing is required • *Disadvantage*: leaks in the system (poor seal or eardrum rupture) cause inaccurate results as He gas volume loss will affect the final concentration • Patients with severe air trapping may require a long time to have all lung units participate in the He dilution process • Because the patient is rebreathing into the same system and total volume must be maintained at a known level, O_2 must be added to the system, and CO_2 must be removed by using a CO_2 absorber (e.g., soda-lime)
N_2 Washout	
• The patient breathes in 1.0 F_{IO_2} for about 7 minutes until the N_2 concentration is nearly 0% • The exhaled gas is collected, and an FRC calculation is made based on the final collected concentration of N_2 is compared to the final collected volume • The test actually measures FRC, so the ERV from an SVC maneuver is used to calculate RV and TLC	• *Advantage*: easy to do as only tidal breathing is required • This "open circuit" technique has no rebreathing; therefore, a CO_2 absorber is not needed • Distribution of ventilation can be determined by the graph produced by this test • *Disadvantage*: leaks in the system affect the accuracy of the result
Body Plethysmography (Body Box)	
• The patient is in a sealed box and breathes into a mouthpiece. • The mouthpiece is at some point closed, and the patient pants against the closed mouthpiece, and the pressure is measured (mouth pressure = alveolar pressure). • Since the volume and pressure in the box is known, and the volume displaced by the patient, and the alveolar pressure is known, Boyle's law can be used to calculate the thoracic gas volume (TGV)	• *Advantages*: quick and accurate and it measures the "trapped" gas caused by air trapping that is not measured by traditional spirometry • *Disadvantage*: claustrophobic patients may not tolerate • It requires specialized equipment

6. Connect the *suction chamber* tubing to the suction outlet.
7. Apply negative pressure until gentle bubbling appears in the suction control chamber.
8. Ensure that the water seal chamber level rises and falls with patient breathing or ventilator cycle (tidal breathing).

Once a pleural drainage system is operating, you should monitor the fluid levels regularly to ensure proper function:

1. If the water seal chamber level is less than 2 cm, refill it.
2. If the suction control chamber level is less than the prescribed suction level, refill it.
3. If the pleural fluid collection chamber fills, replace the unit with a new one.

If you need to transport the patient, make sure the system remains below the patient's chest level, and *do not* clamp the chest tube. This will maintain the water seal and prevent any air from getting into the pleural space.

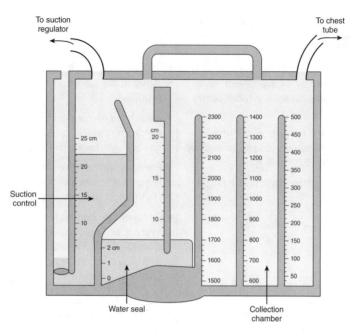

Figure 6-5 Traditional "Wet" Three-Chamber Pleural Drainage System.

If there is no bubbling in the suction control chamber:

1. Check the suction control regulator to confirm that it is on and set to the proper suction pressure.
2. Check the suction chamber tubing for connection leaks or obstructions/kinking; correct any problems.
3. Check the atmospheric vent to ensure that it is open and not obstructed.

If there is *continuous bubbling in the water seal chamber*, there is a leak either at the patient *or* in the drainage system. If the patient has a bronchopleural fistula and is receiving positive pressure, some air leakage is normal. Otherwise, you need to determine the source of the leak and correct it. To determine the source of the leak, briefly pinch the chest tube near its insertion point into the patient. If bubbling in the water seal chamber stops, the leak is at the insertion point or in the patient; if not, the leak is between the patient and the collection system.

1. For an insertion point or patient leak, immediately contact the physician. Patient leaks usually are due to either an outwardly displaced chest tube or an open insertion wound; use a sterile petroleum jelly gauze pad to stop insertion point leaks temporarily.
2. For a collection system leak, check and tighten all tubing connections, apply tape to temporarily seal any tears or holes, and prepare a new drainage unit.

If the water level in the water seal chamber does not fluctuate with breathing (called "tidaling," the drainage system is obstructed. In these cases:

1. Check the collection chamber tubing for kinks or dependent loops; correct any problems if present.
2. "Milk" the tubing connected to the chest tube by compressing and releasing it along its length *toward* the collection chamber (do this regularly to prevent clotting or obstruction).

3. If milking the tubing fails to restore pressure fluctuations in the water seal chamber:
 a. Check the patient for signs of pneumothorax.
 b. Immediately notify the physician of the problem.

Should the patient exhibit clear signs or symptoms of pneumothorax, be sure to notify the physician immediately and obtain both a thoracentesis kit and a tube thoracotomy tray.

Noninvasive Monitoring Devices

The noninvasive monitoring devices you should be most familiar with include pulse oximeters, transcutaneous monitors, and capnography monitors. You select a pulse oximeter to spot check, monitor, or obtain trend data on a patient's oxygen saturation (SpO_2). You select a transcutaneous monitor to provide continuous estimates of arterial blood gases (PO_2 and PCO_2). Details on assessing and interpreting noninvasive oximetry data are provided in Chapter 4.

Pulse Oximeters

Chapter 3 provided details on the setup of pulse oximeters. For monitoring critically ill patients, pulse oximetry readings (SpO_2) should be compared to a simultaneous measure of an ABG O_2 saturation (SaO_2). You can then use the difference between the SaO_2 and SpO_2 to "calibrate" the pulse oximetry reading. **Table 6-37** lists some basic troubleshooting of SpO_2 devices.

Important: just because you get a SpO_2 reading (especially one that you like), does not mean it is correct! Always correlate with other assessment tools and the SaO_2 from an ABG.

Transcutaneous Monitors

Transcutaneous blood gas monitors employ a sensor with miniaturized PO_2 and PCO_2 electrodes like those in lab ABG analyzers, along with a heating element. The heating element "arterializes" the blood by dilating the underlying capillary bed and increasing its blood flow. Oxygen and CO_2 diffuse

Table 6-37 Conditions That Affect the Accuracy of a Pulse Oximeter Readings

Problem	Solution
Device display reads "disconnect"	• Check the probe's connection to the oximeter • Replace the probe (especially if the probe light is not illuminated) • Reposition the probe on the patient as needed. • If bright ambient light appears to be interfering with the reading, shield or cover the probe or reposition it to an unaffected area.
Poor signal (will not read; signal strength indicator has irregular and low amplitude)	• Check probe position; reposition the probe to ensure that the transmitted light is directly opposite the detector. • Try a different site, particularly if the probe has been in place for several hours. • Cold site: warm the probe site and retry. Try a different site. • Poor perfusion: occurs especially in unstable or critical situations. Try a different site that is less peripheral (ear, nose, forehead). Use ABG to determine oxygenation status.
Situations that would warrant to question SpO_2 results	• Fingernail polish/artificial nails/nail jewelry: remove polish, jewelry, or artificial nails. In emergencies, rotate the probe 90 degrees, so it reads sideways through the finger. • Excessive ambient light: shield the probe or change to a site that is not in direct light • CO poisoning: do not use standard pulse oximetry. Use a CO-oximeter. • Intravascular dyes: correlate with ABG SaO_2 before trusting the values

from the capillaries through the skin and into the sensor's contact gel, where their pressures are measured by the electrodes. These pressures are referred to as transcutaneous (tc) partial pressures (i.e., $Ptco_2$ and $Ptcco_2$).

Like lab ABG analyzers, transcutaneous Po_2/Pco_2 monitors require two-point calibration using precision gas mixtures. Failure to calibrate is usually due to a leaking membrane or excessive trapped air under the membrane. In both cases, the calibrating Pco_2 values and the high Po_2 measure will be lower than expected. If a transcutaneous monitor fails to calibrate, you should replace the membrane in the sensor.

To validate transcutaneous readings, the $Ptco_2$ and $Ptcco_2$ should be compared with a concurrently obtained ABG. *For an infant with an anatomic shunt, both the transcutaneous and arterial values must be obtained on the same side.* If the transcutaneous and arterial values differ significantly, poor peripheral circulation is the likely cause. If the patient has good peripheral circulation, but the two readings still differ, try an alternative sensor site. If an alternative sensor site does not provide valid data, replace the membrane and recalibrate the sensor; if the two values still differ significantly, consider another mode of monitoring, such as pulse oximetry or serial ABGs.

Aside from difficulty validating the $Ptco_2$ and $Ptcco_2$ against a patient's arterial values, the most common problem with transcutaneous monitoring is air leaking around the adhesive ring. Air leaks always cause a dramatic fall in $Ptcco_2$. If the leak is large, the $Ptco_2$ and $Ptcco_2$ values will mimic those of room air ($Po_2 \approx 150$ torr; $Pco_2 \approx 0$ torr). In these cases, reapply the sensor using a new adhesive ring.

Capnographs

Capnography is used for ongoing real-time monitoring of ventilation and is extremely accurate in confirming ETT placement after intubation. It can be also be used to evaluate the quality of a resuscitative effort in CPR. Capnographs display a waveform, and capnometry relates to the corresponding numerical $Petco_2$ value. Several problems commonly occur when using capnographs. **Table 6-38** describes these common problems, their likely causes, and the appropriate actions to resolve them.

Table 6-38 Resolving Problems When Using Capnographs

Problem	Cause	Action
CO_2 values are erratic	Mechanically ventilated patients breathing spontaneously	No action needed
	Airway/circuit leak	Check for/correct cuff or ventilator circuit leaks
	Sampling line leak (sidestream units only)	Check for/correct sampling line connections
	Water or sputum blocking the sensor window (mainstream units only)	Clean or replace sensor; recalibrate the device
CO_2 values higher or lower than expected	Physiologic cause	Consider changes in metabolism, ventilation, or cardiac output
	Ventilator malfunction	Check ventilator and patient
	Improper calibration	Recalibrate unit
	Sampling line kinked/clogged (sidestream units only—gives "0" reading)	Unkink/unclog or replace sampling line
	Condensation trap full (sidestream units only)	Empty or replace moisture trap
	BTPS setting OFF (CO_2 values will be falsely high)	Turn BTPS correction ON
BTPS, body temperature, pressure saturated.		

Bronchoscopes and Light Sources

Therapists may assist physicians with bronchoscopy. Key equipment involved includes the broncho-scope itself, its light source, its suction and biopsy valves, and assorted bronchoscopic instruments. Additional equipment typically needed for bronchoscopy includes an oral insertion guide/bite block, specimen-collection devices, a regulated vacuum source and suction supplies, syringes, pulse oxim-eter, O_2 delivery equipment, a BVM resuscitator, saline for lavage, and lidocaine (concentration and amount vary with physician preference).

If the patient is on a ventilator, a special adapter (Bodai adapter) with a bronchoscopy port is required so the bronchoscope can be inserted into the artificial airway without losing ventilation, FIO_2, or PEEP. Troubleshooting of these accessory devices is covered separately in other sections of this chapter. Here we focus on the setup/use of the light source, handling of the bronchoscope, use of the common bronchoscopic instruments, and scope cleaning and disinfection.

Bronchoscope Light Sources

All bronchoscopes require a separate light source. Modern light sources are computerized light-emitting diode (LED) systems, usually controlled via touchscreens.

Troubleshooting

The most common problem with bronchoscope light sources is no light output. To troubleshoot this problem:

- Ensure the AC power cord is properly connected to a power outlet.
- Ensure the power switch is ON (typically will illuminate when on).
- Ensure that any fuses are intact/operating.
- Ensure the light cable is properly seated in the cable port (most units will not provide light output unless the cable is properly seated).
- Check for and correct any error codes that appear on the unit's visual display.
- Check that cooling vents are not obstructed (overheating can cause a safety shutoff).
- If a safety shutoff cannot be deactivated, return the unit for service.

Handling of the Bronchoscope

A fiberoptic bronchoscope is a very delicate instrument. Its outer sheath, filaments in the viewing channel, and objective (distal) lens are very easily damaged. Also, the working channel lining can easily be occluded or ruptured by rigid or sharp instruments. When damage occurs to the fiberoptic filaments, numerous black dots begin appearing in the eyepiece. Damage to the working channel can allow fluid invasion of the scope, causing a foggy image. The possibility of fluid invasion is confirmed by leak-testing the scope during cleaning and disinfection.

To avoid damage to the scope, you must ensure proper handling of the device. Key points in this regard are as follows:

- Avoid letting the distal end strike any hard surface (damages the distal objective lens).
- Avoid forced angulation of the insertion tube (damages the fiberoptic filaments).
- Avoid direct axial twisting of the insertion tube (damages the fiberoptic filaments).
- Use only instruments with external diameters sized adequately for the working channel.
- Keep the proximal portion of the scope as straight as possible during insertion.
- Avoid the use of force when inserting instruments into the working channel.
- Avoid using petroleum-based lubricants for insertion (damage the scope's outer sheath).
- Always replace (do not repair) bronchoscope instruments.
- Always use a bite block whenever the tube is inserted via the mouth or oral ETT.

Also, to avoid endobronchial ignition or fire during laser bronchoscopy, you should ensure that the FIO_2 is kept below 0.40 (if possible) and that alcohol is *not* used to clear the laser tip. Moreover, the physician should make sure that the laser tip is at least 5 mm away from the scope outlet and as far away from the ETT as possible when fired.

If suction appears inadequate during bronchoscopy, first check the vacuum regulator setting and all connections to the scope. If the problem persists, remove and clean or replace the scope's suction valve.

Bronchoscope Instruments

The most common instruments used during bronchoscopy are brushes, biopsy forceps, aspiration needles, grasping forceps, retrieval baskets/snare loops, and balloon catheters. **Table 6-39** summarizes the selection and use of these instruments.

Bronchoscope Cleaning and Disinfection

Because fiberoptic bronchoscopes are a proven source for the spread of infection, you must properly clean, disinfect, and store this equipment after completion of the procedure. The accompanying box (**Box 6-1**) outlines the key elements involved in processing bronchoscopes after use.

Table 6-39 Common Bronchoscope Instruments Used in Pulmonology

Instrument	Use	Comments
Brush	To obtain specimens for cytological or microbiological analysis	Protective sheath avoids contamination during insertion and removal
Biopsy forceps	To obtain specimens for cytological analysis	Must be inserted with bronchoscope tip in neutral position (to avoid damage to operating channel)
Aspiration needle	To obtain specimens for cytological or microbiological analysis	The only technique that allows sampling from *outside* the tracheobronchial tree, such as from lymph nodes
Grasping forceps	To remove foreign bodies	For retrieval of irregular soft objects
Basket/ snare loop	To remove foreign bodies	For retrieval of smooth rounded objects
Balloon catheter	To aid in the removal of foreign bodies lodged deeply in the bronchial tree	Passed beyond the foreign body, inflated then slowly withdrawn to bring object "up" the bronchial tree, where it can be more easily grasped

Box 6-1 Processing of Bronchoscopes After Use

Cleaning

1. While still at the bedside, flush water, saline, or another approved disinfecting solution made for bronchoscopes, through the scope's working channel for 20 seconds.
2. To avoid drying of organic material, immediately transport the scope in a sealed contaminated equipment bag to a processing area.
3. Mechanically clean (e.g., by ultrasonic technology) all reusable accessory instruments and send them for autoclaving.
4. Remove all disposable parts, cap and seal all light/electrical connectors, and place the scope in a cleaning basin.
5. Following the manufacturer's protocol, perform a leak test on the scope (get it repaired if it fails the test).
6. Add enzymatic cleaner to the water and soak the scope for 5 minutes.
7. Using the enzymatic solution, wipe external surfaces with wet gauze and flush the suction channel.
8. Insert an appropriate-size cleaning brush through the working channel and brush all ports until no more visible debris is being removed.
9. Flush the channel again to remove all loosened material.
10. Drain the enzymatic solution from the basin.
11. Rinse all internal and external surfaces with water to prepare the scope for disinfection.

High-Level Disinfection

1. Place the bronchoscope in either an automatic endoscope reprocessor (AER) or a basin used for manual disinfection.
2. Use only disinfectants approved by the U.S. Food and Drug Administration (FDA) that are compatible with the scope; confirm proper disinfectant concentration with each process.
3. Fully immerse the scope in the disinfectant, exposing all surfaces for the proper time (20 minutes or longer for glutaraldehyde); if manually disinfecting the scope, fill the working channel with the disinfectant using a syringe.

Post-Processing

1. After proper immersion time, rinse the scope and its working channel with either sterile or filtered tap water according to the recommendations of the disinfectant supplier.
2. Dry the working channel with 70% alcohol, purged with compressed air.
3. Remove the watertight caps from the scope and hang it vertically in a storage cabinet without attaching any valve.
4. Document the disinfection process (patient ID, date of the procedure, bronchoscopist, model, and the serial number of the scope, and the date of reprocessing).

Modified from Mehta AC, Prakash UB, Garland R, et al. Consensus statement: Prevention of flexible bronchoscopy-associated infection. *Chest.* 2005;128:1742–1755.

Hemodynamic Monitoring Devices

The use and troubleshooting of indwelling vascular catheter systems are discussed in Chapter 3.

T⁴—TOP TEST-TAKING TIPS

You can improve your score on this section of the NBRC exam by reviewing these tips:

- Increased air dilution/decreased F_{IO_2}s occur with low-flow systems when the patient's inspiratory flow, tidal volume, or rate of breathing increase.
- Recommend or apply an air-entrainment mask for unstable patients requiring $< 35\%$ O_2.
- Recommend or apply a heated high-flow nasal cannula for patients with high minute ventilation who require high F_{IO_2}s.
- The air-to-O_2 ratio of an air-entrainment system set to 60% O_2 is 1:1. The ratio for concentrations $< 60\%$ will be less than 1:1 (e.g., 1.7:1 for 50%), with the ratio for concentrations $> 60\%$ more than 1:1 (e.g., 0.6:1 for 70%).
- To set the CPAP pressure in bubble CPAP systems, you vary the depth of the water seal (each cm of depth equal 1 cm H_2O CPAP pressure).
- If using a full oronasal mask for adult CPAP, be sure that it is equipped with a safety inlet valve.
- To confirm a leak-free delivery system when using a bubble humidifier, crimp the tubing at the patient end—the pressure relief should sound.
- Because HMEs require bidirectional flow, they must be placed between the "wye'" connector and the ET or trach tube.
- Intermittent flow or "bubbling" in a heated humidifier tubing circuit indicates partial obstruction with condensate.
- If the aerosol mist disappears during inspiration in a patient receiving O_2 via a large-volume nebulizer and T-piece or mask, the flow is inadequate; boost flow by connecting two or more nebulizers in parallel.
- If you observe residual or caked powder in a dry-powder inhaler, either the patient is not generating enough inspiratory flow during use or is exhaling back into the device.
- The most common problem with nondisposable mesh nebulizers is clogging of the mesh plate with the residual drug, which is easily corrected by cleaning or replacing the device according to the manufacturer's protocol.
- If PEEP is needed when using a bag-valve-mask (BVM), attach a PEEP valve to the device's *expiratory port* and adjust it to the desired level.

- To quickly test a BVM for missing or leaking valves, occlude the patient connector, and then squeeze the bag; if the bag has a relief valve, it should pop off; if there is no relief valve, you should not be able to compress the bag.
- If a BVM pressure pop-off continually activates during use, squeeze the bag more slowly; if this fails to lower airway pressure, consider potential causes (e.g., pneumothorax).
- Refilling time of flow-inflating manual resuscitation devices can be adjusted by changing the input flow, by adjusting the exhalation flow restrictor, and by ensuring proper seal at the interface.
- Select an electrically powered ventilator with volume control, A/C and volume control, or SIMV for patients needing ventilatory support in the home or long-term care setting.
- Any tubing or device (such as an HME) added between the ventilator circuit wye and the patient's airway will increase mechanical deadspace.
- In single-limb NPPV exhaust port breathing circuits, the pressure-monitoring line must be properly connected for the ventilator to function correctly; always check this first if the ventilator is not responding as expected.
- To provide supplemental O_2 to a patient using a home-type electrically powered NPPV bleed O_2 into the circuit to achieve the desired F_{IO_2} (be sure to follow manufacturer's recommendations).
- For patients with hypercapnic respiratory failure requiring NPPV, select a nasal appliance (mask or pillows) to minimize deadspace.
- To avoid condensation impairing their performance, always position ventilator circuit inspiratory HEPA filters before/proximal to any active humidifier.
- To help identify the cause of an unknown problem during ventilatory support, remove the patient from the ventilator and provide equivalent manual support; if this action resolves the problem, you know that the ventilator or circuit was the cause.
- During ventilatory support, leaks will cause low-volume and low-pressure alarms; obstructions will cause low-volume and high-pressure alarms.
- To determine whether a ventilator in volume-control mode is delivering the preset volume, compare the volume setting to that measured *at the ventilator outlet* using a calibrated respirometer.
- To ensure adequate humidification during mechanical ventilation with heated-humidifier/heated-wire systems, always confirm that a few drops of condensation remain at or near the patient connection.
- To help minimize nosocomial infections associated with ventilator circuits, (1) only change circuits when visibly soiled or malfunctioning and (2) avoid unnecessary disconnections.
- If mouth leakage is a problem when using a nasal appliance for NPPV, use a chin strap.
- When using a colorimetric CO_2 detector, ETT position in the lungs is indicated when the color changes from purple to tan/yellow as the patient is ventilated over at least six breaths. If CPR is in progress, be sure compressions are resumed when checking the colorimetric detector.
- If available, capnography should be used to confirm tracheal intubation and to evaluate the quality of a resuscitative effort during CPR.
- A stylet adds rigidity and maintains the shape of an ETT during intubation; a tracheal tube introducer (bougie) is inserted directly into the trachea and used as a guide over which the ETT can be passed.
- If a patient gags or retches when inserting an oropharyngeal airway, remove the device, and maintain the airway by positioning the head/neck; consider a nasopharyngeal airway as an alternative.
- Use/recommend a nasopharyngeal airway to minimize the trauma associated with repetitive nasotracheal suctioning.
- Typical adult ETT insertion length from tip to incisors is 19–21 cm for females and 21–23 cm for males.
- Do *not* recommend a laryngeal mask airway (LMA), or an OPA, for conscious patients who have intact gag reflexes and those with trauma or obstructive lesions in the mouth or pharynx.

- To assess for or allow normal upper airway function in a patient with a fenestrated trach tube, (1) remove the inner cannula, (2) fully deflate the tube cuff, and then (3) plug the outer tube connector.
- To minimize contamination, hypoxemia, and potential lung derecruitment in patients receiving invasive ventilatory support, use an in-line/closed-suction catheter system for suctioning.
- If proper tracheal cuff management is not preventing leakage-type aspiration, recommend replacing the tube with one that can provide continuous aspiration of subglottic secretions.
- Suction pressure always should be set to the lowest level needed to readily remove the patient's secretions and flush them out of the tubing with sterile water.
- To preoxygenate infants before suctioning, increase the F_{IO_2} to 10% above the baseline.
- If the suction regulator is on and set to −120 mm Hg and all connections are tight, but no suction is provided, check to make sure the canister float valve is not blocking vacuum.
- If after setup a blender pressure alarm sounds, verify that both gas sources are at the required inlet pressures (usually $\geq$ 35 psig).
- In general, only a portable O_2 concentrator capable of continuous flow can provide more than 30% O_2, which is needed to provide adequate F_{IO_2} at high altitude (e.g., in airliner cabins).
- If a home-care patient experiences problems with an O_2-conserving device, switch to a nasal cannula at an equivalent liter flow (2–3 times the conserving device rate).
- One pound of liquid O_2 (LOX) equals approximately 344 L of gaseous O_2; a LOX home storage unit filled to 75 lb would provide 75 × 344 or about 26,000 L O_2, enough to last more than a week at a constant flow of 2 L/min (more if using a pulse-dose system).
- If a point-of-care testing (POCT) blood gas analyzer's results are flagged or rejected based on quality control criteria, send the sample to the ABG lab for analysis.
- For spontaneously breathing patients, heliox generally is delivered via either a tight-fitting nonrebreathing mask or a high-flow cannula.
- If heliox is delivered by O_2 flowmeter, you need to apply a correction factor (1.8 for 80/20, 1.6 for 70/30, and 1.4 for 60/40). For example, for every 10 L/min of indicated flow on an O_2 flowmeter delivering an 80% He/20% O_2 mixture, the actual heliox flow is 18 L/min (10 L/min × 1.8).
- To use a respirometer with a one-way breathing valve to measure expired volumes, attach the device to the exhalation side of the valve.
- A portable/screening spirometer should have a volume accuracy of ± 3% or 0.05 L, whichever is greater.
- If the exhaled volume during the last 0.5 sec of a bedside FVC maneuver is still changing, the patient needs to repeat the test and blow out longer.
- If you suspect that a screening spirometer is providing falsely high or low percent normal computations, verify and re-enter correct patient data.
- Continuous bubbling in the water seal chamber of a pleural drainage system indicates a leak; failure of the water level in the water seal chamber to fluctuate with breathing indicates an obstruction. The continuous gentle bubbling of the suction control chamber, though, is normal.
- Never clamp a patient's chest tube during transport; the one-way seal must be maintained.
- Always check a pulse oximeter's displayed rate against an electrocardiogram (ECG) monitor or count the actual pulse rate.
- If you cannot get a good pulse oximetry reading on a patient due to poor peripheral perfusion, consider using an ear sensor or a forehead reflectance sensor.
- If a transcutaneous monitor indicates a sudden drop in P_{tcCO_2} and rapid rise in P_{tcO_2} (in the range of 120–150 torr), the likely problem is air leakage around the adhesive ring.
- Ruling out ventilator disconnection and cardiac arrest, a rapid drop in end-tidal CO_2 levels to 0 torr when using a sidestream capnograph suggests a leak or obstruction in the sampling line.
- Before measurement, all specialty gas analyzers should undergo two-point (high, low) calibration.
- If a bronchoscope light source fails to provide light output, ensure the light cable is properly seated in the cable port.

- To prevent bronchoscope damage, always use a bite block whenever the device is inserted via the mouth or an oral ETT.
- When preparing for a diagnostic bronchoscopy on a patient with a suspected tumor in the right mainstem bronchus, you would obtain both a sterile cytology brush and biopsy forceps.

POST-TEST

To confirm your mastery of each chapter's topical content, you should create a content post-test, available online via the Navigate Premier Access for Comprehensive Respiratory Therapy Exam Preparation Guide, which contains Navigate TestPrep (access code provided with every new text). You can create multiple topical content post-tests varying in length from 10 to 20 questions, with each attempt presenting a different set of items. You can select questions from all three major NBRC TMC sections: Patient Data, Troubleshooting and Quality Control of Devices and Infection Control, and Initiation and Modification of Interventions. A score of at least 70–80% indicates that you are adequately prepared for this section of the NBRC TMC exam. If you score below 70%, you should first carefully assess your test answers (particularly your wrong answers) and the correct answer explanations. Then return to the chapter to re-review the applicable content. Only then should you reattempt a new post-test. Repeat this process of identifying your shortcomings and reviewing the pertinent content until your test results demonstrate mastery.

CHAPTER 7

Ensure Infection Prevention (Section II-B)

Narciso E. Rodriguez

Infection control is a minor topic on NBRC exams, but it is a big part of the respiratory therapist's (RT) job. Most students and clinicians know the basics, such as hand hygiene and isolation procedures. However, the NBRC exams include some areas of infection control with which RTs may not be as familiar, such as equipment disinfection and handling of biohazardous waste. For this reason, candidates should spend a reasonable portion of prep time on this topic, with an emphasis on those areas with which they are least familiar.

OBJECTIVES

In preparing for this section of the NBRC exam content (TMC/CSE), you should demonstrate the knowledge needed to:

1. Adhere to infection prevention policies and procedures.
2. Adhere to disinfection policies and procedures.
3. Properly handle biohazardous materials.

WHAT TO EXPECT ON THIS CATEGORY OF THE NBRC EXAMS

TMC exam: 2 questions; both recall
CSE exam: indeterminate number of sections; however, section II-B knowledge can be tested on CSE Decision-Making sections.

WHAT YOU NEED TO KNOW: ESSENTIAL CONTENT

Key Terms and Definitions

Key terms and definitions necessary to the understanding of infection control are summarized in **Table 7-1**.

ADHERE TO INFECTION CONTROL POLICIES AND PROCEDURES

Centers for Disease Control and Prevention (CDC) Standard Precautions

Standard precautions assume that every patient might be infectious. **Table 7-2** specifies the CDC's recommendations for standard precautions.

Because most hospital-acquired infections occur due to contact between patients and healthcare workers, also known as *direct contact*, good hand hygiene is the best way to help prevent transmission of infections. Good hand hygiene also is part of the CDC respiratory hygiene/cough etiquette guideline, which applies to patients, visitors, and healthcare workers. When caring for patients with signs or symptoms of a respiratory infection, you should wear a mask and maintain good hand hygiene. If you have a respiratory infection, you should avoid direct patient contact, especially with any high-risk patients. If this is not possible, then you should wear a mask while providing care.

Which personal protective equipment (PPE) you use depends on the transmission category under which your patient is receiving care (discussed in the next section). **Table 7-3** outlines the order in which PPE should be applied and removed to avoid cross-contamination.

Table 7-1 Key Terms Used in Infection Control

Term	Meaning
Antiseptic	A chemical that kills microorganisms on living skin or mucous membranes
Bacteriostatic	A descriptive term for chemical agents that inhibit the growth of bacteria but do not necessarily kill them
Cleaning	The physical removal of foreign material (e.g., dirt or organic material), usually with water, detergents, and mechanical action (washing); cleaning generally removes rather than kills microorganisms
Decontamination	The removal of disease-producing microorganisms to leave an item safe for further handling
Disinfection	A general term for the inactivation of disease-producing microorganisms on inanimate objects, usually specified by level type
Disinfection, high-level	The destruction of vegetative bacteria, mycobacteria, fungi, and viruses but not necessarily bacterial spores; some high-level disinfectants can sterilize given adequate contact time
Disinfection, intermediate-level	The destruction of vegetative bacteria, mycobacteria, and most viruses and fungi but not resistant bacterial spores
Disinfection, low-level	The destruction of most vegetative bacteria, some fungi, and some viruses (e.g., hepatitis B and C, HIV) but not mycobacteria or bacterial spores; low-level disinfectants are typically used to clean environmental surfaces
Germicide	A chemical agent capable of killing microorganisms; bactericidal, virucidal, fungicidal, and sporicidal are related terms for chemicals capable of killing these specific categories of microorganisms
Sanitation	A process that reduces microorganisms on environmental surfaces such as tables, beds, and floors to minimize any infectious hazard
Sterilization	The destruction of all forms of microbial life, including bacteria, viruses, spores, and fungi

Transmission-Based Precautions

Transmission-based precautions represent additional measures designed to prevent infection by microorganisms that are transmitted via a particular route. Transmission-based precautions are always used *in combination* with standard precautions. These extra precautions address three routes of transmission:

- *Contact transmission*: the spread of microorganisms by direct or indirect contact with the patient or the patient's environment, including contaminated equipment
- *Droplet transmission*: the spread of microorganisms in the air via large droplets (larger than 5 μm)
- *Airborne transmission*: the spread of microorganisms in the air via small droplet nuclei (5 μm or smaller)

Most NBRC candidates understand that equipment can be a vehicle for contact transmission between patients and that aerosol therapy devices can spread microorganisms via either the droplet or airborne routes. However, the difference between these routes is not always well understood. Because large droplets fall out of suspension quickly, they travel only short distances. Thus, droplet transmission requires close contact, generally 3 feet or less. In contrast, the smaller droplets generated when talking, coughing, or sneezing and during procedures such as suctioning are very stable and, depending on conditions, can travel over long distances, such as between rooms. **Table 7-4** summarizes the CDC's precautions designed to prevent each of these types of transmission, including the most common infections to which they apply.

CDC Central Line Bundle

Indwelling vascular lines—especially those positioned close to the heart or in one of the great vessels—are a significant cause of bloodstream infections. Because such infections are associated with high patient

Table 7-2 Centers for Disease Control and Prevention (CDC) Standard Precautions Recommendations

Component	Recommendations
Hand hygiene	• Perform after touching blood, body fluids, secretions, excretions, or contaminated items. • Perform immediately after removing gloves. • Perform between patient contacts.
Gloves	• Use for touching blood, body fluids, secretions, excretions, or contaminated items. • Use for touching mucous membranes and nonintact skin.
Gown	• Use during procedures and patient-care activities when the contact of clothing/exposed skin with blood/body fluids, secretions, or excretions is anticipated.
Mask, eye protection (goggles, face shield)*	• Use during procedures and patient-care activities likely to generate splashes or sprays of blood, body fluids, or secretions, especially suctioning and endotracheal intubation.
Soiled patient-care equipment	• Handle in a manner that prevents the transfer of microorganisms to others and the environment. • Wear gloves if the equipment is visibly contaminated. • Perform hand hygiene after handling.
Needles and other sharps	• Do not recap, bend, break, or hand-manipulate used needles and sharps. • If recapping is required, use a one-handed scoop technique. • Use safety features when available. • Place used sharps in a puncture-resistant container.
Patient resuscitation	• Use a mouthpiece, bag-valve resuscitator, or other ventilation devices to prevent contact with the patient's mouth and oral secretions.
Patient placement	• Use a single-patient room if the patient is at increased risk of transmission, is likely to contaminate the environment, does not maintain appropriate hygiene, or is at increased risk of acquiring infection or developing adverse outcome following infection.
Respiratory hygiene/cough etiquette	Patients/visitors who are sneezing or coughing should be instructed to: • Cover the mouth/nose when sneezing/coughing. • Use tissues and dispose of them in a no-touch receptacle. • Observe hand hygiene after soiling of hands with respiratory secretions. • In common waiting areas, wear a surgical mask if tolerated or maintain spatial separation of more than 3 feet if possible.

*During aerosol-generating procedures in patients with infections likely to be transmitted via the airborne route (e.g., tuberculosis [TB], severe acute respiratory syndrome [SARS]), wear a fit-tested N95 or higher respirator in addition to gloves, gown, and face/eye protection.

Table 7-3 Sequence for Applying and Removing Personal Protective Equipment (PPE)

Applying PPE	Removing PPE
1. Hair and foot coverings*	1. Hair and foot coverings
2. Gown	2. Goggles or face shield
3. Mask	3. Mask
4. Goggles or face shield	4. Gloves (remove by pulling gloves down from the wrist and turning them inside out)
5. Gloves	5. Gown (remove from the inside out)

*If you touch the floor when donning foot coverings, disinfect hands before proceeding to gown.

Table 7-4 Centers for Disease Control and Prevention (CDC) Transmission-Based Precautions Recommendations

Applicable Infections (Examples)	Precautions
Contact Precautions	
Gastrointestinal infections (including diarrhea of unknown origin and suspected or confirmed *C. difficile* or norovirus infections), wound and skin infections, multidrug-resistant infection or colonization (e.g., methicillin-resistant *Staphylococcus aureus* [MRSA], severe acute respiratory syndrome [SARS])	• Apply standard precautions. • Place the patient in a private room. • Separate clean and dirty supply areas. • Wear clean gloves and gown when entering the room. • Change gloves after contact with any infectious material. • Remove gloves and gown before leaving the room; wash hands immediately or use an alcohol-based rub if hands are not visibly soiled.
Droplet Precautions	
Bacterial meningitis, whooping cough (*Bordetella pertussis*), influenza, mumps, rubella, diphtheria, group A *Streptococcus pneumoniae* infections, SARS, and epiglottitis (due to *Haemophilus influenzae*)	• Apply standard precautions. • Place the patient in a private room (special air handling and ventilation are not needed; the door can stay open). • Separate clean and dirty supply areas. • Wear a surgical mask when within 3 feet of the patient. • Use eye/face protection for an aerosol-generating procedure or contact with respiratory secretions. • Patients transported outside their rooms should wear a mask and follow respiratory hygiene/cough etiquette.
Airborne Precautions	
Tuberculosis [TB], measles (rubeola), chickenpox (varicella-zoster), *Aspergillus* infections, SARS, smallpox (variola)	• Apply standard precautions. • Place the patient in a private negative-pressure airborne infection isolation room (AIIR) with the door closed. • Separate clean and dirty supply areas. • Wear a fit-tested,* N95 respirator certified by the National Institute for Occupational Safety and Health (NIOSH) when entering the room. • Use eye/face protection for an aerosol-generating procedure or contact with respiratory secretions. • Nonimmune healthcare workers should avoid caring for patients with vaccine-preventable airborne diseases (e.g., measles, chickenpox, smallpox). • If airborne precautions cannot be implemented, place the patient in a private room with the door closed; mask the patient. • Patients transported outside their rooms should wear a mask and follow respiratory hygiene/cough etiquette.
*In addition to being fit-tested for a respirator, you need to perform a user-seal check each time you use this device (according to the manufacturer's specifications).	

morbidity and mortality, the CDC has established an evidence-based central line bundle to help prevent them. Although the primary focus is on central lines, application of this bundle to peripheral arterial lines should also help reduce infections associated with those catheters. The accompanying box (**Box 7-1**) summarizes the key recommendations included in the central line bundle.

Protocol for Atypical Viral Infections

Over the past decade, several new viral infections have emerged and raised concerns in the healthcare community. These infections can be difficult to diagnose and treat and have the potential to

Box 7-1 Key Elements in the Centers for Disease Control and Prevention (CDC) Central Line Bundle

Follow Proper Insertion Practices

- Perform vigorous hand hygiene before insertion.

- Adhere to aseptic technique.

- Choose the best site to minimize infections/mechanical complications.

  ○ Avoid the femoral site in adults.

  ○ For central venous pressure (CVP) and pulmonary artery (PA) catheters, use subclavian (not jugular) access.

  ○ Avoid brachial sites for arterial lines in children.

  ○ Use sterile barrier precautions (i.e., mask, cap, gown, sterile gloves, and sterile drape).

  ○ Scrub the skin area for 30 seconds with chlorhexidine 2% in 70% isopropyl alcohol.

  ○ After insertion, cover the site with sterile gauze or sterile transparent dressing.

Handle and Maintain Lines Appropriately

- Comply with hand hygiene requirements.

- Swab access ports with chlorhexidine, povidone-iodine, or alcohol, and access them only with sterile devices.

- Replace dressings that are wet, soiled, or dislodged.

- Perform dressing changes under aseptic technique using sterile gloves.

Review of Status

- Perform daily audits to assess whether the line is still needed.

- Do not routinely replace catheters to minimize infection.

- Promptly remove unnecessary lines.

cause serious widespread epidemics, called pandemics. Examples include avian or bird influenza (an influenza A virus), severe acute respiratory syndrome (SARS), and the Ebola virus.

Influenza A and SARS viruses initially produce common influenza-like symptoms. However, they tend to be much more virulent and can quickly progress to an acute and life-threatening pneumonia and ARDS. For these reasons, all patients who present to a healthcare setting with flu-like symptoms should follow the previously described respiratory hygiene and cough etiquette protocol and be questioned regarding their recent travel history and contact with other sick individuals.

If a patient is suspected of or confirmed as having an atypical influenza-like infection, the CDC currently recommends implementing a protocol that presumes multiple routes of transmission—that is, spread via both contacts and through the air. The protocol thus combines standard, contact, and airborne precautions, which should be continued for 14 days after onset of symptoms or until lab testing indicates that the patient is no longer infected with the suspected virus.

Ebola virus disease (EVD) is a deadly hemorrhagic disease that affects humans and primates. It is caused by an infection with a group of viruses within the genus Ebolavirus. The EVD spreads by *direct contact* with bodily fluids of a person who is sick with or has died from EVD. Splashes to unprotected mucous membranes (for example, the eyes, nose, or mouth) are particularly hazardous. Procedures that can increase environmental contamination with infectious material or create aerosols should be minimized at all times.

In addition, the CDC recommends a combination of measures to prevent transmission of EVD in hospitals:

- Healthcare workers caring for patients with EVD must receive comprehensive training and demonstrate proficiency in EVD-related infection control practices and procedures.

- Personal protective equipment (PPE) must cover the clothing and skin and completely protect mucous membranes when caring for patients with Ebola.
- An onsite manager must supervise all personnel providing care to patients with Ebola at all times.
- PPE donning/doffing procedure must be supervised at each step by a trained observer to make sure the correct protocols are followed.
- Individuals unable or unwilling to adhere to infection control and PPE use procedures should not provide care for patients with Ebola.

Special methods also must be implemented during any aerosol-generating procedures in patients with any of these viral infections. These procedures include aerosol drug delivery, sputum induction, bronchoscopy, suctioning, intubation, and noninvasive and high-frequency oscillatory ventilation. These procedures *should only* be implemented when medically necessary, and then only the needed medical personnel should be present. In these situations, additional guidelines include the following:

- PPE for aerosol-generating procedures should cover the torso, arms, and hands as well as the eyes, nose, and mouth. Consider a surgical hood with an N95 respirator that fully covers the head, neck, and face; for the highest level of protection, use a powered air-purifying respirator (PAPR).
- Perform aerosol-generating procedures in an airborne infection isolation room (AIIR); keep the doors closed, and minimize entry and exit during the procedure.
- Consider sedation during intubation and bronchoscopy to minimize coughing.
- Use high-efficiency particulate air (HEPA) filtration on the expiratory limb of mechanical ventilators.

Adhering to Disinfection Policies and Procedures

High-Level Disinfection (Equipment Processing)

As indicated in **Table 7-5**, different types of equipment pose different infection risks and thus require different levels and methods of disinfection.

Because most respiratory care equipment poses a semicritical infection risk, reusable devices should undergo either sterilization or high-level disinfection via one of the methods specified in the table. Note that some liquid chemical solutions (e.g., glutaraldehyde [Cidex] and ortho-phthalaldehyde [OPA]) can be used to either sterilize or provide high-level disinfection of equipment and—along with pasteurization—are commonly used for heat-sensitive items. The differences in the activity of these solutions reflect the time and temperature variables. For example, high-level disinfection with glutaraldehyde (Cidex) can be achieved in 20 minutes at room temperature, but true sterilization requires a full 10 hours.

When rinsing reusable semicritical equipment after immersion in a liquid disinfectant, you should use sterile water. If this is not feasible, rinse the device with filtered water or tap water, and then rinse with isopropyl alcohol and dry with forced air or in a drying cabinet.

Regarding infection control of specific respiratory care equipment, the following guidelines apply:

- Ventilators
  - Do not routinely sterilize or disinfect the internal machinery of ventilators.
  - Do not routinely change in-use ventilator circuits, attached humidifiers, or heat and moisture exchangers (HMEs), or closed-suction systems; change only if visibly soiled or malfunctioning or as per manufacturer's recommendation.
  - Use only sterile water to fill humidifiers.
  - If using heated humidifiers, use heated-wire circuits to avoid problems with condensate; if condensate does occur, wear gloves to drain and discard as hazardous liquid waste periodically, and then decontaminate hands when done (avoid draining back toward the patient).
  - Always place inspiratory bacterial filters before/proximal to the humidifier.
  - High-level disinfection of nondisposable heating probes is strongly recommended to kill spores if present.

Table 7-5 Infection Risk Categories of Equipment

Description	Example	Processing
Critical Items		
Devices introduced into the bloodstream or other parts of the body	• Surgical devices • Intravascular catheters • Implants • Heart-lung bypass components • Dialysis components • Bronchoscope forceps/brushes	Sterilization For heat-tolerant items: • Steam under pressure (autoclaving) For heat-sensitive items: • Gas or ionized vapor (ethylene oxide, hydrogen peroxide) • Immersion in a liquid chemical sterilant (e.g., glutaraldehyde, ortho-phthalaldehyde)
Semicritical Items		
Devices that contact intact mucous membranes	• Endoscopes/bronchoscopes • Oral, nasal, and tracheal airways • Ventilator circuits/humidifiers • Pulmonary function test (PFT) mouthpieces/tubing • Nondisposable nebulizers • Laryngoscope blades • Nondisposable resuscitation bags • Pressure, gas, or temperature probes	Sterilization or high-level disinfection via either: • Immersion in a high-level liquid disinfectant (e.g., glutaraldehyde, ortho-phthalaldehyde) • Pasteurization (immersion in hot water at > 158°F [70°C] for 30 minutes)
Noncritical Items		
Devices that touch only intact skin or do not contact the patient	• Stethoscopes* • Face masks (external) • Blood pressure cuffs • Ventilators	Detergent washing or exposure to low- or intermediate-level disinfection

*Between patients, wipe down chest piece/diaphragm with 70% alcohol prep pads, ideally keeping visibly wet for at least 10 seconds. Frequent cleaning of tubing in soapy water and headset disinfection with 70% alcohol prep pads also is recommended.

- Large-volume nebulizers (e.g., those used with aerosol masks, T-piece or trach collars)
  - Whenever possible, use prefilled, sterile, disposable nebulizers.
  - If nebulizers are not prefilled, fill with sterile water and discard remaining contents when refilling.
  - Do not drain condensate back into the reservoir or allow it to flow into the airway; use a water trap or drain to collect at a low point in the circuit.
  - Do not handle any internal components; replace if malfunctioning.
  - For nondisposable units, replace with a new sterile or high-level–disinfected unit every 24 hours.
- Small-volume nebulizers (SVNs)
  - Use only sterile fluid for nebulization; dispense fluids aseptically.
  - Whenever possible, use single-dose medications; if using multidose vials, follow manufacturer's instructions for handling.

- Between treatments on the same patient, SVNs should be cleaned, rinsed with sterile water, and air dried.
- Suctioning equipment
  - When using an open-suction system, use a sterile, single-use catheter each time. Follow the strict sterile procedure.
  - Use only sterile solutions to remove secretions from the catheter.
  - Change the suction collection tubing (up to the canister) between patients and according to institutional protocol.
  - Change collection canisters between patients and according to institutional protocol (except in short-term care units).
- Pulmonary function test (PFT) equipment (includes American Thoracic Society recommendations)
  - Do not routinely sterilize or disinfect the internal workings of closed-circuit spirometers; instead, change the mouthpiece and HEPA filter between patients.
  - If any reusable components show breath condensation, sterilize or high-level disinfect them between patients.
  - When using open-circuit devices through which the patient only exhales, disinfect or change only those elements through which rebreathing occurs.
  - Use disposable valves and HEPA filters to isolate nondisposable bedside PFT equipment from each patient; otherwise, these items must be sterilized or undergo high-level disinfection between uses.
  - To protect yourself from infection, always apply standard precautions.
  - Apply airborne precautions if there is potential for exposure to infectious agents transmitted by that route, such as tuberculosis.

Surface Disinfection

Regarding surface disinfection, the following key points apply:

- Noncritical environmental surfaces (e.g., tables, floors) should be cleaned or disinfected regularly, when spills occur, and when these surfaces are visibly soiled.
- Follow manufacturer's instructions for proper use of disinfecting (or detergent) products.
- Detergent and water are adequate for cleaning surfaces in non-patient-care areas.
- Use a low-/intermediate-level disinfectant registered by the U.S. Environmental Protection Agency (EPA) for surface disinfection in patient-care areas either where you are uncertain as to the possible contaminant or where multidrug-resistant organisms may be present.
- In units with high rates of *Clostridium difficile* infection or during an outbreak, use a dilute (5–6%) solution of sodium hypochlorite (e.g., 1:10 dilution of household bleach) for routine surface disinfection.

For decontamination of spills of blood or other potentially infectious materials:

- Use protective gloves and other PPE appropriate for this task.
- If sharps are involved, pick them up with forceps and discard in a puncture-resistant container.
- If the spill contains large amounts of blood or body fluids, first clean the visible matter with disposable absorbent material, and then discard the contaminated materials in appropriate, labeled containment (in some settings, environmental services should be contacted for implementation of the correct spill protocol).
- Disinfect the spill area using an EPA-registered tuberculocidal agent, a registered germicide with effectiveness against HIV or hepatitis B, or freshly diluted sodium hypochlorite solution.
- If sodium hypochlorite is selected, use a 1:100 dilution to decontaminate small spills (e.g., < 10 mL) and a 1:10 dilution for larger spills.

Monitor the Effectiveness of Sterilization Procedures

Mechanical, chemical, and biological techniques can be used to assess the effectiveness of sterilization procedures; generally, they are used together. **Table 7-6** summarizes these monitoring methods.

Table 7-6 Methods to Monitor Sterilization Procedures

Description	Comments
Mechanical Methods	
Assess the *cycle time*, *temperature*, and *pressure* of sterilization equipment.	Correct readings do not ensure sterilization, but incorrect readings might indicate a problem.
Chemical Indicators	
A chemical reaction causes the indicator color to change when the proper sterilizer conditions (e.g., the correct temperature or gas concentration) are achieved.	Indicator changes are visible after processing and, therefore, can provide an immediate warning as to potential problems.
Biological Indicators	
Assess whether sterilization kills bacterial spores impregnated on paper strips that are exposed to growth media and incubated after processing. Biological indicators should be included in every cycle that contains critical items; otherwise, they should be used at least once a week for each sterilizer.	The best method for verifying sterilization; the incubation period requires holding equipment until negative results are confirmed. If mechanical and chemical monitoring indicate proper processing, but culture is positive for growth, recall critical items only.

Proper Handling of Biohazardous Materials

Biohazardous materials include both noninfectious and infectious agents. The materials of most importance to RTs are infectious items such as isolation wastes, blood and blood products, and contaminated sharps and needles. Key recommendations from the CDC for the handling of infectious waste are summarized below:

- Separate infectious and noninfectious wastes at the point of generation; manage isolation wastes using the same methods as for medical wastes from other patient areas.
- Discard and contain all solid infectious wastes except sharps at their point of origin in clearly identifiable leak-proof and tear-/puncture-resistant containers marked with the biological hazards symbol.
- Prevent biohazard bags from coming into contact with sharp objects; if a biohazard bag gets contaminated or punctured, double-bag it.
- To properly handle contaminated sharps:
  - *Never* recap used needles, *never* handle them with both hands, and *never* point them toward the body; rather, use either a one-handed "scoop" technique or a mechanical device for holding the needle sheath.
  - Do *not* remove used needles from disposable syringes by hand, and do not bend, break, or otherwise manipulate used needles by hand.
  - Place all used sharps in an impervious, rigid, puncture-resistant container made for this purpose.
- Liquid wastes (e.g., blood, suction fluids) should be placed in capped or tightly stoppered bottles for transport.
- Most liquid wastes can be either inactivated using governmentally approved treatment technologies or carefully poured down a utility sink drain or toilet.
- When transporting waste or sharp containers, place them within a rigid container lined with plastic bags.

The final disposition of infectious wastes usually involves treatment by either sterilization or incineration, with the solid waste products being buried in a sanitary landfill and liquid or ground-up waste being discharged into a sanitary sewer system.

T⁴—TOP TEST-TAKING TIPS

You can improve your score on this section of the NBRC exam by reviewing these tips:

- High-level disinfection destroys vegetative bacteria, mycobacteria, fungi, and viruses but not necessarily bacterial spores.

- Nondisposable devices introduced into the bloodstream or other parts of the body are categorized as critical items requiring sterilization between uses.
- Nondisposable devices that contact intact mucous membranes (e.g., bronchoscopes, artificial airways, resuscitation bags) are categorized as semicritical items and should either be sterilized or undergo high-level disinfection between uses.
- Sterilization can be achieved with some high-level liquid disinfectants (e.g., Cidex) by prolonging the exposure time.
- When rinsing semicritical equipment after liquid disinfection, use sterile water.
- Large-volume nebulizers are a significant source for the spread of infection; whenever possible, use prefilled, sterile disposable nebulizers, and change these units every day.
- Between treatments on the same patient, small-volume nebulizers should be cleaned, rinsed with sterile water, and air dried.
- Use disposable valves and HEPA filters to isolate nondisposable bedside PFT equipment from each patient.
- To decontaminate spills of blood or other infectious materials, (1) use protective gloves and other PPE as needed, (2) clean the visible matter with disposable absorbent material (discard as hazardous waste), and (3) disinfect the area with an EPA tuberculocidal agent, an EPA germicide effective against HIV or hepatitis B, or freshly diluted sodium hypochlorite (bleach) solution.
- The best method for verifying sterilization is the use of biological indicators.
- If the chemical indicator on the packaging of a sterilized item has not changed color as expected, obtain a replacement item whose indicator is positive for proper processing.
- To properly handle a used hypodermic needle, use either a one-handed "scoop" technique to cap it or a mechanical safety device for holding the needle sheath.
- Most liquid wastes can be either inactivated using state-approved treatment technologies or carefully poured down a utility sink drain or toilet.
- Good hand hygiene is the single best way to help prevent the transmission of infections.
- During aerosol-generating procedures in patients with infections likely to be transmitted via the airborne route (e.g., TB, SARS), wear a fit-tested N95 or higher respirator in addition to following standard precautions.
- Contact precautions should be used for patients with gastrointestinal infections (including diarrhea of unknown origin and suspected or confirmed *C. difficile* infections), wound and skin infections, and multidrug-resistant infection or colonization (e.g., MRSA).
- Droplet precautions are required for patients with bacterial meningitis, whooping cough (*Bordetella pertussis*), influenza, mumps, rubella (German measles), diphtheria, group A *Streptococcus* infections, SARS, and epiglottitis (due to *Haemophilus influenzae*).
- Airborne precautions should be implemented for patients with TB, measles (rubeola), chickenpox (varicella-zoster), *Aspergillus* infections, and atypical pulmonary viral infections (e.g., SARS).
- To help minimize infection when obtaining samples from vascular lines, always comply with hand hygiene requirement; swab access ports with chlorhexidine, povidone-iodine, or alcohol; and access the ports only with sterile devices.
- Patients with atypical viral infections should be managed under combined standard, contact, and airborne precautions in an airborne infection isolation room (AIIR) with the door closed.
- Those caring for patients with atypical viral infections should use PPE that entirely covers the body (at least the upper torso) and consider using a surgical hood with an N95 respirator; make sure ventilators include expiratory HEPA filtration, and recommend sedation during the aerosol-generating procedure (e.g., intubation and bronchoscopy).

POST-TEST

To confirm your mastery of each chapter's topical content, you should create a content post-test, available online via the Navigate Premier Access for Comprehensive Respiratory Therapy Exam Preparation Guide, which contains Navigate TestPrep (access code provided with every new text). You can create multiple topical content post-tests varying in length from 10 to 20 questions, with each attempt presenting a different set of items. You can select questions from all three major NBRC TMC sections: Patient Data, Troubleshooting and Quality Control of Devices and Infection Control, and Initiation and Modification of Interventions. A score of at least 70–80% indicates that you are adequately prepared for this section of the NBRC TMC exam. If you score below 70%, you should first carefully assess your test answers (particularly your wrong answers) and the correct answer explanations. Then return to the chapter to re-review the applicable content. Only then should you reattempt a new post-test. Repeat this process of identifying your shortcomings and reviewing the pertinent content until your test results demonstrate mastery.

Perform Quality Control Procedures (Section II-C)

CHAPTER 8

Narciso E. Rodriguez

The quality of care you provide depends in part on the proper performance of the equipment you use. Quality control (QC) processes help ensure that the devices you use perform as expected. For diagnostic equipment, QC processes ensure accurate measurements. For therapeutic equipment, QC processes ensure proper device function and patient safety. The NBRC expects exam candidates to know the basics of QC as applied to the most common devices used in respiratory care. For this reason, you should plan on spending a reasonable portion of your exam preparation on this topic.

OBJECTIVES

In preparing for the shared NBRC exam content (TMC/CSE), you should demonstrate the knowledge needed to perform quality control procedures for:

1. Blood gas analyzers and hemoximeters
2. Point-of-care analyzers
3. Oxygen and specialty gas analyzers
4. Pulmonary function equipment for testing
5. Mechanical ventilators
6. Noninvasive monitors

WHAT TO EXPECT ON THIS CATEGORY OF THE NBRC EXAMS

TMC exam: 3 questions; 2 recall, 1 application
CSE exam: indeterminate number of questions; however, section II-C knowledge can appear in both CSE Information Gathering and Decision-Making sections.

WHAT YOU NEED TO KNOW: ESSENTIAL CONTENT

Key Terms and Definitions

Basic to your understanding of QC are some key terms, summarized in **Table 8-1**.

Laboratory Blood Gas and Hemoximetry Analyzers

As with most laboratory tests, QC processes for blood gas and hemoximetry analyzers focus on eliminating errors in sample collection and handling (the preanalytical phase), sample measurement (the analytical phase), and results reporting, interpretation, and application (the postanalytical phase). Here we focus primarily on QC during the preanalytical and analytical phases of blood gas and hemoximetry analysis.

Preanalytical Phase

The preanalytical phase involves all sample collection and handling procedures conducted *before* actual analysis. For this reason, you must be proficient with the techniques involved in obtaining blood samples from various sites. Also, to avoid interpretation errors, you must always document the patient's FiO_2, the O_2 delivery device, the mode of ventilation and current settings, and the results of any related assessments made at the time of sampling.

Table 8-1 Key Terms Used in Quality Control (QC)

Term	Meaning
Accuracy	The degree to which a measurement reading coincides with its true value
Analyte	A substance undergoing analysis or measurement
Analytical errors	Result errors due to mistakes made during measurement and analysis
Bias	Systematic inaccuracy—that is, consistently high or low variation from a measure's true value
Calibration	Testing and adjusting an analyzer to provide a known relationship between its measurements and the level or quantity of the substances being analyzed
Calibration verification	Measurement of control media to confirm that the calibration of the analyzer is stable throughout the lab's reportable range
Control charts	A record of the measurements of standard samples used for statistical evaluation of analyzer performance; also referred to as Levy-Jennings charts
Drift	The difference in a given measurement's value between successive analyzer calibrations
Gain	The ratio of the output/response signal of an analyzer to its input signal (the true value) over a range of measurements; equivalent to the calibration slope
Linearity	The change in error over an analyzer's measurement range; the amount of deviation from ideal "straight-line" performance
Mean	The arithmetic average of a group of measurements
Postanalytical errors	Result errors due to mistakes made in data handling, results reporting, or interpretation
Preanalytical errors	Result errors due to mistakes in the collection, handling, or storage of samples before analysis
Precision	The reproducibility or repeatability of an analyzer's results for the same analyte over multiple measurements
Reportable range	The range of values over which a laboratory can verify the accuracy of the measurements
Standard deviation (SD)	A statistical measure indicating the variability of a set of measurements
Statistical QC	The application of statistical analysis and other procedures to detect problems that could invalidate patient results

The most common preanalytical errors affecting blood gas and hemoximetry measurements are air contamination, venous admixture, and continued blood metabolism. As indicated in **Table 8-2**, these errors can yield invalid measurements, which can result in incorrect decisions and potential patient harm. To avoid these problems, you must always strive to ensure that the samples you obtain are free of these common errors.

Analytical Phase

The analytical phase of blood gas and hemoximetry measurement involves three key elements: (1) analyzer calibration and calibration verification, (2) actual sample testing, and (3) ongoing review of QC and proficiency testing results.

Analyzer Calibration and Calibration Verification

During calibration, the response of an analyzer is compared and adjusted to a known standard. The standards used to calibrate blood gas analyzers are precision gases and buffer solutions with known values for pH, P_{CO_2}, and P_{O_2}. Similarly, hemoximeter calibration involves measurement of standard solutions with known values for total Hb, HbO_2, carboxyhemoglobin (COHb), and methemoglobin (MetHb).

Calibration involves adjusting the analyzer to ensure that its response is accurate and linear—in other words, to ensure that the measured value (response) equals the known value (see **Figure 8-1**).

Table 8-2 Common Preanalytical Errors in pH/Blood Gas Analysis and Hemoximetry

Error	Effect	Recognition	Avoidance
Air contamination	• Decreases P_{CO_2} • Increases pH • Variable effect on P_{O_2}/HbO_2%*	• Visible bubbles • Results not consistent with patient condition/setting	• Expel bubbles • Do not mix samples with air bubbles • Cap syringes; seal capillary tubes quickly
Venous admixture	• Increases P_{CO_2} • Decreases pH • Decreases P_{O_2} and HbO_2%	• No pulsations as syringe fills • Results not consistent with patient condition/setting • Blood looks darker	• Do not aspirate sample • Avoid brachial/femoral sites • Use short-bevel needles
Continued metabolism	• Increases P_{CO_2} • Decreases pH • Decreases P_{O_2} and HbO_2%	• Lag time between the collection and analysis of a sample • Results not consistent with patient condition/setting	• Analyze within 30 min if in a plastic syringe (3 min for capillary samples) • Analyze immediately if the patient has high leukocyte/platelet count • If storage > 30 min, use glass syringe chilled to 0 to 4°C

*If the patient's actual Pa_{O_2} is > 150 torr, air contamination will lower the P_{O_2} and HbO_2%; if the actual Pa_{O_2} is < 150 torr, it will raise the measured values.

In this example, the precalibrated response of the analyzer is linear but positively biased. For example, at a known value of 0, the analyzer response is 30; and at a known value of 40, the response is about 80—both clearly inaccurate. Calibration requires adjusting both the offset ("balancing" or "zeroing" the analyzer) and the gain or slope of the instrument. Only after these two adjustments are made can we say that the analyzer is calibrated correctly—that the instrument response will accurately reflect the known value(s).

The method depicted in **Figure 8-1** requires a "two-point calibration," in which two different known values are used. Normal ranges used for two-point calibration of blood gas analyzers are as follows:

$$pH = 6.840 \text{ and } 7.384$$
$$P_{O_2} = 80 \text{ and } 150 \text{ torr}$$
$$P_{CO_2} = 40 \text{ and } 80 \text{ torr}$$

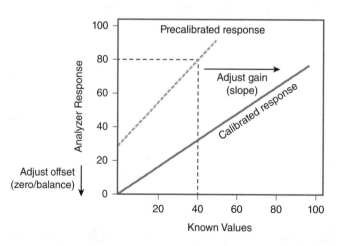

Figure 8-1 Instrument Calibration.

Modern analyzers include automated calibration routines. However, to ensure that the analyzers you use are providing accurate measurements, you must perform a *calibration verification*. Calibration verification involves analysis of prepared *control media*. Control media are analytes that are independently certified to provide a known measurement value when tested. Typically, calibration verification involves analysis of at least *three* different levels of control media spanning the full range of expected results and is conducted at least daily. In addition, calibration verification should be conducted after any instrument maintenance and whenever a question arises regarding instrument performance.

The gold standard for calibration verification of PO_2 and PCO_2 measurements is a procedure called tonometry. *Tonometry* involves exposing and equilibrating liquid media (blood/control solution) to a reference gas with known partial pressures.

Sample Testing

Upon completion of the sample test routine, you report the results. Whenever reporting any analytical test results, you also should provide a brief statement addressing test quality, including any problems encountered with the specimen or its measurement.

The procedure for "running" a blood gas sample is covered in Chapter 3.

Review of QC and Proficiency Testing Results

Comprehensive QC involves recording and continuously monitoring data using accepted statistical methods. To do so, you plot the results of control media analyses on graphs, with a separate chart constructed for each level of control and each analyte reported. The most common plotting format used for statistical QC is the Levy-Jennings chart. As depicted in **Figure 8-2**, a Levy-Jennings chart plots individual values for control media over multiple measurements and compares these values with the mean and standard deviation (SD) of the data. Typically, bounding limits are set to within ± 2 SD. Control measurements that consistently fall within these limits indicate that the analyzer is "in control" and ready for sample measurement. For example, **Figure 8-2** depicts *normal variation* in the measurement of a PCO_2 control value standardized to 40 torr (mm Hg). This variation is considered normal because it consistently falls within the ± 2 SD limits.

Control measurements that fall outside the bounding limits indicate an *analytical error*. **Figure 8-3** depicts this situation, with the observation on day 16 falling well outside the ± 2 SD bounding limit (actually almost greater than 3 SD from the mean). Single irregular values like these are relatively common and are due to *random errors* of measurement that occur with any instrument. If subsequent measures are within the control limits, no remedial action is needed. In contrast, frequent random errors like this one would indicate a lack of precision—that is, poor repeatability of the measurement. Any instrument that demonstrates poor repeatability over time is "out of control." In such cases, you would need to identify the problem, take corrective action, and confirm that the analyzer is back in control before reporting any patient results.

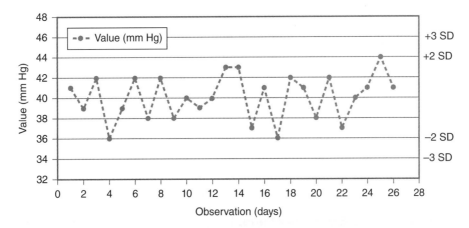

Figure 8-2 Analyzer "in Control": Levy-Jennings Chart for PcO₂ Control Value of 40 Torr. Note that all measures are within the ±2 SD limits. Hence the analyzer is "in control."

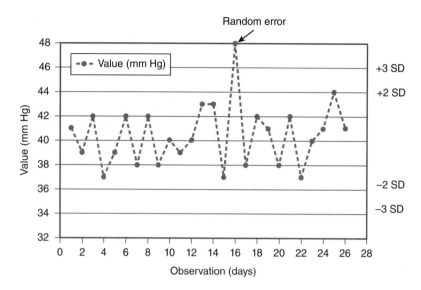

Figure 8-3 Levy-Jennings Chart for Pco$_2$ Showing a Single Random Error in an Analyzer. A single random error noticed on day 16. As long as subsequent measures are in control; no remedial action is needed.

Figure 8-4 demonstrates a different type of error, called *systematic error* or *bias*. Note that beginning with observation 20, there is an upward trend in the reported values for the 40-torr Pco$_2$ control. Over time, this trend shifts the mean above the control value, causing a positive measurement bias. Generally, bias errors are more serious than random errors, indicating either an incorrect procedure or instrument failure. As with recurrent random errors, whenever instrument bias is identified, no patient samples should be analyzed until the problem is corrected.

Table 8-3 compares the common causes and corrective actions for these two types of analytical errors.

Supplementing "in-house" QC procedures is a process called *proficiency testing*. Under proficiency testing requirements, laboratories receive unknown samples from an outside agency on a regular schedule. These samples are analyzed, and the results reported back to the sending agency.

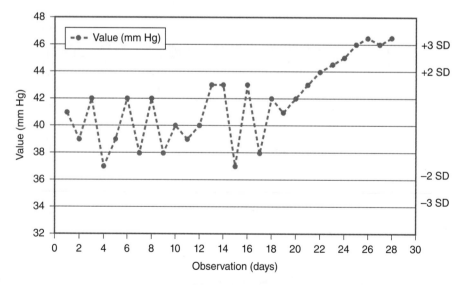

Figure 8-4 Positive Bias Error Over Time: Levy-Jennings Chart for Pco$_2$. Bias errors usually indicate faulty procedure or component failure. The analyzer should not be used until the problem is found and corrected.

Table 8-3 Comparison of Instrument Analytical Errors and Their Correction

Type of Error	Contributing Factors	Corrective Actions
Random errors	• Statistical probability • Contamination of sample • Improper handling of the sample	• Reanalyze control sample after performing a two-point calibration • If repeat quality control (QC) analysis is in control, no further action is needed • If repeat QC analysis is out of control, continue corrective actions according to the manufacturer's recommendations
Bias errors	• Contaminated buffer solutions • Incorrect gas concentrations • Component degradation/failure • Incorrect procedure	• Troubleshoot suspected problem(s) • Repair or replace faulty components • Corrective action(s) continue until an acceptable two-point calibration is achieved and QC sample values are within ± 2 SD of the mean

The agency then compares the results against its own and those of other laboratories using similar instrumentation. Discrepancies must be addressed and remediated for any lab to maintain certification, which is a prerequisite for Medicare/Medicaid reimbursement.

Point-of-Care Analyzers

Point-of-care testing (POCT) involves the collection, measurement, and reporting of selected lab tests at or near the site of patient care. The most common POCT tests that you are likely to perform are for arterial blood gases (ABGs) or combined panels that include ABG measures plus other selected values essential in managing critically ill patients such as electrolytes and blood glucose.

Key QC points applicable to POCT analyzers are as follows:

- Personnel performing POCT tests must have documented competency with the procedures and equipment.
- All POCT results must be auditable/traceable to the patient tested, the instrument and its operator, the date and time of the test, and the process used.
- Complete instrument maintenance records must be maintained.
- In terms of calibration:
  - Most POCT cartridges include solutions for automated calibration.
  - If a POCT device fails to calibrate, rerun the test with a new cartridge.
  - If a second attempt fails, remove the device from service and either obtain a replacement analyzer or send the sample to the central lab.

Most facilities also require that results obtained via POCT analysis regularly be compared with those provided by a calibrated bench-top analyzer. This is done by performing simultaneous analysis of the sample on both instruments ("inter-instrumental comparison"). Based on accumulated data and statistical rules, one can then determine if the POCT results meet the same standards for accuracy and precision as required for regular lab testing. Also, most facilities use proficiency testing to help further ensure the quality of their POCT programs.

Gas Analyzers

Oxygen Analyzers

Most O_2 analyzers use either a Clark electrode (the polarographic type) or a galvanic fuel cell to measure the P_{O_2}. Both types generally are accurate to within $\pm 2\%$ of the actual concentration. Polarographic analyzers require external power to maintain the chemical reaction at the electrode. Galvanic cells do not require external power. However, both types require external power for alarm functions.

Always follow the manufacturer's recommendations to calibrate an O_2 analyzer. However, most O_2 analyzer calibration involves four key steps (this is known as a two-point calibration):

1. Expose the sensor to a source of 100% O_2.
2. After the reading stabilizes, adjust the analyzer to 100%.
3. Remove the sensor from the 100% O_2 source.
4. After restabilization, expose the analyzer to room air and confirm a reading of 21% ($\pm$2%).

A failure to reach either 100% or 21% may indicate a damaged probe or a defective analyzer. **Table 8-4** summarizes the common causes of O_2 analyzer calibration problems and measurement errors and outlines how to correct them.

Other Gas Analyzers

In addition to O_2 analysis, you may use specialty gas analyzers to measure N_2, He, CO, and NO/NO_2 concentrations in the PFT lab or at the bedside. See Chapter 6 for details on the analysis of these gases, as well as the applicable performance standards and calibration methods.

Pulmonary Function Test Equipment

As with the analysis of blood specimens, incorrect PFT results can lead to inappropriate clinical decisions. For these reasons, an effective quality assurance program is required to make certain that PFT data are both accurate and reproducible. An effective PFT quality assurance program must include at least the following elements:

Table 8-4 Troubleshooting Polarographic and Fuel Cell O_2 Analyzers

Problem	Possible Cause	Suggested Solutions
Cannot calibrate to 21% O_2	• Probe not exposed to room air • Bad probe (electrode or cell) • Water condensation on probe membrane • Probe not connected to the analyzer	• Ensure probe is exposed to room air • Recharge/replace the probe • Dry probe membrane • Check and tighten all connections
Cannot calibrate to 100% O_2	• Low battery (polarographic) • Probe not exposed to 100% O_2 • Bad probe (electrode or cell) • Water condensation on probe membrane • Probe not connected to the analyzer	• Replace battery • Ensure probe is exposed to 100% O_2 • Recharge/replace the probe • Dry probe membrane • Check and tighten all connections
Measured %O_2 differs from the expected value	• Low battery • Analyzer not calibrated • O_2 delivery device malfunction • Bad probe (electrode or cell)	• Replace battery • Calibrate analyzer • Confirm delivery device function • Recharge or replace the probe
Analyzer reads 0% O_2	• Low battery • Probe not connected to the analyzer • Dead battery • Dead probe	• Replace battery • Check and tighten all connections • Replace battery • Recharge or replace the probe

Modified from Branson RD, Hess D, Chatburn RL. *Respiratory care equipment* (2nd ed.). Philadelphia: Lippincott; 1998.

- Proper technician training and review
- Accurate spirometry equipment
- Daily spirometer checks
- Individual maneuver validity checks
- Monthly spirometry quality reports
- Documentation of equipment maintenance

The most likely emphasis on the NBRC exams for PFT QC is ensuring the accuracy of the equipment and obtaining accurate results.

Accuracy of PFT Equipment

To ensure the accuracy of PFT equipment, you need to confirm volume and flow values, check the volume and flow linearity, assess system leakage, and validate time measurements. **Table 8-5** summarizes the QC tests used to confirm these measurements, as recommended by the American Thoracic Society (ATS) and the European Respiratory Society (ERS).

If using a volumetric spirometer (bell or bellows systems), you should check it daily for leaks (*before* the volume calibration check) and after any needed cleaning/reassembly activity. To do so, follow these steps:

1. Inject approximately 3 L of room air into the spirometer.
2. Occlude the breathing circuit at the patient interface.
3. Use the manufacturer's recommended method to pressurize the system to 3 cm H_2O.
4. Observe for any change in volume over 1 minute.

Depending on the device, a weight, spring, or rubber band is used to pressurize the system. When pressurized, the system should lose no more than 10 mL/min. Larger losses indicate a leak, which must be corrected before patient testing. Common sources of leaks include loose connections, cracked tubing, and missing or damaged seals.

Volume calibration requires a large-volume (3.0-L) calibration syringe. The ATS volume accuracy standard for diagnostic spirometers is ±3% or ±50 mL, whichever is larger. On computerized systems, you may need to enter the ambient temperature and altitude or barometric pressure before calibration. You also may need to make sure that the body temperature pressure, saturated (BTPS) correction is *deactivated*, otherwise, the calibrating volume will be approximately 10% higher than actual. If the device uses an electronic transducer to measure flow, you also need to zero it before volume or flow calibration. **Figure 8-5** depicts a normal volume calibration graph, showing a percent error computation that falls within the ATS accuracy standard for a 3.0-L calibrating syringe (between 2.91 and 3.09 L).

Table 8-5 Pulmonary Function Test (PFT) Equipment Quality Control

Test	Minimum Interval	Action
Leaks	Daily	3 cm H_2O constant pressure for 1 minute (< 10 mL leak)
Volume	Daily	Calibration check with a 3-L syringe check (±3% or ±50 mL)
Volume linearity	Quarterly	1-L increments with a calibrating syringe over the entire volume range
Flow linearity	Weekly	Test at least three different flow ranges
Time	Quarterly	Mechanical recorder checks with a stopwatch
Software	New versions	Log the installation date and perform a test using a known subject (i.e., a "biological control")
This material has not been reviewed by European Respiratory Society prior to release; therefore the European Respiratory Society may not be responsible for any errors, omissions or inaccuracies, or for any consequences arising there from, in the content. Reproduced with permission of the European Respiratory Society. © European Respiratory Journal Aug 2005, 26 (2) 319–338; DOI: 10.1183/09031936.05.00034805.		

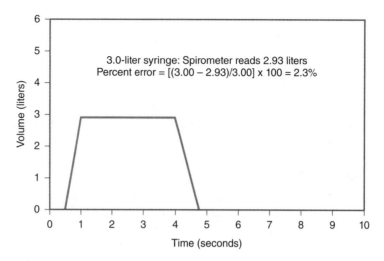

Figure 8-5 Plot of Volume Calibration of a Spirometer Exhibiting Expected Accuracy. Data from the National Institute for Occupational Safety and Health. *NIOSH spirometry training guide—unit three. The quality assurance program.* Publication No. 2004-154c. Atlanta, GA: Centers for Disease Control and Prevention; 2003.

If you obtain a low volume (less than 2.91 L), first repeat the leak check. If you obtain a high volume (more than 3.09 L), recheck the volume/flow zeroing, make sure that BTPS correction is OFF, and confirm that the temperatures of the syringe and spirometer are the same. Do not proceed with patient testing unless you can (1) identify the cause of the inaccurate reading and (2) obtain an accurate volume calibration upon repeat measurement. The gold standard for flow calibration is a computer-controlled air pump that generates standard expiratory waveforms. When using this device, the recommended accuracy standard is ±5% of the reading or ±0.2 L/sec, whichever is greater. An acceptable alternative for flow calibration is to inject the full volume from the 3.0-L syringe into the spirometer using three different time intervals—for example, 0.5 second (about 6 L/sec), 6 seconds (about 0.5 L/sec), and somewhere in between. Volume linearity is confirmed if the recorded volume deviates by no more than 100 mL from the 3.0-L target volume. Computerized spirometers typically include prompted routines to guide you through this process and maintain the appropriate time interval or flow.

You should record the leak test and volume and flow calibration results daily on a QC log. If repeated checks reveal inaccuracies for which you cannot identify any mechanical cause, you will need to recalibrate the device.

Obtaining Valid Test Results

Because forced expiratory maneuvers are technique dependent, obtaining accurate data depends on (1) proper patient instruction and coaching and (2) recognition and correction of patient performance errors. *Your goal is to obtain at least three error-free maneuvers that meet basic acceptability standards.* A forced vital capacity (FVC) maneuver meets acceptability standards if it is free of the following common errors:

- A slow or a false start to the maneuver (back-extrapolated volume ≥ 5% of FVC or 150 mL)
- Coughing during the maneuver
- Breathing during the maneuver
- Variable effort (e.g., prematurely ending exhalation)
- Exhalation time less than 6 seconds

Although many computerized spirometers automatically check the acceptability of each maneuver according to these criteria, the NBRC expects that you can recognize these problems via inspection of the FVC graph. **Table 8-6** depicts the most common validity errors you will encounter when measuring a patient's FVC.

After ensuring acceptability, you need to confirm the reproducibility of the patient's efforts. Efforts are reproducible *if the two largest values for both the FVC and the FEV₁ are within 0.150 L (150 mL) of each other*. If the effort fails to meet both criteria, you must continue testing until either both are met or the patient cannot continue.

Table 8-6 Common Validity Errors Occurring During Measurement of Forced Vital Capacity (FVC)

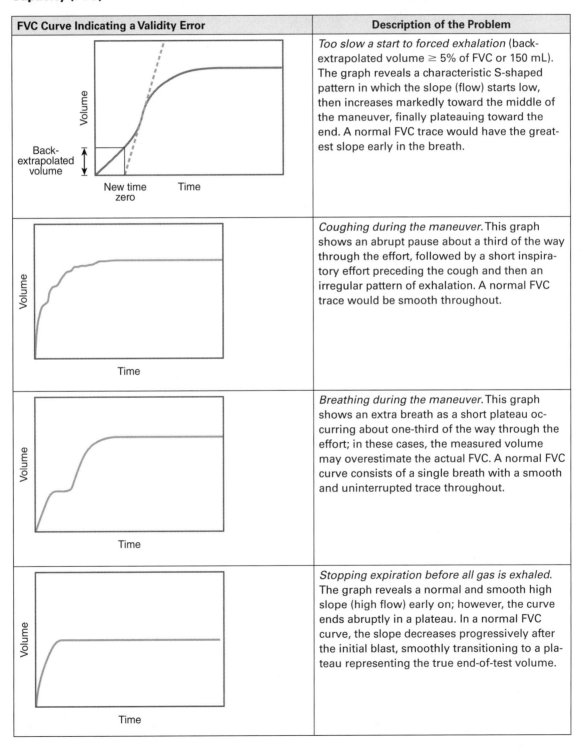

FVC Curve Indicating a Validity Error	Description of the Problem
	Too slow a start to forced exhalation (back-extrapolated volume $\geq$ 5% of FVC or 150 mL). The graph reveals a characteristic S-shaped pattern in which the slope (flow) starts low, then increases markedly toward the middle of the maneuver, finally plateauing toward the end. A normal FVC trace would have the greatest slope early in the breath.
	Coughing during the maneuver. This graph shows an abrupt pause about a third of the way through the effort, followed by a short inspiratory effort preceding the cough and then an irregular pattern of exhalation. A normal FVC trace would be smooth throughout.
	Breathing during the maneuver. This graph shows an extra breath as a short plateau occurring about one-third of the way through the effort; in these cases, the measured volume may overestimate the actual FVC. A normal FVC curve consists of a single breath with a smooth and uninterrupted trace throughout.
	Stopping expiration before all gas is exhaled. The graph reveals a normal and smooth high slope (high flow) early on; however, the curve ends abruptly in a plateau. In a normal FVC curve, the slope decreases progressively after the initial blast, smoothly transitioning to a plateau representing the true end-of-test volume.

Mechanical Ventilators

Ventilator QC involves a procedure called *operational verification*. Operational verification of non-computerized ventilators is performed manually following the manufacturer's recommendations. Most microprocessor-based ventilators include semiautomated self-test programs for operational verification.

Manual Ventilator Operational Verification

Table 8-7 outlines the basic manual operational verification procedure for noncomputerized ventilators, adapted from recommendations disseminated by the Emergency Care Research Institute.

Operational Verification of Computerized Ventilators

Most computer-controlled ventilators perform two types of operational verifications: a power-on-self-test (POST) and an extended self-test (EST). Both QC procedures should be performed according to the manufacturer's recommendations.

A POST generally tests microprocessor function, zeros the sensors, and performs some basic checks related to patient functions, such as leak tests. *You should always confirm a successful POST procedure before applying a ventilator to a patient and whenever you change the circuit.*

Typically, an EST includes the POST, followed by a series of more comprehensive function checks. *You should perform an EST between each application of a ventilator on different patients.* Extended self-testing of ventilators also should be documented in writing, with all records maintained as part of the QC program. Any ventilator that fails self-testing should be taken out of service for repair and replaced with one that has completed operational verification successfully.

Noninvasive Monitors

Pulse Oximeters

Pulse oximeters measure *relative* light intensities, as opposed to absolute values. For this reason, they do not require "true value" calibration, as previously described for blood gas analyzers. Instead, the following simple operational verification procedure is sufficient:

1. Connect the device to a healthy person.
2. Compare the pulse reading with the actual pulse measured manually.
3. Check and confirm a SpO_2 reading of 97–100%.
4. Confirm loss of signal detection by removing the device.

An incorrect pulse rate, SpO_2 below 97%, or failure to detect loss of signal indicates a malfunctioning oximeter that should be taken out of service. **Table 8-8** identifies other common problems with oximeters and their solutions.

Transcutaneous P_{CO_2}/P_{O_2} Monitors

The selection, use, calibration, and troubleshooting of transcutaneous P_{CO_2}/P_{O_2} monitors are covered in Chapter 4. Noteworthy is the fact that this technology has continuously improved over the past several decades, making these systems easier and more reliable to use. In particular, sensors are smaller, require less frequent changing/calibration (twice daily) and membrane replacement (at least every two weeks), operate at lower temperatures (42°C), and can achieve capillary arterialization in as little as 3 minutes.

Capnographs

Chapter 3 reviews the basic procedure for setup and use of capnographs. Here we focus on how to ensure that a capnograph provides accurate data.

To obtain accurate CO_2 measurements with a capnograph, you must properly set up the device, calibrate it, and maintain it while in use. Setup should follow the manufacturer's recommendations.

Table 8-7 Manual Operational Verification of Noncomputerized Ventilators

Component or Function	Operational Verification Procedure (Ventilator Not in Use)
Battery test/power loss alarm	With the unit turned on, disconnect and then reconnect the power source. The machine's battery backup and disconnect alarms should function appropriately.
Fio_2/O_2 analyzer	See the "Gas Analyzers" section in this chapter.
Audible and visual alarms	Gas supply: disconnect the high-pressure O_2 supply hose and, separately, the air hose (if used). The appropriate alarm(s) should result. Reconnect the hoses.
	Low-pressure, low-exhaled-volume, disconnect alarms: connect the ventilator to a test lung and set a stable minute volume; momentarily disconnect the circuit to check for the appropriate activation of all alarms.
	Apnea alarm: connect the ventilator to a test lung with the synchronized intermittent mandatory ventilation (SIMV) rate = 2/min and trigger the ventilator 8–12 times, then cease triggering to confirm appropriate activation of the alarm.
	High-pressure alarm: momentarily occlude the circuit to check for the appropriate activation of all audible and visual alarms.
	Inverse I:E ratio alarm: momentarily adjust the peak flow to create an inverse-ratio condition and confirm appropriate activation of the alarm.
Proximal airway pressure display	Connect the ventilator to a test lung and momentarily disconnect the pressure line or inspiratory limb of the circuit; the pressure display should read zero (±1 cm H_2O). Set the positive end-expiratory pressure (PEEP) level to 10 cm H_2O and trigger several breaths; the pressure display should rise and then return to the appropriate baseline (±1 cm H_2O) at the end of each breath.
PEEP control	Connect the ventilator to a test lung, set a PEEP level of 5 cm H_2O, and trigger several breaths; the pressure display should rise and then return to 5 cm H_2O (±1 cm H_2O) at the end of each breath. Repeat at PEEP = 10 cm H_2O and PEEP = 15 cm H_2O.
Leak tests	Occlusion method: occlude the patient connection, set the pressure limit to its maximum and the peak flow to its minimum, and initiate a 200- to 300-mL breath (adult ventilators). The pressure limit should reach its maximum, and the high-pressure alarm should activate.
	Plateau pressure method: set the inspiratory pause to 2 seconds or longer. When the ventilator triggers, observe the plateau pressure; a drop of 10% or more during the pause indicates a leak.
Modes	Use a test lung to verify proper operation of all ventilator modes.
Ventilator rate (and rate display)	Count the number of breaths delivered during a convenient time interval, timed using a clock or a watch with a second hand. The measured rate should be within one breath per minute of the rate set and rate display.
Delivered volume	Set the ventilator to a specific volume, connect a respirometer to the ventilator outlet, and trigger the ventilator; all measurements should be within $\pm5\%$ of the set volume.
Volume display	Connect a test lung to the circuit, cycle the machine, and compare the measured exhaled tidal volume and minute volume to their respective settings.
Sensitivity	Put the ventilator into an assist mode. Squeeze and release the test lung; an inspiration should result when the airway pressure or flow drops to the set sensitivity level.
Filters	Ensure that a high-efficiency particulate air (HEPA) filter is present on the main inspiratory line.

Modified from the Emergency Care Research Institute. Minimum requirements for ventilator testing. *Health Devices.* 1998;27(9–10):363–364.

Table 8-8 Common Operational Problems with Oximeters and Their Solutions

Problem	Solution
The oximeter continues to "search" but cannot find a pulse, or there is a pulse displayed but no SpO$_2$	• Readjust the sensor or apply it to a new site with better perfusion. • Check and confirm that the detector "windows" are clean. • Remove nail polish if present. • Make sure the sensor is plugged into the monitor. • Check the sensor for damage, and replace if needed.
The heart rate and SpO$_2$ readings fluctuate rapidly	• Usually due to motion artifact (resolved when the patient stops moving). • Use an oximeter with Masimo signal extraction technology (SET).
The oximeter reading seems to be inaccurate	• Check whether the oximeter pulse rate is the same as that determined by a cardiac monitor; if different, the sensor may need to be adjusted or replaced. • Check and confirm that the sensor is shielded from bright light. • Remove nail polish if present. • Check and confirm that the sensor fitting is not too tight (can cause venous pooling/pulsation and falsely low SpO$_2$s).
The SpO$_2$ differs from that provided in a blood gas report	• Remember that an arterial blood gas (ABG) SaO$_2$ value usually is a computed rather than measured value; it is better to compare the SpO$_2$ to a hemoximeter's SaO$_2$ reading. • Use the difference between the SaO$_2$ and SpO$_2$ to "calibrate" the oximeter.

The setup, calibration, and maintenance procedures vary depending on whether the capnograph uses mainstream or sidestream technology.

Capnographs that employ mainstream sensors are used primarily for intubated patients, with the sensor placed at the airway connection. *Placement distal to the airway can result in inaccurate measurements due to rebreathing.* To prevent condensation from affecting the reading, most mainstream sensors are heated. For this reason, you must provide the recommended warm-up time. Accurate readings also require a sensor that is the proper size for the patient.

Capnographs using sidestream technology can be applied to intubated patients but are most useful for monitoring nonintubated patients. Newer low-flow sidestream capnographs that employ disposable nasal sampling cannulas can be used with infants, children, and adults. The primary problem with sidestream systems is occlusion of the sampling tubing with condensate. Manufacturers may address this problem by using water traps, moisture-absorbing filters, and water-absorbing Nafion tubing. Obstruction also can occur if the tube becomes kinked. Use of the recommended condensate prevention methods and proper tube placement can help avoid occlusion of sidestream sampling systems.

Most capnographs automatically zero themselves at start-up and during regular use by aspirating air through a CO$_2$ scrubber. As with ABG analyzer calibration, this one-point method adjusts only the offset (baseline drift) and does not properly correct instrument gain—a step that is required for accurate CO$_2$ readings. To assess and adjust instrument gain, you need to measure a known CO$_2$%. Most capnographs use a precision gas mixture of 5% CO$_2$ for this "high" calibration, equivalent to a PCO$_2$ of 38 torr at sea level/ambient temperature and pressure, dry (ATPD) conditions. Because aspiration through the sampling tube creates a pressure difference that can affect the measurement, sidestream capnograph calibration must be performed using the same setup used on the patient.

Also, as with ABG gas analyzers, to *verify* calibration, you need to confirm accuracy at *three levels* of measurement, usually by adding a high-precision gas with 10% CO$_2$ (PCO$_2$ = 76 mm Hg) to the analysis. Because capnographs are calibrated under ATPD conditions but measure CO$_2$ under BTPS conditions, the calibration routine must account for the difference in values.

T⁴—TOP TEST-TAKING TIPS

You can improve your score on this section of the NBRC exam by reviewing these tips:

- If an O_2 analyzer fails a two-point calibration, replace the probe.
- Water condensate on O_2 analyzer probes can cause inaccurate measurements.
- When submitting an ABG sample for analysis, you must document the patient's FiO_2, the O_2 delivery device, the mode of ventilation, and the results of any related assessments.
- Air contamination of an ABG sample will lower the PCO_2 and increase the pH (effect on PO_2 depends on patient's actual value); continued metabolism will increase the PCO_2 and decrease the pH and PO_2.
- To avoid ABG error caused by continued metabolism, analyze samples in plastic syringes within 30 minutes (3 minutes for capillary samples); if analysis will be delayed by more than 30 minutes, use glass syringes chilled to 0 to 4°C.
- To provide accurate measurement of ABG samples, a blood gas analyzer must undergo frequent two-point calibration of pH, PCO_2, and PO_2.
- In addition to frequent two-point calibration (usually automated), blood analyzers must undergo daily calibration verification using three different levels of control media.
- The typical limits for control media analysis for a blood gas analyzer are ±2 standard deviations (SD); control measurements consistently within these limits indicate that the analyzer is "in control" and ready for use; a control value falling outside ±2 SD indicates an analytical error.
- Frequent control values that *randomly* appear above and below ±2 SD indicate poor repeatability/precision; instruments that demonstrate poor repeatability over time are "out of control" and require correction before analysis of patient samples resumes.
- An upward or downward trend in control values outside the ±2 SD limits represents a *bias* error; bias errors are more serious than random errors, indicating either incorrect procedure or instrument component failure, either of which must be corrected before analysis of patient samples resumes.
- Proficiency testing involves "blind" analysis of samples provided by an external agency; any discrepancies in the analysis must be resolved for the laboratory to maintain certification.
- The best way to validate point-of-care testing (POCT) instrument measurements is to simultaneously analyze the sample on a calibrated bench-top analyzer ("inter-instrumental comparison").
- Volume calibration of a spirometer should be conducted daily using a 3-L syringe with BTPS correction off; the accuracy standard is ±3% or ±50 mL, whichever is larger.
- When measuring forced expiratory volumes and flows, you need to obtain at least three maneuvers that are free of common errors such as a slow or a false start, coughing or breathing during the maneuver, and prematurely ending exhalation.
- After ensuring that the maneuvers are error-free, you also need to confirm the reproducibility of the patient's efforts; efforts are reproducible if the two largest values for both the FVC and the FEV_1 are within 0.150 L (150 mL) of each other.
- To perform a leak test on a ventilator, either use the occlusion method (max pressure limit, low flow, and volume) to verify activation of the high-pressure alarm or verify < 10% drop in pressure during a prolonged inspiratory pause.
- Always confirm a successful power-on-self-test (POST) before applying a ventilator to a patient and whenever you change the circuit; perform an extended self-test between each application of a ventilator on different patients.
- To confirm pulse oximeter function, perform an operational verification check using a normal person as a "biological" control.
- If oximeter readings appear to be inaccurate, (1) check pulse rate against the cardiac monitor, (2) check if the sensor is shielded from bright light, and (3) check if sensor fitting is too tight.
- Capnographs automatically "zero" themselves by aspirating air through a CO_2 scrubber (one-point calibration); two-point calibration requires measuring a known CO_2%, typically a precision gas mixture of 5% CO_2, equivalent to a PCO_2 of 38 torr at sea level, with an expected accuracy of ±0.3%, or a range of 4.7–5.3% (36–40 torr).

POST-TEST

To confirm your mastery of each chapter's topical content, you should create a content post-test, available online via the Navigate Premier Access for Comprehensive Respiratory Therapy Exam Preparation Guide, which contains Navigate TestPrep (access code provided with every new text). You can create multiple topical content post-tests varying in length from 10 to 20 questions, with each attempt presenting a different set of items. You can select questions from all three major NBRC TMC sections: Patient Data, Troubleshooting and Quality Control of Devices and Infection Control, and Initiation and Modification of Interventions. A score of at least 70–80% indicates that you are adequately prepared for this section of the NBRC TMC exam. If you score below 70%, you should first carefully assess your test answers (particularly your wrong answers) and the correct answer explanations. Then return to the chapter to re-review the applicable content. Only then should you reattempt a new post-test. Repeat this process of identifying your shortcomings and reviewing the pertinent content until your test results demonstrate mastery.

CHAPTER 9

Maintain a Patent Airway Including the Care of Artificial Airways (Section III-A)

Albert J. Heuer

Maintaining the airway and caring for artificial airways are critical components of good respiratory care. For this reason, the NBRC devotes a specific section on its exams to this topic. You must be familiar with the many types of artificial airways available and know how to properly place, maintain, troubleshoot, and remove these devices. In addition, because normal airway function depends on proper humidification, you also must be proficient in this area.

OBJECTIVES

In preparing for the shared NBRC exam content (TMC/CSE), you should demonstrate the knowledge needed to:

1. Properly position a patient
2. Recognize a difficult airway
3. Establish and manage a patient's airway using:
   a. nasopharyngeal and oropharyngeal airways
   b. esophageal-tracheal tubes and supraglottic airways (King, LMA)
   c. endotracheal tubes
   d. tracheostomy tubes
   e. laryngectomy tubes
   f. speaking valves
   g. devices to assist with intubation
4. Perform tracheostomy care
5. Exchange artificial airways
6. Maintain adequate humidification
7. Initiate protocols to prevent ventilator-associated infections
8. Perform extubations

WHAT TO EXPECT ON THIS CATEGORY OF THE NBRC EXAMS

TMC exam: 10 questions; 3 recall, 4 application, 3 analysis
CSE exam: indeterminate number of questions; however, section III-A knowledge is a prerequisite to succeed on the CSE, especially on Information Gathering sections.

WHAT YOU NEED TO KNOW: ESSENTIAL CONTENT

Proper Positioning of a Patient

Proper patient positioning is key in emergency airway management. It is important in preventing ventilator-associated pneumonia (VAP) and can help to manage conditions that cause hypoxemia, airway obstruction, or excessive respiratory tract secretions. **Table 9-1** summarizes the conditions requiring special positioning and the rationale for each.

Recognition of a Difficult Airway

A difficult airway occurs when a clinician cannot effectively ventilate a patient with a bag-valve-mask (BVM) device or has trouble with airway insertion. The key to avoiding serious complications

Table 9-1 Conditions Necessitating Special Patient Positions

Condition or Situation	Position	Rationale
Resuscitation	Head-tilt/chin-lift maneuver (all rescuers)	Helps displace the tongue away from the posterior pharyngeal wall
	Jaw-thrust maneuver without head extension (healthcare provider)	Minimizes neck movement in patients with a suspected cervical spine injury
	Recovery position (lateral recumbent) with the patient placed on his or her side and with the lower arm in front of the body	Helps maintain a patent airway and reduces the risk of airway obstruction and aspiration in unresponsive adults with normal breathing and effective circulation
Shock	Elevate the lower extremities (aka modified Trendelenburg)	Mobilizes fluid from the lower extremities to the core during hypotensive episodes. Note that because full Trendelenburg impairs gas exchange and increases the risk of aspiration, it no longer is recommended.
Endotracheal intubation	"Sniffing" position (i.e., neck hyperextended and pillow or towel under the head or shoulders)	Aligns upper airway structures with larynx and trachea, facilitating tube insertion; *not to be used with a suspected cervical spine injury*
Prevent ventilator-associated pneumonia (VAP)	Elevating the head of the bed by 30 degrees or more (unless contraindicated)	Helps prevent gastric reflux aspiration and improves the distribution of ventilation and the efficiency of diaphragmatic action
Acute respiratory distress syndrome (ARDS)	Prone position if severe ARDS (P/F ratio < 150 with Fio_2 > 0.60 and PEEP ≥ 5 cm H_2O)	Recruits collapsed lung units and shifts blood flow away from shunt regions, thereby improving V/Q balance and oxygenation
Unilateral lung disease	Left or right lateral decubitus position with the *good lung down**	Improves oxygenation by diverting blood flow and ventilation to the dependent (good) lung
Postural drainage	Varies according to lobe or segment being drained (see Chapter 10 for details)	Vertical alignment of the lobar or segmental bronchus facilitates drainage into the mainstem bronchi for removal by coughing or suctioning
Directed coughing	Sitting or semi-Fowler's position, with knees slightly flexed, forearms relaxed, feet supported	Aids exhalation and facilitates thoracic compression during coughing

P/F, Pao_2/Fio_2 ratio; PEEP, positive end-expiratory pressure; V/Q, ventilation-perfusion ratio.

*Exceptions to the "keep the good lung down" rule include lung abscess or bleeding, in which the good lung is kept in the upward position to prevent blood or pus from entering the good lung. Likewise, in infants with unilateral pulmonary interstitial emphysema (PIE), the good lung normally is kept on top.

associated with a difficult airway is to recognize the problem quickly, then manage the problem. Chapter 15 reviews the management of lost or obstructed airways. Here we focus on identifying the problem.

Prior knowledge of the patient and situation can help identify the likelihood of difficult airway management. Common patient factors or conditions associated with a difficult airway include the following:

- Micrognathia (small/receding jaw)
- Morbid obesity
- Tonsillar hypertrophy
- Macroglossia (large tongue [e.g., Down syndrome])

- Subglottic stenosis (also seen in Down syndrome)
- Cervical spine kyphosis
- Mediastinal or neck masses
- Large neck circumference
- History of obstructive sleep apnea (OSA)
- Prior tracheostomy or intubation
- Any obstruction causing stridor

Common situations that make airway insertion difficult even with normal anatomy include extreme patient agitation or anxiety, stimulant drug abuse or overdose (e.g., cocaine, methamphetamine), and when uninterrupted compressions must be performed during cardiopulmonary resuscitation (CPR).

Visual inspection of the oropharynx (mouth open, tongue out) also can help predict a difficult airway. **Table 9-2** outlines a common tool used to assess intubation difficulty, the Mallampati classification system. According to this system, patients with a Class III or IV airway will be difficult to intubate.

A similar "grading" scale (Cormack-Lehane) can be used when performing direct laryngoscopy. On this scale, a Grade III view allows visualization of the epiglottis *only*, with Grade IV indicating that the epiglottis cannot be visualized. The likelihood of difficult intubation increases to over 90% with a Grade IV view.

Unfortunately, not all difficult airways can be anticipated in advance. Some are discovered only when attempting BVM ventilation or when intubating via direct laryngoscopy.

The M-O-A-N-S mnemonic can help the clinician predict difficult BVM ventilation. M-O-A-N-S stands for *M*ask seal, *O*besity/Obstruction, *A*ged, *N*o teeth (edentulous), *S*tiff lungs. **Table 9-3** provides details on these factors.

Table 9-2 Mallampati Classification for Predicting Difficult Intubation

Class	Description
I	Can visualize the soft palate, uvula, and pillars/tonsils (easiest intubation)
II	Can visualize the soft palate and portion of the uvula (easy intubation)
III	Can visualize the soft palate and only base of the uvula (difficult intubation)
IV	Can only visualize the hard palate (very difficult intubation)

Table 9-3 M-O-A-N-S Mnemonic for Predicting Difficult Bag-Valve-Mask (BVM) Ventilation

*M*ask seal	A good mask seal requires reasonably normal anatomy, absence of facial hair, no vomitus or excessive blood, a properly sized mask, and the ability of the user to properly secure and seal the mask over the mouth and nose.
*O*besity/ Obstruction	Obesity (body mass index [BMI] > 26) is associated with difficult BVM ventilation. Excessive upper airway tissue and decreased compliance due to the chest wall and abdominal weight restrict inflation. Third-trimester pregnancy creates some of the same problems. Upper airway obstruction also makes BVM ventilation more difficult by increasing both inspiratory and expiratory flow resistance.
*A*ged	As patients age, the general loss of tissue elasticity and the increased incidence of restrictive or obstructive pulmonary disease make BVM ventilation more difficult.
*N*o teeth	Teeth provide a framework that enhances the mask seal. For this reason, edentulousness creates difficulty in creating a seal while providing BVM ventilation.
*S*tiff lungs	"Stiffness" refers to impedance to ventilation as reflected by the need for higher-than-normal inspiratory pressures to ventilate the lungs. This can include conditions that increase airway resistance (such as asthma) and those that decrease lung or thoracic compliance (e.g., pulmonary edema, obesity)

Once BVM ventilation begins, the following signs indicate difficulty with the airway:

- Absent/inadequate chest rise or breath sounds
- Gastric air entry or gastric distention
- Cyanosis or inadequate SpO_2
- Absent or inadequate exhaled CO_2
- Hemodynamic changes associated with hypoxemia or hypercapnia (e.g., hypertension, tachycardia, arrhythmias)

In terms of predicting difficult intubation, the L-E-M-O-N mnemonic is useful. As described in **Table 9-4**, L-E-M-O-N stands for *L*ook externally, *E*valuate external anatomy, *M*allampati classification, *O*besity/*O*bstruction, *N*eck mobility.

Establishing and Managing a Patient's Airway

Insertion of Oropharyngeal (OPA) and Nasopharyngeal Airways (NPA)

The indications, selection, use, and troubleshooting of oropharyngeal and nasopharyngeal airways are covered elsewhere; here we focus on their insertion and management.

The first step in inserting an oropharyngeal or a nasopharyngeal airway is to select the proper size, which is based primarily on patient age (**Table 9-5**). Note that too large or small an airway can

Table 9-4 L-E-M-O-N Assessment for Predicting Difficult Intubation

*L*ook externally	Abnormal facial anatomy (e.g., micrognathia), body habitus (e.g., obesity/large neck), external masses (e.g., goiter), and facial/neck trauma all can make intubation difficult.
*E*valuate external anatomy	Certain *external* anatomic measures help predict ease or difficulty of intubation: (1) the size of the mouth opening, (2) the size of the mandible, and (3) the location of the larynx relative to the base of the tongue.
*M*allampati classification	Mallampati Class I or II predicts easy intubation, Class III predicts difficulty, and Class IV predicts extreme difficulty. *Note*: If the patient cannot fully cooperate with the oral inspection, one should at least attempt to assess the size of the tongue relative to the oropharynx; a large tongue/small oropharynx indicates difficult intubation.
*O*besity/ *O*bstruction	Excessive upper airway tissue in the obese patient makes visualization of the glottis more difficult; any abnormal masses (e.g., tumors), swelling (e.g., edema, hematoma), or tissue trauma also can obstruct the view of the glottis or block the passage of an endotracheal tube (ETT).
*N*eck mobility	Suspected or confirmed cervical spine trauma or cervical collar use prevents the use of the "sniffing" position, making intubation more difficult. So too do many nonacute conditions, such as rheumatoid arthritis, ankylosing spondylitis, and even degenerative joint disease associated with aging.

Table 9-5 Guidelines for Oropharyngeal and Nasopharyngeal Airway Sizing

Patient Age or Size	Oropharyngeal Airway	Nasopharyngeal Airway
Premature infant	40 mm/00	NA
Newborn–1 year	50 mm/0	3 (12-Fr)
1–3 years	60 mm/1	3 (12-Fr)
3–6 years	60 mm/1	4 (16-Fr)
8 years	70 mm/2	5 (20-Fr)
12 years	70 mm/2	5 (20-Fr)
16 years	80 mm/3	6 (24-Fr)
Adult female	80 mm/3	6 (24-Fr)
Adult male	90 mm/4	7 (28-Fr)
Large adult	100 mm/5	8–9 (32- to 36-Fr)

worsen obstruction. To avoid this problem, when using an oropharyngeal airway, tailor the size to the patient by measuring from the corner of the mouth to the angle of the jaw or from the corner of the mouth to the earlobe.

To place and secure the selected oropharyngeal airway:

- Insert the airway either with the distal tip pointing up or from the side, then advance to the base of the tongue.
- Rotate the airway into the midline so that it holds the tongue away from the posterior pharynx.
- Avoid taping over the center or side opening of the airway (may be used to pass a suction catheter).

If after proper insertion of an oropharyngeal airway, the airway obstruction is not relieved:

- Remove and reinsert the airway and confirm that it extends past the base of the tongue.
- Recheck the size of the airway:
  ∘ If the airway is too large/long, it will block the patient's airway.
  ∘ If it is too small/short, it can force the tongue against the posterior pharynx.

To avoid vomiting and aspiration, if the patient gags or otherwise does not tolerate the airway, remove it immediately. *Oropharyngeal airways are not recommended for awake, conscious patients.* Instead, consider a nasopharyngeal airway, or reposition the patient using the head-tilt/chin-lift or jaw-thrust maneuver.

As with the oropharyngeal tubes, sizing of nasopharyngeal airway is based on the patient's age (see Table 9-5). To individually tailor the size, measure from the nares to the earlobe (some devices have an adjustable flange to customize the length). In general, you should select the largest diameter that will pass through the inferior meatus without force.

To place and secure the selected nasopharyngeal airway:

- Before insertion (if time permits), advance a suction catheter to see which meatus is more patent.
- Lubricate the airway with water-soluble jelly before inserting.
- Tilt the patient's head back slightly, and advance the airway without force along the floor of the nasal passage (inferior meatus) until the flange meets the exterior nostril.
- If the tube has a left or right cut bevel (typically labeled "R" or "L"), make sure the bevel faces toward the nasal septum (medially).
- If the patient experiences excessive bleeding or tissue trauma, notify the physician immediately.

If a lubricated nasopharyngeal airway does not pass through the selected nasal passage, the patient may have a deviated septum or nasal polyps. To overcome this problem, insert the airway through the opposite naris. If that is unsuccessful, select and insert a smaller airway.

When suctioning through a nasopharyngeal airway, always lubricate the catheter and secure the airway to prevent it from moving back and forth. If a lubricated catheter does not pass, first check whether mucosal swelling may be compressing the airway. If so, do not try to replace the airway, but instead notify the physician. Otherwise, either remove the airway and reinsert it in the other naris or replace it with a larger one.

Esophageal–Tracheal Tubes and Supraglottic Airways

Oral endotracheal intubation is the procedure of choice in emergencies requiring airway protection and artificial ventilation. However, the NBRC also expects candidates to be proficient with the insertion and management of esophageal–tracheal tubes and supraglottic airways. These airways create a path to the trachea by blocking entrance to the esophagus. Those most likely to appear on the NBRC exams are the Combitube, the King laryngeal tube, and the laryngeal mask airway (LMA). The indications, selection, and use of these specialized airways are covered in Chapter 6. Here we focus on their insertion and management.

Esophageal–Tracheal Combitube (ETC)

As depicted in **Figure 9-1**, the esophageal–tracheal Combitube (ETC) is a double-tube, double-cuff airway. This design ensures adequate ventilation regardless of whether the airway ends up in the

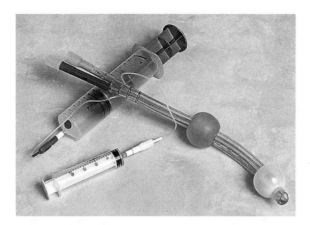

Figure 9-1 Esophageal–Tracheal Combitube. The pharyngeal tube has a large-volume cuff, has ventilation holes distal to the cuff, and terminates in a dead end. The shorter, tracheal/esophageal tube has a regular-volume cuff and beveled opening at its tip. Both cuffs have inflation lines and pilot balloons, ringed insertion markers, and standard 15-mm connectors for attaching equipment at their proximal ends. Accessory equipment provided with the airway includes two inflation syringes (large and small), a suction catheter, and an aspiration deflection elbow (to deflect vomitus should regurgitation occur).

esophagus (the usual location) or the trachea. In either case, the pharyngeal balloon fills the space between the tongue and soft palate, thereby eliminating the need for a mask. If the airway is inserted into the esophagus, the distal cuff seals this passageway, and ventilation occurs via the holes in the pharyngeal tube, below the pharyngeal cuff. If the ETC ends up in the trachea, it functions as an ETT, with the distal cuff sealing the lower airway and preventing aspiration.

The ETC comes in two sizes. The 37-French version is recommended for patients 4 to 5 feet tall, with the 41-French version reserved for taller patients. However, the 37-French ETC generally suffices for patients 4 to 6 feet tall, making it satisfactory for all but the largest patients.

The basic procedure for inserting the ETC is the same for both sizes, except for the cuff inflation volumes. Key steps are outlined in the accompanying box (**Box 9-1**).

Note that most ETCs end up in the esophagus. *This is why initial attempts at ventilation should always be via the blue pharyngeal tube.*

To switch a patient from an ETC to an oral ETT, the airway must be in the esophagus. In this case, gather and prepare all equipment needed for intubation (Chapter 6), and aspirate any stomach contents through the tracheal/esophageal tube. Then deflate the pharyngeal cuff. This will allow for laryngoscopy while the inflated tracheal/esophageal cuff keeps the esophagus occluded. Alternatively, if stomach contents have been aspirated, you can consider removing the ETC before proceeding with tracheal intubation.

Remove the ETC when the patient regains consciousness, begins biting or gagging on the tube, or requires tracheal intubation. Because regurgitation can occur with ETC removal, you must have suction equipment set up for immediate use. Normally, you roll the patient to the side (rescue position) before removing the ETC. You then fully deflate both cuffs until the pilot balloons are completely collapsed and gently remove the tube while suctioning the airway.

King Laryngeal Tube

The King laryngeal tube (King LT) is similar in concept to the Combitube. As shown in **Figure 9-2** upon insertion, the King LT normally ends up in the esophagus. Like the ETC, the King LT uses two cuffs to create a seal between the pharynx and esophagus, where the gas passes through ventilation outlets into and out of the trachea. Unlike the ETC, however, the King LT has only one standard 15-mm connector for ventilation and one cuff inflation line, making it simpler to use and quicker to apply.

Box 9-1 Procedure for Insertion of an Esophageal–Tracheal Combitube (ETC)

1. Suction mouth and oropharynx, and preoxygenate patient.
2. Inflate cuffs with the applicable syringe to confirm integrity, and then fully deflate.
3. Lubricate the tube tip and pharyngeal balloon with a water-soluble lubricant.
4. Place patient's head in a *neutral position,* and pull the mandible and tongue forward.
5. Place the ETC tip in the midline of the mouth, and guide it along the palate and posterior pharynx using a curving motion (do not force tube; if resistance is felt, withdraw tube, reposition the patient's head, and try again).
6. Advance the ETC until the upper teeth or gums are aligned between the two black insertion markers.
7. If unable to insert within 30 seconds, ventilate the patient with O_2 for 1–2 minutes and try again.
8. Inflate the large/small cuffs (41-Fr: 100 mL/15 mL; 37-Fr: 85 mL/12 mL).
9. Begin ventilating through the longer blue pharyngeal tube.
10. If there are good chest rise and breath sounds (or expired CO_2 is detected) without stomach gurgling, continue ventilating through the blue pharyngeal tube.
11. Absence of chest excursions, breath sounds, or expired CO_2 with the presence of stomach gurgling, indicates esophageal placement; in such a case, switch to the clear tracheal/esophageal tube and reconfirm good ventilation.
12. If you cannot ventilate the patient through either tube, the ETC may be inserted too deeply and may be obstructing the glottis; if so, deflate the cuffs and withdraw the tube 2–3 cm at a time while ventilating via connector #1 until breath sounds are heard.
13. If you still cannot provide good ventilation, remove the ETC and reestablish the airway by any alternative means available.
14. Once adequate ventilation is confirmed, secure the airway with tape or a commercially available tube holder, and continue providing essential life support.

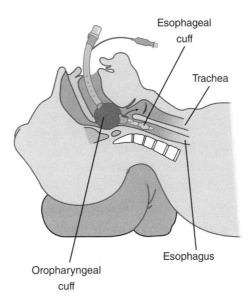

Figure 9-2 King Laryngeal Tube Properly Positioned in Esophagus.

There are two different King LT models: the standard LT and the LT-S. The standard LT tube "dead-ends" at the esophageal cuff, whereas the LT-S model has a gastric access lumen/open distal tip that provides for gastric tube insertion. Both models allow for the passage of either an airway-exchange catheter or fiberoptic endoscope. **Table 9-6** provides the key specifications for the five available sizes of the King LT and LT-S. Note that the LT-S is not available in sizes 2 and 2.5 (smaller children).

The accompanying box (**Box 9-2**) outlines the key steps for preparing, inserting, and removing the King LT.

Table 9-6 King Laryngeal Tubes Specifications

Size	2	2.5	3	4	5
Connector Color	Green	Orange	Yellow	Red	Purple
Patient size	35–45 in. 12–25 kg	41–51 in. 25–35 kg	4–5 feet 122–155 cm	5–6 feet 155–180 cm	> 6 feet > 180 cm
LT OD/ID (mm)	11/7.5	11/7.5	14/10	14/10	14/10
LT-S OD/ID (mm)	–	–	18/10	18/10	18/10
Cuff volume*	25–35 mL	30–40 mL	45–60 mL	60–80 mL	70–90 mL
Cuff pressure	60 cm H_2O	60 cm H_2O	60 cm H_2O	60 cm H_2O	60 cm H_2O

ID, internal diameter; OD, outer diameter.

LT: Maximum-size fiberoptic endoscope: 7.0 mm OD (size 3, 4, 5) and 4.7 (size 2, 2.5); maximum-size airway-exchange catheter: 19-Fr (size 3, 4, 5) and 14-Fr (size 2, 2.5).

LT-S: Maximum-size airway-exchange catheter: 19-Fr; maximum-size fiberoptic endoscope: 6 mm OD.

*Cuff volume varies by patient; ensure that the cuffs are not overinflated. Cuff pressure should be adjusted to 60 cm H_2O or to "just seal" volume.

Box 9-2 Preparation, Insertion, and Removal of the King Laryngeal Tube (LT)

Preparation

- Choose size based on the patient's height or (for small children) weight (see Table 9-6)
- Test cuff inflation system for leakage.
- Apply water-soluble lubricant to the distal tip.
- Position patient.
  - Sniffing position is ideal.
  - Neutral position is acceptable (e.g., for cervical spine precautions).
  - Elevate shoulders/upper back of obese patients.

Insertion

- Hold the airway at the connector with the dominant hand.
- With nondominant hand, hold the mouth open and apply chin lift.
- Use a lateral approach to introduce tip into the mouth.
- Advance the tip behind the base of the tongue while rotating tube back to midline (blue orientation line should face the patient's chin).
- Advance tube until the base of the connector is aligned with teeth or gums (do not use excessive force).
- Inflate the airway cuffs with the appropriate volume/pressure (see Table 9-6).
- Attach the bag-valve device to the airway connector.
- While ventilating the patient, gently withdraw the tube until ventilation becomes easy and free-flowing (large tidal volume with minimal airway pressure).
- Adjust cuff inflation if necessary to obtain a seal of the airway at the peak ventilatory pressure employed.
- If using the LT-S gastric access lumen, lubricate and insert a gastric tube (up to an 18-Fr).

Removal (when protective reflexes have returned)

- Position patient to avoid possible aspiration; be prepared to handle vomitus.
- Suction above cuffs in the oral cavity if indicated.
- *Fully* deflate cuffs (if a 90-cc syringe is not available, multiple withdrawals may be required).
- Carefully withdraw the airway by rotating it out (opposite of insertion motion).

Laryngeal Mask Airway (LMA)

As depicted in **Figure 9-3**, a laryngeal mask airway (LMA) consists of a tube and a mask with an inflatable cuff that is blindly inserted into the pharynx. When properly positioned and with the cuff inflated, the mask seals off the laryngeal opening. This effectively bypasses the esophagus and provides a direct route for bag-valve ventilation via a standard connector.

As with all emergency airways, proper sizing of the LMA is critical. **Table 9-7** provides guidance on LMA selection based on patient size and weight as well as the maximum cuff inflation volume for each size.

Key points related to the use of the LMA are summarized as follows:

- Preparation
  - Choose an LMA appropriate for the patient's size and weight (see Table 9-7).
  - Always have a spare LMA ready for use; ideally, have one size larger and one size smaller available.
  - Fully deflate the cuff by pulling back firmly on the deflating syringe until it forms a smooth wedge shape without wrinkles; insertion with a partially deflated cuff can obstruct the airway.

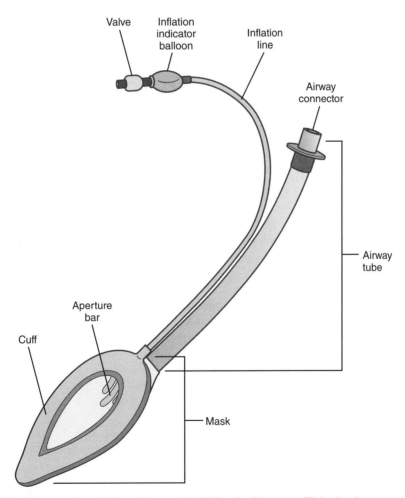

Figure 9-3 Components of the Laryngeal Mask Airway. This device consists of a tube and a mask with an inflatable cuff. The tube provides a standard 15-mm airway connector for attaching equipment. The mask is inflated via an inflation line with a valve and a pilot indicator balloon, much like those used on ETTs. The mask portion fits into the pyriform sinus, over the opening into the larynx. The aperture bars, used mainly in the reusable versions, help prevent the epiglottis from obstructing the inlet to the mask.

Table 9-7 Laryngeal Mask Airway (LMA) Sizes and Maximum Cuff Inflation Volumes

Patient Size	Recommended LMA Size	Maximum Cuff Volume*
Neonate/infant: < 5 kg	1	4 mL
Infants: 5–10 kg	1½	7 mL
Infants/children: 10–20 kg	2	10 mL
Children: 20–30 kg	2½	14 mL
Children: 30–50 kg	3	20 mL
Adults: 50–70 kg	4	30 mL
Adults: 70–100 kg	5	40 mL
Adults: > 100 kg	6	50 mL

*These are maximum volumes that should never be exceeded. The cuff should be inflated to a maximum pressure of 60 cm H_2O.

- Lubricate the posterior side of the mask using a water-soluble lubricant.
- Preoxygenate the patient, and implement standard monitoring procedures.
- Insertion
  - Use the "sniffing position" (head extension, neck flexion) for insertion.
  - Use upward and posterior pressure with the fingers to keep the mask pressed against the rear of the pharynx (palatopharyngeal curve).
  - Avoid excessive force during insertion.
- Inflation
  - Inflate the cuff to 60 cm H_2O; during inflation, avoid holding the tube, as this may prevent the mask from settling into the correct position.
  - Cuff volumes vary according to the size of the patient and LMA; volumes less than the maximum (see Table 9-7) are often sufficient to obtain a seal and achieve a cuff pressure of 60 cm H_2O.
  - During cuff inflation, you should observe a slight outward movement of the tube.
  - Avoid cuff pressures greater than 60 cm H_2O; higher pressures can cause malpositioning or tissue damage.
- Assessing and ensuring correct placement
  - No portion of the cuff should be visible in the oral cavity.
  - Chest expansion during inspiration, good breath sounds, and expired CO_2 indicate correct placement.
  - Malpositioning can cause leakage (decreased tidal volumes/expired CO_2) or obstruction (prolonged expiration and increased peak inflation pressures).
  - If the tube is malpositioned, deflate the cuff and reposition or reinsert the LMA to achieve adequate ventilation.
- Fixation
  - Insert a bite block; avoid oropharyngeal airways because they can cause malpositioning.
  - Apply gentle pressure to the tube while securing it with tape (presses the mask against the esophageal sphincter).
  - Keep the bite block in place until the LMA airway is removed.
- Providing positive-pressure ventilation (PPV)
  - To avoid leaks during manual ventilation, squeeze the bag slowly and try to keep inspiratory pressures below 20–30 cm H_2O.
  - If a leak occurs during PPV:
    - Confirm that the airway is securely taped in place.
    - Readjust the airway position by pressing the tube downward.
    - Resecure the airway in its new position.
    - *Do not only add more air to the cuff* (may worsen leakage by pushing cuff off larynx).

- Troubleshooting
  - If airway/ventilation problems persist, remove the LMA and establish an airway by other means.
  - If regurgitation occurs, do not remove the LMA; instead:
    - Place the patient in a head-down or side-lying (rescue) position and disconnect all ventilation equipment so that gastric contents are not forced into the lungs.
    - Reposition the LMA to ensure its distal end is pressing against the esophageal sphincter.
    - Suction through the airway tube.
    - Prepare for immediate tracheal intubation.
- Removal
  - Consider removing the LMA only after the patient's upper airway reflexes have returned.
  - Prior to removing, gather suctioning and intubation equipment.
  - Avoid suctioning the airway tube with the LMA in place (may provoke laryngospasm).
  - Deflate the cuff and simultaneously remove the device.
  - Verify airway patency and unobstructed ventilation.
  - Perform oropharyngeal suctioning as needed.

Endotracheal Tube

In the NBRC hospital, respiratory therapists (RTs) must be skilled in intubation. For this reason, you can expect to see several questions on this procedure on the NBRC exams. Intubation equipment is covered in Chapter 6, and Chapter 16 discusses assisting physicians with intubation. Here we focus on RTs performing the procedure.

Table 9-8 provides guidelines for ETT sizes and insertion lengths based on patient age and size. You should select an appropriate size tube but have available at least one size larger and one size smaller. Note that *uncuffed* tubes are recommended for premature infants or those weighing less than 3 kg. Otherwise, both cuffed and uncuffed ETTs are acceptable for intubating infants and children. As with adults, if cuffed ETTs are used on infants and children, cuff pressure must be monitored and limited according to manufacturer's specifications (usually no more than 20–30 cm H_2O).

Table 9-8 Endotracheal Tube (ETT) Size Guidelines and Insertion Lengths Based on Patient's Age

Patient Age/Size	ETT ID* (mm)	ETT Insertion Length† (cm)
Premature or < 3 kg	2.5–3.0 uncuffed	9–11
Newborn–1 year	3.0–4.0	11–12
1–3 years	4.0	11–13
3 years	4.5	12–14
5 years	5.0	13–15
6 years	5.5	14–16
8 years	6.0	15–17
12 years	6.5	17–19
16 years	7.0	18–20
Adult female	7.0–8.0	19–21
Adult male	8.0–9.0	21–23
Large adult	8.5+	23+

*ID, internal diameter. For infants and children, you estimate cuffed tube size ID = (age/4) + 3 and uncuffed size ID = (age/4) + 4 (cuffed tubes must be slightly smaller).
†From incisors to tube tip in the trachea; for the nasotracheal route (adults), add 2 cm to the insertion length.

Box 9-3 Key Steps in Adult Orotracheal Intubation

1. Test laryngoscope light and ETT cuff before insertion.
2. Lubricate ETT/stylet.
3. Position patient in sniffing position, and suction oropharynx.
4. Apply topical anesthetic (optional).
5. Hyperoxygenate patient (1–2 min).
6. Insert laryngoscope blade, expose and lift the epiglottis, and visualize vocal cords.
7. Insert ETT between vocal cords until cuff disappears (2–3 cm beyond cords).
8. Inflate the cuff to 20–30 cm H_2O.
9. Provide ventilation and 100% O_2.
10. Observe the patient's breathing, auscultate chest for symmetrical breath sounds, and auscultate epigastrium to confirm the absence of gurgling.
11. Verify tube placement using breath sounds, chest wall movement, and CO_2 detection or capnography.*
12. Secure and stabilize tube; mark and record its length at incisors.
13. Confirm proper tube position in the trachea by x-ray; reposition and resecure as needed.

*During resuscitation, the American Heart Association recommends continuous quantitative waveform capnography for confirmation and monitoring of ETT placement and to assist in recognizing the return of spontaneous circulation (ROSC). If capnography is not available, a CO_2 detector is acceptable.

The accompanying box (**Box 9-3**) outlines the key steps in oral intubation. The nasotracheal route is discouraged because (1) the incidence of VAP, sinusitis, and otitis media is higher; (2) smaller or longer ETTs are required, which increases airway resistance; and (3) necrosis of the nasal septum and naris can occur.

Key considerations related to ETT placement include the following:

- To test the cuff, inflate it and observe for deflation; alternatively, immerse it in sterile water and observe for leaks.
- The average oral tube placement from teeth to tip in adults is 21–23 cm in males and 19–21 cm in females.
- Stomach (epigastric) gurgling sounds indicate esophageal intubation; correct it by immediately deflating the cuff, removing the tube, and reintubating patient. Be prepared to suction oropharynx if vomitus occurs.
- Decreased breath sounds or chest movement on the left suggests intubation of the right mainstem bronchus (left-sided intubation can occur but is much less common); correct this problem by slowly withdrawing the tube until you confirm bilateral breath sounds. Confirm proper position by a chest x-ray.
- If a suction catheter does not pass after placement, the tube may be kinked or displaced out of the trachea; reposition it or reintubate the patient.
- Always provide 1–2 minutes of oxygenation and (if necessary) ventilation between intubation attempts. Intubation attempts should last no more than 20 seconds per attempt.
- If available, use waveform capnography to confirm ETT placement in the lungs; a colorimetric CO_2 detector is an acceptable alternative.
- If using a colorimetric CO_2 detector, ETT placement in the lungs is confirmed by observing a purple to yellow color change over six or more breaths (indicates 2.0–5.0% exhaled CO_2 or about 15–38 torr).
- There are only two ways to confirm proper tube placement above the carina: chest x-ray or fiberoptic laryngoscopy. On x-ray, the ETT tip should be about 4–6 cm above the carina, usually between T2 and T4.
- Because the ETT moves up and down as the patient's head and neck move, you should also consider the head and neck position when reviewing an x-ray for tube placement.
- If the ETT is malpositioned, remove the tape and reposition the tube using the centimeter markings as a guide. Confirm the new position via either a chest x-ray or laryngoscopy.

A variation of a standard ETT is the subglottic version, also known as a Hi-Lo ETT. Subglottic ETTs have an extra-small lumen, with the distal end opening just above the ETT cuff and a proximal end which is connected to continuous, low-level suction (approximately –25 cm H_2O). These tubes are designed to continuously remove secretions that would otherwise accumulate just above the ETT cuff, reducing the likelihood that such secretions could be aspirated into the lungs. Subglottic ETTs are one of the measures used to reduce the risk of ventilator-associated infections, which is discussed later in this chapter.

Tracheotomy Tube

Tracheostomy (trach) tubes are placed through the stoma into the trachea and secured around the neck. Tubes are sized by *internal diameter* (ID) in millimeters using the International Standards Organization (ISO) system. **Table 9-9** provides general guidelines for trach tube selection based on the ISO system. Note that most trach tubes designed for infants and small children (ISO size 5 or smaller) have too narrow an ID to hold an inner cannula.

When a doctor selects a trach tube, primary consideration is given to the outside diameter (OD), especially for cuffed tubes. *A trach tube's OD generally should be no more than two-thirds to three-fourths of the ID of the trachea.* Bigger tubes will impede airflow around the cuff when deflated, whereas smaller tubes may require unacceptably high cuff pressures to achieve an adequate seal.

Key points in the placement and management of standard trach tubes include the following:

- To ease insertion and guard against tears, the cuff should be tapered back by gently "milking" it away from the distal tip as it is deflated.
- The blunt obturator prevents tissue trauma ("snowplowing") during insertion; remove it immediately after insertion, but keep it at the bedside for tube reinsertion.
- If the tube has an inner cannula, slide it into the outer cannula and lock it into place.
  ○ To prevent blockage by secretions, regularly remove and clean the inner cannula.
  ○ Always keep spare inner cannulas at the bedside.
- The flange at the proximal end of some tubes can be adjusted to customize the fit and ensure a proper position in the trachea (needed for severely obese patients or patients with abnormally thick necks).
- Secure the tube using hook-and-loop ties attached to the flange and around the patient's neck (some physicians will use "stay sutures" to secure the tube); ties should be changed as needed for comfort or cleanliness.

Table 9-9 Common Tracheostomy Tube Sizes

Patient Age or Size	ISO Size*	ID Without Inner Cannula (mm)	ID with Inner Cannula (mm)†	Approximate OD (mm)†
Premature infant	2.5	2.5	N/A	4.5
Newborn infant	3.0	3.0	N/A	5.0
	3.5	3.5	N/A	5.5
Toddler/small child	4.0	4.0	N/A	6.0
School-age child	4.5	4.5	N/A	7.0
	5	5	N/A	7.5
Adolescent/small adult	6	6	4–5	8.5
	7	7	5–6	9–10
Adult	8	8	6–7	10–11
	9	9	7–8	11–12
Large adult	10	10	8–9	13–14

*International Standards Organization (ISO) standards require that both the inner diameter (ID) without inner cannula and its outside diameter (OD) in millimeters be displayed on the neck plate.
†Dimensions vary somewhat by the manufacturer.

- To prevent disconnection, accidental decannulation, or tracheal damage, always avoid pulling on or rocking the tube's 15-mm equipment connector.
- As with ETTs, placement of trach tubes should be verified by x-ray or a fiberoptic scope.

Laryngectomy Tube

A laryngectomy involves the surgical removal of the larynx, with the diversion of the trachea to the skin surface of the anterior neck, where a stoma is created for breathing. This procedure creates a permanent separation between the airway and esophagus; that is, *there is no connection between the stoma and upper airway.*

Airways options for laryngectomy patients include the following:

1. Open stoma
2. Laryngectomy tubes (basically an uncuffed small trach tube)
   a. Single cannula type
   b. Double (outer + inner) cannula
   c. Fenestrated tube
3. Laryngectomy button (similar to a trach button)

After the wound heals, many post-laryngectomy patients simply maintain an open stoma. Unfortunately, over time, many patients develop stenosis of the stoma. Laryngectomy tubes and buttons can help prevent stenosis.

Laryngectomy tubes are similar to trach tubes, only shorter and uncuffed. Like trach tubes, laryngectomy tubes include a flange to which ties or a neckband can be attached to secure the tube in place. All laryngectomy tubes also include an obturator that is used for insertion/reinsertion. A 15- or 22-mm connector provides for attachment of accessory devices such as a talking valve or "mini" heat and moisture exchanger (HME; discussed subsequently). In addition to helping prevent stenosis, application of progressively larger tubes can be used to dilate a stoma narrowed by stenosis.

Similar to trach buttons, laryngectomy buttons are short, self-retaining plastic or silicone tubes. Like laryngectomy tubes, laryngectomy buttons can be used to maintain the stoma opening and provide a point of attachment for accessory devices.

Several accessory airway devices are used by patients with laryngectomies. These include various humidification appliances and talking valves (discussed in the following section on speaking valves). Bibs and filters provide a layer of absorbent material (such as foam) that traps expired moisture for re-use during inhalation. Mini-HMEs are smaller versions of those used during mechanical ventilation. All humidification appliances help protect against inhaling particulate matter, with the stoma filters and mini-HMEs also providing some desirable resistance to exhalation that can help prevent alveolar collapse by creating extrinsic positive end-expiratory pressure (PEEP). Stoma filters and mini-HMEs attach directly to an open stoma (using an adhesive base plate) or to a laryngectomy tube or button. To work effectively, all laryngectomy humidification appliances require bidirectional airflow capability.

Key points in managing the airway of patients with a laryngectomy include the following:

- Because there is no connection between the stoma and upper airway, *all airway management (ventilation, oxygenation, intubation, suctioning, aerosol drug delivery, etc.) must be performed via the stoma.*
- Maintenance of a patent airway requires *at least daily* cleaning; steps for the patient with a double (outer + inner) cannula laryngectomy tube include the following:
  - Untie/unhook neckband and remove the whole laryngectomy tube.
  - Inspect the stoma; contact the physician if pus or foul-smelling discharge is present.
  - Remove the inner cannula.
  - Clean the inner and outer cannula with a small brush and soap and water (use hydrogen peroxide to clean crusty, thick mucus).
  - Rinse cannulas with clean water; shake off any excess.
  - Insert obturator in the outer cannula, and lubricate the tip with water-soluble gel.

- Ask the patient to breathe deeply, hold the breath, and then insert the tube into the stoma (avoid tilting the head back because this narrows the stoma).
  - While holding on to the faceplate, remove the obturator.
  - Securely tie the tapes/hook the neckband.
  - Insert the inner cannula, and secure it.
- To prevent aspiration, a protective cover should be used when showering or bathing.
- In the hospital, a bedside sign should identify the patient as a having a laryngectomy and include basic airway safety guidance.
- Should a hospitalized laryngectomy patient exhibit signs of partial or complete airway obstruction:
  - Call for the rapid response team.
  - If present, remove stoma filter, HME, talking valve, and inner cannula.
  - Try to pass a suction catheter; if catheter passes:
    - Suction the trachea.
    - If spontaneous breathing is not restored, provide BVM ventilation with O_2 ***via the laryngectomy tube*** (may require reinsertion of the inner cannula, a tracheostomy tube, or ETT if necessary to maintain patent airway).
  - If the catheter cannot be passed:
    - Remove the laryngectomy tube.
    - Provide BVM ventilation with O_2 via pediatric face mask or LMA applied over the stoma.
    - If obstruction continues, intubate stoma with a small (e.g., 6-mm) ETT.
- If mechanical ventilation is required, the laryngectomy tube should be removed and replaced with a cuffed tracheostomy tube.

Speaking Valves

Speaking valves are used by patients with tracheostomy or laryngectomy tubes/buttons to facilitate phonation/speech. They all consist of a one-way valve that allows inspiration but blocks expiration. With expiration blocked, gas is forced either to pass upward through the larynx (trach patients) or into the esophagus/upper airway through a tracheoesophageal passageway (laryngectomy patients).

For patients with tracheostomy tubes, key pointers in using speaking valves include the following:

- Always suction through the tube and above cuff before attaching the valve.
- Proper use requires that the trach tube cuff is *fully deflated*.
- To provide O_2, use a tracheostomy collar or an O_2 adaptor.
- If patient experiences distress with valve and cuff deflated, likely causes are upper airway obstruction, secretion problems, or too-large tracheostomy tube; remove the valve immediately.
- If used with a ventilator, select volume-control mode and adjust alarms (expiration will not occur through breathing circuit).
- To prevent sticking due to dried secretions, the valve should be cleaned daily in soapy water, rinsed, and air dried.
- Speaking valves should not be worn during sleep because the valve could become clogged and cause obstruction.

There are three main ways that laryngectomy patients can regain the ability to speak: (1) esophageal speech (swallowing/gulping air), (2) voice prosthesis, and (3) use of an electrolarynx device. All methods require forcing air through the throat and mouth, where it causes vibrations. These vibrations are then converted into speech via control of the throat muscles, mouth, and lips. The voice prosthesis is now the most common approach to facilitate speech after laryngectomy and is commonly used in combination with an external speaking valve.

Note also that failure of the prosthesis valve can result in aspiration of liquids into the lungs. Daily cleaning and flushing of the prosthesis can help prevent blockage with food particles and valve failure, as can regular replacement.

Speaking Trach Tubes

By providing a controllable source of gas flow above an inflated cuff, speaking trach tubes allow trach patients to vocalize, even when receiving mechanical ventilation. Key care points include the following:

- If the patient does not need a cuff for airway protection, consider a speaking valve instead.
- The cuff *must be inflated* for vocalization.
- Be sure to separately label gas supply and cuff lines to avoid mix-up (connecting cuff line to a flowmeter will burst cuff).

Providing Tracheotomy Care

Optimal care of patients with trach tubes involves the provision of adequate humidification, suctioning as needed, and regular cuff management. For patients with trach tubes, the NBRC also expects you to be skilled in basic tracheostomy care. In general, you should provide trach care whenever the stoma dressing becomes soiled. Equipment and supplies needed include the following (mostly provided in trach care kits):

- Replacement inner cannula
- Clean trach ties or a replacement hook-and-loop tube holder
- Precut sterile trach dressing (avoid plain gauze pads because fibers can cause additional skin irritation and can be aspirated into the airway)
- Sterile trach brush, basin, cotton-tipped applicators, and gauze pads
- Half-strength hydrogen peroxide
- Sterile normal solution

The basic tracheostomy care procedure is as follows:

1. Remove old dressing, being careful to keep the airway in place.
2. Clean around the stoma site with the hydrogen peroxide and sterile applicators (sterile saline can be used if the peroxide is too irritating).
3. Remove the inner cannula and insert the replacement.
   - Clean the inner cannula in hydrogen peroxide with the trach brush.
   - Rinse the inner cannula thoroughly with sterile saline.
   - Dry the inner cannula using a sterile gauze sponge.
4. Replace the inner cannula.
5. Place a clean trach dressing under the flange.
6. Change the tube ties/holder as necessary (unless there are stay sutures in place, *always have a second person hold the tube in place*).
7. Ensure that the tube is secured in the proper position.

The NBRC exams also may assess your proficiency in caring for patients with fenestrated trach tubes, talking trach tubes, and trach buttons. Here we focus on the care of patients with these specialized tubes. The indications, selection, and use and troubleshooting of these tubes are covered in Chapter 6.

Fenestrated Tracheostomy Tubes

As illustrated in **Figure 9-4**, a fenestrated tube has an opening in the posterior wall of the outer cannula above the cuff. Removal of the inner cannula opens the fenestration. When the cuff is deflated, and the tube's exterior opening can be plugged, air can move freely between the trachea and upper airway through the fenestration and around the cuff. Reinsertion of the inner cannula closes the fenestration, and once the cuff is reinflated, allows for positive-pressure ventilation.

Troubleshooting of fenestrated tubes is similar to that for regular tubes. The most common problem with fenestrated tubes is malpositioning of the fenestration, such as between the skin and the stoma or against the posterior tracheal wall. Tube malpositioning typically causes respiratory distress when the tube is capped and the cuff deflated. In most cases, repositioning the tube under

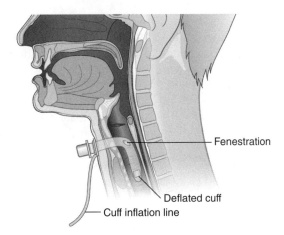

- Fenestration
- Deflated cuff
- Cuff inflation line

Figure 9-4 Fenestrated Tracheostomy Tubes.

bronchoscopic observation solves this problem. Alternatively, if the tube has an adjustable flange, modifying its position can help align the fenestration in the middle of the trachea.

Respiratory distress also can occur if the cuff is not completely deflated before capping the tube. To avoid this problem:

- Always make sure that the cuff is *fully deflated* before capping the tube.
- Attach a warning tag to the tube cap/plug.

If soft tissues obstruct the fenestration, you may feel resistance when inserting the inner cannula. To avoid tissue damage, never force the inner cannula during insertion. If you feel abnormal resistance when placing the inner cannula, withdraw it, and notify the patient's physician immediately.

Tracheostomy Buttons

Key points regarding the use of trach buttons include the following:

- The cannula is slightly flared at the outer end to prevent it from slipping into the trachea.
- The inner end is flanged to keep it in place against the tracheal wall.
- Spacers of various widths are used to adjust the cannula depth.
- A plug can seal the button, forcing the patient to breathe and cough via the upper airway.
- A standard connector can be used for positive-pressure ventilation; however, leakage will occur.
- A one-way speaking valve that blocks expiration can allow the patient to talk, eat, and cough normally.

To ensure continued patency, one should regularly pass a suction catheter through the button. If respiratory distress occurs with an uncapped button, it likely is protruding too far into the trachea and will need to be repositioned by changing the number of spacers. As with fenestrated trach tubes, proper placement is confirmed using fiberoptic bronchoscopy.

Devices That Assist Tube Exchange and Intubation

There are three common types of artificial airway exchanges: (1) endotracheal (ET) tube exchanges, (2) conversion of a supraglottic airway to an ETT, and (3) tracheostomy tube exchanges.

Endotracheal Tube (ETT) Exchange

ETT exchange is indicated for the following:

1. Replacing a damaged ETT
2. Exchanging a smaller ETT for a larger one
3. Exchanging the airway for a specialized ETT (e.g., double-lumen tube)

There are three common methods for ETT exchange: (1) direct laryngoscopy/simple ETT exchange, (2) use of an airway-exchange catheter (AEC), and (3) fiberoptic-assisted ETT exchange. In general, the role of RTs during ETT exchange is that of assistant to the physician and involves preparing and testing the equipment, withdrawing the old tube, securing any guide catheter, confirming replacement tube position, and monitoring the patient during the procedure.

Direct laryngoscopy is the procedure of choice for simple and uncomplicated ETT exchange. However, extubation and reintubation of a critically ill patient are seldom uncomplicated and straightforward. For this reason, if there is any indication whatsoever that the patient may have a difficult airway after ETT removal, methods of airway access other than direct laryngoscopy should be employed.

An *airway-exchange catheter (AEC)* is a device that allows the exchange of one ETT for another without losing airway access. Most AECs also can be used to administer O_2, and some have distal openings and a standard 15-mm adapter, allowing them to serve as a backup airway even after extubation (a ventilating AEC). AECs are available in different sizes and lengths to accommodate different sizes of ETTs. The basic procedure to use an AEC is as follows:

1. Whenever possible, confirm ETT position by bronchoscopy (keep the scope at the bedside for use as a backup rescue device should the exchange fail.
2. Place the lubricated AEC down the ETT, with its tip 2–3 cm above the carina.
3. Fully deflate the old ETT cuff.
4. While securing the catheter in position, remove the old ETT over the AEC.
5. Insert the new ETT over the AEC to the proper depth and inflate its cuff.
6. While carefully securing the new ETT, remove the AEC.
7. Confirm the position of the ETT (bronchoscopy, x-ray, etc.).

When using an AEC, proper equipment and trained personnel should be present to manually ventilate and oxygenate the patient, as well as perform standard endotracheal intubation in the event the attempt to use the ETT is not successful.

Fiberoptic-assisted ETT exchange is another approach in cases involving a suspected or confirmed difficult airway. There are two primary techniques for fiberoptic-assisted ETT exchange: (1) using the bronchoscope as the exchange guide and (2) using the bronchoscope in combination with a specially designed exchange catheter. The procedure for using a bronchoscope as the exchange guide is as follows:

1. Insert a pediatric bronchoscope into the new ETT ("preloading").
2. Using the scope for visual guidance, position the tip of the new tube in the laryngopharynx.
3. The tip of the scope is passed through the glottis and into the trachea alongside the existing tube (requires deflation of the old tube cuff).
4. Once the scope tip is positioned just above the carina, the old tube is removed, followed by threading of the new tube over the bronchoscope into the trachea.
5. Once the new tube is positioned correctly, the bronchoscope is withdrawn.

Note that this method briefly leaves the airway unprotected. To overcome this problem, if sufficient space is available for both tubes to reside together between the cords and in the trachea, some physicians will attempt to place the new tube in the trachea before removing the old one.

The procedure for using a bronchoscope with an exchange catheter is as follows:

1. A pediatric bronchoscope or portable intubating fiberscope is placed *inside* a specially designed 4.7-mm exchange catheter (i.e., the Aintree Intubation Catheter)
2. The catheter-ensleeved bronchoscope is passed through the old ETT ($\geq$ 7 mm ID).
3. Once the bronchoscope tip is positioned just above the carina, the scope is carefully removed, leaving the exchange catheter securely in place.
4. The old ETT is withdrawn around the catheter.
5. Using the catheter as the guide, a new scope preloaded with the replacement ETT is then threaded down into the trachea and positioned above the carina.
6. Once the new tube is securely placed, both the bronchoscope and catheter are withdrawn.

Converting a Supraglottic Airway to an Endotracheal Tube

Although supraglottic airways are adequate for temporary ventilation, they do not adequately protect against aspiration and are not suitable for long-term PPV. **Table 9-10** outlines the five primary options for converting a supraglottic airway to an ETT, the choice of which varies by type of airway.

Tracheostomy Tube Exchanges

Tracheostomy tube exchanges are indicated as follows:

1. To minimize infection risk and granulation tissue formation
2. To replace a damaged tracheostomy tube (e.g., blown cuff)
3. To allow downsizing or switching to a specialty trach tube

The accompanying box (**Box 9-4**) outlines the key points involved in changing a trach tube.

Table 9-10 Converting a Supraglottic Airway to an Endotracheal (ET) Tube

Method	Application
Removing the supraglottic airway and performing standard ET intubation using direct laryngoscopy	For use with *any* supraglottic device
	Not applicable with difficult airway
Performing direct laryngoscopy and intubation while the airway is in place	For use only with Combitube (must be in the esophagus and pharyngeal cuff deflated)
Blindly threading an airway-exchange catheter through the supraglottic airway into the trachea, removing the airway, and then guiding the ETT over the catheter into the trachea	For use only with King laryngeal tube (LT); cannot be used with the laryngeal mask airway (LMA) or Combitube
Blindly inserting an ETT through the supraglottic airway	King LT or LMA only; max 6.0-mm tube through King LT or #3/4 LMA, 7-mm tube through #5 LMA
Using a pediatric or intubating scope within a hollow airway exchange catheter like that previously described for fiberoptic-assisted ETT exchange	For use only with LMA and King LT; cannot be used with Combitube

---

Box 9-4 Key Steps in Changing a Tracheostomy Tube

1. Perform a surgical hand scrub.
2. Follow appropriate barrier precautions, including the use of sterile gloves.
3. Suction the patient before deflating the cuff (first above the cuff, then tracheal aspiration).
4. Remove the new tube from its package, and place it on a sterile field.
5. Check the cuff for leaks; deflate cuff completely while "milking" it away from the distal tip.
6. Attach new, clean tracheostomy ties.
7. Remove the new tube's inner cannula, insert the obturator, and lubricate the tube/obturator tip.
8. Position the patient in semi-Fowler's position with the neck slightly extended.
9. Loosen or untie the old ties, and fully deflate the cuff.
10. Remove any attached supporting equipment.
11. Remove the old tube, and visually inspect the stoma for bleeding or infection.
12. Insert the new tube with a slightly downward and curving motion.
13. Remove the obturator, and insert the inner cannula.
14. Inflate the cuff if ordered, ensure proper placement, and secure tube in place.
15. Restore the patient to the prior level of support.

If any problems are anticipated with recannulation, either recommend or perform the following catheter-guided exchange method:

- If an inner cannula is present in the tube being exchanged, remove it and replace it with a large (14-Fr for adults) suction catheter.
- Be sure that the catheter extends well beyond the tip of the existing tube into the trachea.
- While holding the outer end of the suction catheter by the thumb and index finger, remove the old trach tube over the catheter.
- Slip the new trach tube into the stoma and trachea over the suction catheter.
- Once the new tube is in position, remove the guide catheter and insert the inner cannula.
- Confirm tube position, and restore the patient to the previous level of support.

Management of Tracheal Tube Cuff Leaks

Cuff leaks are among the most common problems with tracheal airways. In patients on a ventilator, a leak in the cuff or pilot tube can cause a loss of delivered volume or an inability to maintain the preset pressure. With both ventilator-managed and spontaneously breathing patients, cuff leaks also can lead to aspiration. Key points you need to address when dealing with leaks include the following:

- Small/slow leaks are evident when cuff pressures decrease between readings.
- Your first step is to try to reinflate the cuff while checking the pilot tube and valve for leaks.
  - If the leak is at the one-way valve, attach a stopcock to its outlet.
  - If the leak is in the pilot tube, place a needle (with stopcock) in the pilot tube distal to the leak. Usually, one of these methods will allow you to reinflate the cuff, stop the leak, and thus avoid reintubation.
- A large cuff leak ("blown cuff") makes it impossible to pressurize the cuff.
  - A patient on a ventilator with a blown cuff will exhibit a decrease in delivered V_T and inspiratory pressure; breath sounds typically decrease, and gurgling may be heard around the tube.
  - A patient with a blown cuff usually requires reintubation; if the blown cuff is on an oral ETT, using a tube exchanger will make reintubation easier.
- Because the signs of partial extubation are similar to those occurring with a blown cuff, do not recommend reintubation until you confirm that a cuff leak is the problem.
- Before presuming a cuff leak, advance the tube slightly and reassess breath sounds. A balloon cuff position at the vocal cord level may cause an airway leak and mimic a blown balloon situation.
- Next, rule out or correct any pilot tube or valve leakage.
- Finally, try to measure cuff pressure.
- If you cannot maintain cuff pressure (confirming a large leak), the patient must be reintubated.

Other Devices That Assist with Intubation and Artificial Airway Exchange

Chapter 6 describes various equipment used in endotracheal intubation, including both standard and video laryngoscopes. Chapter 16 discusses the role of the respiratory therapist in assisting with intubation. In addition to the devices described in this chapter that can be used in placing and exchanging an artificial airway, there has been a recent rise in the use of video laryngoscopes. These devices provide a digitally produced, real-time view of the larynx and the vocal cords on a screen attached to the laryngoscope. They are particularly useful in difficult airway situations to either establish an initial airway or exchange one that is malfunctioning.

Maintain Adequate Humidification

Humidity therapy is indicated either to humidify dry medical gases or to overcome the humidity deficit when bypassing the upper airway. In addition, providing adequate humidification can help mobilize secretions. Heated humidification also can be used to treat hypothermia and bronchospasm caused by inhaling cold air.

Humidification Needs

Table 9-11 specifies the humidification needs by type of therapy. Due to the effectiveness of the nose as a heat and moisture exchanger, temperature and humidity needs are less when delivering medical gases to the upper airway. Indeed, a humidifier normally is *not* needed when delivering O_2 to the upper airways in the following circumstances:

- With low-flow O_2 therapy ($\leq$ 4 L/min)
- Via air-entrainment devices providing less than 50% O_2
- Via O_2 masks in emergencies or for short time periods

In contrast, if a patient's upper airway has been bypassed via intubation, you must overcome the humidity deficit by providing extra heat and humidity. *For this reason, the use of unheated active humidifiers is contraindicated in patients with bypassed upper airways.*

Selecting a Humidification Strategy

Spontaneously Breathing Patients

For patients with intact upper airways with normal secretions receiving low-flow O_2 at flows greater than 4 L/min, a simple, unheated bubble humidifier is satisfactory. For patients with either thick secretions or a tracheal airway, bland aerosol therapy is the most common humidification option. **Table 9-12** itemizes the various airway appliances used to deliver bland aerosol and their best use. As with humidifiers, heat can be added to the nebulizer to increase the water content.

Table 9-11 Humidification Needs by Type of Therapy

Type of Therapy	Temperature Range	Relative Humidity	Minimum H$_2$O Content
O$_2$ Therapy			
Low-flow O$_2$ therapy ($<$ 6–10 L/min) to nose/mouth	20–22°C	50%	10 mg/L
High-flow O$_2$ therapy (e.g., high-flow nasal cannula) to nose/mouth	34–41°C	100%	33–44 mg/L
O$_2$ therapy via tracheal airway (bypassed upper airway)	34–41°C	100%	33–44 mg/L
Mechanical Ventilation			
Invasive ventilation (bypassed upper airway) with active (heated) humidification	34–41°C	100%	33–44 mg/L
Invasive ventilation (bypassed upper airway) with passive humidification (heat and moisture exchanger [HME])	30–35°C	100%	$\geq$ 30 mg/L
Noninvasive ventilation (via mask) with active humidification (heated or unheated humidifier)*	Based on patient comfort, tolerance, adherence, and the underlying condition	50–100%	10–44 mg/L
*Passive humidification (HME) is not recommended for noninvasive ventilation.			

Table 9-12 Selection of Airway Devices for Bland Aerosol Therapy

Airway Devices	Best Use
Aerosol mask	Short-term application to most patients with intact upper airways
Face tent	Patients with intact upper airways who will not tolerate an aerosol mask; also for patients with facial trauma or burns
T-tube	Patients with an ETT or trach tube needing a moderate to high Fio$_2$
Trach mask	Patients with a trach for whom precise or high Fio$_2$ is not needed; ideal when you need to avoid traction on the airway

Patients Requiring Invasive Mechanical Ventilation

All patients receiving ventilatory support via a tracheal airway require a humidifier in the ventilator circuit—either an active heated humidifier or a passive HME. **Figure 9-5** provides an algorithm for determining which device to use. In general, you can begin with an HME unless it is contraindicated (see **Box 9-5**). Because HME performance varies, *be sure that the device you select meets or exceeds the minimum water vapor content of 30 mg/L.* If an HME is contraindicated, start the patient on a heated humidifier.

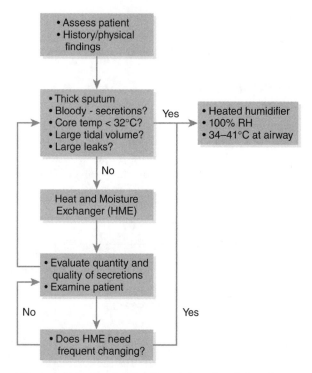

Figure 9-5 Decision Algorithm for Selecting Humidifier Systems for Patients with Artificial Tracheal Airways.

Modified from Branson RD, Davis K, Campbell RS, et al. Humidification in the intensive care unit: Prospective study of a new protocol utilizing heated humidification and a hygroscopic condenser humidifier. *Chest.* 1993;104:1800–1805.

Box 9-5 Contraindications Against Using Heat and Moisture Exchangers (HMEs)

HMEs are contraindicated for patients with any of the following:

- Bloody or thick, copious secretions
- Body temperatures < 32°C (hypothermia)
- High spontaneous minute volumes (> 10 L/min)
- Expired V_T < 70% of delivered V_T (indicating an expiratory leak)
- Acute respiratory distress syndrome (ARDS) receiving low-V_T or hypercapnic respiratory failure
- Noninvasive ventilation via leakage-type breathing circuits

  Should any contraindication arise during patient management, or if you need to change the HME more than four times per day, you should switch to a heated humidifier.

HMEs increase deadspace by 30 to 70 mL. Thus, for infants and small children, you must be sure to select the correct size HME and adjust the V_T to compensate for the deadspace if necessary. HMEs also slightly increase flow resistance through the breathing circuit, which is not a problem for most adults. However, if mucus accumulates in the HME, resistance can increase over time, increasing airway pressures during volume-controlled ventilation and potentially decreasing delivered volumes during pressure-controlled ventilation. You can verify this problem by inspecting the HME and correct it by replacing the device with a new one.

Patients Receiving Noninvasive Mechanical Ventilation

Some patients receiving noninvasive positive-pressure ventilation (NPPV) may also require extra humidification, especially children and infants, those using oral interfaces, or when ambient humidity levels are low. Also, providing humidification during NPPV can improve patient adherence and comfort.

HMEs are contraindicated for patients receiving NPPV. The characteristic one-way flow and large leakage occurring during NPPV impair the performance of these devices. Moreover, the added deadspace and flow resistance that HMEs impose can increase CO_2 levels and the work of breathing.

Because patients breathe through the upper airway during NPPV, a simple, unheated, passover humidifier usually will suffice. However, if supplemental O_2 is being provided or if the patient has problems with secretions retention, consider using a heated humidifier. Likewise, if the patient complains of dryness or discomfort even when using an unheated humidifier, consider heated humidification. To prevent condensation problems with these systems, be sure to place the humidifier *below* both the ventilator and the patient.

Initiate Protocols to Prevent Ventilator-Associated Infections

Ventilator-associated pneumonia (VAP) is a type of infection occurring in patients who have received mechanical ventilation for more than 48 hours. It is a leading cause of death among patients with hospital-acquired infections. Among those who survive, VAP increases ventilator days and prolongs both the intensive care unit (ICU) and overall hospital length of stay. To decrease the incidence of this problem, the Centers for Disease Control and Prevention (CDC) recommends a set of preventive strategies called the VAP bundle. The key components in the VAP bundle are as follows:

- Elevating the head of the bed by 30–45 degrees (unless contraindicated)
- Implementing daily "sedation vacations" and spontaneous breathing trials (SBTs)
- Providing peptic ulcer disease prophylaxis (using sucralfate rather than H_2 antagonists)
- Providing daily oral care with chlorhexidine
- Using subglottic ETTs (Hi-Lo ET Tube) that continuously remove secretions just above the ETT cuff
- Use of in-line or closed-suction catheter system to avoid breaking the ventilator circuit

VAP is associated with gastric reflux aspiration. Elevating the head of the bed helps prevent gastric aspiration, as does ulcer disease prophylaxis. Elevating the head of the bed also improves the distribution of ventilation and the efficiency of diaphragmatic action, which may help prevent atelectasis.

Daily cessation of sedatives can shorten the duration of mechanical ventilation. In conjunction with this sedation vacation, patients should undergo daily SBTs to help wean them from ventilatory support (see Chapter 11 details on weaning). In general, the sooner a patient can be extubated, the lower the risk for VAP. Of course, one needs to be on guard for accidental (self-) extubation when stopping sedatives. To minimize this risk, ensure that the patient is adequately supervised and that restraints devices are used if appropriate.

Other strategies potentially helpful in preventing VAP include general infection control procedures, airway management techniques, equipment maintenance, and oral care.

In terms of *general infection control* procedures, you should always implement both standard precautions *and* any needed transmission-based precautions for patients receiving ventilatory support. This must include rigorous hand hygiene before and after contact with a patient's mucous membranes, respiratory secretions, or related equipment (e.g., ventilator circuit, suction apparatus, ETT).

Airway management techniques that can help decrease the incidence of VAP include the following:

- Avoid intubation whenever possible (*use noninvasive ventilation instead*).
- If intubation is necessary, use the oral route (nasal intubation is associated with sinus infection).
- Maintain tube cuff pressures in the range of 20–30 cm H_2O; *avoid using the minimal leak technique.*
- Aspirate subglottic secretions using tracheal tubes having a suction lumen above the cuff (Hi-Lo ETT).
- Use sterile water or saline to flush suction catheters, only if needed.
- Use an in-line or closed-suction catheter system to avoid breaking the ventilator circuit.
- If delivering nebulized medications, use a T-adapter with a one-way valve in line to avoid breaking the ventilator circuit.

Regarding the use of in-line suction catheters, the American Association for Respiratory Care (AARC) recommends that they are incorporated into VAP prevention protocols. This approach is consistent with the "closed-circuit" concept—that is, the less frequently the ventilator circuit is opened or "broken," the less likely it is that infection will occur.

Also consistent with the closed-circuit concept are specific *equipment maintenance* strategies. To that end, both the CDC and the AARC recommend *against* routine changing of ventilator circuits. Instead, you should change the circuit only when it is visibly soiled or malfunctioning. In terms of humidification, the incidence of VAP does not appear to differ between patients receiving active (heated humidifier) versus passive (HME) support. However, when using heated humidification, the CDC recommends that you regularly drain collected condensate *away from the patient* and properly discard it, ideally without breaking the circuit. If using HMEs, you should place them vertically above the tracheal tube and change them only when they are visibly soiled. Likewise, the use of in-line or closed-suction catheter system is recommended to avoid breaking the ventilator circuit.

Oral care is the last strategy potentially helpful in preventing VAP. Good oral care involves (1) regularly assessing the oral cavity for hydration, lesions, or infections; (2) rotating the oral ETT position at least every 24 hours (or as per the manufacturer's recommendations if using a commercially available ETT holder); (3) providing frequent chlorhexidine rinses and teeth brushing; and (4) applying mouth moisturizer and/or lip balm after oral care.

Perform Extubation

Removal of a tracheal tube should be considered only in the following patients:

- Patients who can maintain adequate oxygenation and ventilation without ventilatory support
- Patients who are at minimal risk for upper airway obstruction
- Patients who have adequate airway protection and are at minimal risk for aspiration
- Patients who can adequately clear pulmonary secretions on their own

The patient's ability to maintain adequate oxygenation and ventilation should be demonstrated via a spontaneous breathing trial. To assess for upper airway obstruction, perform a *cuff-leak test*. To do so, after removing secretions above the tube cuff, fully deflate the cuff and completely occlude the tube at its outlet. If leakage occurs during spontaneous breathing (a "positive" test), then the airway likely is patent. A positive gag reflex and the ability of the patient to raise his or her head off the bed indicate adequate airway protection. In addition, the ability to clear secretions is evident if the patient is alert, coughs deeply on suctioning, and can generate a maximum expiratory pressure (MEP) greater than 60 cm H_2O.

Equipment needed to extubate a patient includes suction apparatus, a BVM resuscitator, a bland aerosol mask setup or nasal cannula, a small-volume nebulizer (SVN) with racemic epinephrine available, and an intubation tray (in case reintubation is required).

Key considerations in performing extubation include the following:

- Place the patient upright if possible (semi-Fowler's position or higher).
- Suction the tube and pharynx to above the cuff.
- Provide 100% O_2 via a bag-valve system for 1–2 minutes after suctioning.

- Fully deflate the cuff and remove the securing tape or device.
- Insert a new catheter into the tracheal tube.
- Simultaneously have the patient cough while you apply suction and quickly pull the tube.
- Provide cool, humidified O_2 via an aerosol mask or a nasal cannula at a higher Fio_2 than before extubation.
- Assess breath sounds, work of breathing, and vital signs.
- If stridor develops, provide cool, humidified O_2 via an aerosol mask, and recommend treatment with aerosolized racemic epinephrine.
- Initiate bronchial hygiene therapy or directed coughing.
- Recommend that the patient be NPO (except for sips of water) for 24 hours.
- Analyze arterial blood gases as needed.

The most serious complication that can occur with extubation is laryngospasm. Should laryngospasm occur, you should initially provide positive-pressure ventilation via a BVM with 100% O_2. If laryngospasm persists, the doctor may need to paralyze the patient with a neuromuscular blocking agent and reintubate.

T⁴ —TOP TEST-TAKING TIPS

You can improve your score on this section of the NBRC exam by reviewing these tips:

- If an adult is unresponsive but has normal breathing and adequate circulation, use the lateral recumbent ("recover") position to help maintain a patent airway and reduce the risk of airway obstruction and aspiration.
- Recommend prone positioning for patients with severe ARDS (P/F ratio < 150 with Fio_2 > 60% and PEEP ≥ 5 cm H_2O); this is most effective if applied for at least 16 hours per day.
- Common patient factors or conditions associated with a difficult airway include severe obesity, macroglossia (large tongue), neck masses (e.g., goiter), and history of OSA.
- Patients with a Mallampati Class III or IV airway (limited or no visualization soft palate or uvula) will be difficult to intubate.
- Predict difficult BVM ventilation using the M-O-A-N-S mnemonic: *M*ask seal, *O*besity/*O*bstruction, *A*ged, *N*o teeth (edentulous), *S*tiff lungs.
- Predict difficult intubation using the L-E-M-O-N mnemonic: *L*ook externally, *E*valuate external anatomy, *M*allampati classification, *O*besity/*O*bstruction, *N*eck mobility.
- If the patient gags or otherwise does not tolerate an oropharyngeal airway, remove it immediately and consider a nasopharyngeal airway instead.
- If you have difficulty passing a nasopharyngeal airway, insert it through the opposite naris; if that is unsuccessful, try a smaller size airway.
- The best way to initially confirm ETT placement in the lungs is via continuous waveform capnography.
- The average oral tube length from teeth to tip in adults is 21–23 cm in males and 19–21 cm in females.
- After intubation, decreased breath sounds or chest movement on the left suggest right mainstem intubation; correct this problem by slowly withdrawing the tube until you hear bilateral breath sounds.
- If after insertion of a Combitube and initiating ventilation via the longer blue pharyngeal tube you observe no breath sounds or expired CO_2 and hear gurgling over the epigastrium, switch to the clear tracheal/esophageal tube.
- Remove a supraglottic airway (e.g., Combitube, King LT) whenever a patient regains consciousness, begins biting or gagging on the tube, or requires tracheal intubation (King LT allows passage of airway exchange catheter to aid intubation); position patient to avoid possible aspiration, and be prepared for regurgitation!
- Before insertion, be sure to fully deflate an LMA cuff; after insertion, inflate the cuff to 60 cm H_2O and assess for a good seal.
- To avoid leaks during manual ventilation of a patient with an LMA, squeeze the bag slowly, and try to keep inspiratory pressures below 20–30 cm H_2O.

- A tracheostomy tube's outside diameter generally should be no more than 2/3 to 3/4 the diameter of the trachea; bigger tubes will impede airflow around the cuff when deflated, whereas smaller tubes may require unacceptably high cuff pressures to get an adequate seal.
- In laryngectomy patients, there is no connection between the stoma and upper airway; therefore, *all* airway management (ventilation, oxygenation, intubation, suctioning, aerosol drug delivery, etc.) must be via the stoma or its artificial airway (tube or button).
- If a laryngectomy patient exhibits signs of partial or complete airway obstruction, (1) remove all accessories except the laryngectomy tube; (2) try to pass a suction catheter and suction the trachea; (3) if catheter passes but spontaneous breathing is not restored. Provide BVM ventilation with O_2 via the laryngectomy tube; (4) if the catheter cannot be passed, remove the laryngectomy tube and provide BVM with O_2 via either a pediatric face mask or an LMA applied over the stoma.
- If a trach patient with a speaking valve in place and the tube cuff deflated experiences respiratory distress, the likely causes are upper airway obstruction, retained secretions, or a too-large trach tube; in any case, remove the valve immediately.
- For laryngectomy patients with a tracheoesophageal voice prosthesis who want to use a speaking valve, recommend a fenestrated laryngectomy tube.
- When changing trach tube ties or holders, always have a second person (or the patient) hold the tube in place to avoid inadvertent decannulations.
- The procedure for "plugging" a fenestrated trach tube is as follows: (1) deflate the cuff, (2) removal the inner cannula (opens the fenestration), and (3) plug the tube; always make sure the cuff is fully deflated before plugging the tube, and always attach a warning tag to the tube cap/plug.
- If a patient with an unplugged trach button exhibits respiratory distress, the button probably is protruding too far into the trachea and will need repositioning with spacers.
- To allow a trach patient with a speaking trach tube to vocalize, you must inflate the cuff.
- Recommend ETT exchange to (1) replace a damaged ETT, (2) exchange a smaller ETT for a larger one, or (3) exchange a regular ETT for a specialized one (e.g., double-lumen tube).
- To exchange an ETT using airway-exchange catheter (AEC): (1) introduce the lubricated AEC down the ETT until its tip is 2–3 cm above the carina; (2) deflate the old ETT cuff, and then pull the old tube out over the AEC; (3) insert the new ETT over the AEC to the proper depth and inflate its cuff, and (4) while securing the new ETT, remove the AEC.
- When using an AEC, proper equipment and trained personnel should be present to manually ventilate and oxygenate the patient, as well as perform standard endotracheal intubation in the event the attempt to use the ETT is not successful.
- For patients with a supraglottic airway who require airway protection or long-term positive-pressure ventilation, recommend converting the airway to an ETT.
- If any problems are anticipated with changing a trach, either recommend or perform the exchange by (1) inserting a 14-Fr suction catheter through the old tube, (2) removing the old tube over the catheter, then (3) using the catheter to guide insertion of the new tube.
- Because the signs of partial extubation are similar to those occurring with a blown ETT cuff, do not recommend reintubation until you confirm that a cuff leak is the problem.
- Video laryngoscopes provide a digitally produced real-time view of the larynx, on a screen attached to the laryngoscope. These devices are particularly useful in difficult airways situations to either establish an initial airway or exchange one which is malfunctioning.
- For patients with either thick secretions or a tracheal airway, bland aerosol therapy via aerosol mask/face tent (intact upper airway) or T-tube/trach mask (ETT or trach) is the most common humidification option.
- Apply or switch to active heated humidification in patients receiving ventilatory support who (1) exhibit bloody, thick, or copious secretions; (2) have high spontaneous minute volumes (> 10 L/min); or (3) have a body temperature < 32°C.
- In patients receiving invasive mechanical ventilation with active heated humidification, the goal is an airway temperature of 34–41°C with 100% relative humidity (at least 33–44 mg/L absolute humidity).

- Do not use HMEs with (1) ARDS patients receiving low V_T ($<$ 6 mL/kg), (2) patients in hypercapnic respiratory failure, and (3) patients receiving noninvasive positive-pressure ventilation (NPPV).
- To help prevent ventilator-associated pneumonia (VAP), (1) keep the head of the patient's bed elevated by 30–45° (unless contraindicated); (2) recommend daily "sedation vacations" and spontaneous breathing trials; (3) maintain tube cuff pressures in the range of 20–30 cm H_2O, avoiding the minimal leak technique; (4) consider or recommend use of tracheal tubes that provide for suctioning of subglottic secretions; and (5) use an in-line or closed-suction catheter system to avoid breaking the ventilator circuit.
- Recommend extubation only for patients who have passed a spontaneous breathing trial, are at minimal risk for upper airway obstruction (+ leak test), have adequate airway protection (+ gag reflex), and can clear pulmonary secretions on their own (usually requires an MEP $>$ 60 cm H_2O).
- If stridor develops after extubation, recommend treatment with aerosolized racemic epinephrine.

POST-TEST

To confirm your mastery of each chapter's topical content, you should create a content post-test, available online via the Navigate Premier Access for Comprehensive Respiratory Therapy Exam Preparation Guide, which contains Navigate TestPrep (access code provided with every new text). You can create multiple topical content post-tests varying in length from 10 to 20 questions, with each attempt presenting a different set of items. You can select questions from all three major NBRC TMC sections: Patient Data, Troubleshooting and Quality Control of Devices and Infection Control, and Initiation and Modification of Interventions. A score of at least 70–80% indicates that you are adequately prepared for this section of the NBRC TMC exam. If you score below 70%, you should first carefully assess your test answers (particularly your wrong answers) and the correct answer explanations. Then return to the chapter to re-review the applicable content. Only then should you reattempt a new post-test. Repeat this process of identifying your shortcomings and reviewing the pertinent content until your test results demonstrate mastery.

Perform Airway Clearance and Lung Expansion Techniques (Section III-B)

CHAPTER 10

Albert J. Heuer

Many patients require assistance in removing bronchopulmonary secretions and lung recruitment to improve ventilation and gas exchange. In this section of the NBRC exam, you will be tested on this type of therapy, including postural drainage, percussion, and vibration, as well as suctioning, mechanical devices, and assisted coughing. Also included in this section are questions on hyperinflation techniques and inspiratory muscle training.

OBJECTIVES

In preparing for the NBRC exam content (TMC/CSE), you should demonstrate the knowledge needed to:

1. Perform postural drainage, percussion, and vibration.
2. Clear secretions via nasotracheal and oropharyngeal suctioning.
3. Perform airway clearance using mechanical devices.
4. Ensure that patients can properly perform assisted cough techniques.
5. Administer hyperinflation therapy to prevent or treat atelectasis.
6. Ensure appropriate inspiratory muscle training techniques.

WHAT TO EXPECT ON THIS CATEGORY OF THE NBRC EXAMS

TMC exam: 5 questions; 2 recall, 2 application, 1 analysis
CSE exam: indeterminate number of questions; however, section III-B knowledge is a prerequisite to succeed on the CSE, especially on Information Gathering sections.

WHAT YOU NEED TO KNOW: ESSENTIAL CONTENT

Selecting the Best Approach

Airway clearance therapy involves a variety of methods. Important factors in determining which methods to use are the patient's age, preexisting conditions, and personal preference. **Table 10-1** indicates the recommended techniques, which can be used alone or in combination to treat the most common disorders that require secretion clearance. This information is based on a combination of research evidence and the expectations of the NBRC hospital.

Airway clearance often is ordered by protocol, giving you discretion as to the selection and implementation of therapy and its evaluation. **Figure 10-1** provides a sample algorithm for an airway clearance protocol that directs your decision making based on the patient's diagnosis, the volume of sputum produced, and the ability to cough.

Postural Drainage, Percussion, and Vibration

Postural drainage, percussion, and vibration (PDPV) techniques help loosen and clear secretions from a patient's respiratory tract. These methods can help reduce infection, enhance ventilation, and improve both pulmonary function and gas exchange. Although research supports the use of PDPV for the conditions noted in Table 10-1, the NBRC hospital may expect you to consider its use for additional conditions, including those that increase the likelihood of secretion retention, mucus plugging, and atelectasis, especially if combined with the inability to ambulate and a weak cough.

230

Not all patients can undergo this rigorous procedure. **Table 10-2** summarizes the contraindications, hazards, and complications of PDPV.

The accompanying box (**Box 10-1**) outlines the key elements in the PDPV procedure. As indicated, you should monitor the patient's clinical status before, during, and after the therapy. Your monitoring of patients should include their overall appearance, vital signs, breathing pattern, and

Table 10-1 Airway Clearance Techniques

Condition	Recommended Technique
Cystic fibrosis, bronchiectasis	
Infants	PDPV
3–12 years old	PEP, PDPV, HFCWO
> 12 years old	PEP, PDPV, HFCWO
Adult, living alone	PEP, HFCWO
Asthma (with mucus plugging)	PEP, PDPV, HFCWO
COPD exacerbation (with retained secretions)	PDPV, PEP, FET/DC, suction
Neuromuscular disease (muscular dystrophy, myasthenia, poliomyelitis)	I-E, FET/DC, suction
Postoperative without complications	Early mobility and ambulation
Uncomplicated pneumonia	None

COPD, chronic obstructive pulmonary disease; FET/DC, forced expiratory technique/directed cough; HFCWO, high-frequency chest wall oscillation; IPV, intrapulmonary percussive ventilation; I-E, insufflation–exsufflation; PDPV, postural drainage, percussion, and vibration; PEP, positive expiratory pressure.

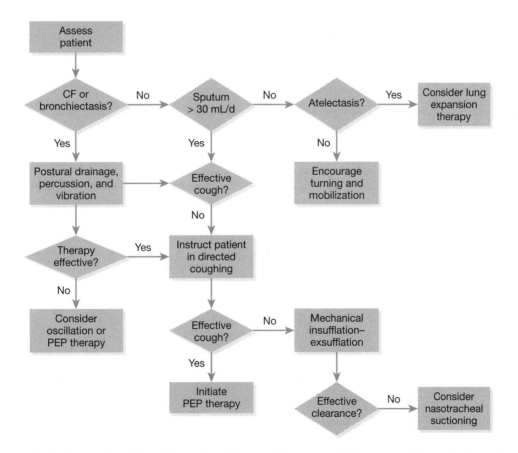

Figure 10-1 Example Algorithm for Airway Clearance Therapy. CF, cystic fibrosis; PEP, positive expiratory pressure.

Modified from Burton GG, Hodgkin JE, Ward J. *Respiratory Care: A Guide to Clinical Practice* (4th ed.). Philadelphia: J. B. Lippincott; 1997.

Table 10-2 Contraindications, Hazards, and Complications of Postural Drainage, Percussion, and Vibration (PDPV)

Contraindications	Hazards and Complications
• Intracranial pressure (ICP) > 20 mm Hg	• Hypoxemia
• Head and neck injury until stabilized	• Increased ICP
• Active hemorrhage with hemodynamic instability	• Acute hypotension
• Recent spinal surgery	• Pulmonary hemorrhage
• Active hemoptysis	• Pain or injury to muscles, ribs, or spine
• Empyema or large pleural effusion	• Vomiting and aspiration
• Bronchopleural fistula	• Bronchospasm
• Pulmonary edema	• Dysrhythmias
• Pulmonary embolism	
• Rib fracture	
• Uncontrolled airway at risk for aspiration	

Box 10-1 Key Elements in the Postural Drainage, Percussion, and Vibration Procedure

- Verify and evaluate order or protocol; determine lobes/segments to be drained by reviewing x-rays results, progress notes, and diagnosis; scan chart for any possible contraindications.
- Coordinate therapy (before meals/tube feedings or 1–1½ hours later and with pain medication, as needed).
- Assess vital signs, breath sounds, SpO_2, color, level of dyspnea, and ability to cooperate.
- Instruct patient in diaphragmatic breathing and coughing.
- Position patient for drainage, beginning with most dependent zones first.
- Maintain the position for 10–15 minutes as tolerated.
- Perform percussion/vibration over identified areas.
- Encourage maintenance of proper breathing pattern.
- Encourage and assist patient with coughing; examine (collect) sputum.
- Reassess patient's response and tolerance; modify as needed.
- Reposition patient and repeat the procedure as indicated and tolerated.
- Return patient to a comfortable position and reassess.
- Document outcomes.

Modified from Scanlan CL, West GA, von der Heydt PA, Dolan GK. *Respiratory Therapy Competency Evaluation Manual.* Boston: Blackwell Scientific; 1984.

---

pulse oximetry. If the patient shows any signs of distress, you should stop the treatment, remain with and monitor the patient, and promptly notify the nurse and physician.

Figure 10-2 depicts the positions commonly used during PDPV, which align the affected area in the "up" position. With such positioning, gravity can help move secretions toward the large airways for removal. For example, to drain the posterior segment of the lower lobes, you would place the patient in the prone position with the foot of the bed raised by 18 inches. However, it should be noted that the positions depicted may need to be modified due to specific conditions or situations. For example, because patients with cystic fibrosis are at higher risk for gastroesophageal reflux, it is generally recommended that they no longer be placed in a head-down position during PDPV.

Percussion and vibration are applied to the affected area using cupped hands to deliver rapid, repetitive thumps to the chest wall over the targeted segment(s). As described subsequently, you can also use equally effective mechanical devices such as pneumatic or electrical percussors. Your selection of percussion method should be guided by patient preference, convenience, and availability.

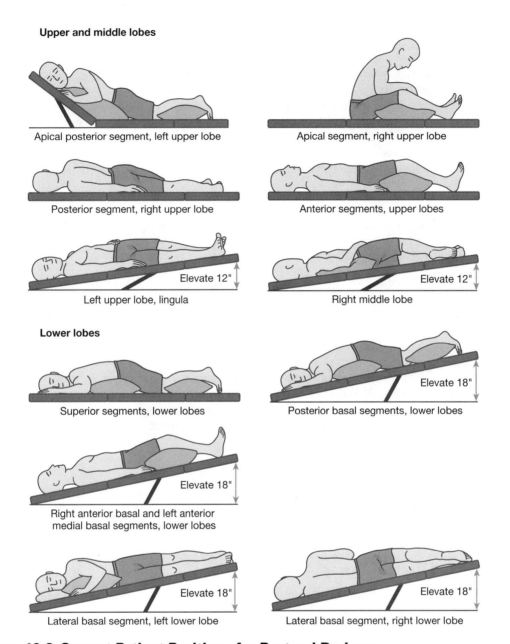

Upper and middle lobes

Apical posterior segment, left upper lobe

Apical segment, right upper lobe

Posterior segment, right upper lobe

Anterior segments, upper lobes

Left upper lobe, lingula — Elevate 12"

Right middle lobe — Elevate 12"

Lower lobes

Superior segments, lower lobes

Posterior basal segments, lower lobes — Elevate 18"

Right anterior basal and left anterior medial basal segments, lower lobes — Elevate 18"

Lateral basal segment, left lower lobe — Elevate 18"

Lateral basal segment, right lower lobe — Elevate 18"

Figure 10-2 Correct Patient Positions for Postural Drainage.

Modified from Potter PA, Perry AG. Patient positions for postural drainage. In Kozier BJ, Erb G, Berman AJ, Snyder S. *Fundamentals of Nursing: Concepts, Process, and Practice* (4th ed.). St. Louis, MO: Mosby; 1997. Courtesy of Elsevier Ltd.

Vibration involves a rapid shaking motion performed against the chest wall over the affected area during expiration. It may be performed manually, with a mechanical device or with beds equipped to do so.

Instead of or in addition to the intermittent application of PDPV, some critical care units use turning and rotation protocols to help prevent retained secretions, as well as bed sores. This procedure involves rotating the patient's body around its longitudinal axis. Turning can be done manually (with pillows or a foam wedge) or using a specially equipped bed.

To assess the effectiveness of PDPV, you should monitor several indicators. Changes in chest x-rays and vital signs, including Spo$_2$, can all be monitored noninvasively. Sputum production and auscultation also provide a good gauge to determine effectiveness. In general, when the sputum production drops below 30 mL/day, and the patient can generate an effective spontaneous cough, PDPV is no longer indicated and should be discontinued.

Suctioning

If assisted coughing techniques and the use of adjunct devices prove ineffective, you may need to consider suctioning. Suctioning is used as needed on all patients with artificial tracheal airways. Also, patients with certain neuromuscular disorders or those with conditions that increase the volume or viscosity of secretions may require suctioning.

Chapter 6 provides details on the selection, use, and troubleshooting of suctioning equipment, including both vacuum systems and suction apparatus. Here we focus on the procedures used to remove retained secretions.

Several clinical clues indicate the need for suctioning:

- Presence of a weak, loose cough
- Auscultation revealing rhonchi
- Direct observation of secretions in the mouth or oropharynx
- Tactile fremitus (vibrations felt on the chest wall)
- Patient feedback suggesting retained secretions

For patients receiving mechanical ventilation, an increase in peak pressure (volume-control ventilation) or a decrease in delivered volume (pressure-control ventilation) may indicate the presence of secretions. Less specific indications for excessive secretions include a deterioration in SpO_2 or arterial blood gases and a chest x-ray suggesting atelectasis.

Suctioning can be dangerous. Potential hazards and complications associated with the various suctioning methods include oxygen desaturation/hypoxemia, tissue trauma/bleeding, bronchospasm, cardiac dysrhythmias, hypertension or hypotension, cardiac or respiratory arrest, increased intracranial pressure (ICP), and infection. Careful implementation of safety measures before, during, and after the procedure, as well as careful monitoring throughout, can minimize these potential risks. In most cases, the danger associated with not clearing retained secretions far outweighs these potential hazards.

Oropharyngeal Suctioning

Oropharyngeal suctioning involves the removal of secretions, vomit, or food particles from the oral cavity and pharynx. For this reason, you usually use a rigid catheter with a larger-diameter lumen, such as a Yankauer suction tip (**Figure 10-3**). With a Yankauer tip, you can reach the back of the oropharyngeal cavity and remove both secretions and particulate matter.

Suctioning via a Tracheal Airway

Two general methods are used for suctioning of patients with tracheal airways: open suctioning and closed ("in-line") suctioning. Open suctioning is performed using a suction kit and sterile technique; it requires disconnecting the patient from supporting equipment. Closed suctioning employs a closed in-line catheter system; it requires neither sterile technique nor disconnecting the patient from support. The accompanying box (**Box 10-2**) outlines the essential elements common to these methods.

When setting vacuum pressure, you should select the lowest level needed to remove the secretions effectively. For centrally piped vacuum systems, the recommended starting range for adults is between –100 and –120 mm Hg; the initial range for children is –80 to –100 mm Hg. Negative pressure applied to the infant airway generally should be limited to –60 to –80 mm Hg.

To ensure that there is adequate space for gas to flow around the catheter and prevent atelectasis, always select a suction catheter that occludes less than 50% of the ETT internal diameter (ID) (less than 70% in infants). **Table 10-3** provides general guidelines for selecting suction catheters with tracheal tubes in the 2.5- to 9.5-mm ID range.

Alternatively, you can quickly estimate the correct catheter size in French units (Fr) by doubling the internal diameter of the tracheal tube and selecting the next smallest catheter size. For example, to suction a patient with a 6.0-mm tracheal tube:

$$2 \times 6 = 12$$

Next smallest catheter size = 10-Fr

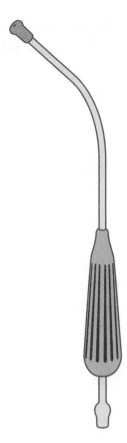

Figure 10-3 Yankauer Suction Tip.

Box 10-2 Key Elements in the Tracheal Suctioning Procedure

- Perform suctioning only when indicated, not routinely.

- Decontaminate hands and apply standard/transmission-based precautions.

- Assess patient oxygenation continuously via SpO_2.

- Preoxygenate and postoxygenate patients with 100% O_2 (10% above baseline for neonates) for at least 30–60 seconds.

- Use an in-line/closed-suction system on patients receiving ventilatory support.

- Select a catheter that occludes less than 50% of the endotracheal tube (ETT) internal diameter (less than 70% in infants).

- Maintain sterile technique with open suctioning; maintain asepsis with the in-line/closed technique.

- Use the lowest vacuum pressure needed to evacuate secretions.

- Limit the duration of suctioning to less than 15 seconds.

- Use shallow suctioning (insert the catheter just beyond the tube tip—about 2 cm in adults).

- Do not routinely lavage the patient with saline (its use is controversial).

- Immediately terminate the procedure if a serious adverse event is observed.

- Restore patient to prior status.

- Assess and document outcomes.

Modified from Scanlan CL, West GA, von der Heydt PA, Dolan GK. *Respiratory Therapy Competency Evaluation Manual.* Boston: Blackwell Scientific; 1984.

Table 10-3 Guidelines for Selection of Suction Catheter Size

Tracheal Tube (ID, mm)	Suction Catheter (OD, Fr)
2.5–3.0	5
3.0–4.0	6
4.0	6
4.5	8
5.0	8
5.5	10
6.0	10
6.5	12
7.0	12
8.0	14
8.5	16
9.0	16
> 9.0	16
8.5–9.5	16
ID, inner diameter; OD, outer diameter.	

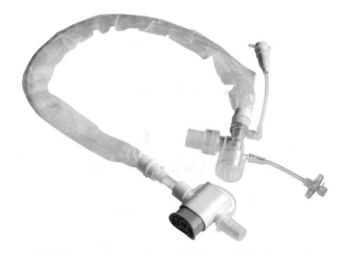

Figure 10-4 Closed-Suction System.

Courtesy of medisize, www.medisize.com.

Figure 10-4 depicts the key components of an in-line/closed-suction system for use on ventilator patients (a separate model is available for spontaneously breathing patients with trach tubes).

A common problem in intubated patients is leakage of subglottic secretions past the tracheal tube cuff. These secretions can contaminate the lower respiratory tract and are thought to contribute to the development of ventilator-associated pneumonia (VAP). For this reason, many VAP protocols call for continuous aspiration of subglottic secretions (CASS). As depicted in **Figure 10-5**, this is accomplished using specially designed ETTs that incorporate a suction port just above the cuff. You connect this port via a suction line to a standard wall vacuum unit and set it to apply continuous low suction, usually –20 to –25 mm Hg. To avoid any confusion over the various connecting lines (e.g., cuff inflation line, feeding lines), you should clearly label the CASS suction port.

Nasotracheal Suctioning

Nasotracheal suctioning is the method most commonly used to clear secretions in patients who do not have artificial airways and cannot cough effectively. In general, this method should be considered

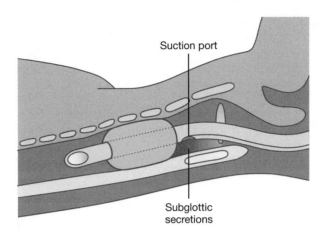

Figure 10-5 Endotracheal Tube Designed for Continuous Aspiration of Subglottic Secretions.

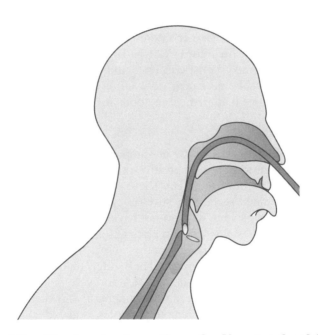

Figure 10-6 Patient Positioning for Insertion of a Nasotracheal Suction Catheter.

only when other efforts to remove secretions have failed. Contraindications to nasotracheal suctioning include occluded nasal passages; nasal bleeding; epiglottitis or croup (both absolute contraindications!); upper respiratory tract infections; nasal, oral, or tracheal injury or surgery; a coagulopathy or bleeding disorder; and laryngospasm or bronchospasm.

With a few exceptions, nasotracheal suctioning is similar to open tracheal suctioning. Many protocols specify that patients should blow their noses and rinse their mouths and throats with an antiseptic mouthwash before the procedure to minimize the risk of spreading nasopharyngeal bacteria into the lungs. To avoid airway trauma, lubricate the catheter with a sterile, water-soluble jelly before insertion. If frequent suctioning is required, you can minimize trauma by using a nasopharyngeal airway. In this case, lubricate the catheter with sterile water, not water-soluble jelly.

To increase the likelihood of the catheter entering the trachea, have the patient assume a modified sniffing position while sitting upright or in a Fowler's position (**Figure 10-6**), with the neck slightly hyperextended and the tongue displaced forward. If the patient cannot displace the tongue, you can manually pull it forward using a gauze pad. You should then advance the catheter slowly during inspiration (to ensure abduction of the vocal cords). In most patients, vigorous coughing confirms that you have passed through the vocal cords and are in the trachea.

Assessment

The effectiveness of suctioning can be assessed by the amount of secretions removed, as well as by changes in breath sounds, vital signs, and oxygenation. For a patient being mechanically ventilated in the volume-control mode, removal of retained secretions usually reduces peak airway pressures, whereas patients receiving pressure-control ventilation may experience an increase in delivered volume. Ultimately, the benefits of airway clearance, including suctioning, may be seen in improved aeration on the chest x-ray and an overall improvement in clinical status.

Mechanical Devices to Facilitate Secretion Clearance

Several mechanical devices may be used to aid clearance of secretions, all of which can appear on NBRC exams. Note that irrespective of the device used, effective secretion clearance still requires the rigorous implementation of airway clearance therapy, including directed coughing.

Handheld Percussors and Vibrators

Handheld mechanical percussors and vibrators are used to aid secretion clearance in children and adults (for infants, use small percussion cups or a percussion "wand"). You adjust the force to achieve the desired impact, using the higher frequencies (20–30 Hz) for vibration. As compared with manual "clapping," these devices deliver more consistent rates and impact force and do not cause user fatigue. They also are useful when home caregivers cannot perform manual percussion. However, these devices are no more effective than manual methods for facilitating secretion clearance.

High-Frequency Chest Wall Oscillation

High-frequency chest wall oscillation (HFCWO) or compression systems consist of an inflatable vest and an air-pulse generator that produces rapid positive-pressure bursts. You can adjust both the pulse strength and frequency, typically from 5 to 20 Hz. These systems are used primarily on patients with chronic conditions causing retained secretions, such as cystic fibrosis and bronchiectasis. They are particularly useful for home-care patients who do not have caregiver support.

To assemble and use a chest wall oscillation system, follow these steps:

1. Select the appropriate-size vest or wrap and fit it snugly to the patient during deep inhalation.
2. Connect the air hoses to the air-pulse generator and vest.
3. Select the mode, frequency, pressure, and treatment time, and ensure the system is plugged into a functional electrical outlet (a remote control is available for independent patient use).

If a vest system fails to oscillate, make sure that the remote control is on; if oscillation is inadequate after adjustment, check all tubing connections and the vest's fit.

Vibratory Positive Expiratory Pressure (PEP) Devices

PEP therapy is another method used to aid secretion clearance. PEP therapy also can be used to help prevent or treat atelectasis and to reduce air trapping in asthma and chronic obstructive pulmonary disease (COPD). When used in conjunction with a nebulizer, some PEP devices can facilitate bronchodilator administration as well.

PEP therapy should not be used on patients who cannot tolerate any increased work of breathing, are hemodynamically unstable, or suffer from bullous emphysema, high intracranial pressure, untreated pneumothorax, sinusitis, epistaxis, or middle ear problems.

There are three types of PEP devices, as summarized in **Table 10-4**. All of these devices typically generate between 6 and 25 cm H_2O pressure during exhalation and allow unrestricted inspiration. **Figure 10-7** depicts the two most common vibratory PEP devices: the Flutter valve and Acapella.

Because PEP therapy is no more effective than other methods of airway clearance, you should select the approach that best meets the patient's needs and preferences. Because some PEP devices

Table 10-4 Vibratory Positive Expiratory Pressure (PEP) Devices

Type of PEP Device	Mechanism to Generate PEP	Example
Flow resistor	The patient exhales against a fixed orifice (size is based on patient age and expiratory flow)	TheraPEP® system
Threshold resistor	The patient exhales against an adjustable counterweight, spring-loaded valve, or reverse Venturi	EZPap* Threshold PEP device
Vibratory PEP	The patient exhales against a threshold resistor with an expiratory valve oscillating at 10–30 Hz	Flutter valve Quake®† Acapella® Aerobika®

*The EZPap device also provides positive pressure on inspiration.

†Pressure oscillations with the Quake device are generated by rotating a crank that opens and closes the expiratory orifice.

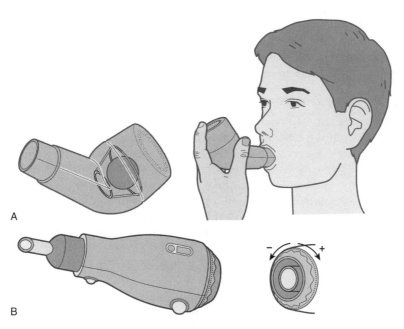

A

B

Figure 10-7 The Pipe-Shaped Flutter Valve and Acapella Device. (A) The pipe-shaped Flutter valve contains a steel ball that sits atop a cone-shaped orifice covered by a perforated cap. When a patient exhales through the mouthpiece, the weight of the ball creates expiratory pressures between 10 and 25 cm H_2O. Due to the angle of the orifice, the ball rapidly rises and falls, which creates the pressure oscillations. Flutter-valve PEP levels increase when the device is raised above horizontal and with higher expiratory flows. **(B)** The Acapella device uses a counterweighted lever and magnet to produce PEP and airflow oscillations. As exhaled gases pass through the device, flow is intermittently blocked by a plug attached to the lever, producing the vibratory oscillations. PEP levels are adjusted using a knob located at the distal end of the device. To increase PEP, this knob is turned clockwise.

are flow sensitive, your selection may also need to take into account the patient's flow capabilities. If the goal is to help mobilize retained secretions, then a vibratory PEP device probably is the best choice. If concurrent aerosol therapy is indicated, all devices except the Flutter valve and Threshold PEP device provide adaptors for attaching a nebulizer.

Key considerations in applying PEP therapy include the following:

1. The patient should sit upright or in a semi-Fowler's position, with the abdomen unrestricted.
2. Initially set PEP to its lowest level, as per the manufacturer's recommendations (e.g., the largest orifice, the lowest spring tension or flow).
3. Slowly increase the PEP to between 10 and 20 cm H_2O as per the manufacturer's recommendations (e.g., a smaller orifice, increased spring tension or flow, higher device angle [for the Flutter valve]).
4. With vibratory PEP, vibrations should be felt over the central airways during exhalation.
5. Have the patient perform sets of 10–20 slow, moderately deep inspirations with short breath-holds followed by active (but not forced) exhalations (I:E ratio = 1:3 to 1:4).
6. After each cycle of 10–20 breaths, assist the patient with the appropriate directed coughing technique/airway clearance therapy.
7. Repeat the cycle four to eight times, not to exceed a total session time of 20 minutes.

If a PEP device fails to generate pressure, the most likely problem is a leak, which is easily corrected by tightening all connections. Unexpectedly high pressures also can occur in these devices if the outlet port is obstructed—for example, by the patient's hand or bedding. To overcome this problem, make sure the outlet port remains open.

Home-care patients should be taught to properly maintain their PEP device according to the manufacturer's recommendations. Most PEP devices can be cleaned in warm, soapy water, followed by a good rinse and complete air-drying.

Intrapulmonary Percussive Ventilation

Mechanical compressions also can be applied internally via a technique called intrapulmonary percussive ventilation (IPV). IPV treatment is similar to intermittent positive-pressure breathing (IPPB) therapy, except that high-frequency (100–300/min) percussive bursts of gas are provided during breathing. Percussion is manually activated via a button and adjusted to ensure visible/palpable chest wall vibrations. Typically, saline solution (normal or hypertonic) is aerosolized during the IPV procedure, with the device requiring a fill volume of 20 mL. As with vest systems, patients can use IPV independently, and the treatment has the added benefit of providing aerosolized drug delivery. If an IPV device fails to properly function, make sure that there is an adequate source of gas pressure and that all connections are leak-free.

The Metaneb® System

The Metaneb system combines airway clearance and lung expansion with the ability to simultaneously deliver aerosolized medication. This device has two modes. In the continuous high-frequency oscillation (CHFO) mode, the aerosol is delivered while oscillating the airways with adjustable pulses of positive pressure. In the continuous positive expiratory pressure (CPEP) mode, airway pressure is combined with positive airway pressure while the aerosol is delivered. A typical Metaneb therapy session lasts approximately 10 minutes of alternating between the two modes and can be used in-line with ventilator protocol.

Insufflation–Exsufflation

Insufflation–exsufflation (I-E), also known as cough assist, involves the application of alternating positive and negative pressure to the airway to help increase expiratory flows and remove secretions. **Figure 10-8** depicts the device used for I-E. I-E is indicated for patients with weak cough effort (expiratory pressures less than 60 cm H_2O), such as those with neuromuscular conditions causing respiratory muscle weakness. Contraindications include a history of bullous emphysema, susceptibility to pneumothorax, and recent barotrauma.

I-E can be applied to spontaneously breathing patients via a mask or mouthpiece and via a standard 15-mm adaptor for those patients with tracheal airways. The inspiratory and expiratory time and pressure can be manually adjusted or preset for models with auto mode. Key elements in the procedure are summarized in the following box (**Box 10-3**). Newer and automated cough-assist devices provide airway oscillations to enhance airway clearance and secretion removal.

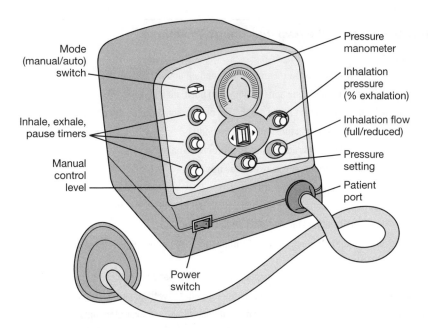

Figure 10-8 Cough-Assist or Mechanical Insufflation–Exsufflation Device. The mask and large-bore tubing attach to the patient port. The power switch turns the unit on and off. The mode switch toggles between automatic and manual modes. The pressure setting varies the inhalation and exhalation pressures together, and the inhalation pressure knob adjusts this value to a percentage of the exhalation pressure. Inhalation flow can be switched between full and reduced. Three timers allow adjustment of the inhalation, exhalation, and pause time. A pressure manometer calibrated in cm H_2O displays the pressure changes.

Box 10-3 Key Elements in the Insufflation–Exsufflation (I-E) Procedure

- Test equipment by turning it on, occluding the circuit, and toggling between inhalation and exhalation.

- Connect the circuit interface to the patient's airway.

- Set inhalation pressure between 15 and 40 cm H_2O and exhalation pressure between 35 and 45 cm H_2O (the lowest effective pressures should be used).

- Administer four to six cycles of insufflation and exsufflation.

- Remove visible secretions from airway or tubing.

- Reassess patient.

- Return the patient to prescribed support therapy.

- Document outcomes.

Assisted Cough

A cough is a natural mechanism for the clearance of airway secretions. A normal cough has three phases: (1) deep inspiration, (2) compression against a closed glottis, and (3) explosive exhalation. Often, patients have trouble with one or more of these phases.

Box 10-4 Key Elements in the Assisted Cough Technique

- Assess patient.
- Explain and demonstrate the procedure and confirm patient understanding.
- Position patient in semi-Fowler's position (or side-lying position) with knees bent.
- Instruct patient in the effective use of the diaphragm and demonstrate cough phases.
- Demonstrate how to splint incision (postoperative patients).
- Encourage deep inspiration, inspiratory hold, and forceful exhalation.
- Observe, correct common errors, and reinstruct as needed.
- Modify technique as appropriate:
    - Coordinating cough sessions with pain medication (postop patients)—to decrease pain
    - Splinting the incision site (postop patients)—to decrease pain
    - Using the forced expiratory technique or "huff cough"—to decrease pain (postop) or prevent airway collapse (patients with COPD)
    - Applying abdominal thrust/lateral chest compression—for patients with expiratory muscle weakness
    - Using manually assisted bag-valve inspiration—for patients with inspiratory muscle weakness
    - Using insufflation–exsufflation—for patients with inspiratory and expiratory muscle weakness
- Reassess patient, and repeat the procedure as indicated and tolerated.
- Collect and examine sputum.
- Return patient to a comfortable position.
- Document outcomes.

The accompanying box (**Box 10-4**) outlines the key elements involved in assisted coughing, including the modifications that may be needed for patients with ineffective cough.

Key instructions for assisting a patient with the forced expiratory technique/huff cough include the following:

1. Take three to five moderately deep breaths, inhaling through the nose, exhaling through pursed lips, and using diaphragmatic breathing.
2. Take a deep breath and hold it for 1–3 seconds.
3. Perform three short, forced exhalations with the mouth and glottis open ("keep your throat open"; the patient should make a huffing or "ha-ha-ha" sound on exhalation).
4. Follow each effort with a period of relaxed, controlled, diaphragmatic breathing (step 1).
5. As tolerated, perform three to five cycles of huffing and relaxation.

Key steps in applying the abdominal thrust/lateral chest compression include the following:

1. Assess for contraindications:
   - Abdominal thrust—pregnant women
   - Lateral chest compression—patients with osteoporosis or flail chest
2. Place the patient in supine or semi-Fowler's position with the knees bent.
3. Have the patient take a moderately deep breath (or have an assistant provide a mechanically assisted deep breath) followed by a short breath-hold.
4. Select/apply the appropriate technique:
   - Abdominal thrust (epigastric pressure)
       - Place the heels of hand(s) underneath the ribs in the epigastric region (making sure to avoid the xiphoid area).
       - Synchronize application of inward/upward pressure with the patient's expiratory cough effort.
   - Lateral chest compression (thoracic squeeze):
       - Spread your hands laterally around the anterior lower rib cage and upper abdomen (costophrenic angle).
       - Synchronize application of inward/upward pressure with the patient's expiratory cough effort.
5. Reassess patient and repeat the procedure as indicated and tolerated.

To provide a mechanically assisted deep breath, you can use an IPPB machine or a modified bag-valve device. To modify the bag-valve device to generate enough volume, you would include a one-way valve between the mask or mouthpiece and the bag outlet, allowing for successive delivery of two to three stroke volumes without exhalation. Alternatively, insufflation–exsufflation can be used with these patients (discussed earlier in this chapter).

The forced expiratory technique (FET) or "huff cough" is an alternative to the explosive exhalation normally created by compression of air against a closed glottis. The FET method consists of two or three forced exhalations, or huffs, with the glottis open, followed by a rest period. This process is repeated until the secretions have been mobilized and cleared. The FET is best suited for postoperative patients for whom explosive exhalation is very painful and patients with COPD who are prone to airway closure during regular coughing.

Hyperinflation Therapy

Incentive Spirometry

Incentive spirometry (IS) uses simple disposable indicator devices to help patients perform slow, deep breaths accompanied by a breath-hold (a sustained maximal inspiration). To perform IS, the patient must be able to cooperate and ideally generate an inspiratory capacity that is at least one-third of the predicted values. Discomfort due to pain is the primary hazard of IS.

The accompanying box (**Box 10-5**) summarizes the key points to keep in mind when administering incentive spirometry. Chapter 6 provides details on the selection, use, and troubleshooting of incentive spirometry equipment.

Because current evidence indicates that IS provides little to no benefit for patients undergoing thoracic or upper abdominal surgery, it is no longer recommended for routine prophylactic use in postoperative patients. Instead, early mobilization and ambulation are considered the primary means of reducing postoperative complications and promoting airway clearance.

After preliminary patient instruction and confirmation of proper breathing technique, you should encourage the patient to increase the volume goal. Other key points that can help ensure effective outcomes with IS include the following:

- If ordered for a surgical patient, initial instruction ideally should occur preoperatively.
- To accurately measure volumes, attach a one-way breathing valve and respirometer to the IS device.
- If the patient cannot cooperate or cannot generate an IC greater than 33% of predicted, recommend either IPPB or intermittent CPAP therapy as alternatives.

Box 10-5 Key Elements in the Incentive Spirometry Procedure

- Verify and evaluate order or protocol; review chart for pertinent information.
- Coordinate therapy with other therapies and with pain medication, as needed.
- Assess vital signs, breath sounds, SpO_2, color, level of dyspnea, and ability to cooperate.
- Instruct the patient in the proper method:
  - Full inspiratory capacity (IC) with 5- to 10-second breath-hold
  - Adequate recovery time between breaths to avoid hyperventilation
  - Perform 6–10 times per hour
- Have the patient confirm understanding via a return demonstration.
- Assist patient in splinting any thoracic/abdominal surgical incisions to minimize pain.
- Measure the achieved volume.
- Assist the patient with coughing; observe for any sputum production.
- Notify appropriate personnel, and make recommendations or modifications to the patient care plan.
- Document outcomes.

Modified from Scanlan CL, West GA, von der Heydt PA, Dolan GK. *Respiratory Therapy Competency Evaluation Manual.* Boston: Blackwell Scientific; 1984.

- If the patient also has retained secretions, recommend the addition of airway clearance therapy to the regimen.
- Recommend discontinuation when adequate volumes are being achieved (> 60–70% of the predicted IC) and clinical signs indicate the resolution of atelectasis (e.g., improvement in breath sounds and oxygenation).

Intermittent Positive-Pressure Breathing Therapy

IPPB is the application of positive-pressure breaths to a patient as a short-duration treatment modality. IPPB is indicated as follows:

- To improve lung expansion in patients who cannot use other methods, such as IS
- In rare situations, to provide short-term ventilatory support

Table 10-5 specifies the major contraindications and hazards associated with IPPB.

IPPB machines are either pneumatic or electrically powered pressure-cycled devices. Pneumatic IPPB devices typically are driven by oxygen and use air entrainment to enhance flow and lower the Fio_2. Electrically powered devices use a small compressor to deliver room air to the patient. All IPPB devices provide user control over the peak inspiratory (cycling) pressure and incorporate a small-volume nebulizer to deliver aerosolized drugs. Some devices provide additional control over the sensitivity or trigger level, inspiratory flow and flow waveform, and expiratory flow (i.e., expiratory retard). Airway interfaces common to all IPPB devices include mouthpieces, flanged mouthpieces, masks, and 15-mm ETT adaptors. Flanged mouthpiece or masks are used for patients unable to maintain a seal with a simple mouthpiece.

Except for the Fio_2 control, which device you use to deliver IPPB is less important than your skill in its application. Key points in ensuring effective IPPB therapy include the following:

- After assembly, confirm proper operation of the equipment.
  - Manually trigger the device/confirm that it cycles off when the circuit is obstructed (if not, check for leaks in the tubing connections).
  - If the device includes a rate control, make sure it is off.
  - If delivering inhaled medications, make sure that the nebulizer is on and that aerosol is being produced
- Assess the patient before therapy (vital signs and breath sounds).
- Record the relevant outcome measure at baseline:
  - Tidal volume and inspiratory capacity for treating atelectasis
  - Peak flow or $FEV_1\%$ for bronchodilator therapy
- Adjust the initial setting:
  - Sensitivity approximately –2 cm H_2O
  - Cycle pressure 10–15 cm H_2O with moderate flow

Table 10-5 Contraindications and Hazards/Complications Associated with Intermittent Positive-Pressure Breathing (IPPB)

Contraindications	Hazards/Complications
• Tension pneumothorax (untreated)*	• Increased airway resistance/work of breathing
• Intracranial pressure (ICP) > 15 mm Hg	• Barotrauma, pneumothorax
• Hemodynamic instability	• Nosocomial infection
• Recent facial, oral, or skull surgery	• Hyperventilation or hypocarbia
• Tracheoesophageal fistula	• Hyperoxia when oxygen is the gas source
• Recent esophageal surgery	• Gastric distention
• Active hemoptysis	• Impedance of venous return
• Radiographic evidence of bleb	• Air trapping, auto-PEEP, overdistended alveoli
*The only absolute contraindication. PEEP, positive end-expiratory pressure.	

- Have patient maintain a tight seal with a mouthpiece (apply nose clips, mouth flange, or mask as needed).
- Instruct patient to inhale slightly until the breath triggers; measure and note inspired volumes.
- Adjust the sensitivity as needed to facilitate triggering.
- Adjust the pressure and flow until the V_T is 1½ to 2 times the baseline as tolerated.
- Instruct the patient to avoid forceful exhalation and breathe slowly.
- Reassess the patient's vital signs, breath sounds, and IC and expiratory flows.
- Observe for adverse reactions.

In terms of FiO_2, you should try to match it to the patient's O_2 therapy prescription, if any. With pneumatic units, you can deliver either 100% O_2 or an air mixture with a FiO_2 varying between 0.40 and 0.60. The air-mix control also affects the amount and pattern of inspiratory flow. In the air-mix modes, flow is higher, and the pattern of flow more normal (decelerating ramp). When the air mix is off, the available flow is less. Also, some devices set to deliver pure source gas provide a less desirable square-wave (constant) flow pattern.

To provide a precise FiO_2 with a pneumatically powered IPPB unit, you must attach it to an O_2 blender and set the device to deliver pure source gas (turn off air mix). Moderate but inexact O_2 concentrations can be achieved with electrically powered IPPB units by bleeding 100% O_2 into the delivery circuit.

Chapter 6 provides details on the troubleshooting of IPPB.

Continuous Positive Airway Pressure

An alternative to the use of IPPB therapy for lung expansion is the delivery of continuous positive airway pressure (CPAP) or bilevel noninvasive positive-pressure ventilation (NPPV) via a noninvasive ventilator with mask interface. Among the various therapies for treating postoperative atelectasis, CPAP has proven to be the most effective, especially in patients who are hypoxemic (P/F ratio < 300) but do not have a problem with retained secretions. In these patients, CPAP can decrease the incidence of intubation and pneumonia. Typically, a CPAP level of 5 to 10 cm H_2O is ordered to be applied every 4 to 6 hours for up to 30 minutes per treatment session. If using bilevel NPPV, the pressure support level above the CPAP pressure is adjusted to provide a tidal volume of 8 to 10 mL/kg.

In case studies, high-flow nasal cannula devices have also has been shown to help manage postoperative atelectasis. Such devices provide up to 60 L/min of flow through a special nasal cannula at a FiO_2 of up to 100%. Although they are mainly used to deliver humidified oxygen to patients with moderate hypoxemia, the high flows delivered to the airway also provide some level of CPAP and may help prevent or treat atelectasis.

Breathing Exercises and Inspiratory Muscle Training

Breathing Exercises

There are two types of inspiratory breathing exercises: diaphragmatic (abdominal) breathing and lateral costal breathing. Both are intended to promote effective use of the diaphragm, with less emphasis on the accessory muscles. As an added benefit, inspiratory breathing exercises can improve the efficiency of ventilation by increasing V_T and decreasing the rate of breathing.

Key steps in teaching diaphragmatic breathing include the following:

1. Place the patient in a semi-Fowler's position, with forearms relaxed and knees bent.
2. Position your hand on the patient's upper abdomen, below the xiphoid.
3. Encourage the patient to inhale slowly through the nose and "push out" against your hand.
4. Provide progressive resistance to the abdominal movement until end-inspiration.
5. Repeat this exercise (with rest as needed) until satisfactory movement is achieved.

In teaching patients, you should first demonstrate this technique on yourself while explaining both the "why" and "how" to the patient. Your goal is to get patients to perform these exercises on their own. In the rehabilitation setting, patients can create resistance using a small weight (about 5 lb) placed over the upper abdomen and progressively increase the load as the diaphragm becomes stronger.

Lateral costal breathing exercises are a good alternative to the diaphragmatic method, especially for patients who have undergone abdominal surgery. The technique is similar to that used in teaching diaphragmatic breathing, but with the resistance applied by both hands "cupping" the lower rib edges. As you apply increasing resistance during inspiration, you instruct the patient to slowly "breathe around the waist" and push out against your hands.

The expiratory breathing technique is also important, especially for patients with COPD. Exhalation through pursed lips increases "back-pressure" in the airways during exhalation and can help lessen air trapping and prolong expiratory times, thereby decreasing the rate of breathing. In combination, these effects can improve ventilation and may help diminish dyspnea. Patients should aim for an expiratory time that is at least two to three times longer than inspiration.

Inspiratory Muscle Training

Inspiratory muscle training (IMT) can help COPD patients manage their dyspnea, increase their exercise tolerance, and enhance their health-related quality of life. IMT also may improve diaphragm function in patients with certain neuromuscular disorders and may aid in weaning ventilator-dependent patients.

There are two types of IMT devices: flow and threshold resistors. Both are similar in concept to the resistors used to deliver PEP therapy. However, with IMT, the patient inhales against the resistor. Spring-loaded threshold resistors are preferred for IMT because they can be adjusted to a specific negative pressure, which ensures a constant muscle load independent of flow.

Key points needed to ensure effective outcomes with IMT include the following:

- Before implementing IMT, train the patient in proper diaphragmatic breathing.
- Measure the patient's maximum inspiratory pressure (MIP or PI_{max}) with a calibrated manometer.
- Encourage slow breathing (fewer than 10–12 breaths/min) through the device with minimal initial resistance.
- Once the patient becomes accustomed to the device, slowly increase resistance until the inspiratory pressure is 30% or more of the MIP/PI_{max}.
- After confirming the load setting and the patient's ability to perform the procedure, instruct the patient to perform 10- to 15-minute exercise sessions once or twice per day.
- Encourage the patient to maintain a detailed treatment log, including session dates and durations.
- If the MIP does not improve, interview the patient and inspect the log to determine why (usually noncompliance).

Table 10-6 summarizes IMT parameter recommendations from various sources. Note that patients will progressively lose any health-related benefit if they cease training.

Table 10-6 Recommended Inspiratory Muscle Training (IMT) Parameters

Parameter	Consideration	Recommendation
Mode	Type of device	Threshold or flow resistor (calibrated threshold preferred; if using a flow resistor, attach a manometer to the device's monitoring port)
Intensity	Load against which the person is exercising	Minimum of 30% of PI_{max} (lower initial intensity may be needed with COPD patients); increase PI_{max} by 5% per week as tolerated
Frequency/ duration	Number of sessions/ day	1–2 sessions per day, depending on patient exercise tolerance
	Length of sessions	Total of 30 minutes per day (divided over 1–2 sessions); initial sessions may need to be limited to 3–5 minutes
	Number of days/week	4–6 days of sessions per week according to patient tolerance
	Weeks of training	Continue indefinitely to maintain training benefits; functional improvement usually requires at least 5 weeks of training

T⁴—TOP TEST-TAKING TIPS

You can improve your score on this section of the NBRC exam by following these tips:

- Most PDPV positions involve positioning the affected area in the "up" position to permit gravity to help move secretions toward the large airways for removal.
- Contraindications for performing postural drainage, percussion, and vibration (PDPV) include the following: intracranial pressure (ICP) > 20 mm Hg, many head and neck injuries, active hemorrhage, hemodynamic instability, recent spinal surgery, active hemoptysis, and empyema.
- Always remember that the effectiveness of airway clearance and lung expansion therapy can be assessed through an improvement in breath sounds, vital signs, oxygenation, and overall appearance.
- In general, when the sputum production drops below 30 mL/day, and the patient can generate an effective spontaneous cough, PDPV is no longer indicated and should be discontinued.
- When deciding on a suction catheter size for a patient with an artificial airway, suction catheters that occlude less than 50% of the ETT internal diameter (less than 70% in infants) should be selected. For example, a maximum catheter size of 8-Fr should be used for a 5.0 ETT, a 12-Fr catheter should be used for a 7.0 ETT, and a 14-Fr catheter should be used for an 8.0 ETT.
- In general, suction pressures should never exceed –120 mm Hg for adults, –100 mm Hg for children, and –80 mm Hg for infants, and applying suction to the airway for more than 15 seconds for each attempt should be avoided.
- In-line/closed-suctioning techniques should be strongly considered in patients receiving continuous mechanical ventilation, especially those requiring high FiO_2s and positive end-expiratory pressure (PEEP).
- Potential hazards and complications associated with the various suctioning methods include oxygen desaturation/hypoxemia, tissue trauma/bleeding, bronchospasm, cardiac dysrhythmias, hypertension or hypotension, cardiac or respiratory arrest, increased ICP, and infection.
- Remember to preoxygenate a patient with a FiO_2 of 100% (10% above the baseline FiO_2 in neonates) for at least 30–60 seconds before each suction attempt and monitor the patient carefully during and immediately after the procedure, especially oxygenation via pulse oximetry.
- Handheld percussors and vibrators, as well as high-frequency chest wall oscillation, are viable alternatives to manual chest physical therapy.
- A forced expiratory technique (FET) or "huff cough" is an alternative for patients who cannot generate the explosive exhalation usually created by compression of air against a closed glottis.
- A patient performing a FET/huff cough should be coached to do three to five cycles as follows: take a deep breath and hold it for 1–3 seconds; perform three short forced exhalations with the mouth and glottis open; make a huffing or "ha-ha-ha" sound on exhalation; and follow each effort with a period of relaxed, controlled diaphragmatic breathing.
- If the goal is to help mobilize retained secretions and the patient can generate enough inspiratory and expiratory flows, then a vibratory PEP device (e.g., flutter valve) should be strongly considered.
- If a patient cannot generate sufficient flows but may benefit from vibratory PEP, then intrapulmonary percussive ventilation (IPV) should be considered. IPV involves the application of high-frequency (100–300/min) mechanical compressions applied internally during breathing.
- As an alternative to IPV, the Metaneb system combines airway clearance and lung expansion with the ability to simultaneously deliver aerosolized medication. The two modes combine aerosol therapy with either continuous high-frequency oscillation or adjustable pulses of positive pressure.

- For airway clearance, mechanical devices such as mechanical insufflators–exsufflators, percussors, and PEP devices can be used in addition to or as an alternative to PDPV.
- Insufflation–exsufflation (I-E) involves alternating positive and negative pressures up to 40–50 cm H_2O and is indicated for patients with weak cough effort, such as those with neuromuscular conditions causing respiratory muscle weakness.
- Contraindications for I-E include a history of bullous emphysema, susceptibility to pneumothorax, and recent barotrauma.
- To perform IS, the patient must be able to cooperate and ideally generate an inspiratory capacity that is at least one-third of the predicted values. If the patient needs hyperinflation but IS is not suitable, then other hyperinflation techniques should be considered, such as IPPB or CPAP.
- Contraindications to IPPB therapy include untreated tension pneumothorax, ICP > 15 mm Hg, hemodynamic instability, recent facial or oral surgery, tracheoesophageal fistula, recent esophageal surgery, active hemoptysis, and radiographic evidence of bleb.
- An alternative to the use of IPPB therapy for lung expansion is the delivery of continuous positive airway pressure (CPAP) or bilevel positive pressure ventilation via a noninvasive ventilator with mask interface for up to 30 minutes every 4–6 hours.
- Breathing exercises and inspiratory muscle training may help patients with chronic lung problems, such as COPD, by increasing the efficiency of ventilation and exercise tolerance, as well as enhancing their health-related quality of life.
- Inspiratory muscle training (IMT) generally involves inhalation and exhalation through flow or threshold resistors to build the strength and endurance of respiratory muscles. IMT can help COPD patients manage their dyspnea, increase their exercise tolerance, and enhance their health-related quality of life.
- Closely monitor a patient before, during, and immediately following airway clearance and lung expansion therapy, as well as when performing breathing exercises and IMT. If an adverse reaction occurs during therapy, stop the treatment, stay with and monitor the patient, and notify the nurse and physician.

POST-TEST

To confirm your mastery of each chapter's topical content, you should create a content post-test, available online via the Navigate Premier Access for Comprehensive Respiratory Therapy Exam Preparation Guide, which contains Navigate TestPrep (access code provided with every new text). You can create multiple topical content post-tests varying in length from 10 to 20 questions, with each attempt presenting a different set of items. You can select questions from all three major NBRC TMC sections: Patient Data, Troubleshooting and Quality Control of Devices and Infection Control, and Initiation and Modification of Interventions. A score of at least 70–80% indicates that you are adequately prepared for this section of the NBRC TMC exam. If you score below 70%, you should first carefully assess your test answers (particularly your wrong answers) and the correct answer explanations. Then return to the chapter to re-review the applicable content. Only then should you reattempt a new post-test. Repeat this process of identifying your shortcomings and reviewing the pertinent content until your test results demonstrate mastery.

CHAPTER 11

Support Oxygenation and Ventilation (Section III-C)

Narciso E. Rodriguez

Supporting oxygenation and ventilation is "job number #1" for respiratory therapists (RTs). This chapter includes critical NBRC topical content on treating hypoxemia and initiating, optimizing, and discontinuing both invasive and noninvasive ventilatory support.

OBJECTIVES

In preparing for the shared NBRC exam content (TMC/CSE), you should demonstrate the knowledge needed to:

1. Initiate and adjust oxygen therapy.
2. Minimize hypoxemia.
3. Initiate and adjust mask or nasal CPAP.
4. Initiate and adjust mechanical ventilation settings.
5. Recognize and correct patient–ventilator dyssynchrony.
6. Utilize ventilator graphics.
7. Perform lung recruitment maneuvers.
8. Liberate patient from mechanical ventilation.

WHAT TO EXPECT ON THIS CATEGORY OF THE NBRC EXAMS

TMC exam: 15 questions; 1 recall, 5 application, and 9 analysis
CSE exam: indeterminate number of questions; however, section III-C knowledge is a prerequisite to succeed on both Information Gathering and Decision-Making sections.

WHAT YOU NEED TO KNOW: ESSENTIAL CONTENT

Initiating and Adjusting Oxygen Therapy

Recommend starting O_2 therapy whenever a patient exhibits one or more of the following signs or symptoms of hypoxemia:

- Tachypnea or tachycardia
- Dyspnea
- Cyanosis
- Hypertension or peripheral vasoconstriction
- Disorientation/confusion, headache, or somnolence

You should also suspect hypoxemia in cases in which poor oxygenation is common, such as in postoperative patients and those suffering from carbon monoxide or cyanide poisoning, shock, trauma, or acute myocardial infarction (MI). Documented hypoxemia exists regardless of the patient's condition when the adult patient's Pao_2 is less than 60 torr or the arterial saturation is less than 90%. Due to the potential hazards of oxygen therapy, the threshold for hypoxemia for infants is lower and generally is defined as a Pao_2 of less than 50 torr in such patients.

You normally treat suspected or documented hypoxemia by administering oxygen. However, when hypoxemia is caused by shunting, O_2 therapy alone is insufficient to remedy it. You know that hypoxemia is due to significant shunting when the P/F ratio drops below 200 or you cannot maintain adequate arterial oxygenation on 50% or more oxygen (i.e., $Pao_2 \leq 50$ torr on $Fio_2 \geq 0.50$). In these cases, the recommended treatment is typically continuous positive airway pressure (CPAP) or positive end-expiratory pressure (PEEP), as discussed elsewhere. An additional method that can help raise the Pao_2 level in patients suffering from refractory hypoxemia is to use patient positioning to decrease shunting.

The following guidelines apply to titrate O_2 therapy:

- In otherwise healthy patients, adjust the flow and Fio_2 to the lowest level needed to maintain normal oxygenation (i.e., Pao_2 of 80–100 torr with saturation $\geq 92\%$).
- If you cannot maintain normal oxygenation on less than 50% oxygen, accept a $Pao_2 \geq 55$–60 torr with a $Sao_2/Spo_2 \geq 88\%$.
- When treating patients with carbon monoxide poisoning, cyanide poisoning, acute pulmonary edema, shock, trauma, or acute MI in emergency settings, provide the highest possible Fio_2.
- For patients with chronic hypercapnia, aim to keep the Pao_2 in the range of 55–60 torr to prevent depression of ventilation (O_2-induced hypoventilation).
- In low birth weight or preterm neonates at risk for retinopathy of prematurity (ROP), your goal should be a Pao_2 in the range of 50–80 torr.

Minimizing Hypoxemia

Patient Positioning

Patient positioning can be used to alter the distribution of ventilation and perfusion, thereby improving oxygenation without raising the Fio_2. Patient positioning may also decrease the incidence of pneumonia in certain patients. **Table 11-1** describes positioning techniques you need to be familiar with and their appropriate use.

Table 11-1 Patient Positioning Techniques to Minimize Hypoxemia

Use/Recommend	Comments
Semi-Fowler's Position (Head of the Bed Elevated 30 Degrees or More)	
To minimize ventilator-associated pneumonia in patients receiving mechanical ventilation	• Use on all ventilator-supported patients unless contraindicated • Helps prevent aspiration • Improves the distribution of ventilation • Enhances diaphragmatic action
Lateral Rotation Therapy	
To prevent or minimize respiratory complications associated with immobility in bedridden patients	• Employs a bed or air mattress system that automatically turns the patient from side to side • Improves drainage of secretions within the lung and lower airways • Increases the functional residual capacity (FRC) by increasing the critical opening pressure to the independent lung
Keeping the Good Lung Down	
To improve oxygenation in patients with unilateral lung disease	• The patient is positioned in the left or right lateral decubitus position with the *good lung down.* • Improves oxygenation by diverting most blood flow and ventilation to the dependent (good) lung • Exceptions in which the good lung is kept up include (1) lung abscess or bleeding and (2) unilateral pulmonary interstitial emphysema (PIE) in infants

Use/Recommend	Comments
Prone Positioning ("Proning")	
To improve oxygenation in patients with ARDS and refractory hypoxemia	• Improves oxygenation by shifting blood flow to better-aerated regions; may also improve diaphragmatic action • Facilitated by devices that support the chest and pelvis, leaving the abdomen freely suspended • Trial recommended for patients with acute respiratory distress syndrome (ARDS) if oxygenation is inadequate on $Fio_2 \geq 0.6$ and PEEP ≥ 10 cm H_2O • Not all patients will benefit; an increase in $Pao_2 > 10$ torr in the first 30 minutes is a good indicator of success • Should be maintained for a minimum of 12 hours at a time, as tolerated • Not recommended for patients whose heads cannot be in a face-down position, for those who have circulatory problems, for those with a fractured pelvis, and for those who are morbidly obese or for those at high risk for needing cardiopulmonary resuscitation • Major risks include extubation and dislodgement of intravascular catheters

Preventing Procedure-Associated Hypoxemia

Hypoxemia is a potential complication of many respiratory therapy procedures (e.g., postural drainage, suctioning, exercise testing) and can worsen in patients with acute lung injury or acute respiratory distress syndrome (ARDS) whenever ventilator disconnection occurs. General guidelines for avoiding procedure-associated hypoxemia include the following:

- Ensure that the patient is adequately oxygenated before any risky procedure.
- Always monitor the patient's Spo_2 before, during, and after any risky procedure.
- If a patient develops hypoxemia during a procedure, the following apply:
  ○ For mild hypoxemia (Spo_2 drops by more than 4–5% but remains ≥ 88–90%), increase the Fio_2.
  ○ For moderate to severe hypoxemia (Spo_2 drops below 88–90%), immediately terminate the procedure and administer 100% O_2.

Suctioning is a particular case because it involves both the removal of oxygen and reduction of lung volume. Key pointers for preventing hypoxemia due to suctioning include the following:

- Always preoxygenate the patient with 100% O_2 (10% increase from baseline for neonates) for 30–60 seconds.
- Set suction pressure at the lowest level needed to effectively clear secretions.
- Limit each attempt to no more than 10–15 seconds.
- If the patient is receiving invasive ventilatory support for hypoxemic respiratory failure/ARDS, prevent ventilator disconnection by using either of the following:
  ○ An in-line/closed catheter system (ideal)
  ○ A bronchoscope ventilator adapter (swivel adapter with self-sealing port)
- If available, use the 100% O_2 button provided on the intensive care unit (ICU) ventilator.
- Recommend or implement a lung recruitment maneuver after any suctioning episode likely to have caused a reduction in lung volume (e.g., loss of PEEP).

Initiating and Adjusting Mask or Nasal CPAP

CPAP involves *spontaneous breathing at an elevated baseline pressure*. CPAP is indicated to treat obstructive sleep apnea and acute cardiogenic pulmonary edema, as well as to treat hypoxemic respiratory failure/infant respiratory distress syndrome (IRDS) and apnea of prematurity in neonates.

To avoid confusion, we refer to elevated baseline pressures during invasive mechanical ventilation as PEEP and apply the term *expiratory positive airway pressure* (EPAP) for elevated baseline pressures during noninvasive ventilation. Assembly and troubleshooting of CPAP and noninvasive systems are covered in Chapter 6. Here we focus on the procedures involved in the application of simple CPAP.

Key points related to the application of CPAP for sleep apnea include the following:

- Counsel patients regarding maintaining good sleep habits, ensuring a comfortable sleep environment, and avoiding factors that can interfere with sleep.
- Have patients select the mask option with which they are most comfortable; confirm good fit and minimal leakage.
- Set CPAP level by prescription or auto-CPAP (maximum 15 cm H_2O).
- Assess effectiveness by apnea-hypopnea index (AHI), with optimum control indicated by an AHI < 5/hour.
- If the patient cannot tolerate CPAP, assess and recommend equipment or interface alternatives to improve tolerance—for example, various mask options, humidification, ramp feature, auto-titration, pressure relief (aka C-flex, expiratory pressure relief [EPR], bilevel positive airway pressure [BiPAP]).

Key points related to the application of CPAP to treat cardiogenic pulmonary edema include the following:

- Avoid this method if systolic blood pressure (BP) < 90 mm Hg, acute MI, Glasgow ≤ 8, or need for intubation.
- Select/use a CPAP or noninvasive positive-pressure ventilation (NPPV) device capable of providing 100% O_2.
- Start therapy at 10 cm H_2O and 100% O_2; titrate pressure/Fio_2 to maintain Spo_2 > 90%.
- Switch to bilevel ventilation with backup rate if hypopnea or hypercapnia is evident.

Key points related to the application of CPAP to neonates and infants include the following:

- Avoid this method in infants with a congenital diaphragmatic hernia, tracheoesophageal (T-E) fistula, choanal atresia, severe cardiovascular instability, or hypercapnic respiratory failure ($Paco_2$ > 60 torr, pH < 7.25).
- Recommend insertion of an orogastric tube to prevent gastric distention.
- For bubble systems, use sterile H_2O (add 0.25% acetic acid for infection control).
- Set the flow to 5–10 L/min (continuous-flow systems, e.g., bubble CPAP).
- Start therapy at 4–6 cm H_2O, 40–50% O_2.
- Adjust to maintain Spo_2 87–93%, minimize chest retractions and grunting, and improve aeration (as indicated by chest x-ray).
- Switch to ventilatory support if Pao_2 < 50 torr on CPAP > 7 cm H_2O and Fio_2 > 0.60 or hypercapnic respiratory failure develops.

Initiating and Adjusting Mechanical Ventilation

Chapter 6 covers the selection of ventilators and related equipment. Chapter 8 reviews procedures for verifying proper ventilator function.

Here we focus on selecting the appropriate ventilator mode, setting initial parameters, and making basic adjustments to ensure adequate ventilation and oxygenation. **Box 11-1** outlines key elements in initiating mechanical ventilation.

Initiating and Adjusting Invasive Mechanical Ventilation

Selecting the Mode

The NBRC expects candidates to be proficient with all common invasive ventilator modes. For invasive ventilatory support, the NBRC uses a simplified classification system that is based on whether the control variable is volume (volume control [VC]) or pressure (pressure control [PC]) and whether only machine breaths are provided (assist/control [A/C]) or spontaneous breaths are incorporated (synchronized intermittent mandatory ventilation [SIMV]). Applying this system yields *four* basic combinations you are likely to be tested on the NBRC exams: VC, A/C; VC, SIMV; PC, A/C; and PC, SIMV. Of course, you also will be assessed on your knowledge of pressure support (PS) and PEEP as "add-ons" to a primary mode. Although they are less common, you also may see a few questions on advanced or dual modes such as pressure-regulated volume control (PRVC) and airway pressurerelease ventilation (APRV).

Table 11-2 describes each of these modes of ventilation and "add-ons," specifies their appropriate use, and defines their advantages and disadvantages. In NBRC scenarios, you generally should start an intubated patient in respiratory failure on *full ventilatory support*, with the ventilator initially responsible for the full minute volume and workload. Full ventilatory support modes include A/C (VC or PC) and normal-rate SIMV (VC or PC), usually with PS or dual-mode ventilation, which is a hybrid combination of VC and PC, such as the PRVC available in the Maquet Servo-I ventilator. If, however, the physician wants to avoid intubation but still provide a patient with ventilatory support, you should select or recommend noninvasive ventilation (NIV).

Box 11-1 Key Elements in Initiating Mechanical Ventilation

- Verify and evaluate order or protocol; scan chart for indications and precautions.
- Evaluate the patient's vital signs, breath sounds, and applicable monitored parameters (e.g., electrocardiogram [ECG], Spo_2).
- Connect the ventilator to an emergency electrical outlet and applicable gas supply (usually 50 psi air and O_2).
- Turn on the ventilator, test circuit, and verify proper ventilator function.
- Select appropriate ventilator mode and settings, including initial alarm parameters.
- Analyze and confirm Fio_2 (if appropriate).
- Connect the patient to the ventilator, and confirm ventilation (chest rise, return tidal volume, breath sounds).
- Reassess the patient, including comfort, oxygenation, ventilation, mechanics, and hemodynamics.
- Adjust ventilator settings (including alarms) to ensure adequate ventilation and oxygenation and patient–ventilator synchrony.
- Record pertinent data in the patient's record and departmental records.
- Notify appropriate personnel and make any necessary recommendations or modifications to the care plan.

Data from Scanlan CL, West GA, von der Heydt PA, Dolan GK. *Respiratory Therapy Competency Evaluation Manual.* Boston: Blackwell Scientific; 1984.

Table 11-2 Invasive Mechanical Ventilation Modes

Description	Recommend or Use	Advantages	Disadvantages
Pure Control Mode (Patient Triggering Not Allowed)			
• Rate fixed by ventilator setting • No patient triggering • All machine (mandatory) breaths • Provides full support • May control either volume (VC) or pressure (PC)	• When full support is needed but the rate and pattern must be controlled, or patient effort eliminated; examples include inverse I:E ratio ventilation and permissive hypercapnia	• Rate, ventilatory pattern, and Paco$_2$ are controlled • Eliminates work of breathing (as long as the patient makes no efforts) • Allows for "abnormal" patterns such as inverse I:E ratio	• Poorly tolerated • Patient efforts cause asynchrony ("fighting the ventilator") and increased work of breathing (WOB) • May require heavy sedation or neuromuscular paralysis

(continues)

Table 11-2 Invasive Mechanical Ventilation Modes (*continued*)

Description	Recommend or Use	Advantages	Disadvantages
Assist/Control (A/C)			
• The ventilator provides a guaranteed rate, which the patient can exceed by triggering additional machine breaths • All machine (mandatory) breaths • Provides full ventilatory support (no spontaneous breaths) • Can be VC or PC	• When full ventilatory support is needed but the patient's breathing rate results in acceptable Pa_{CO_2}	• The patient controls his or her own breathing rate (above set rate) and Pa_{CO_2} level • May avoid the need for sedation or paralysis • Guaranteed rate if patient's rate falls	• Hyperventilation can occur at high triggering rates (due to anxiety, fear, pain, brain injury, fever, or hypoxemia) • Asynchronous breathing due to trigger, flow, or cycle problems; may increase WOB and O_2 consumption • May worsen auto-PEEP in COPD/asthma patients
Synchronous Intermittent Mandatory Ventilation (SIMV)			
• The patient breathes spontaneously between machine breaths • Provides full support at normal rates (partial at lower rates) • Machine breaths may be VC or PC • Spontaneous breaths may be pressure supported	• When full support is needed but the patient's rate causes hyperventilation on A/C • Ventilator weaning (being replaced by SBTs on T-tube, CPAP, or BiPAP)	• Allows graded support adjustments • Spontaneous breathing allowed; patient controls rate and pattern • Decreased need for sedation • Less "fighting" of ventilator • Lower mean pressures than with A/C	• Hypoventilation is a hazard at low rates (if adequate minute volume is not ensured) • Asynchrony can still occur during both machine and PS breaths
Pressure-Regulated Volume Control (PRVC)			
• Pressure-control A/C ventilation in which the pressure limit automatically adjusts breath to breath (according to patient mechanics) to maintain a set target tidal volume	• For patients requiring the lowest possible pressure and a guaranteed consistent V_T • For patients requiring variable inspiratory flow • For patients with changing C_{rs} or Raw	• Lower PIP than VC or PC, A/C; lower incidence of barotrauma • Pressure automatically adjusts to changing C_{rs} and Raw • Near-constant V_T • The patient controls rate and minute ventilation • Automatic decrease in ventilatory support as the patient improves • Decelerating flow pattern (improves oxygenation)	• Variable patient effort results in variable V_T and possible asynchrony • Severe increase in Raw or decrease in C_{rs} may result in high/unsafe PIP or reduced V_T • When patient demand increases, pressure level may diminish when support is most needed • As the pressure drops, P_{mean} drops, possibly causing hypoxemia • May cause/worsen auto-PEEP • Ventilator unable to differentiate between patient-caused *vs* machine-generated increases on Raw (e.g., wet filters)

Description	Recommend or Use	Advantages	Disadvantages
Airway Pressure-Release Ventilation (APRV)			
• Equivalent to CPAP with intermittent releases in pressure to baseline • Technically, time-triggered, pressure-limited, time-cycled ventilation with spontaneous breathing at the high- and low-pressure levels • Often referred to as "inverted IMV" (based on graphic appearance)	• For patients with acute lung injury, especially when $P_{plat} > 30$ cm H_2O • For patients with refractory hypoxemia due to collapsed alveoli • For patients with massive atelectasis	• Lower PIP/P_{plat} than VC, PC A/C • Less hemodynamic impact than A/C • Reduced risk of lung injury • Allows for spontaneous breathing throughout the ventilatory cycle • Improves V/Q matching and oxygenation • May decrease VD_{phys} and lower minute ventilation needs • Reduces the need for sedation/paralysis	• V_T delivery depends on C_{rs}, Raw, and patient effort • Provides partial support only (relies on spontaneous breathing to help remove CO_2) • Caution should be used with hemodynamically unstable patients • Auto-PEEP is usually present (and desired!) • Asynchrony can occur if spontaneous breaths are out of phase with release time
Pressure Support (PS) as Sole Mode			
• Patient-triggered, pressure-limited, flow-cycled spontaneous breaths • Provides full support only if pressure level yields normal V_T ("PSV_{max}") • V_T depends on pressure level and patient effort	• To overcome the imposed work of breathing caused by artificial airways (low PSV) • To boost the spontaneous V_T of patients receiving SIMV or CPAP • To incrementally lower support levels (for weaning)	• The patient controls the rate of breathing, inspiratory time, and flow • Results in a lower rate, higher V_T, less muscle activity, and lower O_2 consumption than pure spontaneous breathing (CPAP) • Improves respiratory muscle conditioning; facilitates weaning	• Without backup rate (SIMV), hypoventilation can occur • Variable V_T and minute ventilation • Unless rise time and flow cycle can be adjusted, asynchrony can occur • In COPD patients, flow cycling to end-inspiration may either require active effort or be prolonged (due to air-trapping)

A/C, assist control; BiPAP, bilevel positive airway pressure; COPD, chronic obstructive pulmonary disease; CPAP, continuous positive airway pressure; C_{rs}, respiratory system compliance (lung + thorax); IMV, intermittent mandatory ventilation; PC, pressure control; PEEP, positive end-expiratory pressure; PIP, peak inspiratory pressure; P_{mean}, mean airway pressure; P_{plat}, plateau pressure; PSV, pressure support ventilation; Raw, airway resistance; SBT, spontaneous breathing trial; V/Q, ventilation–perfusion ratio; VC, volume control; VD_{phys}, physiologic deadspace; V_T, tidal volume.

In terms of using VC or PC for mandatory breaths, in the NBRC hospital, *either option is satisfactory as long as the volume or pressure setting helps minimize the likelihood of barotrauma* by delivering 6–8 mL/kg V_T of predicted body weight (PBW). **Table 11-3** compares the basic advantages and disadvantages of volume and pressure control of mandatory breaths. *To help avoid or worsen lung injury, patients requiring plateau pressures higher than 30 cm H_2O during VC ventilation should probably be switched to pressure control at a safe pressure limit (i.e., 30 cm H_2O or less).*

Initiating Invasive Mechanical Ventilation

Table 11-4 outlines the typical settings used to initiate A/C or SIMV ventilation for adult patients. In terms of tidal volumes, the NBRC generally expects an initial setting of 6–8 mL/kg of PBW for

Table 11-3 Comparison of Volume Control and Pressure Control of Mandatory Breaths

Breath Control	Advantages	Disadvantages
Volume control (VC)	• Maintains constant V_T with changes in C_{rs} and Raw • Changes in C_{rs} and Raw easy to detect by monitoring PIPs	• Airway pressures can rise as C_{rs} falls and Raw increases, risking barotrauma • Fixed flow pattern (square) can cause asynchrony
Pressure control (PC)	• Variable decelerating flow pattern aids patient synchrony • Less risk of barotrauma with decreasing C_{rs} or increasing Raw	• V_T varies with changes in C_{rs} and Raw • Changes in C_{rs} and Raw difficult to detect • Changes in tidal volume and minute ventilation must be monitored closely

C_{rs}, respiratory system compliance (lung + thorax); PIP, peak inspiratory pressure; Raw, airway resistance; V_T, tidal volume.

Table 11-4 Typical Initial Settings for Full Ventilatory Support of Adults

Parameter	Typical Settings
Tidal volume (VC or PRVC)	• 6–8 mL/kg PBW; keep $P_{plat} \leq$ 30–35 cm H_2O • 4–6 mL/kg in ARDS (ARDS protocol)
Pressure limit (PC)	• 20–30 cm H_2O to achieve expired V_T as above
Rate	• 8–24/min (up to 35/min if using low-V_T strategy)
Trigger/sensitivity	• Pressure triggering: 1–2 cm H_2O below baseline • Flow triggering: 1–3 L/min below baseline
Flow, I-time, I:E	• Set to achieve I:E $\leq$ 1:1 (e.g., 1:2, 1:3) and prevent auto-PEEP by allowing proper E-time
Flow waveform	• VC: square or decelerating with flow enough to prevent scalloping (flow starvation) of inspiratory pressure curve (use flow compensation if available) • PC: adjust rise time to achieve pressure plateau without spiking (too much flow)
Pressure support (SIMV only)	• 5–10 cm H_2O as needed to overcome artificial airway resistance and maintain an acceptable spontaneous rate ($<$ 25/min) and work of breathing
Fio_2	• Initially 60–100% if Sao_2 or Pao_2 data not available • Then as needed to maintain $Pao_2 \geq$ 60 torr or $Sao_2 \geq$ 92% • ARDS: Fio_2/PEEP combinations (ARDS protocol)
PEEP	• Initially 5–10 cm H_2O, then as needed to maintain $Sao_2 \geq$ 92% with $Fio_2 \leq$ 50% • ARDS: Fio_2/PEEP combinations (ARDS protocol) • As needed to balance auto-PEEP

ARDS, acute respiratory distress syndrome; E-time, expiratory time; PBW, predicted body weight; PC, pressure control; PEEP, positive end-expiratory pressure; P_{plat}, plateau pressure; PRVC, pressure-regulated volume control; SIMV, synchronized intermittent mandatory ventilation; VC, volume control.

most patients, *except those with acute hypoxemic respiratory failure*, in accordance with the National Heart, Lung, and Blood Institute (NHLBI) ARDS protocol. To compute the PBW, use the applicable gender-specific formula:

$$\text{Male PBW (kg)} = 50 + 2.3[\text{height (in.)} - 60]$$

$$\text{Female PBW (kg)} = 45.5 + 2.3[\text{height (in.)} - 60]$$

For example, the PBW for a male patient who is 6 feet (72 in.) tall would be calculated as follows:

$$PBW\ (kg) = 50 + 2.3\ [72 - 60]$$

$$PBW\ (kg) = 50 + 27.6$$

$$PBW\ (kg) = 78\ kg$$

Using 8 mL/kg for this patient would yield a starting volume of approximately 625 mL. Note that using PBW (versus actual weight) is necessary to avoid excessive volumes. Based on this understanding, if this 6-foot-tall patient weighs 120 kg (265 lb), *we would still apply a V_T in the range of 600–800 mL*, and definitely *not* 1200 mL!

APRV is a different mode with unique settings. As depicted in **Figure 11-1**, patients in APRV breathe spontaneously at a high baseline pressure termed P_{high} (the inflation pressure, equivalent to CPAP). However, after a set time interval termed T_{high}, this pressure is released or allowed to drop down to a lower deflation pressure termed P_{low}. This drop in pressure causes the patient to exhale, which facilitates CO_2 removal, with the length of this release termed T_{low}. P_{low} generally is set in the range of 0–8 cm H_2O, with P_{high} set to provide an inflation volume of 4–8 mL/kg PBW but kept below 30–35 cm H_2O. Initially, T_{high} is set in the range of 3–5 seconds, with T_{low} typically adjusted to between 0.2 and 0.8 seconds, resulting in approximately 10–20 inflation/deflation cycles per minute. The initial FiO_2 settings for APRV are the same as for traditional full-support modes. However, it is important to note that because of the nature of APRV, it should only be used on patients who can spontaneously trigger enough breaths to maintain adequate minute ventilation. Pressure-supported breaths can be added to both the P_{high} and P_{low} levels to improve CO_2 removal.

Adjusting Invasive Mechanical Ventilation

In adjusting ventilator settings, your primary goals are to (1) achieve acceptable arterial blood gases (ABGs) and (2) maximize patient comfort and patient–ventilator synchrony. To achieve acceptable ABGs, you should focus on normalizing the pH, assuring adequate oxygenation, and optimizing PEEP. To maximize patient comfort and synchrony, you must be able to detect and correct asynchrony, should it occur (covered in a subsequent section).

Normalizing the pH

To normalize the pH, you adjust the minute ventilation, which alters the $Paco_2$. **Table 11-5** outlines the methods commonly used to alter pH and $Paco_2$ for the various ventilator modes. In most cases, the goal is a pH between 7.35 and 7.45. However, depending on the patient's underlying problem, you may allow the pH to go as low as 7.25 or as high as 7.50. Note also that in normalizing the pH of some patients, the resulting $Paco_2$ may be abnormal. For example, in a patient with chronic obstructive pulmonary disease (COPD) who has chronic CO_2 retention (compensated respiratory acidosis),

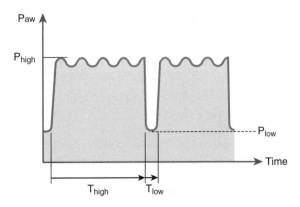

Figure 11-1 Representative Pressure-Versus-Time Graph for Airway Pressure-Release Ventilation.

Table 11-5 Altering the pH and Paco$_2$ of Adult Patients Receiving Ventilatory Support

Mode	To Decrease Paco$_2$/Increase pH	To Increase Paco$_2$/Decrease pH
Volume Control		
A/C	• Increase set rate (keep ≤ 24/min) • Increase set V$_T$ (keep P$_{plat}$ < 30–35 cm H$_2$O)	• Decrease set rate (keep ≥ 8/min) • Add mechanical deadspace • Decrease V$_T$ if > 8 mL/Kg
SIMV	• Increase set rate (keep ≤ 24/min) • Increase set V$_T$ (keep P$_{plat}$ < 30 cm H$_2$O) • Add/increase pressure support	• Decrease set rate (keep ≥ 6-8/min) • Decrease set V$_T$ • Decrease pressure support
Pressure Control		
A/C	• Increase set rate (keep ≤ 24/min) • Increase ΔP (PIP – PEEP)	• Decrease set rate (keep ≥ 6–8/min) • Decrease ΔP (PIP – PEEP)
SIMV	• Increase set rate (≤ 24/min) • Increase ΔP (PIP – PEEP) • Add/increase pressure support	• Decrease set rate (≥ 6–8/min) • Decrease ΔP (PIP – PEEP) • Decrease pressure support
APRV	• Increase release frequency (↓T$_{high}$) • Increase ΔP (P$_{high}$ – P$_{low}$)	• Decrease release frequency (↑T$_{high}$) • Decrease ΔP (P$_{high}$ – P$_{low}$)

A/C, assist control; APRV, airway pressure release ventilation; PEEP, positive end-expiratory pressure; PIP, peak inspiratory pressure; SIMV, synchronized intermittent mandatory ventilation.

a normal pH may be achieved with Paco$_2$ levels of 55 torr or higher. In contrast, in a patient with severe (uncorrected) diabetic ketoacidosis and respiratory failure, a normal pH may be achieved only via hyperventilation—that is, with a lower-than-normal Paco$_2$.

Because you alter the minute ventilation to adjust the pH, you can do so by changing the rate or the delivered V$_T$. In all modes (except CPAP), the base machine rate is set. In VC modes, the delivered V$_T$ is set. In PC modes, you alter the delivered V$_T$ by increasing or decreasing the driving pressure, termed ΔP (PIP – PEEP). The following guidelines apply to making such changes:

- In most modes, to adjust the pH, you first adjust the set rate, keeping it in the range of 8–24/min (up to 35/min in acute lung injury).
- If rate adjustments alone do not normalize the pH, then you alter the delivered V$_T$.
- In altering the delivered V$_T$, try to keep it between 4 and 8 mL/kg PBW with the P$_{plat}$ ≤ 30–35 cm H$_2$O.
- If the pH remains below 7.30 and the rate, delivered V$_T$, and P$_{plat}$ are at their recommended high limits, consider permissive hypercapnia (allowing the Paco$_2$ to rise as long as the pH remains above 7.20–7.25).

Normalizing Oxygenation

To ensure normal oxygenation, you need to do the following:

1. Adjust/maintain an acceptable Pao$_2$ and Sao$_2$.
2. Check and confirm an acceptable Hb content (≥10 g/dL).
3. Check for and confirm adequate circulation.

For most patients, acceptable ABG values for oxygenation are Pao$_2$ ≥ 65 torr and Sao$_2$ ≥ 92%. Note, however, that in patients with either COPD or ARDS, we can accept Pao$_2$ values as low as 55 torr as long as we keep the arterial saturation at or above 88%.

General guidelines for initial adjustment of Pao$_2$/Sao$_2$ are as follows:

- If an acceptable Pao$_2$/Sao$_2$ can be maintained on less than 50% O$_2$, normalize oxygenation by altering the Fio$_2$.

- If an acceptable Pao_2/Sao_2 cannot be maintained on less than 50% O_2, normalize oxygenation by altering the baseline pressure (PEEP, CPAP, P_{low}).
- If Pao_2/Fio_2 ratio is 200 or less or if 50% or more O_2 with PEEP of 12 cm H_2O or more cannot provide acceptable Pao_2/Sao_2 values, you should recommend the NHLBI ARDS protocol.
- When oxygenation improves, first decrease Fio_2 until it is 0.50 or less, and then lower PEEP.

Optimizing PEEP

Deciding when to apply PEEP is easy; determining how much PEEP to use is difficult. The problem is that too little PEEP may not prevent alveolar collapse, whereas too much can cause overdistension and worsen preexisting lung injury. "Optimal" PEEP represents the end-expiratory pressure level that maximizes patient benefits while minimizing risks.

Currently, there are several ways to determine optimal PEEP, any of which might appear on the NBRC exams. These different methods define optimal PEEP as the pressure level that does the following:

1. Maximizes O_2 delivery to the tissues
2. Yields the highest static (respiratory system) compliance (C_{rs})
3. Provides the maximum volume change for a given ΔP
4. Prevents alveolar collapse
5. Maximizes the average expired tidal %CO_2

Method 1 is based on the fact that oxygen delivery to the tissues depends on the cardiac output (CO) and the arterial O_2 content (Cao_2):

$$\textbf{O}_2 \textbf{ tissue delivery} = \textbf{CO} \times \textbf{Cao}_2$$

In general, as PEEP levels rise, so does the patient's arterial O_2 content (good!). However, the higher the PEEP level, the greater the potential negative impact on cardiac output (bad!). Based on these relationships, PEEP is optimized when the desired increase in CaO_2 is not offset by decreases in CO.

Because this method requires serial measurements of cardiac output (via pulmonary artery [PA] catheter or noninvasive means) and ABGs, it is not commonly used and thus not frequently tested on the NBRC exams. Instead, the NBRC may substitute arterial blood pressure as an indicator of cardiac output, with SpO_2 measurements used instead of ABGs. Using these data, optimum PEEP is the one needed to maintain the $SpO_2 \geq 88-90\%$ *without lowering the patient's blood pressure*. Also based on this approach, you would "back off" any increase in PEEP that significantly lowers the patient's blood pressure.

Methods 2 through 4 all use respiratory mechanics to determine optimal PEEP. Common to these methods is the fact that bedside estimates of respiratory mechanics require (1) complete relaxation of the patient's respiratory muscles *and* (2) adequate time under static conditions of zero flow for airway and alveolar pressures to equilibrate (at least 2–3 seconds). For these reasons, getting accurate data can be challenging and sometimes may require sedation or paralysis.

Method 2 involves raising PEEP while simultaneously measuring the patient's static compliance during VC ventilation. An example of this type of PEEP study as it might appear on the NBRC exams is as follows:

PEEP (cm H_2O)	V_T (mL)	PIP (cm H_2O)	P_{plat} (cm H_2O)
0	600	30	20
5	600	36	24
10	600	41	27
15	600	45	33
20	600	49	41

First, you can disregard the peak pressure (PIP)—it is there to confuse you. What you are interested in is the difference between the plateau pressure and the positive end-expiratory pressure: P_{plat} − PEEP. *Because the tidal volume is constant, the smaller this difference, the greater the compliance (Remember: C[RS] = V_T/[P_{plat} − PEEP]).* This relationship is demonstrated here:

P_{plat} (cm H_2O)	PEEP (cm H_2O)	PIP (cm H_2O)	C_{rs} (mL/cm H_2O)
20	0	20	30
24	5	19	32
27	10	17	35
33	15	18	33
41	20	21	29

Based on this method, the optimal PEEP for this patient would be 10 cm H_2O, the level yielding the highest static compliance (35 mL/cm H_2O).

What if the patient is receiving PC ventilation? In this case, you can use method 3, which applies the same basic concept as just discussed. With this method, however, *rather than maintain a constant volume, you maintain a constant* ΔP (PIP − PEEP), typically 15–25 cm H_2O. You then assess the exhaled V_T, with the largest increase representing the optimal PEEP. For obvious reasons, this approach is called the *equal pressure method.* An example of the equal pressure method for determining optimal PEEP as it might appear on the NBRC exams is as follows:

PEEP (cm H_2O)	PIP (cm H_2O)	V_T (mL)
5	20	390
10	25	410
15	30	430
20	35	380

Using method 3, the optimal PEEP for this patient is 15 cm H_2O, corresponding to the maximum volume change for a given ΔP (430 mL).

The last approach for establishing optimal PEEP is to determine the minimum pressure needed to prevent alveolar collapse. One of two methods can be used to make this determination: (1) plotting a static pressure-volume curve or (2) titrating PEEP *down* after a recruitment maneuver. Here we cover only the use of static pressure-volume curves to determine optimum PEEP. The decremental PEEP method is covered in this chapter's section on recruitment maneuvers.

Figure 11-2 depicts an idealized pressure-volume curve for a patient, obtained by recording the *static* pressure at each of several gradual increases in volume. Although this measurement can be performed manually (with a "super" syringe), some newer ventilators provide an automated routine to obtain the relevant data. Key points are as follows:

- The slope of any line on this graph equals compliance ($\Delta V/\Delta P$).
- The curve exhibits a characteristic "S" shape:
  ○ Low slope (low compliance) at low pressures and volumes—indicates that high pressures are needed to open collapsed alveoli
  ○ A steep slope (high compliance) at moderate volumes/pressures—is equivalent to the "sweet spot" for safe and efficient volume exchange
  ○ A low slope (low compliance) at high pressures and volumes—indicates that the limits of elastic expansion have been reached (i.e., overdistention is occurring [beak sign])

As indicated in Figure 11-2, the minimum pressure needed to prevent alveolar collapse corresponds to the lowest pressure needed to *exceed* the pressure required to open collapsed alveoli. This point is called the *lower inflection point* or LIP. Once measured, PEEP typically is set 2–3 cm H_2O above the LIP.

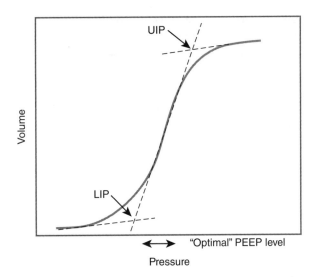

Figure 11-2 Idealized Static Pressure-Volume Curve of the Respiratory System. The points at which the slope of the curve changes are called inflection points (mathematically extrapolated from tangents of the curve). Optimal PEEP is the lowest pressure needed to exceed the lower inflection point (LIP). UIP, upper inflection point, representing the changeover from high compliance to low compliance at high lung volume.

Method 5 uses volumetric capnography to measure the average tidal CO_2 concentration or $VTCO_2$. As the PEEP level rises and additional perfused alveoli are recruited, the $\%VTCO_2$ also increases. On the other hand, if the PEEP level is high enough to overdistend the alveoli, deadspace increases, lung perfusion is impeded, and the $\%VTCO_2$ will begin to fall. Using this method, optimum PEEP is reached just before the $\%VTCO_2$ begins to fall. Note that this approach can be used by itself to determine optimum PEEP or in conjunction with methods 2–4.

Noninvasive Positive Pressure Ventilation (NPPV/BiPAP)

NPPV is the delivery of assisted mechanical ventilation without the need for an artificial tracheal airway. Because intubation is not required, NPPV provides many advantages over invasive support, but it also has significant limitations (**Table 11-6**).

The predominant mode of NPPV is bilevel positive airway pressure (BiPAP). BiPAP provides patient or machine-triggered (back up rate), pressure-limited breaths with positive pressure maintained throughout the expiratory phase.

BiPAP: Basic Requirements, Indications, and Contraindications

Unlike invasive ventilatory support, *BiPAP requires that the patient has control over his or her upper airway function, can manage secretions, and is cooperative and motivated.*

Indications for BiPAP include the following:

- To avoid intubation of patients in hypercapnic respiratory failure (e.g., COPD)
- To avoid reintubation of patients after extubation
- To treat patients with acute cardiogenic pulmonary edema
- To treat patients with sleep apnea (especially central sleep apnea)
- To support patients with chronic hypoventilation syndromes
- To alleviate breathlessness and fatigue in terminally ill patients

There are several situations or conditions in which BiPAP generally should *not* be used to support ventilation. These include the following:

- Respiratory or cardiac arrest
- pH < 7.20

Table 11-6 Advantages and Limitations of Noninvasive Ventilation

Advantages	Limitations
• Avoidance of intubation-related trauma	• Can be used only in cooperative patients
• Preservation of airway defenses	• Does not provide direct airway access
• Lower incidence of nosocomial pneumonia	• Increases the risk of secretion retention
• Permits normal speech and eating*	• Increases the risk of aspiration
• Reduces the need for sedation	• Increases the risk of pressure sores
• Facilitates the weaning process	• Requires more caregiver time (initially)
• Shorter duration of ventilation/length of hospital stay	
• Reduces costs	
*By removing interface for a short period of time.	

- Uncooperative patient
- Excessive airway secretions
- Need for airway protection, high risk for aspiration
- Upper airway obstruction
- Hemodynamic instability/hypotension
- Uncontrolled arrhythmias
- Active upper gastrointestinal bleeding
- Facial burns or trauma
- Nausea and vomiting

Note that BiPAP is similar to CPAP with pressure support (CPAP+PS) during invasive ventilation but with some key distinctions. When using CPAP+PS, the PS level is the pressure above CPAP. Thus, a CPAP+PS order for "5+10 cm H_2O" would mean a CPAP pressure of 5 cm H_2O, *on top of which* you would add 10 cm H_2O PS, with the resulting PIP being 15 cm H_2O with a driving pressure (ΔP) of 15 − 5, or 10 cm H_2O.

With BiPAP, you independently set two pressure levels: the peak or *IPAP* pressure (inspiratory positive airway pressure) and the baseline or *EPAP* pressure (expiratory positive airway pressure—equivalent to CPAP). So, an order for "BiPAP 5/10 cm H_2O" looks similar to the CPAP+PS order but results in a PIP (=IPAP) of 10 cm H_2O and a ΔP of only half as large (i.e., 10 − 5 = 5 cm H_2O).

Initiating and Adjusting BiPAP

Table 11-7 outlines the typical initial settings and basic ways to adjust BiPAP. Additional key pointers related to its application include the following:

- Always confirm that the patient is alert and has intact upper airway function/secretions control.
- Position the patient in a high semi-Fowler's (sitting) position if possible.
- Choose the best interface (generally an oronasal or "full" face mask for acute respiratory failure).
- Establish initial settings (Table 11-7).
- Hold the interface in place (without strapping) until the patient becomes accustomed to it.
- Keep IPAP levels less than 20–25 cm H_2O (esophageal opening pressure) to avoid gastric insufflation.
- Assess for improvement in blood gases, resolution of dyspnea, tachypnea, and accessory muscle use.
- Adjust ventilation (Pa_{CO_2}, pH) via IPAP and ΔP.
- Adjust oxygenation (Pa_{O_2}/Sa_{O_2}) via Fi_{O_2} and EPAP.
- If any factor that is a contraindication to BiPAP develops, or if oxygenation or ventilation worsens, consider intubation and conventional invasive mechanical ventilation.

Table 11-7 Initial Settings and Basic Adjustments for Bilevel Positive Airway Pressure (BiPAP)

Parameter	Initial Settings and Basic Adjustments
Tidal volume	Function of patient effort and ΔP (IPAP – EPAP); aim for 6–8 mL/kg
Pressure limit	Initial IPAP = 10–15 cm H_2O; adjust to normalize pH/$Paco_2$
Rate	Patient determined but set backup rate of at least 8/min
Trigger/sensitivity	If adjustable: 1–2 cm H_2O below baseline pressure or 1–3 L/min below baseline flow
Flow, I-time, or I:E	N/A for spontaneous breaths; in timed modes, start with %I-time in the 20–30% range
Flow waveform	If adjustable, set rise time to achieve the pressure plateau without spiking (left "dog-ear")
Fio_2	As needed to maintain Pao_2 ≥ 65 torr or Sao_2 ≥ 92%
PEEP	Initial EPAP = 5 cm H_2O; adjust to maintain Pao_2 ≥ 65 torr or Sao_2 ≥ 92% (to avoid changing the $Paco_2$ keep ΔP constant)
To adjust pH/$Paco_2$	To ↓ $Paco_2$ or ↑ pH: ↑ IPAP or increase ΔP (also ↑ mandatory rate if low patient rate) To ↑ $Paco_2$ or ↓ pH: ↓ IPAP or decrease ΔP
To adjust Pao_2/Sao_2	If simple V/Q imbalance and Fio_2 < 0.50, raise Fio_2 If shunting is present (Pao_2 ≤ 50 torr and Fio_2 ≥ 0.50), increase EPAP (to avoid altering the $Paco_2$, keep ΔP constant) When oxygenation improves, first decrease Fio_2 until ≤ 0.50, and then lower EPAP (to avoid altering the $Paco_2$, keep ΔP constant)

EPAP, expiratory positive airway pressure; IPAP, inspiratory positive airway pressure; PEEP, positive end-expiratory pressure; V/Q, ventilation–perfusion ratio.

The NBRC questions on BiPAP typically focus on adjusting IPAP and EPAP settings to alter ventilation or oxygenation. Example problems like those commonly appearing on these exams include some of the following:

Problem 1: Patient on 10/5 cm H_2O IPAP/EPAP—you need to improve oxygenation *only*.
Solution: Increase both IPAP and EPAP equally—to 12/7 cm H_2O (increased of 2 cm H_2O equally). This keeps ΔP constant (does not change ventilation), but the increase in baseline pressure may help improve oxygenation.
Problem 2: Patient on 10/5 cm H_2O IPAP/EPAP—you need to increase ventilation *only*.
Solution: Increase *only* the IPAP—to 15 cm H_2O. This will increase ΔP (increasing ventilation), but because the baseline pressure remains unchanged, it will not have a major effect on oxygenation. Alternative, if oxygenation is stable (and patient comfort is an issue), you could also decrease the EPAP (e.g., 2 cm H_2O) to 3 cm of H_2O. This will also increase the ΔP.
Problem 3: Patient on 10/5 cm H_2O IPAP/EPAP—you need to improve oxygenation *and* increase ventilation.
Solution: Increase both IPAP and EPAP but increase IPAP more than EPAP—increase IPAP to 15 cm H_2O and EPAP to 7 cm H_2O. This will increase ΔP (increasing ventilation) while also raising the baseline pressure, which may also help improve oxygenation.

Initiating and Adjusting High-Frequency Ventilation

High-frequency ventilation (HFV) is mechanical ventilation at frequencies between 150 and 900 breaths per minute, with tidal volumes as small as 1–2 mL/kg (significantly less than the anatomic deadspace). Gas transport at such low volumes likely involves various mechanisms, including bulk convection, "pendelluft effect," shear-type dispersion, and molecular diffusion. Because less pressure is transmitted to the distal airways and alveoli, HFV may decrease the risk of ventilator-associated lung injuries such as barotrauma and bronchopulmonary dysplasia (BPD) in neonates. HFV also may improve gas exchange in the presence of air leaks (e.g., persistent pneumothoraces, PIE).

HFV is indicated primarily for patients with hypoxemic respiratory failure who have not responded to more conventional methods of improving oxygenation. Common scenarios include patients with severe IRDS or ARDS, with or without an air-leak syndrome. Additional indications specific to neonates include BPD, meconium aspiration syndrome (MAS), PIE, congenital diaphragmatic hernia (CDH), and pulmonary hypoplasia. Relative contraindications include hypotension/unstable cardiovascular status, the presence of air trapping/dynamic hyperinflation, and (among neonates) intracranial hemorrhage. Moreover, based on current evidence, HFV should not be applied if conventional ventilation can provide adequate patient support. It should not also be used as rescue therapy. Recent studies have shown a transient improvement in oxygenation but an increase in mortality among ARDS patients.

The two primary modes of HFV in current use are high-frequency oscillation ventilation (HFOV) and high-frequency jet ventilation (HFJV). Gas delivery during HFOV is driven by an oscillating rubber diaphragm, much like a stereo speaker. Because the diaphragm pushes gas forward *and* draws gas back through the circuit, both *inspiration and exhalation are active processes (unlike conventional ventilation).* Gas delivery during HFJV is controlled by an interrupter valve that rapidly opens and closes, causing intermittent "jets" or bursts of gas to be applied to the airway. With HFJV, inspiration is active, but *exhalation is passive.*

In the United States, the CareFusion (Sensormedics) 3100A is the most common HFOV device used with infants and small children (a separate model, the 3100B, is available for larger children and adults). The Bunnell LifePulse is the most commonly used device to deliver HFJV, with its application limited to infants and small children. Unlike the free-standing CareFusion HFOV device, the Bunnell LifePulse *always* is used in conjunction with a conventional ventilator, which provides the background PEEP, FiO_2 and intermittent mandatory ventilation (IMV) breaths as needed for alveolar recruitment and stabilization.

A variation of these two modes of ventilation is high-frequency *percussive* ventilation (HFPV). HFPV is delivered via a pneumatically powered, pressure-limited, time-cycled, high-frequency flow interrupter and provides small tidal volumes with 300 to 700 oscillations per minute. In addition to providing ventilatory support, the unique gas flow creates percussive-like pressure waves that also help mobilize pulmonary secretions, further facilitating gas exchange. HFPV is less commonly used than HFOV or HFJV and is available via the Percussionaire VDR volume diffusive ventilator.

Table 11-8 compares HFOV and HFJV ventilation as delivered by these two different ventilators, including commonly recommended initial settings used on neonates, the parameters typically monitored, and how to adjust ventilation and oxygenation. In terms of adjusting ventilation or $PaCO_2$, the *primary* control variable for both HFOV and HFJV is ΔP or the difference between the high and low oscillation/jet pressures. As with conventional ventilation, changes in frequency also can affect ventilation but with lesser effect. Interestingly, frequency changes during HFOV affect CO_2 elimination in a manner opposite to that observed during conventional ventilation—that is, decreasing the HFOV frequency tends to lower the $PaCO_2$, whereas increasing the HFOV frequency tends to raise the $PaCO_2$. In terms of adjusting oxygenation, the *primary* control variables during both HFOV and HFJV are the mean airway pressure (P_{mean}) and FiO_2.

Setting and Adjusting Ventilator Alarms

Ventilator alarms indicate potential ventilator malfunction or untoward changes in patient status. Most ventilator malfunction alarms are preprogrammed, whereas those warning of changes in patient status typically are set by the clinician. **Table 11-9** summarizes some of the most common alarms found in a patient–ventilator system, their recommended settings, and their possible causes.

In general, all noninvasive positive pressure ventilators used in the acute care setting must have a low-pressure/disconnect and power failure alarm. Most have a separate apnea alarm, and some include high-/low-volume and high-pressure alarms. Clinicians should respond to these alarms in the same manner as with invasive ventilatory support, with the emphasis always on ensuring adequate patient ventilation and oxygenation.

Table 11-8 Comparison of High-Frequency Ventilation Modes (Neonatal Application)

HFOV (CareFusion 3100A)	HFJV (Bunnell LifePulse)
Description	
Rapid "push-pull" of small volumes applied to airways via oscillating diaphragm (active inspiration and exhalation)	Rapid application of small bursts of gas to the airways via an interrupter valve (active inspiration with passive exhalation)
Ventilator Control Variables (Ranges)	

Frequency: 3–15 Hz; 180–900/min
%I-time: 30–50%
Bias flow: 0–40 L/min
Power/amplitude: 1–10
P_{mean}: 3–45 cm H_2O
FiO_2: 0.21–1.0 via external blender
	Jet ventilator
	  Frequency: 240–660/min; 6–11 Hz
	  PIP: 8–50 cm H_2O
	  I-time: 0.02–0.034 sec
	  FiO_2: 0.21–1.0; via external blender
	Companion (standard) ventilator
	  PEEP: varies by device and patient
	  FiO_2: 0.21–1.0 to match jet ventilator
	  IMV breaths: varies by device and patient

Circuit	
External blender and heated humidifier system controls FiO_2 and conditions source gas Specialized three-valve circuit delivers source gas, controls P_{mean}, and limits applied pressure	External blender and heated cartridge-type humidifier controls FiO_2 and conditions source gas External box with electronically controlled "pinch valve" to provide gas bursts Special adapter placed between standard ventilator circuit "Y" and endotracheal tube; provides jet port and pressure-monitoring adapter
Typical Initial Settings for Neonates	

Frequency: 10–15 Hz
%I-time: 33% (I:E 1:2)
Bias flow: 10–20 L/min
Power/amplitude: 2–4*
P_{mean}: 10–20 cm H_2O†
FiO_2 as needed for adequate PaO_2/SaO_2
(Note: the larger the patient, the lower the frequency and the higher the applied bias flow, amplitude, and P_{mean})
	Jet ventilator
	  Frequency: 420/min (7 Hz)
	  PIP: 0–2 cm H_2O < PIP on CMV
	  I-time: 0.02 sec
	Standard ventilator
	  PEEP:
	    7–12 cm H_2O or
	    2–4 cm H_2O < P_{mean} on CMV
	  FiO_2 as needed for adequate PaO_2/SaO_2
	  IMV breaths:
	    Frequency: 0–3/min
	    I-time: 0.4–0.6 sec
	    PIP: 20–50% < HFJV PIP

Monitored Parameters	
Frequency %I-time P_{mean} ΔP	PIP ΔP P_{mean} PEEP Servo pressure‡ I:E ratio

(continues)

Table 11-8 Comparison of High-Frequency Ventilation Modes (Neonatal Application) (*continued*)

HFOV (CareFusion 3100A)	HFJV (Bunnell LifePulse)
Adjusting Paco₂ (Ventilation)	
To raise $Paco_2$	To raise $Paco_2$
$\downarrow$ power/amplitude (ΔP)	$\downarrow$ PIP (ΔP)
$\uparrow$ frequency	$\uparrow$ frequency
To lower $Paco_2$	To lower $Paco_2$
$\uparrow$ power/amplitude (ΔP)	$\uparrow$ PIP (ΔP)
$\downarrow$ frequency	$\downarrow$ frequency
$\uparrow$ %I-time	
Adjusting Pao₂ (Oxygenation)	
To increase Pao_2/Sao_2	To increase Pao_2/Sao_2
$\uparrow$ P_{mean}	$\uparrow$ P_{mean} ($\uparrow$ PIP + PEEP, keep ΔP = K)
$\uparrow$ Fio_2	$\uparrow$ Fio_2
$\uparrow$ %I-time	$\uparrow$ I-time
To decrease Pao_2/Sao_2	$\uparrow$ frequency ($\uparrow$ I:E)
$\downarrow$ Fio_2	To decrease Pao_2/Sao_2
$\downarrow$ P_{mean}	$\downarrow$ P_{mean} ($\downarrow$ PIP + PEEP, keep ΔP = K)
	$\downarrow$ Fio_2

CMV, conventional mechanical ventilation; HFJV, high-frequency jet ventilation; HFOV, high-frequency oscillation ventilation; Hz, hertz or cycles per second, 1 Hz, 60 breaths/min; %I-time, percent of total cycle time devoted to inspiration; IMV, intermittent mandatory ventilation; K, constant; ΔP, difference between high and low oscillation or jet applied pressures; PEEP, positive end-expiratory pressure; PIP, peak inspiratory pressure; P_{mean}, mean airway pressure.

*Adjust to get chest "wiggle."

†Set 1–5 cm H_2O higher than P_{mean} on volume-control (VC) or pressure-control (PC) ventilation.

‡Pressure needed to maintain the desired PIP; rough indicator of changes in pulmonary mechanics.

Table 11-9 Clinical Alarms Commonly Used During Adult Mechanical Ventilation

Alarm	Recommended Alarm Parameters	Possible Causes
Ventilator Malfunction Alarms		
Loss of power	Preprogrammed	• Accidental power cord disconnection • Backup battery failure • Tripped circuit breaker • Institutional power failure
Gas supply loss	Preprogrammed	• Failure to connect gas lines to high pressure 50 psi outlets • Gas lines connected to the low-pressure outlet (e.g., flowmeters) • High-pressure line failure
O₂ analyzer alarm	Usually preprogrammed ($\pm$5–6% of set Fio_2)	• Gas source failure (air or O_2) • Analyzer needs calibration or replacement • Sudden changes in delivered Fio_2 (e.g., 100% O_2 button activated for suctioning)

Alarm	Recommended Alarm Parameters	Possible Causes
Temperature	Usually preprogrammed ±2°C set temperature; not to exceed 41°C	• Dry water chamber • Tubing condensation • Defective wiring, probes, and chamber • Heater malfunctioning • Environmental temperature changes in the room • High minute ventilation and high ventilator flow
Patient Status Alarms		
Apnea delay alarm	20 seconds	• Sedation/anesthesia • Low metabolic rate • Low set respiratory rate (< 3/min)
Low-pressure alarm	8 cm H_2O or 5–10 cm H_2O below PIP (use PIP of pressure supported breaths during SIMV)	• Disconnection • Airway/circuit leaks • Alarm set above PIP of pressure supported breath • Improved compliance and resistance
High-pressure limit	50 cm H_2O or 10–15 cm H_2O above PIP (use mechanical breaths' PIPs during SIMV)	• Increased resistance/decreased compliance • Airway obstruction (partial/complete) • Cough/secretions, mucus plugs • Patient–ventilator asynchrony • Anxiety, restlessness, pain • Alarm set below PIP of pressure supported breath
Low PEEP/CPAP	3–5 cm H_2O below set PEEP	• Disconnection • Airway/circuit leaks • Malfunctioning PEEP valve
Low exhaled V_T	100 mL or 10–15% below set V_T or spontaneous V_T during SIMV and CPAP	• Disconnection • Airway/circuit leaks • Pulmonary leaks (bronchopleural fistula) • Shallow spontaneous breathing • Coughing • Patient-ventilator asynchrony
Low $\dot{V}e$	4–5 L/min or 10–15% below minimum SIMV or A/C set $\dot{V}e$	• Same causes as "low exhaled V_T" • Sedation/anesthesia • Low metabolic rate
High $\dot{V}e$	10–15% above baseline $\dot{V}e$	• Increased metabolic rate (e.g., fever) • Tachypnea • Anxiety, restlessness, pain • Patient waking up from anesthesia/sedation

A/C, assist control; CPAP, continuous positive airway pressure; PEEP, positive end-expiratory pressure; PIP, peak inspiratory pressure; SIMV, synchronized intermittent mandatory ventilation.

Modified from Shelledy DC. Initiating and adjusting ventilatory support. In Kacmarek R, Stoller JK and Heuer AJ, eds. *Egan's Fundamentals of Respiratory Care* (11th ed.). St. Louis, MO: Mosby; 2016.

Utilizing Ventilator Graphics

The ventilator graphics display incorporated into most critical care ventilators provides the following essential monitoring capabilities:

- Checking/confirming and fine-tuning ventilator function
- Assessing patients' respiratory mechanics
- Evaluating patients' responses to therapy
- Troubleshooting patient–ventilator interaction

There are two major types of ventilator graphics: scalar (time-based) and X-Y (loops). As depicted in **Figure 11-3**, scalar graphics plot pressure, volume, and flow on the y-axis against time on the x-axis. Most ventilators allow you to change the time scale (sweep speed) when displaying scalar graphics. Changing the time scale by selecting a faster speed gives you a closer look at individual breath waveforms, whereas selecting a slow sweep speed can help you identify trends.

Table 11-10 provides guidance on the uses of scalar graphics, and **Figures 11-4** through **11-6** provide scalar graphic representations likely to appear on the NBRC exams, along with their clinical implications.

X-Y or loop graphics simultaneously display two variables plotted on the x- and y-axes. The two most common loop graphics are pressure (x-axis) versus volume (y-axis) and volume (x-axis) versus flow (y-axis). **Figure 11-7** depicts a representative X-Y plot of volume versus pressure.

Table 11-11 provides guidance on the use of loop graphics. **Figures 11-8** through **11-10** provide common loop graphic representations likely to appear on the NBRC exams, along with their clinical implications.

Figure 11-8 is a graphic representation of the pressure needed to deliver a particular volume; this helps you to assess compliance and resistance "at a glance." As mentioned earlier in this chapter, compliance is given by the slope of the curve. The higher the slope (loop A), the higher the compliance (compare to loop C, where higher pressure is required to deliver a smaller V_T—i.e., a lower

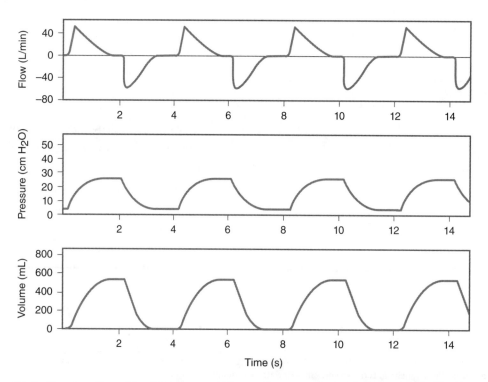

Figure 11-3 Scalar Graphic Display of Flow, Pressure, and Volume Versus Time.
The flow and pressure waveform indicate pressure-control ventilation with 4 cm H_2O PEEP.

Table 11-10 Common Uses for Scalar Graphics

Display	Uses
Flow versus time	• To identify the presence of auto-PEEP (see Figure 11-4) • To assess/adjust PC, PS rise time • To assess/adjust PC inspiratory time (see Figure 11-5) • To identify asynchrony
Pressure versus time	• To confirm PIP and PEEP level • To visually assess mechanics using PIP – P_{plat} ($\approx$ Raw) and P_{plat} – PEEP ($\approx C_{rs}$) • To identify asynchrony
Volume versus time	• To identify leaks (see Figure 11-6) • To identify asynchrony
PC, pressure control; PS, pressure support; PEEP, positive end-expiratory pressure; PIP, peak inspiratory pressure.	

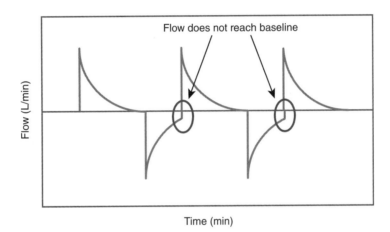

Figure 11-4 Flow-Time Graphic Showing Auto-PEEP.
Expiratory flow does not return to baseline before the
next breath indicating gas-trapping (circles).

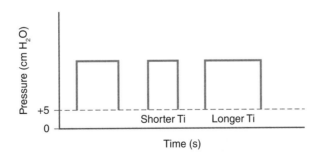

**Figure 11-5 Pressure–Time Graphic of
PCV**. Pressure remains constant during
inspiration, but the time (T_i) to deliver the
pressure has changed.

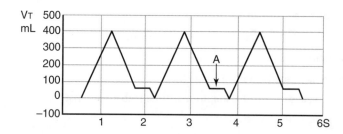

Figure 11-6 Volume–Time Graphic Showing Volume Loss. Note that the expired volume does not return to baseline.

Reproduced from Burns SM, ed. *AACN Protocols for Practice: Noninvasive Monitoring* (2nd ed.). Sudbury, MA: Jones & Bartlett Publishers; 2006.

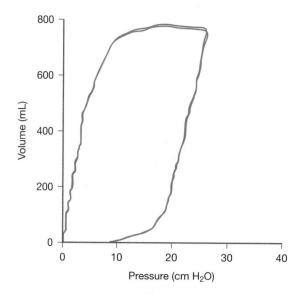

Figure 11-7 X-Y Loop Graphic Display of Pressure-Volume Loop During Mechanical Ventilation. The right-side upswing is the inspiratory portion, with the downswing to the left being the expiratory return to baseline pressure (in this example 0 cm H_2O).

Table 11-11 Common Uses for X-Y Loop Graphics

Display	Uses
Pressure-volume loop	• Assess overall mechanics of breathing (see Figure 11-8) • Identify overdistention ("beak sign") (see Figure 11-9) • Assess trigger work • Adjust PSV levels • Identify asynchrony
Volume–flow loop	• Assess bronchodilator response (see Figure 11-10) • Identify the presence of auto-PEEP • Identify leaks
PSV, pressure support ventilation.	

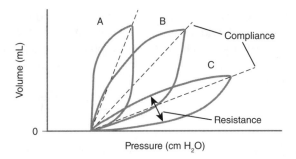

Figure 11-8 Compliance/Resistance. Graphic representation of the pressure needed to deliver a certain volume; helps to assess compliance and resistance "at a glance." The higher the slope (loop A), the higher the compliance. The thinner the loop (loop C), the less airway resistance.

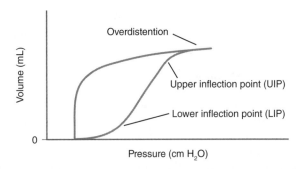

Figure 11-9 P-V Loop Indicating Overdistention During a Positive-Pressure Breath. Beyond the upper inflection point (UIP), small changes in volume result in very large increases in pressure, making the loop appear like the beak of a bird ("beak sign"), indicating airway overdistention (excessive V_T being delivered).

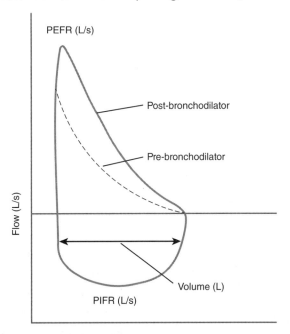

Figure 11-10 Bronchodilator Response. Note the peak expiratory flow rate (PEFR) improvement after a bronchodilator treatment has been given.

slope indicates lower compliance). Airway resistance (Raw) is assessed by the width of the loop. The thinner the loop (C), the less Raw. A wider loop (B) indicates increased Raw.

As indicated in Tables 11-10 and 11-11, ventilator graphics are particularly helpful in identifying the presence and type of patient–ventilator asynchrony. The next section reviews the common types of asynchrony and their graphic appearance.

Correcting Patient–Ventilator Asynchrony (aka Dyssynchrony)

Patient–ventilator asynchrony occurs when there is a lack of coordination between the patient's ventilatory needs and the support provided by the ventilator. There are three major categories of patient–ventilator asynchrony: trigger, flow, and cycle. Because asynchrony is associated with increased duration of mechanical ventilation and intensive care unit (ICU) length of stay, RTs need to be proficient in identifying the type of asynchrony and how to correct it.

Table 11-12 describes the three major types of trigger asynchrony, how to identify them, and the possible actions that can be used to correct these common problems. **Figures 11-11** through **11-13** provide example graphic displays for each type of flow asynchrony.

Table 11-13 describes the two major types of flow asynchrony, how to identify them, and applicable corrective actions. **Figures 11-14** and **11-15** provide example graphic displays for each type of flow asynchrony.

Performing Lung Recruitment Maneuvers

Lung recruitment maneuvers (RMs) are designed to increase the pressure gradient responsible for lung expansion temporarily; that is, the *transpulmonary pressure gradient* ($P_{alv} - P_{pl}$). The goal is to reopen unaerated or poorly aerated alveoli by increasing the end-expiratory lung volume and FRC. An increase in lung volume can improve gas exchange, especially oxygenation. An RM can also increase compliance and thus decrease the spontaneous work of breathing. Keeping previously collapsed alveoli aerated also can help avoid the stress associated with their repetitive opening and closing, which is a cause of ventilator-associated lung injury. Last, by increasing the number of aerated alveoli, an RM (*followed by optimizing PEEP*) may help prevent overdistention and thus minimize the incidence of high-volume/high-pressure injuries (i.e., barotrauma). Although RMs can help

Table 11-12 Trigger Asynchrony

Type	What to Look For	Corrective Actions
Ineffective trigger	Pressure, flow scalars show delayed or absent response to the effort (see Figure 11-11)	Increase sensitivity Switch to flow triggering Reduce/counteract auto-PEEP Reduce sedation
Autocycling	Extra breaths triggered without patient effort, usually caused by circuit condensate or leaks (see Figure 11-12)	Decrease sensitivity Switch to flow triggering Correct leaks Drain condensate and change filters
Double triggering	Two consecutive machine breaths triggered without an interval between them (see Figure 11-13)	Increase inspiratory flow (VC) Increase set V_T (VC) Increase inspiratory time (PC) Increase (shorten) rise time (PC) Increase pressure level (PS) Decrease %cycling criteria (PS)
PC, pressure control; PS, pressure support; PEEP, positive end-expiratory pressure; VC, volume control.		

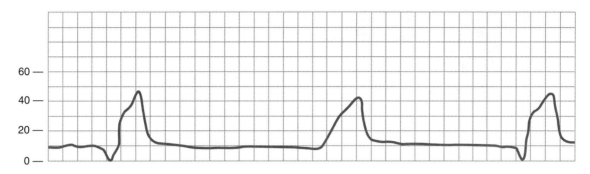

Figure 11-11 Ventilator Graphic Showing Inappropriate Sensitivity. Note that the patient must drop the pressure 10 cm H_2O below the baseline to trigger the first and third breaths.

Reproduced from Burns SM, ed. *AACN Protocols for Practice: Noninvasive Monitoring* (2nd ed.). Sudbury, MA: Jones & Bartlett Publishers; 2006.

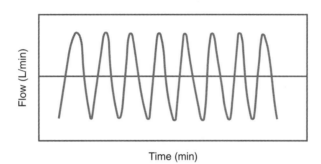

Figure 11-12 Autocycling. Extra breaths triggered without patient effort, usually by circuit condensate or leaks.

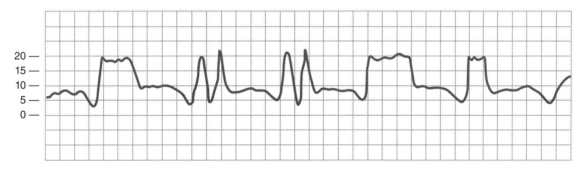

Figure 11-13 A Graphical Display of Patient–Ventilator Asynchrony Showing Double Triggering. Double triggering can be observed on breaths 2 through 5.

restore physiologic function, there currently is no evidence that their use affects clinical outcomes (e.g., morbidity or mortality).

Indications and Contraindications

Patients for whom an RM may be considered are those receiving ventilatory support who exhibit significant hypoxemia that is not fully responsive to O_2 therapy due to intrapulmonary shunting. Using the P/F ratio as a guide, this would include those being managed for acute lung injury/ARDS with P/F ratios < 200–300. For these patients, an RM may be conducted as follows:

1. Early in the course of the disorder to help prevent further lung injury (barotrauma)
2. As a preliminary maneuver preceding an optimum PEEP study

Table 11-13 Flow Asynchrony

Type	What to Look For	Corrective Actions
Inadequate flow	Figure 11-14 showing "scalloping" (concavity) in pressure scalar of assisted breaths during inspiration (A) and on flow scalar during volume ventilation (B)	Increase flow (VC) Change flow pattern (VC) Switch VC to PC Increase set PIP (PC) Increase (shorten) rise time (PC) Check for/correct cause of increased patient ventilatory demand
Excessive flow	Pressure peak is achieved too early (PC) or upward spike seen on inspiratory flow (VC) (see Figure 11-15)	Reduce inspiratory flow (VC) Reduce set PIP (PC) Reduce (lengthen) rise time (PC)
PC, pressure control; PIP, peak inspiratory pressure; VC, volume control.		

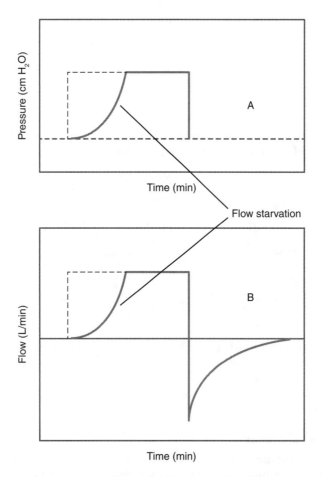

Figure 11-14 Graphs Showing Inadequate Flow.
"Scalloping" seen in pressure waveform of assisted breaths during inspiration **(A)** and on flow waveform during volume ventilation **(B)**.

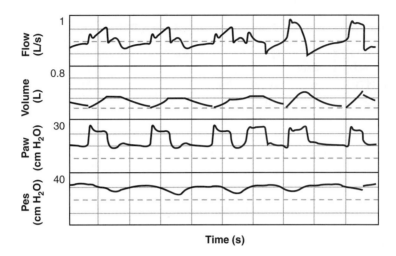

Figure 11-15 Excessive Flow. Pressure peak is achieved too early (PC) or upward spike seen on inspiratory flow (VC). Reproduced from Kallet RH, Campbell AR, Dicker RA, et al. Work of breathing during lung-protective ventilation in patients with acute lung injury and acute respiratory distress syndrome: a comparison between volume and pressure-regulated breathing modes. *Respir Care* 2005;50(12):1623-1631.

3. To restore lung volume after the loss of PEEP (i.e., after disconnection from the ventilator or open suctioning)

4. As salvage therapy for life-threatening hypoxemia that is unresponsive to other interventions

Because an RM can decrease cardiac output and tissue perfusion (due to high intrathoracic pressures), RMs should only be conducted on hemodynamically stable patients, most commonly defined as those having a mean arterial pressure ≥ 60–65 mm Hg that has not required recent alterations in vasoactive or inotropic drug dosing.

Because RMs also can increase intrathoracic pressure and cause barotrauma, they generally are contraindicated in the following situations:

1. Hemodynamic instability (mean arterial pressure ≤ 60–65 mm Hg)
2. Untreated pneumothorax or active air leak (bubbling) through a chest tube
3. Bullous lung disease (COPD)
4. Increased intracranial pressure (ICP) and intracranial bleeding
5. Massive intrapulmonary hemorrhage
6. Recent chest trauma/flail chest or pulmonary contusion
7. Consolidating lung disease (e.g., atelectasis, pneumonia)

Methods

Until recently, the most commonly used RM was the sustained inflation technique, in which CPAP of 40 cm H_2O is applied to the airways for up to 40 seconds (the "40/40" method). The protocol currently in favor involves the application of pressure-control ventilation with a brief application of high-level PEEP, as outlined in the accompanying box (**Box 11-2**).

Box 11-2 Example RM Protocol (Pressure Control with PEEP)

1. Confirm hemodynamic stability and absence of contraindications.
2. Have patient sedated if necessary.
3. Assess for auto-PEEP and correct before continuing.
4. Adjust high-pressure alarm to 50–55 cm H_2O.
5. Set FiO_2 to 1.0.
6. Set inspiratory time and rate appropriate for the patient (avoiding auto-PEEP).
7. Increase PEEP to 20 cm H_2O and PIP to 40 cm H_2O ($\Delta P = 20$ cm H_2O).*
8. Apply for 1 to 3 minutes based on patient tolerance.
9. Terminate if any of the following occur:
   - Mean arterial pressure falls below 60–65 mm Hg.
   - SpO_2 drops by more than 4%.
   - Heart rate rises above 140/min or falls below 60/min.
   - New air leaks (through a chest tube) become apparent.
   - New cardiac arrhythmias develop.
10. Assess results (see following Assessment section).
11. If not successful, repeat at PEEP = 25 cm H_2O, PIP = 45 cm H_2O (as tolerated)

*Depending on the protocol, PEEP may be increased either incrementally or in a single step.

Recruitment Assessment

You know that an RM is successful with the following results (compared to before the maneuver):

- Oxygenation improves—for example:
  - An increase in SaO_2 of $\geq$ 4–5%
  - An increase in P/F ratio $\geq$ 20%
  - The same PaO_2/SaO_2 achieved at a lower FiO_2
- Respiratory system compliance increases—for example:
  - Increased V_T for same pressure (PC), or
  - Same V_T at lower inspiratory pressures (VC)

Optimizing PEEP After RMs

Following any recruitment maneuver, you must titrate the PEEP level back down *to the minimum needed to prevent alveolar collapse.* This method for optimizing PEEP is termed a *decremental* PEEP study. The basic steps in conducting a decremental PEEP study are outlined in the accompanying box (**Box 11-3**). **Figure 11-16** demonstrates a decremental PEEP study conducted after an RM at 24 cm H_2O PEEP. Note that like the assessment of respiratory mechanics "on-ventilator," this procedure may require sedation because patient effort can invalidate compliance measurements.

Liberating a Patient from Mechanical Ventilation

Conventional Invasive Ventilation

Patients receiving conventional invasive mechanical ventilation for respiratory failure should undergo a weaning assessment whenever the following criteria are met:

1. Evidence for some reversal of the underlying cause of respiratory failure
2. Adequate oxygenation (e.g., P/F $\geq$ 150–200, PEEP $\leq$ 5–8 cm H_2O, FiO_2 $\leq$ 0.4–0.5)
3. pH $\geq$ 7.25
4. Hemodynamic stability (no myocardial ischemia or significant hypotension)
5. Capability to initiate an inspiratory effort

Box 11-3 Decremental PEEP Titration Following a Recruitment Maneuver (RM)

1. Immediately following the RM, switch to VC ventilation with V_T = 4–6 mL/kg PBW.
2. Begin lowering the PEEP from the previously established RM level (e.g., 20–25 cm H_2O).
3. Allowing 3–5 minutes between each step (for equilibration), measure C_{rs} ($V_T/[P_{plat} - PEEP]$).
4. Decrease the PEEP in steps of 2 cm H_2O and remeasure C_{rs}.
5. Continue lowering the PEEP until you obtain the highest C_{rs} (*requires observing at least one decrease in C[RS] from the peak value*).*
6. Repeat the recruitment procedure.
7. Set the PEEP to *2 cm H_2O higher than that needed to obtain the highest C[RS]*.
8. Return ventilation to pre-RM settings with the new optimized PEEP.
9. After 20–30 minutes, analyze blood gases.

C_{rs}, respiratory system compliance (lung + thoracic).

*The decrease in C_{rs} from its peak indicates that the critical closing pressure of some lung units has been reached; *the optimum PEEP must be set above this level.*

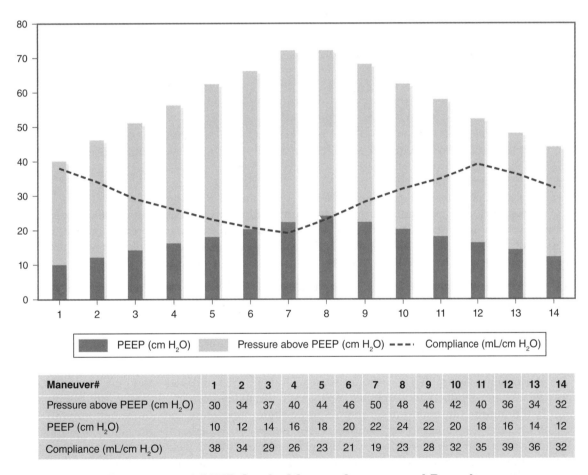

Maneuver#	1	2	3	4	5	6	7	8	9	10	11	12	13	14
Pressure above PEEP (cm H_2O)	30	34	37	40	44	46	50	48	46	42	40	36	34	32
PEEP (cm H_2O)	10	12	14	16	18	20	22	24	22	20	18	16	14	12
Compliance (mL/cm H_2O)	38	34	29	26	23	21	19	23	28	32	35	39	36	32

Figure 11-16 Decremental PEEP Study After an Incremental Recruitment Maneuver (RM). Decremental PEEP study conducted after an RM at 24 cm H_2O PEEP. Note that as PEEP is lowered by 2 cm H_2O (after maneuver 8), the compliance steadily increases until a peak value of about 39 mL/cm H_2O is reached at a PEEP of 16 cm H_2O. Any further decrease in PEEP will cause compliance to fall. In this example, the optimum PEEP is +2 cm H_2O above the level needed to obtain the highest C_{rs} (i.e., 16 + 2 = 18 cm H_2O). In concept, this is the lowest baseline pressure needed to prevent alveolar collapse.

Daily *spontaneous breathing trials (SBTs)* provide the quickest route for discontinuing mechanical ventilation. Tracking measures such as vital capacity and maximum inspiratory pressure (MIP)/negative inspiratory force (NIF) while the patient is receiving ventilatory support can provide useful insights into weaning potential. However, a carefully monitored SBT provides the most valid information for deciding whether a patient can stay off the ventilator.

Spontaneous breathing modes used in SBT weaning protocols include (1) straight T-tube breathing, (2) CPAP, (3) pressure support, and (4) CPAP plus pressure support. Based on current evidence, no one approach appears to be better than the others. However, the provision of CPAP during weaning can help improve breath triggering in patients who experience auto-PEEP, and PS helps to overcome the additional work of breathing imposed by the artificial airway. Chapter 9 of this text includes a decision-making algorithm for a typical spontaneous breathing trial protocol.

SBT protocols vary somewhat by institution and unit—for example, surgical versus medical ICU. All such protocols involve an initial assessment of the patient to ensure that he or she is ready to wean, using criteria such as those delineated previously. The next step normally is the application of a brief (2–5 minutes) supervised period of carefully monitored spontaneous breathing. During this "screening" phase, you assess the patient's breathing pattern, vital signs, and comfort level. If the patient tolerates the screening phase, you continue the SBT for at least 30 minutes but no more than 120 minutes.

Objective physiologic measures indicating a successful SBT include the following:

- Acceptable gas exchange:
  - $SpO_2 \geq$ 85–90% or $PaO_2 \geq$ 50–60 torr
  - pH $\geq$ 7.30
  - Increase in $PaCO_2 \leq$ 10 torr
- Stable hemodynamics:
  - Heart rate < 120–140/min; change < 20%
  - Systolic blood pressure < 180–200 mm Hg and > 90 mm Hg; change < 20%
  - No vasopressors required
- Stable ventilatory pattern;
  - Respiratory rate $\leq$ 30–35/min
  - Change in respiratory rate < 50%

If these objective indicators are not met, you should return the patient to a sufficient level of ventilatory support to maintain adequate oxygenation and ventilation and prevent muscle fatigue. Even when the patient meets these physiologic measures, you may need to discontinue the SBT if you note one or more of the following subjective indicators of intolerance or failure:

- Change in mental status (e.g., somnolence, coma, agitation, anxiety)
- Onset or worsening of discomfort
- Diaphoresis
- Signs of increased work of breathing:
  - Use of accessory respiratory muscles
  - Thoracoabdominal paradox

If a patient fails an SBT, you should work with the physician to determine the cause(s). Once these factors are identified and corrected, you should resume performing an SBT every 24 hours.

If the patient can maintain acceptable physiologic parameters and can tolerate the SBT for its full duration, you can consider extubation. The decision of whether to proceed with extubation should be a separate consideration, based on an assessment of the patient's airway patency and protective reflexes. Chapter 9 provides details on when and how to extubate a patient.

Noninvasive Ventilation

There are no standard guidelines for weaning a patient from NPPV. However, there is general agreement on the following key points:

- Patient readiness to wean:
  - Condition underlying need for NPPV mostly resolved
  - Acceptable vitals: respiratory rate < 25/min; heart rate < 110/min

- ○ IPAP $<$ 15 cm H_2O, EPAP $<$ 10 cm H_2O
  - ○ Compensated pH $>$ 7.35
  - ○ $Spo_2 >$ 90% on $<$ 50%
- Weaning procedure:
  - ○ The procedure should initially be conducted during daytime hours.
  - ○ Wean by incrementally extending the time periods off the ventilator.
  - ○ Use periods off the ventilator for meals, fluid replenishment, airway clearance therapy, and skin care.
  - ○ After successful daytime weaning, provide at least one additional night of support.
  - ○ Weaning is complete when the patient can maintain adequate oxygenation and ventilation off the ventilator with an acceptable work of breathing.

ARDS Weaning Protocol

The NHLBI ARDS protocol follows these basic principles but uses a progressive transitioning from CPAP to pressure support to true unassisted spontaneous breathing. Details on this portion of the ARDS protocol are provided in the accompanying box (**Box 11-4**).

Weaning from HFOV

Weaning from HFOV focuses mainly on oxygenation needs. As oxygenation improves in the adult HFOV patient, you should first lower the Fio_2 to 0.40, then slowly reduce P_{mean} by 2–3 cm H_2O every 4–6 hours until it is 20 cm H_2O or less. At this point, you should consider switching the patient to pressure control at a pressure limit $\leq$ 30 cm H_2O and PEEP of 10–12 cm H_2O. After that, weaning should follow a standard SBT protocol, as previously described.

Box 11-4 NHLBI ARDS Protocol: Weaning Component

Criteria Indicating Readiness for a Spontaneous Breathing Trial (SBT)

- $Fio_2 \leq$ 0.40 and PEEP $\leq$ 8 cm H_2O, or $Fio_2 \leq$ 0.50 and PEEP $\leq$ 5 cm H_2O
- PEEP and $Fio_2 \leq$ previous day's settings
- Acceptable spontaneous breathing efforts of the patient (decrease ventilator rate by 50% for 5 minutes to detect effort)
- Systolic BP $\geq$ 90 mm Hg without vasopressors
- No neuromuscular blocking agents or blockade

Procedure

Initiate an SBT of up to 120 minutes with $Fio_2 <$ 0.5 and PEEP $<$ 5 cm H_2O:
1. Place patient on T-piece, trach collar, or CPAP $\leq$ 5 cm H_2O with PS $<$ 5 cm H_2O.
2. Assess for tolerance as follows for up to 2 hours:
   a. $Spo_2 \geq$ 90% and $Pao_2 \geq$ 60 torr
   b. Spontaneous $V_T \geq$ 4 mL/kg PBW
   c. Respiratory rate $\leq$ 35/min
   d. pH $\geq$ 7.3
   e. No respiratory distress (distress = 2 or more of the following)
      - HR $>$ 120% of baseline
      - Marked accessory muscle use
      - Abdominal paradox
      - Diaphoresis
      - Marked dyspnea
3. If tolerated for at least 30 minutes, consider extubation.
4. If not tolerated, resume pre-weaning settings.

Data from National Heart, Lung, and Blood Institute, ARDS Clinical Network. *Mechanical ventilation protocol summary.* 2008.

T⁴—TOP TEST-TAKING TIPS

You can improve your score on this section of the NBRC exam by following these tips:

- Never withhold supplemental oxygen from a patient who needs it.
- Suspect hypoxemia in situations such as postoperative patients and those suffering from carbon monoxide or cyanide poisoning, shock, trauma, or acute myocardial infarction.
- Use CPAP or PEEP to treat refractory hypoxemia ($Pao_2 \leq 50$ torr with $Fio_2 \geq 0.5$).
- In patients with either COPD or ARDS, Pao_2 values as low as 55 torr are acceptable as long as we can keep the arterial saturation at or above 88%.
- In general, do not use NPPV for patients who do not have control over the upper airway or cannot manage their secretions.
- To improve oxygenation in patients with unilateral lung disease, position the patient in the left or right lateral decubitus position with *the good lung down.*
- If the patient cannot tolerate CPAP, assess and recommend equipment or interface alternatives to improve tolerance—for example, various mask options, humidification, ramp feature, auto-titration, pressure relief (aka C-flex, EPR), BiPAP.
- All noninvasive positive-pressure ventilators used in the acute care setting must have a low-pressure/disconnect and power failure alarm.
- Whenever possible, avoid plateau pressures > 30 cm H_2O during mechanical ventilation.
- Do not use or recommend high-frequency oscillation ventilation for patients with obstructive lung disease.
- When initiating mechanical ventilation, either VC or PC for mandatory breaths are acceptable as long as the volume or pressure setting helps minimize the likelihood of barotrauma by delivering 6–8 mL/kg V_T of PBW.
- When initiating mechanical ventilation, always use a high Fio_2 (0.60–1.0) until an ABG can be obtained.
- Adjust ventilator settings by (1) monitoring arterial blood gases and (2) maximizing patient comfort and patient–ventilator synchrony.
- Except with ARDS patients, when initiating mechanical ventilation, set the initial V_T to 6–8 mL/kg PBW when targeting volume, or set the pressure limit to 20–30 cm H_2O when targeting pressure.
- "Optimal" PEEP represents the end-expiratory pressure level that maximizes patient benefits while minimizing risks.
- Usually, patient–ventilator asynchrony occurs when there is a lack of coordination between the patient's ventilatory needs and the support provided by the ventilator.
- High-frequency jet or oscillatory ventilation should be considered for patients with low lung compliance and hypoxemic respiratory failure, such as those with ARDS.
- Because an RM can decrease cardiac output and tissue perfusion, RMs should only be conducted on hemodynamically stable patients, most commonly defined as those having a mean arterial pressure $\geq$ 60–65 mm Hg that has not required recent alterations in vasoactive or inotropic drug dosing.
- Lung recruitment maneuvers (e.g., periodic PEEP of 40 for 40 seconds) can be combined with optimal PEEP to help enhance oxygenation in mechanically ventilated patients who are otherwise difficult to oxygenate.
- To adjust a patient's $Paco_2$/pH during mechanical ventilation, always change the rate first; change the V_T/pressure limit only if rate changes exceed the recommended adult limits (8–24 breaths/min and up to 35/min for adults with ARDS).
- BiPAP requires that the patient has control over his or her upper airway function, can manage secretions, and is cooperative and motivated.
- Unless contraindicated, always use an oronasal/"full" face mask when initiating NPPV for patients with acute respiratory failure.
- To avoid esophageal opening/gastric distention, always keep IPAP levels below 20–25 cm H_2O during NPPV̇.

- Whenever a patient's cardiac output or blood pressure falls when the PEEP level is raised, decrease PEEP back to its prior setting.
- Daily spontaneous breathing trials (SBTs) provide the quickest route for discontinuing mechanical ventilation.
- Spontaneous breathing modes used in SBT weaning protocols include (1) straight T-tube breathing, (2) CPAP, (3) pressure support, and (4) CPAP plus pressure support.
- If a patient fails an SBT, you should work with the physician to determine the cause(s). Once these factors are identified and corrected, you should resume performing an SBT every 24 hours.
- When treating patients with carbon monoxide poisoning, cyanide poisoning, acute pulmonary edema, shock, trauma, or acute myocardial infarction in emergency settings, always provide the highest possible Fio_2.

POST-TEST

To confirm your mastery of each chapter's topical content, you should create a content post-test, available online via the Navigate Premier Access for Comprehensive Respiratory Therapy Exam Preparation Guide, which contains Navigate TestPrep (access code provided with every new text). You can create multiple topical content post-tests varying in length from 10 to 20 questions, with each attempt presenting a different set of items. You can select questions from all three major NBRC TMC sections: Patient Data, Troubleshooting and Quality Control of Devices and Infection Control, and Initiation and Modification of Interventions. A score of at least 70–80% indicates that you are adequately prepared for this section of the NBRC TMC exam. If you score below 70%, you should first carefully assess your test answers (particularly your wrong answers) and the correct answer explanations. Then return to the chapter to re-review the applicable content. Only then should you reattempt a new post-test. Repeat this process of identifying your shortcomings and reviewing the pertinent content until your test results demonstrate mastery.

Administer Medications and Specialty Gases (Section III-D)

CHAPTER 12

Albert J. Heuer

Administering medications and specialty gases is an important function for respiratory therapists (RTs). In terms of medications administered via aerosol, there are now several dozen specific preparations with which the NBRC expects candidates to be familiar. In addition, the NBRC expects candidates to be able to match the delivery system to both the drug and the patient. Moreover, although specialty gas administration is less commonly performed than aerosol drug delivery, candidates must know the basics regarding application and modification of heliox and inhaled nitric oxide systems.

OBJECTIVES

In preparing for this section of the NBRC exams (TMC/CSE), you should demonstrate the knowledge needed to:

1. Select among and recommend various aerosolized drug preparations.
2. Apply selected inhaled drug category characteristics to optimize their administration.
3. Select and use or teach the use of various aerosol drug delivery systems.
4. Select and administer drugs via endotracheal instillation.
5. Administer heliox and inhaled nitric oxide (NO).

WHAT TO EXPECT ON THIS CATEGORY OF THE NBRC EXAMS

TMC exam: 4 questions; 1 recall, 3 application
CSE exam: indeterminate number of questions; however, section III-D knowledge is a prerequisite to succeed on the CSE, especially on Information Gathering sections.

WHAT YOU NEED TO KNOW: ESSENTIAL CONTENT

Aerosolized Drug Preparations

Table 12-1 provides details on the most common drugs you may administer by aerosol, including their generic and brand names, available preparations, recommended adult doses, and frequency of administration.

Special Considerations That Apply to Selected Inhaled Drug Categories

Antimicrobials

Regarding the use of inhaled *antimicrobials*, keep in mind the following key points:

- Aerosolized antibiotics (Colistin, Cayston, TOBI) are generally indicated only in patients with cystic fibrosis (CF) and suspected or confirmed *Pseudomonas aeruginosa* (gram-negative) pulmonary infections.
- If the patient is receiving several inhaled medications, the recommended order is bronchodilator first, followed by mucolytic, then airway clearance therapy, then steroids, and finally the aerosolized antibiotic.

Table 12-1 Medications Commonly Administered by the Inhalation Route

Generic Name	Brand Name(s)	Delivery and Preparation	Adult Dose and Frequency
Antimicrobials			
Antibiotics			
Best Use: Treatment of *Pseudomonas* infections in cystic fibrosis (CF) and other gram-negative respiratory infections not responsive to other therapies.			
Colistimethate polymyxin E	Colistin; Coly-Mycin	SVN 150-mg vials (powder); add 2 mL sterile H_2O	37.5–150 mg q8–q12
Tobramycin	TOBI	SVN 300 mg in 5-mL saline unit dose	300 mg q 12 h for 28 days, then 28 days off
Tobramycin	TOBI Podhaler	28-mg dry powder capsules	4 capsules 2× daily for 28 days
Cayston	Aztreonam	SVN 75-mg unit dose vial reconstituted with 1 mL 0.17% saline	3× daily for 28 days, then 28 days off
Antivirals			
Best Use: Treatment of uncomplicated influenza A and B			
Zanamivir	Relenza	DPI (5 mg/blister)	10 mg (2 blisters) 2× daily for 5 days
Pulmonary Vasodilators *Note*: Though the NBRC exam matrix includes pulmonary vasodilators here, between antimicrobials and bronchodilators, they are discussed later in this chapter following another pulmonary vasodilator, inhaled nitric oxide			
Bronchodilators			
Adrenergic Bronchodilators			
Short-Acting β-Agonists (SABAs)			
Best Use: Fast symptom relief ("rescue inhalers")			
Albuterol	Proventil	SVN 0.5%	0.5 mL q 4–6 h
	Ventolin	MDI (90 mcg/puff)	2 puffs q 4–6 h
		DPI (200 mcg/cap)	1 cap q 4–6 h
Bitolterol	Tornalate	SVN 0.2%	1.25 mL 3–4× daily
		MDI (37 mcg/puff)	2 puffs q 6 h
Epinephrine	Adrenalin	SVN 1% (1:100)	0.25–0.5 mL prn
Levalbuterol	Xopenex	SVN 0.31, 0.63, or 1.25 mg	3.0-mL unit dose tid
	Xopenex HFA	MDI (45 mcg/puff)	2 puffs q 4–6 h
Metaproterenol	Alupent	SVN 5%	0.2–0.3 mL q 4–6 h
	Metaprel	MDI (650 mcg/puff)	2–3 puffs q 4–6 h
Pirbuterol	Maxair	MDI (200 mcg/puff)	2 puffs q 4–6 h
Racemic epinephrine	Vaponefrin Micronefrin	SVN 2.25%	0.25–0.5 mL prn
Terbutaline	Bricanyl	DPI (500 mcg/puff)	2 puffs q 4–6 h

(continues)

Table 12-1 Medications Commonly Administered by the Inhalation Route (*continued*)

Generic Name	Brand Name(s)	Delivery and Preparation	Adult Dose and Frequency
Long-Acting β-Agonists (LABAs)			
Best Use: Maintenance/control of asthma* and COPD			
Formoterol	Foradil	DPI (25 mcg/cap)	1 cap 2× daily
	Perforomist	SVN (20 mcg)	2× daily
Salmeterol	Serevent	MDI (25 mcg/puff)	2 puffs 2× daily
	Serevent Diskus	DPI (50 mcg/blister)	1 blister 2× daily
Arformoterol	Brovana	SVN (15 mcg/2 mL vial)	1 vial 2× daily
Olodaterol	Striverdi Respimat	Slow-mist MDI (2.5 mcg/puff)	2 puffs 1× daily
Indacaterol	Arcapta	DPI (75 mcg/cap)	1 cap daily
Anticholinergic Bronchodilators			
Short-Acting Anticholinergics			
Best Use: Fast symptom relief (alone or combined with SABAs)			
Ipratropium bromide	Atrovent	SVN 0.2%	2.5 mL 3–4× daily
	Atrovent HFA	MDI (17 mcg/puff)	2 puffs q 6 h
Long-Acting Anticholinergics			
Best Use: Maintenance treatment of bronchospasm in COPD			
Tiotropium bromide	Spiriva HandiHaler	DPI (18 mcg/capsule)	2 inhalations daily
	Spiriva Respimat	Slow-mist MDI (2.5 mcg/puff)	2 puffs daily
Aclidinium bromide	Tudorza Pressair	DPI (400 mcg/puff)	2 inhalations daily
Glycopyrrolate	Seebri Neohaler	DPI (15.6 mcg/capsule)	2 inhalations daily
Umeclidinium bromide	Incruse Ellipta	DPI (62.5 mcg/puff)	1 inhalation daily
Adrenergic + Anticholinergic Combinations			
Short-Acting Combinations			
Best Use: Fast symptom relief, especially exacerbations of asthma			
Ipratropium bromide + albuterol	DuoNeb	SVN 0.5 mg ipratropium + 2.5 mg albuterol	3 mL unit dose
	Combivent	DPI ipratropium 18 mcg/puff + albuterol 90 mcg/puff	2 inhalations/day
	Combivent Respimat	Slow-mist MDI ipratropium 20 mcg/puff + albuterol 100 mcg/puff	1 puff 4× daily
Long-Acting Combinations			
Best Use: Maintenance/control of bronchospasm in COPD			
Umeclidinium bromide + vilanterol	Anoro Ellipta	DPI 62.5 mcg umeclidinium + 25 mcg vilanterol	1 inhalation daily
Indacaterol + glycopyrrolate	Utibron Neohaler	DPI 27.5 mcg indacaterol + 15.6 mcg glycopyrrolate	2 inhalations daily

Generic Name	Brand Name(s)	Delivery and Preparation	Adult Dose and Frequency
Mucolytics & Proteolytics			
Best Use: Facilitate clearance of airway secretions			
N-Acetylcysteine Cystine	Mucomyst	SVN 10/20% (4-, 10-, 30-mL vials)	3–5 mL 20% solution or 6–10 mL 10% solution 3–4× daily
Dornase alpha	Pulmozyme	SVN 2.5-mL single-use ampule (1.0 mg/mL)	1 ampule/day
Hypertonic saline	Hypersal	SVN 3–7%	With bronchodilator
Inhaled Steroids			
Best Use: Long-term control of asthma symptoms			
Beclomethasone dipropionate	QVAR	MDI (40 mcg/puff)	2 puffs 2× daily
		MDI (80 mcg/puff)	2 puffs 2× daily
Budesonide	Pulmicort Flexhaler	DPI (90 mcg/puff)	2 puffs 2× daily
		DPI (180 mcg/puff)	2 puffs 2× daily
Ciclesonide	Alvesco	MDI (80/160 mcg/puff)	1 puff daily
Flunisolide	Aerobid	MDI (250 mcg/puff)	2 puffs 2× daily
Fluticasone hemihydrate	Aerospan	MDI (80 mcg/puff	1–2 puffs 2× daily
Fluticasone propionate	Flovent HFA	MDI (44/110/220 mcg/puff)	2 puffs 4× daily
Fluticasone furoate	Arnuity Ellipta	DPI (100/200 mcg/blister)	1 inhalation daily
Mometasone furoate	Asmanex	DPI (110/220 mcg/puff)	1 or 2 inhalations daily
Steroid + Adrenergic Combinations			
Best Use: Maintenance/control of asthma			
Fluticasone + salmeterol	Advair Diskus	DPI 100 mcg fluticasone + 50 mcg salmeterol	1 inhalation 2× daily
		DPI 250 mcg fluticasone + 50 mcg salmeterol	1 inhalation 2× daily
		DPI 500 mcg fluticasone + 50 mcg salmeterol	1 inhalation 2× daily
Fluticasone + salmeterol	Advair HFA	MDI 45 mcg fluticasone + 21 mcg salmeterol	1 inhalation 2× daily
		MDI 115 mcg fluticasone + 21 mcg salmeterol	1 inhalation 2× daily
		MDI 230 mcg fluticasone + 21 mcg salmeterol	1 inhalation 2× daily
Budesonide + formoterol	Symbicort	MDI 80 mcg budesonide + 4.5 mcg formoterol	2 puffs 2× daily
		MDI 160 mcg budesonide + 4.5 mcg formoterol	2 puffs 2× daily

(*continues*)

Table 12-1 Medications Commonly Administered by the Inhalation Route (*continued*)

Generic Name	Brand Name(s)	Delivery and Preparation	Adult Dose and Frequency
Mometasone + formoterol	Dulera	MDI 100 mcg mometasone + 5 mcg formoterol	2 puffs 2× daily
		MDI 200 mcg mometasone + 5 mcg formoterol	2 puffs 2× daily
Fluticasone + vilanterol	Breo Ellipta	DPI 100 mcg fluticasone + 25 mcg vilanterol	1 inhalation daily
Mast Cell Stabilizers			
Best Use: Maintenance/control of asthma			
Cromolyn sodium	Intal	MDI (1 mg/puff)	2–4 puffs 4× daily
		SVN (20 mg/2 mL ampule)	1 ampule 4× daily
Nedocromil	Tilade	MDI (1.75 mg/puff)	2–4 puffs 2× daily

DPI, dry-powder inhaler; mcg, microgram; MDI, metered-dose inhaler; SVN, small-volume nebulizer.

*LABAs should *not* be used for relief of acute bronchospasm and should always be prescribed in combination with an inhaled corticosteroid in patients with asthma.

Adrenergic Bronchodilators

Regarding the use of the β-*agonist* bronchodilators, keep the following key points in mind:

- All β-agonists have some cardiovascular and central nervous system (CNS) effects; in general, you should recommend those with the least β_1 (cardiac) and most β_2 (bronchodilation) effects (e.g., albuterol or its isomer levalbuterol).
- Short-acting β-agonists (SABAs) are best used as relievers of bronchospasm; long-acting β-agonists (LABAs) and steroids should be used to control reactive airway disease.
- If also administering steroids, mucokinetics, or anti-infective agents by inhalation, always give the bronchodilator first.
- In acute exacerbations of asthma, repeat the standard dose every 20 minutes (up to three times) or provide continuous nebulization until symptoms are relieved.
- Considerations for LABAs include the following:
  - May increase the risk of severe exacerbations/death in some patients with asthma
  - Should only be used in combination with inhaled steroids in these patients
  - Should not be recommended or used to treat acute exacerbations of asthma
- For maintenance therapy of bronchospasm in patients with chronic obstructive pulmonary disease (COPD), consider a LABA (e.g., salmeterol), a long-acting anticholinergic (e.g., tiotropium), or a LABA plus long-acting anticholinergic combination (e.g., umeclidinium + vilanterol).

Mucolytics

In administering *mucolytics*, you need to be aware of the following issues:

- All mucolytics are irritating to the airway; to prevent bronchospasm, always precede treatment with a bronchodilator.
- Mucolytics should be administered in combination with airway clearance therapy to facilitate removal of secretions.

Inhaled Steroids

In terms of administration of inhaled steroids, you need to remember the following essentials:

- Inhaled steroids control inflammation and are the first-line drugs for mild, persistent asthma.
- Except for budesonide (Pulmicort), common inhaled steroid preparations are all intended for use in a metered-dose inhaler (MDI) or dry-powder inhaler (DPI); therefore, the proper patient technique is critical.
- Rinsing the mouth after therapy is essential to prevent pharyngitis and oral candidiasis.
- Use of spacers or valved holding chambers with MDI-delivered steroids minimizes pharyngeal deposition and the incidence of pharyngitis and candidiasis.

Aerosol Drug Delivery Systems

As noted in Table 12-1, various delivery devices are used to administer medications via the inhalation route. These include small-volume nebulizers (SVNs), MDIs (including breath-actuated and slow-mist systems), DPIs, and electronic nebulizers (ultrasonic and vibrating mesh systems). **Table 12-2** compares the advantages and disadvantages of these devices.

Table 12-2 Advantages and Disadvantages of Aerosol Drug Delivery Systems

Advantages	Disadvantages
Metered-Dose Inhaler (MDI)	
• Convenient	• Patient activation/coordination required
• Low cost	• High percentage of pharyngeal deposition
• Portable	• Has the potential for abuse
• No drug preparation required	• Difficult to deliver high doses
• Difficult to contaminate	• Not all medications formulated for MDI delivery
MDI with Valved Holding Chamber or Spacer	
• Less patient coordination required	• More complex for some patients
• Less pharyngeal deposition	• More expensive than MDI alone
• No drug preparation	• Less portable than MDI alone
	• Not all drugs formulated for MDI delivery
Breath-Actuated MDI	
• Less patient coordination required	• Requires high inspiratory flow
• Suitable for use with limited hand dexterity	• More expensive than MDI alone
• No drug preparation	• Not ideal for mechanical ventilation
	• Not all drugs formulated for this device
Slow/Soft-Mist MDI (Respimat; Boehringer Ingelheim)	
• Enhanced medication deposition and delivery	• More complex for some patients (e.g., coordinating the medication release button, accidental removal of transparent base)
• No drug preparation	• More expensive than MDI alone
	• Not suitable for mechanical ventilation
	• Not all drugs formulated for this device

(continues)

Table 12-2 Advantages and Disadvantages of Aerosol Drug Delivery Systems (*continued*)

Advantages	Disadvantages
Dry-Powder Inhaler (DPI)	
• Less patient coordination required • Breath activated • Breath-hold not required • Can provide accurate dose counts	• Requires high inspiratory flow • Some units are a single dose • Can result in pharyngeal deposition • Not all medications formulated for DPI delivery • Difficult to deliver high doses • Cannot be used for drug delivery during mechanical ventilation
Small-Volume Nebulizer (SVN; Jet Nebulizer)	
• Less patient coordination required • Can provide high doses/continuous therapy • Nebulizes both solutions and suspensions • Inexpensive/disposable	• Wasteful (large residual volume) • Drug preparation required • Contamination possible if not cleaned carefully • Not all medications formulated for SVN delivery • Pressurized gas source required • Long treatment times
Electronic Drug Nebulizers (Compact Ultrasonic and Vibrating Mesh Devices)	
• Create a fine-particle mist that is ideal for lower respiratory tract delivery • Do not require propellants/compressor system • Small residual volume/less waste • Small, silent, and portable • Can aerosolize small volumes, eliminating the need for diluent (may require dose reduction) • Add no flow/volume to the ventilator circuit • Fast nebulization rate/shorter duration of treatments • Mesh nebulizers do not heat or degrade medication and are thus suitable for solutions, suspensions, proteins, and peptides	• Expensive • Prone to electrical or mechanical failure; requires backup • Batteries need to be replaced/recharged periodically • Patients need training in device assembly/disassembly • Aerosol production can be position dependent • Nondisposable vibrating mesh plates require regular cleaning and have limited life span/require replacement • Ultrasonic not recommended for aerosolizing suspensions, and transducer heat can degrade some drugs

Selection of Aerosol Drug Delivery System

Figure 12-1 outlines a general algorithm for selecting an aerosol drug delivery system for spontaneously breathing patients. As indicated in this figure, you first must determine the available formulations for the prescribed drug. Given that some drugs are available only in a single formulation (such as DPI only), your choice in these cases will be limited to that system. For example, Advair (fluticasone propionate and salmeterol) is available only in a DPI formulation, Cayston® (aztreonam—an antibiotic used to treat *Pseudomonas aeruginosa* infection) is approved for administration only via specific electronic (vibrating mesh) nebulizers, and olodaterol (a long-acting β-agonist) is prepared only for delivery via a proprietary slow-mist MDI system (Striverdi Respimat). Given the cost and complexity of electronic nebulizers, their use generally is limited to administering formulations that require them and for delivery of these drugs to patients receiving mechanical ventilation. Details on aerosol drug delivery to patients via mechanical ventilation circuits are provided later in this chapter.

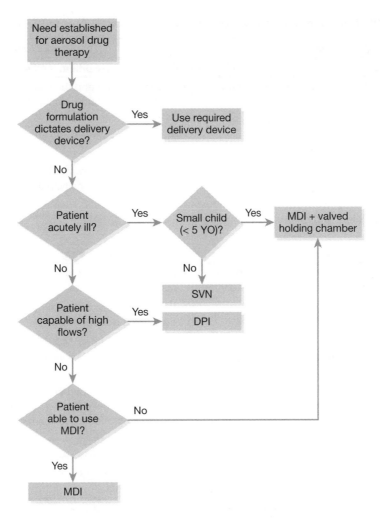

Figure 12-1 Basic Selection of Aerosol Drug Delivery Devices for Spontaneously Breathing Patients. In many cases, the drug formulation will dictate the choice. Otherwise, assessment of the patient's acuity, age, inspiratory flows, and ability to properly use an MDI will determine the best device to use on a patient. If several different devices qualify, patient preference should be the deciding factor.

If multiple formulations of a medication are available, you should assess the patient to determine the best delivery system. In general, SVN administration should be reserved for acutely ill adults who cannot use either a DPI or an MDI. Most infants and small children should receive aerosolized drugs via an MDI with a holding chamber and mask (an SVN is an alternative if tolerated). If an adult who is not acutely ill has difficulty properly coordinating MDI actuation with breathing, you should consider adding a holding chamber. A breath-actuated MDI is an alternative for such patients. Patients prescribed steroids by MDI should use either a spacer or a holding chamber to minimize pharyngeal deposition. DPIs are ideal for maintenance therapy in outpatient adults, larger children, and adolescents who can generate enough inspiratory flow to carry the powder into the lungs.

Aerosol drug delivery is both patient and device dependent. **Table 12-3** outlines the optimal technique and key therapeutic issues involved in spontaneously breathing patients' use of the common aerosol delivery devices.

Table 12-3 Optimal Technique and Therapeutic Issues in Using Aerosol Delivery Devices

Optimal Technique	Therapeutic Issues
Metered-Dose Inhaler (MDI) for β_2 Agonists, Steroids, Cromolyn Sodium, and Anticholinergics	
• The patient should open the mouth wide and keep the tongue down • Actuate during 3- to 5-second deep inhalation, followed by 10-second breath-hold • Holding MDI 2 inches away from the open mouth may enhance lung deposition • Use the closed-mouth method only if (1) the patient cannot use the open-mouth technique, (2) a spacer is not available, and (3) the drug is not a steroid	• Young children and the elderly may have difficulty coordinating inhalation with device actuation • Patients may incorrectly stop inhalation at actuation • To reduce the amount of drug swallowed and absorbed systemically, patients should rinse the mouth with water
Spacer or Valved Holding Chamber (VHC) for Use with MDIs	
• Slow (30 L/min or 3–5 sec) deep inhalation, followed by 10-second breath-hold immediately following actuation • Actuate only once into the spacer/VHC per inhalation • Face mask (if used) should fit snugly and allow 3–5 breaths/actuation • Rinse plastic VHCs once a month in water with diluted dishwashing detergent and let air-dry	• Indicated for patients having difficulty properly using an MDI • Simple spacers still require coordinated actuation; VHCs are preferred • A face mask allows MDIs to be used with small children but reduces lung deposition by 50% • Because spacers and VHCs decrease oropharyngeal deposition, they can help reduce the risk of topical side effects such as thrush • Use antistatic VHCs or rinse plastic non-antistatic VHCs with dilute household detergents to enhance efficacy and delivery to the lungs
Breath-Actuated MDI for β_2 Agonists	
• Maintain a tight seal around the mouthpiece and slightly more rapid inhalation than with a standard MDI, followed by a 10-second breath-hold	• Useful for patients who cannot coordinate inhalation with actuation, such as the elderly • Patients may incorrectly stop inhalation at actuation • Cannot be used with spacers or VHCs
Slow-Mist MDI/Respimat for Various Single and Combined Adrenergic and Anticholinergic Preparations	
• Set the device spring by rotating the base until it clicks • Snap open the mouthpiece cap • Breathe out slowly and fully • Seal lips tightly around the mouthpiece, being sure to avoid covering the air vents • While taking in a slow, deep breath, press the dose release button • Hold the breath for 10 seconds if able • Exhale slowly after breath-hold • Close mouthpiece cap	• Enhanced medication deposition and delivery • More complex for some patients (e.g., coordinating the medication release button, accidental removal of transparent base) • More expensive than MDI alone • Not all drugs formulated for this device • Cannot be used with spacers or VHCs

Optimal Technique	Therapeutic Issues
Dry-Powder Inhaler (DPI) for β_2 Agonists, Steroids, and Anticholinergics	
• Do not use with a spacer or VHC • Lips must be tightly sealed around the mouthpiece to avoid loss of drug • After loading, most DPIs must be held horizontal to avoid loss of drug • Requires rapid (60 L/min or 1–2 sec), deep inhalation • The patient must exhale to room (not back into the device) • Children younger than 4 years may not generate enough flow to use this device	• The dose is lost if the patient exhales into the device after loading • Exhaling into device may cause clogging due to moisture caking and powder residue • Rapid inhalation increases deposition in large airways • To reduce the amount of drug absorbed systemically, the patient should rinse the mouth with water • The device should never be washed or rinsed in water • Between uses, the device should always be capped and stored in a dry place
Small-Volume Nebulizer (SVN) for β_2 Agonists, Steroids, Cromolyn Sodium, and Anticholinergics	
• Slow tidal breathing with occasional deep breaths • Use a tightly fitting face mask for those patients who are unable to use a mouthpiece • Avoid using the "blow-by" technique (i.e., holding the mask or open tube near the infant's nose and mouth)	• Less dependent on the patient's coordination and cooperation • As effective as MDI + VHC for bronchodilators delivery to patients with mild to moderate exacerbations of asthma • More wasteful and time-consuming than other methods • Output depends on the device, fill volume, and driving gas flow • Use of a face mask reduces lung deposition by 50% • Bacterial infections can occur if the SVN is not cleaned properly

Drug Delivery with Ventilators, Continuous Positive Airway Pressure (CPAP) Devices, and Breathing Circuits

Drug Delivery During Mechanical Ventilation

Depending on the drug, available equipment, and protocol, you will use an SVN, MDI, or electronic (ultrasonic or vibrating mesh) nebulizer to deliver aerosolized drugs to patients on ventilators. The accompanying box (**Box 12-1**) provides general guidelines for incorporating aerosol drug systems in ventilator circuits.

Drug Delivery with CPAP/Bi-Level Positive Airway Pressure (BiPAP) to Infants and with Intermittent Positive-Pressure Breathing (IPPB)

It is common to have to deliver inhaled medications to patients to patients receiving CPAP, BiPAP, and other single-limbed breathing circuits. In general, the T-adaptor for the SVN or MDI adaptor should be located near the mask or other patient interface. For SVNs, the gas source (air vs O$_2$) used to drive the nebulizer and flow should approximate the Fio$_2$ being delivered to the patient through the circuit. In other words, if a patient is on a high Fio$_2$ on the BiPAP device, the oxygen should be used to drive the nebulizer.

For neonates and infants, a blender should be used to obtain a precise Fio$_2$ for the gas driving the nebulizer, and pulse oximetry should be continuously monitored to minimize oxygen risks

---

Box 12-1 Guidelines for Incorporating Drug Aerosol Systems in Ventilator Circuits

1. If a heated humidifier is in use, recommend increasing the dose of the prescribed drug.*
2. If a heat and moisture exchanger (HME) is in use, remove the HME before aerosol administration (traps aerosol particles).
3. If using flow triggering, set the trigger level to 2 L/min (high-bias flow dilutes the aerosol/increase washout during expiration).
4. Be sure that an *expiratory* high-efficiency particulate air (HEPA) filter is in place (to prevent drug residue from entering the ventilator).
5. Use an in-line chamber or spacer with MDIs.
6. Placement
   - In dual-limb circuits, place the MDI/SVN in the *inspiratory* limb, about 6 inches from the wye connector.
   - In dual-limb circuits *without heated humidity*, place mesh nebulizer between wye and ETT/trach tube.
   - In dual-limb circuits *with a heated humidifier* being used, place the mesh nebulizer at or near the inlet (dry side) to the humidifier.
   - In single-limb circuits (e.g., home care ventilators), place the nebulizer between the patient and the exhalation port.
7. Use manual (MDI) or automated means (SVN) to synchronize aerosol generation with the start of inspiration.†
8. If continuous flow is used with SVN, adjust the ventilator volume or pressure limit to compensate (*need not be done with MDIs or electronic nebulizers*).
9. Upon completion of the treatment, remove the nebulizer from the circuit, reconnect the HME, return the ventilator settings and alarms to previous values, and confirm proper function.

*Bypassing a heated water humidifier can increase aerosol delivery by as much as 40%. However, the effect of dry, cool gas (even for short intervals) on the patient's respiratory tract mucosa can be of concern. Also, failure to reconnect the humidifier might have more dire consequences.

†Synchronous flow to an SVN from the ventilator must meet the SVN manufacturer's specifications.

---

to such patients. Essentially all IPPB circuits include a nebulizer for delivering medications, and the manufacturer's instructions should be followed when using them.

Endotracheal Instillation

Selected drugs can be administered as liquids or "instilled" directly into the lungs via a tracheal airway. You may be asked to instill lidocaine, epinephrine, atropine, or naloxone ("L-E-A-N") in emergencies when IV access is not available (some add vasopressin to the list). Guidelines for endotracheal instillation of these agents include the following:

- Make sure the dose administered is 2–2.5 times greater than the IV dose.
- Dilute the drug dose with 10 mL of sterile water or saline for injection.
- Put the patient in a supine position (not Trendelenburg).
- Halt chest compressions.
- Instill the drug through a catheter that passes beyond the endotracheal tube (ETT) tip.
- Immediately after instillation, provide 5–10 rapid inflations via a bag-valve resuscitator.

The only other respiratory agent you may be asked to administer by endotracheal instillation is surfactant. Surfactant preparations are administered prophylactically to infants at high risk of developing respiratory distress syndrome (RDS) or as rescue therapy for those infants with clinical evidence of RDS. When administering surfactant to these patients, be sure to do the following:

- Recommend a chest x-ray before instillation to confirm ETT position.
- Suction the infant before administration if necessary.
- Monitor the patient's SpO_2 and electrocardiogram (ECG) continuously.
- Use a 5-Fr feeding tube or suction catheter to instill the solution.
- Insert the instillation catheter up to, but not past, the tip of the ETT.

- Split the dose in half and instill half a dose into each dependent bronchus (turning the infant from side to side).
- Administer the dose as rapidly as tolerated.
- After administration, manually ventilate the infant for 1–2 minutes.
- Carefully monitor blood gases and chest wall movement during the first 3 hours after dosing.
- Adjust the ventilator settings and Fio_2 as appropriate (the patient may transiently require higher levels of ventilatory support).
- If possible, avoid suctioning for 6 hours following instillation.

Helium-Oxygen (Heliox) Therapy

The value of helium in respiratory care is based on its low density. Breathing a heliox mixture decreases the driving pressure needed in ventilation, particularly in large airways. Hence, heliox can help reduce the work of breathing associated with large airway obstruction. Major indications for this therapy include acute upper airway obstruction, reversible obstructive disorders, post-extubation stridor, and croup.

Chapter 6 discusses the equipment and setup needed for applying heliox to spontaneously breathing patients, heliox generally is delivered using premixed cylinders of 80%, 70%, or 60% He in 20%, 30% or 40% O_2, respectively, either via a tight-fitting nonrebreathing mask with the flow high to meet or exceed the patient's minute ventilation and peak inspiratory flow requirements or via a high-flow nasal cannula. For infants with bronchiolitis, heliox can be administered via an oxyhood. However, the heat loss and hypothermia associated with helium's high thermal conductivity has limited its use for such young patients, with preference now being given to using a high-flow nasal cannula in this population.

Heliox can also be delivered to patients receiving invasive ventilatory support via a cuffed tracheal airway. As specified in Chapter 6, only a ventilator approved by the U.S. Food and Drug Administration (FDA) for heliox delivery should be used for this purpose. At this time, heliox is not recommended for use in conjunction with noninvasive positive-pressure ventilation (NPPV).

Heliox administration also has been combined with jet-nebulized bronchodilator therapy to treat severe acute obstructive disorders such as status asthmaticus, especially when standard therapy fails. Nebulization with heliox may improve the delivery and deposition of aerosolized drugs in such patients and result in better clinical improvement compared with using air as the carrier gas. Note that flows need to be increased by 50–100% when using heliox to power drug nebulizers. Moreover, because the inhaled aerosol mass and particle size produced by commonly used SVNs vary substantially, no general guidelines other than using higher flows can be provided for this application.

Irrespective of the delivery method, all patients receiving heliox should be closely monitored, and an oxygen analyzer with active alarms should always be used to measure the Fio_2 being delivered to the patient continuously. Once heliox is in use, you may need to modify or troubleshoot the therapy. **Table 12-4** summarizes the major situations where such changes may be appropriate.

Inhaled Nitric Oxide Therapy

Inhaled nitric oxide (INO) is a potent pulmonary vasodilator. Because it relaxes the capillary smooth muscle of the pulmonary vessels, this therapy can reduce intrapulmonary shunting, improve arterial oxygenation, and decrease both pulmonary vascular resistance and pulmonary artery pressures.

After several years of testing, inhaled NO was approved for the treatment of term and near-term (more than 34 weeks' gestation) neonates with hypoxemic respiratory failure associated with persistent pulmonary hypertension of the newborn (PPHN). Inhaled NO has also been used in adults to treat pulmonary hypertension associated with acute respiratory distress syndrome (ARDS), although to date, no significant improvement in long-term clinical outcomes has been shown in such patients.

Although INO can be administered to spontaneously breathing patients via a nasal cannula or a mask, it is more commonly applied to patients receiving mechanical ventilation. The delivery systems include storage cylinders containing NO (800 parts per million [ppm]) delivered via an injector placed

Table 12-4 Common Modifications for Heliox Therapy

Problem/Situation	Possible Cause(s)	Recommended Modification(s)
A patient receiving 80/20 heliox mixture has symptoms of moderate hypoxemia and $SpO_2 < 90\%$	Insufficient FiO_2 delivery to the patient	Analyze the FiO_2 to ensure prescribed concentration is being delivered; if confirmed, consider recommending a mixture with a higher FiO_2 (e.g., 70/30)
A patient receiving heliox via non-rebreathing mask at 10 L/min, but reservoir bag completely collapses during inspiration	Insufficient input flow	Use a flow adequate to keep the bag inflated throughout the breathing cycle; if using standard O_2 flowmeter, apply appropriate conversion factor; consider high-flow cannula administration
Less effective cough and secretion clearance	Lower density heliox inhibits expulsive phase of coughing	Wash out heliox with air–O_2 mixture before coughing
Excessive heat loss and hypothermia for infant receiving heliox via oxyhood	Higher thermal conductivity associated with helium	Warm and humidify gas and closely monitor patient
Variability in medication (bronchodilator) delivery when using heliox	Variability in particle size and deposition due to lower-density gas	Use only nebulizers approved for heliox and monitor patient response to therapy
A patient receiving heliox via invasive ventilation exhibits signs of volume loss or ventilatory insufficiency	Excessive volume loss from insufficient air in ETT cuff or failure to use conversion factors to adjust ventilator settings	Add air to cuff to ensure an adequate seal; if airway seal adequate, make sure ventilator is approved for heliox delivery and conversion factors applied to adjust settings
Evidence of lung overdistention ("beaked" pressure-volume graphic) in a patient receiving heliox through a ventilator	Excessive volume delivery and lung distention because of failure to account for lower-density gas	Use conversion factors to adjust settings, confirm the use of an approved ventilator; closely monitor patient

in the inspiratory side of the ventilator circuit, near its outlet. Also included is a sensor that measures the ventilator's inspiratory flow. To achieve the desired NO dose, the injection rate is automatically adjusted in proportion to the measured gas flow. The recommended initial dose of INO is 20 ppm but can often be quickly reduced to 5–6 ppm.

When NO comes in contact with oxygen, a toxic by-product known as nitrogen dioxide (NO_2) is produced. INO delivery equipment is designed to limit the contact time between these two gases, thereby minimizing the production of NO_2. Nitric oxide, NO_2, and O_2 concentrations are continuously analyzed through a sampling line connected near the distal end of the circuit near the patient's airway. Alarms are used to detect and warn of excessive levels of NO or NO_2 or undesired changes in the FiO_2. NO_2 levels should not exceed 2–3 ppm.

In many cases, the benefits of increased oxygen saturation and decreased pulmonary artery pressure may be seen soon after initiating INO therapy. Treatment may be continued for up to 14 days. Factors to consider when preparing to withdraw therapy are as follows:

- Reduce the NO concentration to the lowest effective dose, ideally 5–6 ppm or less.
- Ensure that the patient is hemodynamically stable.
- Verify patient tolerance of a FiO_2 of 40% or less and a positive end-expiratory pressure (PEEP) of 5 cm H_2O or less.
- Monitor the patient closely during withdrawal of therapy.
- Prepare to provide hemodynamic support if required.

Table 12-5 Common Modifications for Inhaled Nitric Oxide (INO) Therapy

Problem/Situation	Possible Cause(s)	Recommended Modification(s)
Immediately after initiating INO therapy, nitrogen dioxide (NO_2) levels steadily rise above 2–3 ppm	Failure to flush system during setup	Flush system with 100% oxygen before initiating therapy
NO therapy initiated at 20 ppm, but no clinical improvement is seen	Improper equipment setup	Ensure equipment is properly set up and functioning
	Poor or paradoxical response	Recommend alternative (pharmacologic) therapy
INO therapy is started with an initial dose of 6 ppm, but no clinical improvement is seen	The initial dose is too low	Recommend an increase in the initial dose, up to 20 ppm, and monitor the patient closely
Analyzed INO level drops to 0	NO supply tank is empty	Check NO tank pressure and switch or replace NO cylinder
NO, NO_2, and O_2 analyzer readings suddenly drop to 0	Obstructed or disconnected sample line	Check/reconnect gas sampling line, and replace the in-line sampling line filter
NO, NO_2, and O_2 analyzer readings altered during bronchodilator therapy via SVN	Alteration of the prescribed gas mixture by nebulizer flow	Recommend bronchodilator therapy via MDI or mesh nebulizer (no additional flow)
	Disruption of the circuit by nebulizer insertion	Add MDI adaptor to circuit
NO_2 level exceeds 2–3 ppm	NO_2 analyzer malfunction	Check and recalibrate NO_2 analyzer
	Excessive contact time between INO and O_2	Check the proper setup of all equipment
During weaning or immediately after withdrawing INO, the patient becomes hemodynamically unstable or hypoxemic	Patient not tolerating weaning from NO	If weaning is ongoing, recommend that patient be returned to original INO dosage
	Rebound effect	If INO was recently withdrawn, recommend increased Fio_2 and hemodynamic support (vasopressors), consider reinstituting INO therapy, and closely monitor patient

At the recommended doses, INO has been shown to have minimal toxicity and adverse side effects. Nevertheless, although they remain quite rare, hazards include excessive methemoglobin levels, worsening of congestive heart failure, and rebound effect (reoccurrence of hypoxemia/pulmonary hypertension) soon after the withdrawal of therapy. Inhaled NO is also contraindicated in some patients, most notably in neonates with certain cardiovascular anomalies, such as coarctation of the aorta. **Table 12-5** summarizes instances when modifications to this therapy should be recommended.

Other Inhaled Pulmonary Vasodilators

In addition to the medical gas nitric oxide, some medications can be aerosolized to treat pulmonary hypertension and associated hypoxemia. Among them are iloprost (Ventavis), treprostinil (Tyvaso), and epoprostenol (Flolan). These medications all dilate pulmonary arterial vascular beds and decreases platelet aggregation; thus, they can reduce intrapulmonary shunting and improve oxygenation. They have been used to treat spontaneously breathing patients with chronic pulmonary hypertension and, more recently, mechanically ventilated patients with acute pulmonary hypertension, secondary acute lung injury, ARDS, or other similar conditions. **Table 12-6** summarizes their indications, delivery system/dose, and adverse effects.

Table 12-6 Aerosolized Pulmonary Vasodilators

Medication	Indications	Delivery System and Recommended Inhaled Dose	Adverse Effects
Iloprost (Ventavis)	Primarily spontaneously breathing patients with pulmonary hypertension	2.5–5 mcg, 6–9 times daily via I-Neb nebulizer	Cough, headache, hypotension
Treprostinil (Tyvaso)	Primarily spontaneously breathing patients with pulmonary hypertension	1.74 mg in 2.9-mL ampule, 4 times daily via Tyvaso Inhalation System, an ultrasonic pulse-dose device	Headache, hypotension, bleeding (especially if taking anticoagulants)
Epoprostenol (Flolan)	Mechanically ventilated patients with acute pulmonary hypertension, secondary acute lung injury, or acute respiratory distress syndrome (ARDS)	50 nanogram/kg/min via infusion syringe and Aerogen vibrating mesh nebulizer, at the inlet side of the humidifier Titrate down to 10 nanograms/kg/min as tolerated	Headache, hypotension, bleeding (especially if taking anticoagulants)

T⁴—TOP TEST-TAKING TIPS

You can improve your score on this section of the NBRC exam by reviewing these tips:

- Because of their cardiovascular and CNS effects, in general, you should recommend a β adrenergic bronchodilator with the least β_1 (cardiac) and most β_2 (bronchodilating) effects.
- Rinsing of the mouth and use of spacers or valved holding chambers with MDI-delivered steroids minimizes pharyngeal deposition and the incidence of pharyngitis and candidiasis.
- Remove the HME before administering aerosolized medications to mechanically ventilated patients.
- When instructing patients on MDI/spacer use, always remember to tell them to maintain a tight lip seal, and, after actuating, to breathe in slowly (30 L/min or 3–5 sec) and deeply, followed by 10-second breath-hold, then a slow exhalation.
- Consider recommending a valved holding chamber, spacer, or breath-actuated MDI setup for patients having difficulty properly using an MDI.
- Aerosolized antibiotics (Colistin, Cayston, TOBI) are generally indicated only in patients with cystic fibrosis (CF) and suspected or confirmed *Pseudomonas aeruginosa* (gram-negative) pulmonary infections.
- All mucolytics are irritating to the airway; to prevent bronchospasm, always precede treatment with a bronchodilator.
- When directly instilling medications down an endotracheal tube, make sure the dose administered is 2–2.5 times greater than the IV dose, and dilute the drug dose with 10 mL of sterile water or saline for injection; immediately after instillation, provide 5–10 rapid inflations via a bag-valve resuscitator.
- Remember the "L-E-A-N" mnemonic for lidocaine, epinephrine, atropine, or naloxone, which can be instilled down the endotracheal tube in emergencies when IV access is not available.
- Heliox can help decrease the work of breathing associated with large airway obstruction, such as in acute upper airway obstruction, reversible obstructive disorders, post-extubation stridor, and croup.
- Inhaled nitric oxide (NO) is a potent pulmonary vasodilator that can be used in doses from 5 to 20 PPM to reduce intrapulmonary shunting, improve arterial oxygenation, and decrease both pulmonary vascular resistance and pulmonary artery pressures.
- As a less costly alternative to INO, aerosolized medications such as iloprost (Ventavis), treprostinil (Tyvaso), and epoprostenol (Flolan) can dilate pulmonary vessels and improve intrapulmonary shunting and oxygenation.

POST-TEST

To confirm your mastery of each chapter's topical content, you should create a content post-test, available online via the Navigate Premier Access for Comprehensive Respiratory Therapy Exam Preparation Guide, which contains Navigate TestPrep (access code provided with every new text). You can create multiple topical content post-tests varying in length from 10 to 20 questions, with each attempt presenting a different set of items. You can select questions from all three major NBRC TMC sections: Patient Data, Troubleshooting and Quality Control of Devices and Infection Control, and Initiation and Modification of Interventions. A score of at least 70–80% indicates that you are adequately prepared for this section of the NBRC TMC exam. If you score below 70%, you should first carefully assess your test answers (particularly your wrong answers) and the correct answer explanations. Then return to the chapter to re-review the applicable content. Only then should you reattempt a new post-test. Repeat this process of identifying your shortcomings and reviewing the pertinent content until your test results demonstrate mastery.

Ensure Modifications Are Made to the Respiratory Care Plan (Section III-E)

CHAPTER 13

Narciso E. Rodriguez

Beyond providing initial respiratory care to patients, the respiratory therapist (RT) often must recommend modifications to the care plan based on the patient's response and changes in clinical status. This chapter reviews both, when and how to modify the respiratory care plan.

OBJECTIVES

In preparing for the shared NBRC exam content (TMC/CSE), you should demonstrate the knowledge needed to ensure modifications are made to the respiratory care plan in the following areas:

1. Treatment termination and discontinuation based on patient response
2. Recommendations on:
   a. Starting treatment based on patient response
   b. Treatment of pneumothorax
   c. Adjustment of fluid balance and electrolyte therapy
   d. Insertion or change of artificial airway
   e. Extubation and liberation from mechanical ventilation
   f. Consultation from a physician specialist
3. Recommendations for changes on
   a. Patient position
   b. Oxygen and humidification therapy
   c. Airway clearance and hyperinflation
   d. Mechanical ventilation parameters and settings
4. Recommendations for pharmacologic interventions
   a. Bronchodilators, anti-inflammatory drugs, and mucolytics and proteolytics
   b. Aerosolized antibiotics and antimicrobials
   c. Inhaled pulmonary vasodilators
   d. Cardiovascular drugs
   e. Aerosolized antibiotics and antimicrobials
   f. Sedatives and hypnotics, narcotic antagonists, analgesics, and neuromuscular blocking agents
   g. Diuretics and surfactants
   h. Changes to drug, dosage, frequency or concentration

WHAT TO EXPECT ON THIS CATEGORY OF THE NBRC EXAMS

TMC exam: 18 questions; 1 recall, 7 application, and 10 analysis
CSE exam: indeterminate number of questions; however, exam III-E knowledge is a prerequisite to success on Decision-Making sections.

WHAT YOU NEED TO KNOW: ESSENTIAL CONTENT

Recommendations

Termination of Therapy Based on an Adverse Response and Patient Safety

The RT should terminate or recommend discontinuing therapy based on a patient's condition or response when either (1) a patient's safety or well-being appears to be in jeopardy or (2) the goals/objectives of the therapy have been achieved.

Regardless of the type of respiratory therapy intervention, patient safety is paramount. Anytime an adverse patient response is noted, the RT should immediately ensure that the therapy is stopped, notify the nurse and doctor, and carefully monitor and help stabilize the patient. For example, if signs of an allergic reaction such as hives, swelling, or redness are noticed after a new medication is started, the RT should immediately recommend that the medication be stopped, the medical emergency team (MET) be alerted, and the patient be closely monitored.

Regarding patient safety, the RT must prescreen all patients for potential contraindications and hazards before therapy. If any major contraindications exist, the RT should not initiate the therapy. Instead, the RT should contact the prescribing physician for guidance on whether to proceed with the therapy or provide an alternative.

In the absence of contraindications, the RT should proceed with the therapy while monitoring the patient before, during, and after treatment for adverse effects. The most common adverse effects to be on guard for include the following:

- Patient complaints of:
  - Dyspnea
  - Pain
  - Dizziness
- Marked changes in vital signs (20% above or below initial baseline or outside of critical limits)
- Development or worsening of a cardiac arrhythmia
- Development of cyanosis, pallor or diaphoresis
- A greater than 4% drop in SpO_2 or any fall $< 90\%$
- Severe paroxysmal coughing
- Any changes in the patient's level of consciousness or responsiveness
- Nausea/vomiting
- Development/worsening of wheezing or stridor
- A marked decrease in the intensity of breath sounds
- Hemoptysis

In addition to these general adverse effects, the RT must be familiar with those *specific* to each therapy administered (e.g., increased heart rate for β-adrenergic medications).

If a serious adverse effect is observed during therapy, the RT should always follow the "triple-S rule" (**S**top, **S**tay, **S**tabilize):

- **S**top therapy.
- **S**tay with and monitor the patient.
- **S**tabilize the patient by providing oxygen therapy; and if necessary, call for assistance.

If an adverse effect occurs in a hospital, immediately notify the nurse and physician. If the adverse effect appears life-threatening, call for either a MET (rapid-response team [RRT]) or a "code blue," as indicated. If this occurs at an alternate care site such as homecare or nursing home, dial 911 and call for help.

Another reason for discontinuing therapy is if the goals/objectives have been achieved. For example, if a post-op patient receiving incentive spirometry can achieve an inspiratory capacity at or near his predicted value and the chest x-ray is clear, the therapy is no longer needed, and it should be discontinued.

Starting Treatment Based on Patient Response

A good respiratory care plan begins with careful identification and assessment of the patient's problem(s). Once the patient's problem(s) are identified, the RT should then plan to provide or recommend those therapies most consistent with the problem(s) at hand. **Table 13-1** summarizes common findings in respiratory patients (*Objective Data*), the problem(s) that these findings usually indicate (*Assessment*), and the types of therapy that should be provided or recommended (*Recommendations*).

Treatment of a Pneumothorax

A pneumothorax is a serious condition that can be life-threatening, especially if the gas in the thorax is under positive pressure (tension pneumothorax). Clinical signs indicating a tension pneumothorax include the following:

- Sudden respiratory distress/increased work of breathing
- Decreased chest expansion on the affected site
- Decreased or absent breath sounds on the affected site
- Tracheal deviation *away* from the affected site

Table 13-1 Initial Treatment Recommendations in Respiratory Patients

Objective Data	Assessment (Most Likely Problems)	Recommendations
Airway		
Wheezing	• Bronchospasm • Congestive heart failure (CHF) • Airway inflammation	• Bronchodilator therapy* • Diuretics* • Anti-inflammatory (steroids)*
Inspiratory stridor	• Laryngeal edema (e.g., post-extubation or infection) • Tumor/mass • Inhalation injury • Foreign-body aspiration (FBA)	• Cool mist/racemic epinephrine • Diagnostic bronchoscopy
Rhonchi/tactile fremitus	Secretions in large airways	Airway clearance therapy
Cough		
Weak cough	• Poor secretion clearance • Neuromuscular weakness	• Airway clearance therapy • Suctioning • Mechanical insufflation–exsufflation
Secretions		
Amount: > 30 mL/day	Excessive secretions	• Airway clearance therapy • Suctioning
Yellow/opaque sputum	Acute airway infection	• Treat underlying cause • Antibiotic therapy*
Frothy, pink secretions	Pulmonary edema	• Treat underlying cause (e.g., CHF) • Positive airway pressure (CPAP/BiPAP) • Oxygen therapy • Medications (including positive inotropes and diuretics)*

Objective Data	Assessment (Most Likely Problems)	Recommendations
Lungs		
Dull percussion note, bronchial breath sounds	Infiltrates, atelectasis, consolidation	• Lung expansion therapy • O_2 therapy if hypoxemia
Opacity on chest x-ray	Infiltrates, atelectasis, consolidation	• Lung expansion therapy • O_2 if hypoxemia
Hyperresonant percussion, decreased breath sounds	Lung hyperinflation (COPD, asthma, FBA)	• Treat COPD/asthma symptoms • Foreign-body removal by bronchoscopy if necessary
Pleural Space		
Hyperresonant percussion, decreased breath sounds, respiratory distress	Tension pneumothorax	• Evacuate air (chest tube, needle decompression) • Lung expansion therapy
Dull percussion	Pleural effusion (CHF, infections, lung tumor)	• Chest tube, diuretics, thoracentesis • Lung expansion therapy
Acid-Base Balance/Ventilation		
$\downarrow pH = \dfrac{HCO_3^-}{\uparrow Paco_2}$	Acute ventilatory failure	Mechanical ventilation[‡]
$\downarrow pH = \dfrac{\Uparrow HCO_3^-}{\uparrow Paco_2}$	Chronic ventilatory failure	Disease management to prevent exacerbations; low-flow O_2 if hypoxemia
$\uparrow pH = \dfrac{\uparrow HCO_3^-}{Paco_2}$	Metabolic alkalosis	• Hypokalemia—give potassium[‡] • Hypochloremia—give chloride[‡]
$\downarrow pH = \dfrac{\downarrow HCO_3^-}{Paco_2}$	Metabolic acidosis	• Lactic acidosis—give O_2 • Increase cardiac output • Give HCO_3^{-}[‡]
Oxygenation		
$Pao_2 < 60$ torr or $Spo_2 < 90\%$ on room air or low-moderate Fio_2	• Moderate hypoxemia • V/Q imbalance	• Provide for O_2 therapy • Treat the underlying cause
$Pao_2 < 60$ torr on $Fio_2 > 0.60$ or P/F < 100–200	• Severe hypoxemia • Large physiologic shunt	• O_2 therapy • PEEP/CPAP

[‡]indicates physician ordered; ↑ indicates primary increase; ↓ indicates primary decrease; ⇑ indicates compensatory increase; BiPAP, bi-level positive airway pressure; COPD, chronic obstructive pulmonary disease; CPAP, continuous positive airway pressure; FBA, foreign body aspiration; PEEP, positive end-expiratory pressure; Tx, treatment; V/Q, ventilation–perfusion ratio.

- Hyperresonant percussion note on the affected side
- Absence of lung markings and radiolucency on the chest x-ray
- A sudden increase in airway pressure (volume control mode) or decrease in V_T (pressure control mode) during mechanical ventilation

If a pneumothorax is suspected, the RT should recommend (1) obtaining a stat chest x-ray and (2) placing the patient on 100% O_2 (helps reabsorb the gas). If the patient is receiving positive-pressure ventilation, recommend changing the settings to minimize peak inspiratory pressures (e.g., decrease PIP, lower PEEP, lower V_T). For chest tube troubleshooting, refer to Chapters 6 and 16.

If a *tension* pneumothorax is suspected and the situation appears life-threatening, recommend either immediate needle decompression or insertion of a chest tube on the affected side. See Chapter 15 for responding to tension pneumothorax and Chapter 16 for details on assisting a physician with chest tube insertion.

Adjustment in Fluid Balance

The normal fluid intake and output (I/O) for adults is 2–3 liters/day. Maintaining the balance between intake and output is essential to maintain proper metabolic functions. **Table 13-2** lists the signs most commonly associated with alteration of fluid balance and some common management strategies that can be recommended.

Adjustment of Electrolyte Therapy

Monitoring electrolyte concentrations is also very important in critically ill patients and patients with abnormal fluid balance. **Table 13-3** lists the most common causes of abnormal serum levels of the three electrolytes that are typically measured (Na^+, K^+, and Cl^-) and provides some suggested actions the RT can recommend for their treatment.

Insertion or Change of Artificial Airways

In some instances, the RT should recommend the insertion or modification of an artificial airway based on patient assessment. **Table 13-4** summarizes the major indications for insertion of an artificial airway. The various airway equipment used in respiratory care is detailed in Chapter 6. Procedures for inserting artificial airways and the care of such devices are discussed in Chapters 9 and 16.

Common modifications and troubleshooting when managing artificial airways that the RT can perform or suggest are described elsewhere. Some changes involving artificial airways may require a physician's order; such changes often relate to the size, type, or other major feature of the artificial airway. **Table 13-5** outlines the most common situations warranting such recommendations.

Table 13-2 Common Signs of Fluid-Balance Alteration and Management Strategies

Alteration	Common Signs	Recommended Management Strategies
Dehydration (negative fluid balance)	• Dry mucous membranes • Hypotension • ↓ Urine output • ↓ Skin turgor • ↑ Hematocrit • Thick and tenacious secretions • ↓ Central venous pressure (CVP) • ↓ Pulmonary artery wedge pressure (PAWP)	• Increase IV fluid intake • Minimize sensible and insensible water loss • Heated humidification during mechanical ventilation • Administer mucolytics for thick secretions • In critically ill patients, insert a CVP or pulmonary artery (PA) catheter to monitor fluid status • Avoid the use of diuretics
Overhydration (positive I/O)	• Pedal edema • Pulmonary edema • Hepatomegaly • Jugular venous distention • ↓ Hematocrit • ↑ CVP • ↑ PAWP	• Restrict and closely monitor fluid intake (IV and orally) • Initiate diuretic therapy • Administer inotropic agents if heart failure is suspected • Implement dialysis if renal failure is present • Insert a CVP or PA catheter to monitor fluid status if indicated

↑, increased; ↓, decreased; CVP, central venous pressure; PA, pulmonary artery; PAWP, pulmonary artery wedge pressure.

Table 13-3 Causes of Abnormal Electrolytes and Recommendations for Their Treatment

Electrolyte	Causes of Low Serum Levels (*Hypo-*)	Causes of High Serum Levels (*Hyper-*)	Recommendations
Sodium (Na^+)	• Diuresis • Overhydration • Antidiuretic hormone abnormalities • Acute/chronic renal failure	• Fluid loss • Diabetes • Antidiuretic hormone abnormalities • Acute/chronic renal failure	• Treat the underlying cause • Monitor fluid balance • Electrolyte replacement therapy • Dialysis
Potassium (K^+)	• Vomiting • Nasogastric suction • Diarrhea • Diuretics • Renal disease • Metabolic alkalosis • Continuous albuterol nebulization	• High-potassium diet • Renal failure • Metabolic acidosis • Red blood cell hemolysis	• Treat the underlying cause • Monitor fluid balance • Electrolyte replacement therapy • If K^+ is low and patient on diuretics, use a "K^+-sparing" agent (e.g., amiloride or spironolactone) • If K^+ is high, administer high-dose aerosolized albuterol or a "K^+-wasting" agent (e.g., Lasix)
Chloride (Cl^-)	• Severe vomiting • Chronic respiratory acidosis • Renal disease • Burns • Nasogastric suction • Metabolic alkalosis	• Prolonged diarrhea • Metabolic acidosis • Respiratory alkalosis • Renal disease • Thyroid gland disease	• Treat the underlying cause • Monitor fluid balance • Electrolyte replacement therapy

Table 13-4 Indications for Artificial Airways

Artificial Airway	Indications
Oropharyngeal airway (OPA)	Stabilize tongue to facilitate ventilation and relieve obstruction (unconscious patients)
Nasopharyngeal airway (NPA)	Facilitate frequent nasal suctioning and ventilation in conscious patients
Laryngeal mask airway (LMA)	Facilitate short-term artificial ventilation; an alternative during difficult intubations
Endotracheal tube (oral)	Facilitate airway protection, artificial ventilation (up to 2 weeks), and secretion clearance
Endotracheal tube (nasal)	In the presence of oral or mandibular trauma or pathology, facilitate airway protection, artificial ventilation, and secretion clearance
Tracheostomy tube (cuffed, unfenestrated)	Facilitate long-term airway protection, artificial ventilation, and secretion clearance; improve oral care when the artificial airway is indicated; improve weaning attempts
Tracheostomy tube (cuffed, fenestrated)	Same indications for standard tracheostomy tube, with the added benefit of permitting phonation (speaking) and testing upper airway patency and control
Tracheostomy tube (uncuffed)	Maintain patent airway (e.g., in obstructive sleep apnea); provide secretion clearance and permit supplemental oxygenation and humidification for a patient with a bypassed upper airway
Tracheostomy button	Maintain patent airway (e.g., in obstructive sleep apnea); provide secretion clearance and permit supplemental oxygenation and humidification for a patient with a bypassed upper airway

Table 13-5 Recommending Modifications for Artificial Airways

Problem/Situation	Possible Cause(s)	Recommendation(s)
Clinical evidence of impending respiratory failure	Inadequate oxygenation (e.g., pneumonia) and ventilation (e.g., neuromuscular disease)	Immediate intubation
Clinical evidence of inadequate airway protection	Diminished neurologic function (e.g., drug overdose); airway injury, facial trauma, or burns	Immediate intubation
Difficult intubation	Glottis located anteriorly or excessive epiglottic tissue; incorrect laryngoscope blade/endotracheal tube (ETT) size; patient agitated or anxious	Repositioning the patient's airway, rapid-sequence intubation (RSI), inserting laryngeal mask airway (LMA), or performing fiberoptic intubation and video-assisted laryngoscopy; selecting correctly sized ETT and laryngoscope blade or sedating the patient
Excessive ETT cuff leak despite air being added to the pilot balloon	Blown ETT cuff; broken/defective pilot balloon or pilot tube; too small ETT size; ETT too high (cuff at the vocal cord level)	Reintubation with proper-size tube (e.g., 8.0–9.0 for average adult male/female) Use an ETT exchanger Deflate cuff and reposition ETT Pilot balloon repair kit
Intubation indicated in the presence of facial or mandibular trauma or pathology	Oral intubation contraindicated	Nasal intubation or tracheotomy
Oral ETT in place but the need for long-term ventilation exists	Failed weaning attempts Need for long-term secretion management	Tracheostomy
Trach tube in place but patient with good upper airway control wishes to talk	Improvement in patient condition	Deflate cuff and attach speaking valve; alternatively, use "talking" trach tube
Need to maintain an airway without an indication for artificial ventilation	Obstructive sleep apnea or upper airway pathology (tumor or scarring); excessive secretion production	Uncuff trach tube or tracheostomy button
The patient has an artificial airway, but a suction catheter cannot be passed	Partial airway obstruction; suction catheter too large	Use a smaller catheter; in case of patient compromise, recommend immediate extubation if ETT being used or change the inner cannula if trach tube being used
Artificial airway no longer indicated	Improvement in patient condition	Extubation or decannulation
Need for mechanical ventilation in a patient with unilateral lung disease	Unilateral lung infections, localized tumors, lobectomy, pneumonectomy	Double-lumen ETT

Liberation (Weaning) from Mechanical Ventilation

Once mechanical ventilation is initiated, the treatment plan should aim to successfully remove the patient from ventilatory support as soon as possible. The traditional bedside parameters used in assessing ventilation and ventilatory mechanics, such as vital capacity (Vc) and negative inspiratory force (NIF)/maximum inspiratory pressure (MIP), are still used in the NBRC exams to assess a patient's readiness to wean, but recent evidence-based guidelines now recommend different criteria.

According to these guidelines, the RT should recommend that patients on mechanical ventilation undergo daily weaning assessment whenever the following criteria are met:

- Evidence indicating at least some reversal of the underlying cause of respiratory failure
- Adequate oxygenation (e.g., $Pao_2/Fio_2 \geq 150–200$, positive end-expiratory pressure [PEEP] $\leq 5–8$ cm H_2O, and $Fio_2 \leq 0.4–0.5$)
- pH ≥ 7.25
- Hemodynamic stability (no myocardial ischemia or significant hypotension)
- The ability to initiate an inspiratory effort

Once these criteria are met, weaning should begin, usually with an initial short (30–120 minutes) spontaneous breathing trial (SBT) during which the RT should monitor the patient's respiratory pattern (rate, V_T, rapid shallow breathing index [RSBI]), adequacy of gas exchange (Spo_2, arterial blood gases [ABGs], and capnography), hemodynamic stability, and subjective comfort. The use of synchronized intermittent mandatory ventilation (SIMV) as a weaning mode is no longer recommended (see **Figure 13-1**).

A daily sedation interruption or sedation vacation should be performed for all mechanically ventilated patients stable enough to tolerate being off sedation. This will allow a more accurate assessment of the patient's readiness for extubation (including a neurologic assessment) and may facilitate the daily SBT. If the SBT is not tolerated, it is recommended to return the patient to previous settings.

Extubation

The decision to extubate a patient who successfully completes an SBT should be made separately from the weaning assessment (see Figure 13-1). A patient is ready for extubation if the following conditions are met:

1. The upper airway is patent.
2. The airway can be adequately protected, indicated as follows:
   - Positive gag reflex
   - The ability of the patient to raise his or her head off the bed
   - Presence of cough reflex

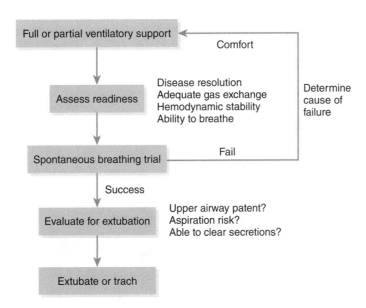

Figure 13-1 An Evidence-Based Approach to Ventilator Discontinuation and Extubation.

3. Adequate artificial airway cuff leak (no signs of significant anatomic airway swelling)
4. Secretions can be effectively cleared, indicated as follows:
   - Deep cough when suctioned
   - If alert, maximum expiratory pressure [MEP] > 60 cm H_2O and/or peak cough flow > 60 L/min

Recommending Consultation from a Physician Specialist

In certain clinical scenarios, the RT may want to recommend consultations from specialties other than a pulmonary physician to address the complex issues surrounding the care of the pulmonary patient. Those recommendations are not limited to a physician only but to a variety of healthcare specialties involved in the care of these patients. **Table 13-6** lists those clinical situations that may warrant those recommendations and the locations where the care is provided.

Recommendations for Changes

Changes in Patient Position

Table 13-7 summarizes when it may be appropriate to recommend changing a patient's position.

Table 13-6 Situations in Which to Recommend Additional Consultation from a Specialty

Clinical Situation	Specialty	Location of Service
Patient with muscle weakness after being bedridden for a long period of time due to prolonged or chronic pulmonary condition (e.g., COPD exacerbation, mechanical ventilation, neuromuscular condition)	Physical therapy, Occupational therapy	Hospital, acute and subacute location, standalone rehab clinics, and patient's home or location
Patient unable to swallow and speak properly after extubation/decannulation due to prolonged mechanical ventilation and/or artificial airway	Speech-Language Therapist	Hospital, acute and subacute locations
A hospitalized child with acute or chronic conditioning needing additional support	Child Life Specialist	Hospital, acute and subacute rehab locations
Pulmonary patient being discharged home with additional medical needs (e.g., COPD, neuromuscular conditions)	Case Manager, Licensed Social Worker, Discharge Planner	Hospital, acute and subacute rehab locations
Pulmonary patients with an acute or chronic condition needing a special diet, specific caloric intake, management of feeding devices, and fluid management (e.g., COPD, CF, neuromuscular, burns, patient with permanent or temporary feeding tubes)	Dietitian and Nutritionist specialist	Hospital, acute and subacute location, standalone rehab clinics, and patient's home or location
Asthmatic patient with uncontrolled allergic asthma	Pulmonary Allergist Specialist Dietitian and Nutritionist specialist	Hospital, clinic, or private practice
The patient appears excessively anxious or depressed	Psychiatrist or Social Worker	Hospital, clinic, or private practice

Table 13-7 Recommending Modifications in Patient Position

Clinical Situation	Recommended Position Change
General dyspnea	Semi-Fowler's position (consider recommending other therapy, such as supplemental O_2)
Orthopnea (dyspnea while supine) generally associated with CHF	Semi-Fowler's or high Fowler's position (consider recommending other therapy, such as supplemental O_2 and diuretics)
Perform postural drainage on a patient with increased ICP or at risk for aspiration	Avoid Trendelenburg (head-down) position; consider rotating the patient laterally to approximate this position
Perform postural drainage on an immobile, bedridden patient	Recommend rotation/vibration bed
Perform IPPB/PEP or oscillation therapy	Semi-Fowler's or Fowler's (avoid slouching); supine is acceptable for patients who are unable to tolerate an upright position
Mechanically ventilated patient with unilateral disease (e.g., consolidation, atelectasis)	Place the patient in "good-lung-down" position
Mechanically ventilated patient with poor oxygenation despite high Fio_2 and PEEP	Consider prone positioning or kinetic therapy bed
Chest tube insertion	The involved side should be slightly elevated, with the arm flexed over the head
Thoracentesis	Patient sitting on the edge of the bed, leaning forward over a pillow-draped bedside table, arms crossed, with an assistant in front for stability
Immobile patient at risk for bedsores (decubitus ulcers)	Change position (side to side) every 2 hours; use decubitus mattress
Perform CPR on a patient in bed	Place a "compression board" under the patient's back or put the bed in "CPR" mode

CHF, congestive heart failure; CPR, cardiopulmonary resuscitation; ICP, intracranial pressure; IPPB, intermittent positive-pressure breathing; PEEP, positive end-expiratory pressure; PEP, positive expiratory pressure.

Changes in Oxygen Therapy

Chapter 11 describes the features and appropriate uses of various O_2 delivery devices. When possible, an O_2 therapy protocol should be used to make recommendations regarding O_2 therapy management. **Figure 13-2** is an example of such a protocol. An O_2 therapy protocol allows the RT to modify therapy independently based on preapproved clinical criteria. However, in the absence of such protocols, the RT may be limited to recommend changes in input flow, delivery device, or Fio_2 to meet the patient's needs. **Table 13-8** outlines some of the common clinical situations that would warrant recommended changes in O_2 therapy.

Changes in Humidification

Humidity and aerosol therapy are a common task for the RT. Humidification of dry medical gases is particularly important in those patients receiving long-term oxygen therapy or noninvasive ventilatory support and those with bypassed upper airways. **Table 13-9** outlines some of the common clinical situations that would warrant recommended changes in humidification therapy.

Changes in Airway Clearance Therapy

The primary indication for airway clearance therapy is to assist patients in clearing retained secretions. The various indications for and methods used to aid secretion removal are detailed in Chapter 10.

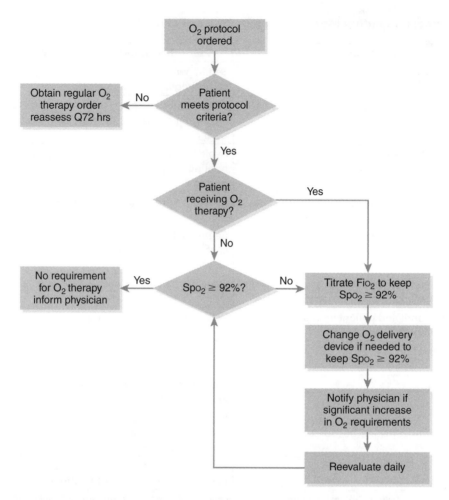

Figure 13-2 Example of an O₂ Therapy Protocol. Note that a full therapy protocol also would include patient inclusion criteria and specifications for equipment selection.

Table 13-8 Recommending Changes in Oxygen Therapy

Problem/Clinical Situation	Possible Cause(s)	Recommendation(s)
The patient remains hypoxemic after initiation of nasal O₂ therapy	The patient is a mouth breather	Switch to an air-entrainment mask or simple mask
	Cannula nasal prongs are blocked with secretions	Clean or replace the cannula
	The patient needs higher FiO_2	Contact the physician for an order to increase or use higher FiO_2 as permitted per protocol
	O₂ device connected to air	Ensure that the device is connected to an O₂ flowmeter and that the flowmeter is turned on
	Bubble humidifier being used	Check for leaks and tighten connections
A patient with chronic obstructive pulmonary disease (COPD) becomes lethargic and disoriented soon after being placed on a nasal cannula at 5 L/min	Oxygen-induced hypoventilation	Recommend that the input flow be reduced to 2 L/min or switch to an air-entrainment system at 24–28% O₂; continue to monitor the patient closely and notify the nurse

Problem/Clinical Situation	Possible Cause(s)	Recommendation(s)
The physician orders oxygen via a simple mask with an input flow of 2 L/min for an adult patient	Physician unaware of the risk of CO_2 rebreathing at low flows with O_2 masks and enclosure devices	Recommend that the input flow be increased to a minimum of 5 L/min to ensure "washout" of exhaled CO_2 or change to a nasal cannula device
A patient on a simple mask at 5 L/min complains that the mask is confining and interferes with his ability to eat	The patient cannot eat with mask on	Recommend that the device be switched to a nasal cannula with a flow of 4–6 L/min during meals, which will deliver an equivalent Fio_2
A nasal cannula at 2 L/min is in use on a patient with a high or unstable minute ventilation who requires a Fio_2 of 0.28	Standard nasal cannula not suitable for patients with high/variable minute volume	Recommend a high-flow device such as a 28% air-entrainment mask, which can meet the patient's inspiratory flow needs and maintain a stable Fio_2
A patient on a 40% air-entrainment system has a Spo_2 of 89%	Insufficient Fio_2 to correct hypoxemia	Recommend that the Fio_2 be increased accordingly, and monitor the patient's response closely
	Insufficient device flow to meet patient's inspiratory flow needs and maintain a stable Fio_2	Recommend adding a second aerosol nebulizer in tandem or bleeding in supplemental O_2 to increase the total output flow of the system
A patient on a simple mask at 10 L/min has a Pao_2 of 212 torr	Too much Fio_2 being delivered to the patient	Recommend a reduction in Fio_2—for example, switching to a nasal cannula at about 5 L/min (Fio_2 of about 0.40)
The patient feels claustrophobic with the aerosol mask in use	Confining feeling imposed by mask	Switch to a face tent or nasal cannula as tolerated.
After you switch an adult patient from a simple mask to a nonrebreathing mask, the Spo_2 only increases from 83% to 87%	Inability to meet high inspiratory flow demands at high Fio_2	Recommend a high-flow nasal cannula at 20–40 L/min, titrate Fio_2 to the desired Spo_2
	Alveolar shunting	Consider mask continuous positive airway pressure (CPAP) with high Fio_2
The patient has facial injury or burns, but the order is for 40% aerosol	Mask may cause irritation or further damage to the face	Switch to a face tent
Air-entrainment aerosol mask delivers higher Fio_2 than set	Obstruction of entrainment ports with bedding, clothing, or other items	Remove obstructions and monitor patient
	Obstruction caused by condensate rainout in the tubing	Recommend a water trap to drain tubing condensation
Non-/partial rebreather mask bag fails to remain inflated	Insufficient input flow	Increase flowmeter setting
	O_2 tubing disconnect/ obstruction	Ensure that tubing is correctly connected to the flowmeter and check for kinks
A physician orders a nonrebreathing mask for a "code blue" patient in respiratory arrest	Nonrebreathing masks do not provide additional ventilation	Immediately recommend a bag-valve-mask (BVM) that can provide 100% O_2 and can be used to ventilate the patient effectively
A patient in the emergency department (ED) is having a myocardial infarction and is on a nasal cannula at 6 L/min	Myocardial ischemia/infarction present requiring high Fio_2	Recommend a nonrebreathing mask with an input flow enough to keep the reservoir bag from collapsing through the breathing cycle
A victim of a house fire with a Spo_2 of 98% is placed on a nasal cannula at 5 L/min	Spo_2 cannot detect carbon monoxide hemoglobin saturations on suspected smoke inhalation victims	Place the patient in the highest possible Fio_2 (usually a nonrebreather mask) and perform a CO-oximetry test. Consider hyperbaric oxygen therapy, if available

(continues)

Table 13-8 Recommending Changes in Oxygen Therapy (*continued*)

Problem/Clinical Situation	Possible Cause(s)	Recommendation(s)
Signs of atelectasis on chest x-ray in a patient receiving high Fio_2	Nitrogen-washout atelectasis	Use the lowest possible Fio_2; implement alveolar recruitment techniques
An oxygen dependent home-care patient who desires greater mobility, but whose activity is limited due to a stationary oxygen concentrator	Limited activity and mobility. Negative physical and psychosocial consequences.	Recommended a portable oxygen concentrator.
An infant or child receiving 50% O_2 in an isolette must be removed for a special procedure	The infant will breathe room air and become hypoxemic	Consider a simple mask that can be easily set up but is not easily dislodged
The Spo_2 of an infant receiving CPAP via nasal prongs drops during episodes of crying	Decrease in Fio_2 due to mouth breathing associated with crying	Collaborate with the nurse to address reasons for crying (e.g., hunger).
		If crying and decrease in Spo_2 continue, consider an enclosure such as an oxy-hood with the same Fio_2

Table 13-9 Recommending Changes in Humidification Therapy

Problem/Clinical Situation	Possible Cause(s)	Recommendation(s)
Patient on a 4-L/min nasal cannula complains of nasal or mouth dryness	Insufficient humidity causing drying of mucosa	Add a humidifier, particularly if the input flow of nasal cannula is $\geq$ 4 L/min
Insufficient aerosol mist from the end of the T-piece of an intubated patient on a T-piece aerosol	Inability to meet high inspiratory flow demands	Recommend adding a second aerosol nebulizer in tandem, or switch to a high-output jet nebulizer (Misty Ox)
	Obstruction caused by condensate rainout in the tubing	Recommend a water trap to drain tubing condensation
A patient develops mild stridor after extubation	Subglottic tissue edema caused by the endotracheal (ET) tube cuff	Provide cool aerosol therapy via an aerosol mask
A patient on a 40% air-entrainment mask complains of too much dryness	Dry gas being delivered to the patient at high flows	Connect a large-volume aerosol nebulizer to the air-entrainment port of the air-entrainment mask
A patient receiving noninvasive positive pressure support complains of dryness and wants to refuse therapy due to discomfort	Cold, dry gas being delivered to the patient at very high flows	Add a blow-by humidifier and *never* use heat and moisture exchangers (HMEs) during noninvasive positive pressure therapy
RT notes that a patient receiving mechanical ventilation with an HME has developed very thick secretions	The use of HME may be contraindicated for this patient	Add heated humidity; HMEs are contraindicated in patients with thick secretions

In general, recommendations for changes in airway clearance therapy may be appropriate considering preexisting conditions (e.g., increased intracranial pressure), recent procedures (e.g., surgery), patient demographics (e.g., age), or an adverse reaction to the therapy (e.g., hypoxemia). Modifications involve one or more of the following: (1) altering the duration of therapy, (2) changing the positions used, or (3) using a different airway clearance strategy. The accompanying box (**Box 13-1**) provides common examples of when to recommend such modifications.

Changes in Hyperinflation Therapy

The equipment used for hyperinflation therapy and the procedure are discussed in more detail in Chapter 10.

Changes for Incentive Spirometry

Incentive spirometry (IS) involves the use of a simple device to promote lung expansion. The success of this therapy depends heavily on patient cooperation and participation. Although IS therapy is relatively simple, sometimes modifications are needed to achieve clinical objectives. **Table 13-10** summarizes common problems and situations that may occur with IS, their likely causes, and modifications that may help resolve the problems.

Table 13-10 Common Modifications for Incentive Spirometry

Problem/Situation	Possible Cause(s)	Recommended Modification(s)
No volume or flow recorded on the device, despite an inspiratory effort from the patient	Equipment assembled incorrectly, tubing or mouthpiece disconnected, patient exhaling instead of inhaling	Recheck equipment assembly and tube/mouthpiece connection, replace the unit, and reinstruct patient
The patient cannot generate enough inspiratory effort to record volume or flow	Insufficient patient instruction, patient unable to follow directions or generate enough inspiratory effort, pain	Reinstruct patient, coach patient to breathe in more deeply, consider another modality (e.g., intermittent positive-pressure breathing [IPPB]). Coordinate pain medication schedule with the nurse
Mild lightheadedness, dizziness, tingling fingers	Hyperventilation	Coach patient to breathe normally and pause between maneuvers
Patient not showing clinical improvement, despite the proper implementation of therapy	Incorrect diagnosis; consider diagnosis other than atelectasis or hypoventilation (e.g., pneumonia)	Call a physician and recommend additional or alternative treatment (e.g., antibiotics, IPPB, Metaneb)
The patient cannot achieve enough flow to activate the incentive indicator	An obstructive disorder that prevents the patient from generating the flow needed to use a flow-oriented device Muscle weakness	Recommend a volume-oriented device or one designed for patients with obstructive disorders; consider another modality (e.g., IPPB, Metaneb)

Box 13-1 Examples of Airway Clearance Therapy Modification

- Shorten the duration of a given postural drainage position for patients who become anxious or otherwise do not tolerate the therapy.

- Discourage strenuous coughing for stroke patients or those otherwise predisposed to increased intracranial pressure (ICP). Instead, instruct these patients to use a "huff" cough, or sit them up until the cough subsides.

- For patients at risk for hypoxemia, provide supplemental O_2, and monitor the Spo_2 throughout the procedure.

- If an adverse event (e.g., hypoxemia, bronchospasm, dysrhythmias) occurs, stop the therapy, return the patient to the original position, administer supplemental O_2, monitor the patient closely, contact the physician, and recommend an alternative strategy.

- Coordinate pain medication schedules for those patients complaining of pain.

Changes for Intermittent Positive-Pressure Breathing

Intermittent positive-pressure breathing (IPPB) therapy involves the application of positive pressure to the airway during inhalation to hyperinflate the lungs, help treat or prevent atelectasis, or aid in secretion clearance and can be used to enhance the deposition of aerosolized drugs. The initiation of IPPB therapy, contraindications, and hazards are discussed elsewhere, but **Table 13-11** outlines the common problems encountered when administering IPPB therapy, along with the recommended modifications to correct these problems.

Changes in Mechanical Ventilation Parameters and Settings

During mechanical ventilation, a host of changes may be necessary to properly manage a patient, many of which require a physician's order. Nevertheless, whenever is appropriate according to patient clinical assessment and needs, the RT should recommend changes aimed at enhancing oxygenation and ventilation, adjusting flow and I:E ratios, changing modes and improving patient synchrony.

Enhancing Oxygenation

During mechanical ventilation, arterial oxygenation is affected mainly by two parameters: the Fio_2 and the PEEP level. The following recommendations apply to adjusting the Fio_2 and PEEP level:

- If hyperoxia is present ($Pao_2 > 100$ torr), lower the parameter (Fio_2 or PEEP) that is potentially *most* dangerous to the patient at that moment.
- If Pao_2 or Sao_2 is low (< 60 torr or $< 90\%$), hypoxemia is present.
  - Increase the Fio_2 if it is less than 0.60.
  - Increase PEEP if $Fio_2 \geq 0.60$.

According to these recommendations, if a patient on 10 cm H_2O PEEP and a Fio_2 of 0.75 has a Pao_2 of 175 torr, the high Fio_2 is of most concern (O_2 toxicity) and should be lowered. In contrast, if

Table 13-11 Common Modifications for Intermittent Positive-Pressure Breathing (IPPB) Therapy

Problem/Situation	Possible Cause(s)	Recommended Modification(s)
Pressure does not rise after triggering	Major leak/poor airway seal	Fix any circuit leaks, coach patient to achieve a tight mouth seal, use nose clips, consider a flanged lip seal or mask;
The machine does not cycle off at end-inspiration	A major leak or poor airway seal	See modifications above
	IPPB valve malfunction	Troubleshoot/clean IPPB valve
Insufficient measured exhaled V_T (one-third or more than the patient's predicted inspiratory capacity [IC])	Insufficient pressure setting on the machine	Gradually increase the pressure to achieve targeted V_T Check for leaks and proper setup
Mild dizziness, lightheadedness, and paresthesia (tingling in the extremities)	Hyperventilation	Coach patient to breathe more slowly (fewer than 8–10 breaths/min) and pause between breaths; lower set pressure
Clinical evidence of worsening hypoxemia (e.g., decreasing Spo_2)	Inadequate Fio_2	Switch to a device capable of high Fio_2
		Provide 100% O_2 (turn off air mix)
	Patient–machine asynchrony	Coach patient to "breathe with the machine"
		Adjust flow for desired I:E ratio
Patient not showing clinical improvement, despite the proper implementation of therapy	Incorrect diagnosis; consider diagnosis other than atelectasis or hypoventilation (e.g., pneumonia)	Call a physician and recommend additional or alternative treatment (e.g., antibiotics)

a patient receiving 18 cm H_2O PEEP and a FiO_2 of 0.45 has a PaO_2 of 150 torr, the high PEEP level is of most concern (barotrauma) and should be lowered.

Likewise, the parameter chosen to increase depends on the cause of the hypoxemia. To decide between adding PEEP or increasing FiO_2, follow the "60-60 rule" to determine the cause and treatment of hypoxemia:

- If PaO_2 > 60 torr on FiO_2 < 0.6, the problem is mainly a ventilation-perfusion (V/Q) imbalance that will respond to a simple increase in FiO_2.
- If PaO_2 < 60 torr on FiO_2 > 0.6, the problem is shunting, and PEEP/continuous positive airway pressure (CPAP) must be added or increased.
- Alternatively, a "50-50 rule" can also be applied.

In addition to managing the FiO_2 and PEEP levels, the RT can also recommend different lung recruitment maneuvers to improve the patient's oxygenation in situations where ARDS and severe atelectasis are suspected. A list of recruitment maneuvers that can be recommended as well as methods to determine the "best" or optimal PEEP levels are discussed in detail in Chapter 11.

Improving Alveolar Ventilation

The presence of abnormal alveolar ventilation can be confirmed via an ABG report showing an abnormal pH due to an abnormal $PaCO_2$. A low $PaCO_2$ can be normalized by decreasing the V_E. Conversely, a high $PaCO_2$ can be restored to normal levels by increasing the V_E. To estimate how much the V_E should be increased or decreased, use the following formula:

$$\text{New } V_E = \text{current } V_E \times \frac{\text{current } PaCO_2}{\text{desired } PaCO_2}$$

In applying this formula, be careful in specifying the desired $PaCO_2$. *The goal should be the $PaCO_2$ that normalizes the pH.* Although in most situations, this means a normal $PaCO_2$ of 40 torr, this may not always be the case. For example, in a patient with COPD who develops ventilatory failure "on top" of a compensated respiratory acidosis (acute-on-chronic), the desired $PaCO_2$ could be substantially higher than normal.

The minute ventilation can be changed by changing either the respiratory rate or the delivered V_T. Exactly how to change V_E depends on the mode of ventilation in use. Note that if the patient's V_T is properly set (6–8 mL/kg predicted body weight [PBW] with a plateau pressure less than 30 cm H_2O), rate changes are the preferred method to alter V_E. Refer to Chapter 11 for detailed guidance on how to increase or decrease V_E for the most common modes of ventilation.

Changes in the I:E Ratios and Flow

During mechanical ventilation in the assist-control (A/C) mode, the I:E ratio can be controlled and altered. Precise control is possible only in the pure control mode (no patient triggering allowed), but adjustments also can be made when some machine breaths are patient triggered.

Factors affecting the I:E ratio during A/C ventilation include any parameter that alters either the I-time or E-time. During volume-control A/C (VC, A/C), I-time is a function of the set flow and volume—that is, I-time = volume (L) ÷ flow (L/sec). During pressure-control A/C (PC, A/C), the I-time usually is set by the clinician. In both modes, the E-time is simply the time remaining between each breath cycle, as determined by the I-time and frequency (f) of machine breaths and the patient. **Table 13-12** provides an example I:E ratio computations for both volume- and pressure-control A/C. More details in time-related computations can be found on the accompanying website for the textbook.

Note that on some ventilators and in some modes, the time parameter set or monitored is the %I-time (also called the *duty cycle*). %I-time is computed as follows:

$$\%tI = \frac{tI}{Ttot} \times 100$$

Table 13-12 Example I:E Ratio Computations

Mode	Ventilator Settings	I-Time	Cycle Time (60 ÷ f)	E-Time	I:E Ratio
VC, A/C	V_T = 500 mL Flow = 60 L/min (1 L/sec) Rate (f) = 20/min	0. 5 L ÷ 1.0 L/sec = 0.5 sec	60 ÷ 20 = 3.0 sec	3.0 – 0.5 = 2.5 sec	0.5 ÷ 2.5 = 1:5
PC, A/C	PIP = 30 cm H_2O I-time = 2.0 sec Rate (f) = 10/min	Set = 2.0 sec	60 ÷ 10 = 6.0 sec	6.0 – 2.0 = 4 sec	2.0 ÷ 4.0 = 1:2

Box 13-2 Determination of Inspiratory Flow Setting During Volume-Control Ventilation

Example: An apneic patient receiving volume-control A/C ventilation at a rate of 15/min has a V_T of 600 mL. The physician orders an I:E ratio of 1:4. Which inspiratory flow should you set to achieve these parameters?

First, compute the minute volume:

$$V_E = 15 \times 600 = 9000 \text{ mL/min} = 9.0 \text{ L/min}$$

Next, convert the I:E ratio into percent inspiratory time:

$$\%I\text{-time} = I\text{-time} \div (I\text{-time} + E\text{-time}) = 1 \div (1 + 4) = 20\%$$

Last, compute the inspiratory flow needed (be sure to use the decimal equivalent for %I-time):

$$\text{Needed flow} = 9.0 \div 0.20 = 45 \text{ L/min}$$

Based on this formula, the example I:E ratios and their %I-time equivalents are as follows:

I:E Ratio	%I-Time
1:4	20
1:3	25
1:2	33
1:1	50
2:1	67

Knowing the %I-time allows quick computation of the needed inspiratory flow during volume-control ventilation using the following formula:

$$\dot{V}_{insp} = \frac{\dot{V}_E}{\% tI}$$

See the accompanying box (**Box 13-2**) for an example of this computation.

More frequently, the RT will need to *decrease or lower* a patient's I:E ratio. This situation occurs commonly when providing mechanical ventilation to patients with severe expiratory airflow obstruction. During spontaneous breathing, these patients typically exhibit prolonged E-times and *low* I:E ratios, such as 1:4 or 1:5. If similar ratios are not provided during mechanical ventilation, air trapping or auto-PEEP will occur. If auto-PEEP is present and the I:E ratio is high (e.g., 1:1 or 1:2), the first step usually is to adjust the settings to allow enough time for complete exhalation. To do so requires decreasing the I:E ratio to a value more normal for these patients, such as 1:4 or 1:5. The I:E ratio can be decreased by increasing the E-time and decreasing the I-time. Methods to do so are summarized in **Table 13-13**.

Modifying Ventilator Modes and Techniques

In many situations, a change in ventilator mode or mode settings may be required. **Table 13-14** summarizes the most common situations warranting such recommendation.

Table 13-13 Methods for Decreasing the I:E Ratio During Assist-Control (A/C) Ventilation

Clinical Situation	Goal	Volume Control	Pressure Control
Ventilator asynchrony due to tachypnea, high set RR, auto-PEEP, air-trapping, agitation	Increase E-time	• Decrease set respiratory rate • Switch to low-rate SIMV	• Decrease set respiratory rate • Switch to low-rate SIMV
	Decrease I-time	• Increase inspiratory flow • Decrease tidal volume	• Decrease I-time and %I-time

PEEP, positive end-expiratory pressure; RR, respiratory rate; SIMV, synchronized intermittent mandatory ventilation.

Table 13-14 Recommending Ventilator Mode and Mode Changes

Clinical Situation	Recommended Mode or Change
Full ventilatory support is needed, but the rate and breathing pattern must be controlled (e.g., hyperventilation syndrome)	Volume- or pressure-control assist-control (A/C) mode with sedative and paralytic
Full ventilatory support upon ventilator initiation; failed weaning attempt	Volume- or pressure-control A/C mode or normal-rate synchronized intermittent mandatory ventilation (SIMV)
Full ventilator support is needed, but total respiratory rate results in hyperventilation (respiratory alkalosis) on A/C mode	Switch to volume or pressure control normal-rate SIMV, add deadspace, or recommend sedation if the patient is agitated
To overcome the imposed work of breathing caused by artificial airways or ventilator circuit	Add/increment pressure-support (PS) level or implement automatic tube compensation (if available)
To boost spontaneous tidal volume in patients with muscle weakness in SIMV or spontaneous modes	Increase RR (SIMV only) Add/increment PS level
To overcome tachypnea or low spontaneous tidal volume during SIMV with signs of increased work of breathing	Increase RR (SIMV only) Add/increment PS level
To reduce airway pressures (plateau pressure) in patients with low lung compliance (acute respiratory distress syndrome [ARDS]) on volume-control A/C	Switch to pressure control A/C with a maximum peak inspiratory pressure (PIP) of less than 30 cm H_2O
To support ventilation and oxygenation in patients with ARDS if National Heart, Lung, and Blood Institute (NHLBI) protocol fails	Consider high-frequency ventilation modality or airway pressure release ventilation (APRV)
To avoid intubation of patients requiring short-term ventilatory support due to exacerbations of chronic obstructive pulmonary disease (COPD)	Provide noninvasive positive-pressure ventilation (NPPV)
To avoid reintubation of patients who develop mild to moderate hypercapnia after extubation	Provide NPPV
To avoid reintubation of patients who develop mild to moderate hypoxemia after extubation	Recommend high-flow nasal cannula at 20–40 L/min and titrate Fio_2 as needed
To avoid or minimize atelectasis associated with low-volume lung protection strategies	Switch to APRV, apply lung recruitment maneuvers, and increase or add PEEP

Other Recommendations Related to Ventilator Settings

Other ventilator modifications that can be recommended are those designed to minimize ventilator-induced lung injury. Related lung-protective strategies that the RT can recommend are the following:

- Volume-control ventilation with low tidal volumes (4–6 mL/kg of PBW)
- Volume-control ventilation with low plateau pressures (≤ 30 cm H_2O)
- Pressure-control ventilation with peak inspiratory pressure (PIP) ≤ 30 cm H_2O

- "Dual-mode" ventilation (e.g., pressure-regulated volume control [PRVC])
- Airway pressure release ventilation (APRV)
- High-frequency percussive ventilation

These techniques can be recommended in conjunction with *permissive hypercapnia*. Permissive hypercapnia is a ventilation strategy in which a higher-than-normal $Paco_2$ is accepted in exchange for the lower risk of lung injury associated with smaller V_T or PIPs. In general, hypercapnia/respiratory acidosis can be accepted until the pH falls below 7.25–7.30, at which point recommend either an increase in rate or administration of sodium bicarbonate.

A final area in which the RT might recommend special ventilator settings involves specific clinical conditions. Patients with a clinically significant bronchopulmonary fistula who do not ventilate or oxygenate well on other settings may respond well to high-frequency ventilation (e.g., HFOV, jet ventilation, or percussive ventilation). Likewise, patients on a ventilator who are particularly at risk for developing atelectasis may be candidates for "open-lung" techniques such as recruitment maneuvers involving the periodic use of PEEP levels as high as 20–30 cm H_2O for a short period of time.

Recommending Pharmacologic Interventions

There are clinical situations when RTs should recommend that drug therapy should be initiated or modified. This section summarizes the most frequent pharmacologic agents used in the NBRC exams.

Initiation or Changes of Bronchodilators, Anti-Inflammatory Agents, and Mucolytics and Proteolytic Drugs

Table 13-15 summarizes the most common clinical situations when the RT should recommend that drug therapy should be initiated for bronchodilators, anti-inflammatory agents, and mucolytics and proteolytic drugs.

Table 13-15 Common Situations in Which to Recommend Drug Therapy for Bronchodilators, Anti-Inflammatory Agents, and Mucolytics and Proteolytic Drugs

Clinical Situation	Recommendation(s)
Acute airway obstruction associated with asthma or a similar condition (relievers)	Short-acting β-agonist (SABA) such as albuterol; consider continuous nebulization and systemic steroids such as prednisone
Maintenance medication for asthma management (controllers)	Depending on the level of control: • An inhaled corticosteroid (ICS; e.g., fluticasone) • A long-acting β-agonist (LABA) in combination with an ICS (e.g., salmeterol/fluticasone [Advair Diskus]) • A leukotriene inhibitor (e.g., montelukast [Singulair]) • A mast-cell stabilizer, such as cromolyn sodium (Intal)
Chronic airway obstruction associated with COPD	For relief of flare-ups: • A SABA For control/maintenance, one of the following: • An ICS (e.g., budesonide, fluticasone, mometasone) • A LABA (e.g., salmeterol [Serevent], formoterol [Foradil], arformoterol [Brovana], indacaterol [Arcapta]) • A long-acting anticholinergic/long-acting muscarinic antagonist (LAMA) (e.g., tiotropium [Spiriva], aclidinium [Tudorza, Pressair], glycopyrronium [Seebri]) • An ICS+LABA combo (e.g., salmeterol/fluticasone [Advair], formoterol/budesonide [Symbicort], formoterol/mometasone [Dulera], fluticasone/vilanterol [Breo]) • A LABA+LAMA combo (e.g., umeclidinium/vilanterol [Anora])

Clinical Situation	Recommendation(s)
Retained, thick/tenacious secretions	• Acetylcysteine (Mucomyst) • Dornase alpha (Pulmozyme), • Hypertonic saline 3–7% (Hypersal) if cystic fibrosis or bronchiectasis is present
Need to increase the volume of secretions for sputum induction	An aerosolized nebulizer treatment with 3–10% hypertonic saline solution

Table 13-16 Indications and Common Recommendations for Antimicrobial Drugs

Clinical Situation	Recommendation(s)
Refractory gram-negative infection of the respiratory tract, especially *Pseudomonas*	Inhaled tobramycin (Tobi), aztreonam (Cayston), or polymyxin E (Colistin)
Treatment or prevention of influenza	Influenza vaccine for prevention and treatment with an anti-influenza agent such as oseltamivir (Tamiflu) or zanamivir (Relenza)
Prevention of pneumococcal pneumonia and pneumococcal infections in elderly and immunocompromised patients	A polyvalent pneumococcal vaccine with scheduled revaccination for high-risk populations

Antimicrobials Drugs

Table 13-16 lists three common recommendations for antimicrobial drugs commonly found on the NBRC exams.

Pulmonary Vasodilators

Pulmonary vasodilators are indicated for pulmonary arterial hypertension (PAH) and neonates presenting with persistent pulmonary hypertension of the newborn (PPHN) at birth. Both conditions have a high level of morbidity and mortality, even with the appropriate pharmacologic management.

Depending on severity and symptoms, the following pulmonary vasodilator agents can be recommended:

- Inhaled nitric oxide (INO)
- Inhaled prostacyclin (e.g., treprostinil [Tyvaso] or iloprost [Ventavis])
- Aerosolized epoprostenol (Flolan)—off-label use in critical care situations only
- Combined oral and inhaled vasodilator therapy

When INO is in use, the following recommended modifications may be warranted:

- Wean the delivered dose in small increments at a time (3–5 ppm) to avoid a rebound effect.
- If an increase in MetHg occurs (>1.5%), recommend a decrease in the inhaled NO dosage as tolerated, and continue to monitor.
- If upper airway is intact or the patient is extubated, recommend the use of a nasal cannula system to deliver the inhaled NO.

When delivering an inhaled prostacyclin agent, the following recommendations should be considered:

- Using the proper delivery device as recommended by the manufacturer
- Avoiding healthcare worker exposure by using expiratory filters and placing the patient in a negative-pressure room
- Titrating dosage and frequency according to patient response

Cardiovascular Drugs

See Chapter 15 for indications and recommendations related to advanced cardiovascular life support (ACLS) drugs.

Sedatives, Hypnotics, Analgesics, and Neuromuscular Blocking Agents

Although the RT cannot independently initiate sedation, paralytics, or muscle relaxant therapy, the RT can recommend that sedatives, neuroleptics/antipsychotics, analgesics, and paralytics be used in specific circumstances. **Table 13-17** includes the major indications for these drugs.

There are special considerations for the RT while recommending these agents. The most common ones are listed in the accompanying boxes (**Boxes 13-3, 13-4,** and **13-5**).

Table 13-17 Most Common Recommendations for the Use of Sedatives, Analgesics, Paralytics, and Antipsychotic Agents

Clinical Situation	Recommendation(s)
Need to anesthetize a patient's airway before a bronchoscopy	Topical/aerosolized lidocaine (1%, 2%, or 4%) or Cetacaine spray before the procedure
Patient agitation and ventilator–patient asynchrony	• Sedation with midazolam (Versed), clonidine (Catapres), propofol (Diprivan), or dexmedetomidine hydrochloride (Precedex) • If the situation requires paralysis (e.g., high intracranial pressure [ICP]), recommend a nondepolarizing agent (e.g., cisatracurium [Nimbex])
Facilitate minor invasive procedures or for procedures requiring "moderate" sedation	• Sedation with barbiturates, such as thiopental (Pentothal), or benzodiazepines, such as diazepam (Valium), lorazepam (Ativan), or midazolam (Versed) • Others: etomidate (Amidate), ketamine (Ketalar), propofol (Diprivan)
Significant pain affecting patient management, long-term control of chronic pain, any surgical procedures likely to generate pain and suffering	• Opioid analgesics, such as morphine, codeine, fentanyl (Sublimaze), hydrocodone, hydromorphone (Dilaudid), meperidine (Demerol), or oxycodone (OxyContin)
Hallucinations or intensive care unit (ICU) psychosis affecting patient management	Neuroleptic/antipsychotics, such as haloperidol (Haldol) or chlorpromazine (Thorazine)
Respiratory depression induced by opioids	Opioid antagonist, such as naloxone (Narcan), to reverse respiratory depression
Difficult intubation and/or rapid-sequence intubation (RSI), facilitate "control-mode" ventilation, muscle relaxation during surgery, facilitate patient–ventilator synchrony, decrease ICP, reduce oxygen consumption	Sedation with midazolam (Versed) and possibly paralytics/neuromuscular blocking agents (e.g., depolarizing—succinylcholine [Anectine]; nondepolarizing—cisatracurium [Nimbex], pancuronium [Pavulon], rocuronium [Zemuron], vecuronium [Norcuron])

Box 13-3 Special Considerations When Recommending Sedatives

- Sedatives decrease anxiety and produce amnesia, *but they do not alleviate pain.*

- Concerns include long half-lives/drug accumulation (resulting in prolonged effects) and cardiac depression.

- Cardiac depression is seen mainly with midazolam or propofol (Diprivan). In this situation, recommend dexmedetomidine hydrochloride (Precedex).

- Benzodiazepine action can be quickly reversed with flumazenil (Romazicon).

- Propofol (Diprivan) is often the sedative of choice in the intensive care unit (ICU) for minor invasive procedures. It has a rapid onset and a half-life of less than 30 minutes.

- A single IV dose (2–5 mg) of midazolam (Versed) may be used to facilitate other respiratory procedures such as intubation and bronchoscopy.

- Propofol and midazolam should be used with caution because they often cause hypotension and respiratory depression.

- As an alternative to propofol and midazolam, dexmedetomidine (Precedex) can be recommended for sedation because it has been reported to have less effect on blood pressure and respiratory drive.

Box 13-4 Special Considerations When Recommending Analgesic Agents

- Morphine is the drug of choice for patients with stable cardiovascular status. Gastrointestinal (GI) side effects are common.

- For patients with unstable cardiovascular status, the histamine-associated hypotension that morphine may cause can be avoided by using fentanyl (Sublimaze) or hydromorphone (Dilaudid).

- Because opioid analgesics can depress respiration, spontaneously breathing patients should be monitored for the adequacy of ventilation.

Box 13-5 Special Considerations When Recommending Paralytics/Neuromuscular Blocking Agents

- There are two classes of neuromuscular blocking agents: nondepolarizing (inhibit acetylcholine) and depolarizing (prolong depolarization of the postsynaptic receptors).

- The depolarizing agents (e.g., succinylcholine [Anectine]) have a short duration of action and are used for short-term paralysis during intubation.

- The nondepolarizing agents produce prolonged paralysis and are used for controlled mechanical ventilation (e.g., pancuronium [Pavulon], vecuronium [Norcuron], and cisatracurium [Nimbex]).

- Paralytics should never be used unless the patient is receiving full ventilatory support, with properly set disconnect alarms.

- Paralytics have *no sedative or analgesic effects*. For this reason, paralytics *must always* be administered with a sedative and, in the presence of pain, an analgesic.

Diuretics and Surfactant Agents

For pulmonary edema associated with congestive heart failure (CHF) and peripheral edema due to right heart failure, a quick-acting loop diuretic such as furosemide (Lasix) and possibly an inotropic medication such as digoxin are recommended. However, for a patient with low serum potassium (< 3.5 mEq/L), a potassium-sparing diuretic such as amiloride (Midamor) should be recommended instead.

Exogenous surfactant therapy has an established role in the management of neonatal respiratory distress syndrome (RDS). The use of surfactant for the treatment or prophylaxis of neonatal RDS results in a reduction in the risk of morbidity and mortality of the neonate.

The following recommendations apply to surfactant delivery:

- Recommend exogenous surfactant therapy for a premature newborn having difficulty breathing or with clinical signs of infant respiratory distress syndrome (IRDS).
- Recommend the *prophylactic* administration of surfactant rather than "rescue" administration, especially in infants of < 30 weeks' gestation, because it decreases the risk of pneumothorax, pulmonary interstitial emphysema, and neonatal mortality.
- Recommend using *multiple doses* of surfactant if required because this method has advantages over a single-dose approach.

Examples of exogenous surfactant agents are beractant (Survanta), calfactant (Infasurf), and poractant alfa (Curosurf).

Recommending Changes to Drug, Dosage, or Concentration

There are a few special situations in clinical practice and on the NBRC exams in which knowing what pharmacologic agent to use is essential to stabilize the patient and treat the underlying condition appropriately. **Table 13-18** lists some of these scenarios.

Table 13-18 Common Modifications to Drug Dosage or Concentration

Clinical Situation	Recommendation(s)
Patient heart rate increases by more than 20% or another unwanted side effect occurs during or after a short-acting β-agonist (SABA) bronchodilator treatment	Stop treatment, monitor patient, notify nurse and doctor, recommend dose reduction or consideration of a drug with minimal B$_1$ side effects (e.g., levalbuterol)
A SABA bronchodilator is prescribed and indicated, but the patient has a recent history of uncontrolled atrial fibrillation, significant tachycardia, or other dysrhythmias	Consider drug with minimal B$_1$ side effects (e.g., levalbuterol), or anticholinergic bronchodilator (e.g., ipratropium bromide)
A physician orders an incorrect drug dosage (e.g., 25 mg albuterol or 0.5 mL Atrovent) to be given via small-volume nebulizer (SVN) every 6 hours	Contact a physician immediately for order clarifications whenever a medication dosage appears incorrect
Prophylactic asthma management in patients age 2 years or younger	Montelukast (Singulair—the only leukotriene inhibitor approved for young children) or cromolyn sodium (Intal—a mast-cell stabilizer)
2 mL of 20% acetylcysteine is ordered, but only 10% acetylcysteine is available	Administer 4 mL (twice the volume) of the more diluted 10% acetylcysteine
Physician orders acetylcysteine, but the patient is at risk for bronchospasm	Add a SABA bronchodilator to prevent bronchospasm
Post-extubation stridor and airway edema	Racemic epinephrine (0.5 mL of 2.25% solution in 3 mL of normal saline)
Hemostasis occurs during a bronchoscopy procedure due to suspected tissue trauma	Epinephrine (10% solution) recommended to produce vasoconstriction

T⁴—TEST-TAKING TIPS

- Whenever an adverse patient response is noted, the RT should immediately stop the therapy, notify the nurse and doctor, and carefully monitor and stabilize the patient.
- If a serious adverse effect during therapy is observed, always follow the "triple-S" rule: stop the therapy, stay with and monitor the patient, and stabilize the patient.
- When troubleshooting wheezing, also consider CHF and foreign-body aspirations as possible causes.
- Clinical signs of a tension pneumothorax usually include sudden respiratory distress, increased work of breathing, unilateral chest expansion, decreased or absent breath sounds on the affected site, tracheal deviation away from the affected site, and hyperresonant sound when percussing the affected side. Additionally, a mechanically ventilated patient with a tension pneumothorax will exhibit a sudden increase in airway pressure (volume control mode) or decrease in V$_T$ (pressure-control mode).
- If a tension pneumothorax is suspected and the situation appears life-threatening, recommend either immediate needle decompression or insertion of a chest tube on the affected side.
- Recommend a nasopharyngeal airway to stabilize the tongue to facilitate ventilation and relieve obstruction in unconscious patients.
- To facilitate airway protection, secretion clearance, and mechanical ventilation for up to 2 weeks, recommend an oral ETT.
- Recommend a nasal ETT only in the presence of oral or mandibular trauma or pathology.
- For long-term airway protection, artificial ventilation, and secretion clearance, use a tracheostomy tube.
- Recommend rapid-sequence intubation for patients with clinical signs of impending respiratory failure or inadequate airway protection.
- If a difficult intubation is expected, recommend one or a combination of the following: (1) repositioning the patient's airway, (2) initiating rapid-sequence intubation (RSI), (3) inserting

a laryngeal mask airway (LMA), (4) performing fiberoptic intubation and/or video-assisted laryngoscopy, (5) selecting correctly sized ETT and laryngoscope blade, (6) sedating the patient.

- When there is a need for mechanical ventilation in a patient with unilateral lung disease, recommend the use of a double-lumen ETT.
- Once mechanical ventilation is initiated, begin the weaning process as soon as possible.
- For patients on a ventilator who are particularly at risk for developing atelectasis or ARDS, recommend "open-lung" techniques such as recruitment maneuvers and optimal PEEP to improve oxygenation and ventilation.
- For patient–ventilator asynchrony, always consider and recommend measures to address both patient-related causes, such as airway obstruction and anxiety, and machine-related causes, such as inappropriate trigger sensitivity or inspiratory flow.
- In a patient with a bronchopulmonary fistula or any airway-leak syndrome who does not ventilate or oxygenate well on conventional ventilation, recommend high-frequency ventilation or jet ventilation.
- A daily sedation interruption or sedation vacation together with a spontaneous breathing trial (SBT) should be performed for all mechanically ventilated patients stable enough to tolerate such measures.
- The decision to extubate a patient who successfully completes an SBT should be made separately from the weaning assessment.
- Recommend extubation only if (1) the upper airway is patent, (2) the airway can be adequately protected (as indicated by positive gag reflex and ability of the patient to raise his or her head off the bed), and (3) secretions can be effectively cleared (as indicated by deep cough when suctioned and an MEP > 60 cm H_2O).
- Avoid Trendelenburg (head-down) position in a patient with increased ICP or at risk for aspiration.
- In general, place the patient in the "good-lung-down" position when ventilating patients with unilateral disease (e.g., consolidation, atelectasis).
- Place a compression board under the patient's back or put the bed in "CPR" mode during CPR.
- When a patient is a mouth breather, recommend using an enclosure device such as an entrainment mask or simple mask to deliver oxygen therapy.
- Recommend that the input flow is reduced to 2 L/min, or switch to a 24% or 28% air-entrainment system to avoid O_2-induced hypoventilation in COPD patients.
- To avoid CO_2 rebreathing at low flows with O_2 masks and enclosure devices, recommend that the input flow is increased to a minimum of 5 L/min.
- If a patient has high or unstable minute ventilation, recommend a high-flow device such as an air-entrainment mask, which can meet the patient's inspiratory flow needs and maintain a stable Fio_2.
- Always recommend the highest possible Fio_2 for a patient with myocardial ischemia or infarction.
- Humidification of dry medical gases is particularly important in those patients receiving long-term oxygen therapy or noninvasive ventilatory support and those with bypassed airways.
- Provide cool aerosol therapy via aerosol mask if a patient develops stridor after extubation to relieve subglottic tissue edema caused by the ETT.
- If a patient receiving noninvasive support complains of dryness and wants to refuse therapy due to discomfort, add a blow-by humidifier, and never use HMEs during noninvasive therapy.
- Switch to active (heated) humidification if any contraindications for the use of an HME, such as retained secretions, are suspected.
- Stop postural drainage in the head-down position if the patient begins coughing vigorously. Sit the patient up and stabilize the situation before continuing with therapy.
- Consider recommending a laryngeal mask airway (LMA) as an alternative to intubation in the presence of a difficult airway.

- If a patient performing incentive spirometry (IS) develops mild lightheadedness, dizziness, and tingling fingers, the likely cause is hyperventilation, and the patient should be coached to breathe normally and pause between maneuvers.
- If the pressure does not rise after triggering during IPPB therapy, the possible cause is a major leak/poor airway seal. To address the problem for spontaneously breathing patients, check and fix any leaks, ensure a tight mouth seal, or use a mask or nose clips. For patients with an artificial airway, check cuff pressure and tube connection, and adjust the terminal flow, if available.
- To enhance oxygenation during mechanical ventilation, increase the Fio_2 if the $Pao_2 > 60$ torr on $Fio_2 < 0.6$, to address an apparent V/Q imbalance. However, if the $Pao_2 < 60$ torr on $Fio_2 > 0.6$, the problem is shunting, and PEEP/CPAP must be added or increased.
- During mechanical ventilation, a high $Paco_2$ can be normalized by increasing the V_E. To estimate how much to increase or decrease the V_E, the following formula can be used:

$$\text{New } V_E = \text{current } V_E \times \frac{\text{current } Paco_2}{\text{desired } Paco_2}$$

- When attempting to minimize air trapping/auto-PEEP in mechanically ventilated patients, recommend that the E-time can be increased by decreasing the rate or switching to low-rate SIMV. Alternatively, to address this problem, the I-time can be shortened by increasing the inspiratory flow or decreasing the tidal volume.
- When full ventilator support is needed, but total respiratory rate results in hyperventilation (respiratory alkalosis) on A/C mode, recommend switching to volume- or pressure-control normal-rate SIMV, add deadspace, or recommend sedation if the patient is agitated.
- To boost spontaneous tidal volume in patients with muscle weakness or signs of increased work of breathing during SIMV or spontaneous modes, recommend adding or increasing the pressure-support level.
- To avoid intubation of patients requiring short-term ventilatory support due to exacerbations of COPD or reintubation of patients who develop mild hypercapnia after extubation, recommend noninvasive positive-pressure ventilation (NPPV).
- To avoid reintubation of patients who develop mild to moderate hypoxemia after extubation, recommend high-flow nasal cannula at 20–40 L/min, and titrate Fio_2 as needed.
- To support ventilation and oxygenation in patients with ARDS when other conventional ventilator strategies fail, consider recommending high-frequency ventilation (HFOV, jet or percussive ventilation) or airway pressure-release ventilation (APRV).
- To avoid or minimize atelectasis associated with low-volume lung protection strategies, recommend switching to APRV, apply lung recruitment maneuvers, and add or increase PEEP.
- Consider recommending pulmonary vasodilators such as inhaled nitric oxide (NO), aerosolized prostacyclin (e.g., treprostinil [Tyvaso], iloprost [Ventavis], or epoprostenol [Flolan]) for patients with pulmonary arterial hypertension (PAH), for neonates with persistent pulmonary hypertension of the newborn (PPHN), or for patients with hypoxemia secondary to ARDS or acute lung injury.
- For acute asthma or status asthmaticus, recommend a short-acting β-agonist (SABA) such as albuterol; consider continuous nebulization and systemic steroids such as prednisone.
- Maintenance medications for asthma management should include controllers such as an inhaled corticosteroid (e.g., fluticasone); a mast-cell stabilizer (e.g., cromolyn sodium); a leukotriene inhibitor, such as montelukast (Singulair); and/or a long-acting β-agonist (LABA) in combination with an inhaled steroid, such as salmeterol/fluticasone.
- If a patient's heart rate increases by more than 20% or another unwanted side effect occurs during or after a SABA bronchodilator treatment, stop the treatment, monitor the patient, notify the nurse and doctor, and recommend dose reduction or a drug with minimal β_1 side effects (e.g., levalbuterol).
- For post-extubation stridor due to airway edema, racemic epinephrine (0.5 mL of 2.25% solution in 3 mL of normal saline) should be recommended, along with close monitoring.

- Patient agitation and ventilator–patient asynchrony can be pharmacologically managed with sedation from agents such as midazolam (Versed), propofol (Diprivan), or dexmedetomidine hydrochloride (Precedex).
- Moderate to severe pain should be treated with opioid analgesics, such as morphine, codeine, fentanyl (Sublimaze), or hydrocodone.
- To facilitate short-term procedures requiring patient paralysis, such as intubation, a depolarizing paralytic (e.g., succinylcholine [Anectine]) should be recommended.
- Patient paralysis during mechanical ventilation is better achieved by longer-acting nondepolarizing paralytics: cisatracurium (Nimbex), pancuronium (Pavulon), rocuronium (Zemuron), or vecuronium (Norcuron).
- Before pharmacologically paralyzing a patient, the patient should first be adequately sedated.
- The influenza vaccine should be recommended for the prevention of influenza, especially in the elderly and immunocompromised. Viral infections such as influenza can also be treated with antiviral medications (e.g., oseltamivir [Tamiflu] or zanamivir [Relenza]).
- Bacterial pneumococcal pneumonia and pneumococcal infections are best prevented with a polyvalent pneumococcal vaccine but can be treated with antibiotics to which the microbe is sensitive.
- For pulmonary edema associated with CHF and peripheral edema due to right heart failure, a quick-acting loop diuretic, such as furosemide (e.g., Lasix), and possibly an inotropic medication, such as digoxin, are recommended.
- For a patient needing diuresis but who also has low serum potassium (< 3.5 mEq/L), a potassium-sparing diuretic such as amiloride (Midamor) should be recommended.
- Exogenous surfactant therapy should be recommended to reduce the work of breathing and in the overall management of neonatal respiratory distress syndrome (RDS).

POST-TEST

To confirm your mastery of each chapter's topical content, you should create a content post-test, available online via the Navigate Premier Access for Comprehensive Respiratory Therapy Exam Preparation Guide, which contains Navigate TestPrep (access code provided with every new text). You can create multiple topical content post-tests varying in length from 10 to 20 questions, with each attempt presenting a different set of items. You can select questions from all three major NBRC TMC sections: Patient Data, Troubleshooting and Quality Control of Devices and Infection Control, and Initiation and Modification of Interventions. A score of at least 70–80% indicates that you are adequately prepared for this section of the NBRC TMC exam. If you score below 70%, you should first carefully assess your test answers (particularly your wrong answers) and the correct answer explanations. Then return to the chapter to re-review the applicable content. Only then should you reattempt a new post-test. Repeat this process of identifying your shortcomings and reviewing the pertinent content until your test results demonstrate mastery.

Utilize Evidence-Based Principles (Section III-F)

Albert J. Heuer

CHAPTER 14

Respiratory therapists (RTs) rely on the results of research, also known as evidence, to help guide how they perform or recommend therapeutic and diagnostic procedures. As a result, the NBRC exams are highly reflective of questions and scenarios that are based on research evidence. In addition, the NBRC expects that exam candidates have basic knowledge of the types of research designs and how to locate and utilize evidence-based resources. This chapter summarizes major types of research categories, explains how to find commonly used evidence-based guidelines, and provides examples of how research evidence can be effectively applied in respiratory care. An adequate understanding of these principles can help RTs optimize patient care and assist candidates in performing well in related aspects of the NBRC exam(s).

OBJECTIVES

In preparing for the shared NBRC exam content (TMC/CSE), you should demonstrate knowledge related to locating, evaluating, and applying evidence-based or clinical practice guidelines in assessing a patient's physiologic state and making recommendations related to the patient's care plan. Such research-based evidence includes the following:

1. ARDS Network (ARDSNet)
2. National Asthma Education and Prevention Program (NAEPP)
3. Global Initiative for Chronic Obstructive Lung Disease (GOLD)
4. The American Association for Respiratory Care (AARC) Clinical Practice Guidelines and other related guidelines available from the AARC

WHAT TO EXPECT ON THIS CATEGORY OF THE NBRC EXAMS

TMC exam: 6 questions; 0 recall, 2 application, 4 analysis
CSE exam: indeterminate number of questions; however, exam III-F knowledge is a prerequisite to success on CSE Information Gathering and Decision-Making sections.

WHAT YOU NEED TO KNOW: ESSENTIAL CONTENT

Types of Evidence

Various types of research are used to shape the clinical interventions applied in medicine and more specifically in respiratory care. However, not all research evidence is the same, and some types support clinical practice more strongly than others. The relative strength of various types of research is illustrated in the research hierarchy depicted in **Figure 14-1**. The strongest evidence is shown at the top.

The types of research designs are described below and are presented in order from strongest to weakest in terms of scientific rigor:

- *A meta-analysis* thoroughly examines several valid studies on a topic, and mathematically combines the results using accepted statistical methodology to report the results as if it were one large study.
- *Systematic reviews* focus on a clinical topic and answer a specific question. An extensive literature search is conducted to identify studies with sound methodology. The studies

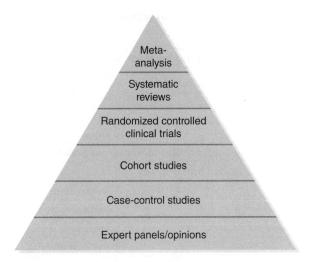

Figure 14-1 Evidence-Based Research Hierarchy.

are reviewed and assessed for quality, and the results are summarized according to the predetermined criteria of the review question.

- *Randomized controlled clinical trials (RCTs)* are carefully planned experiments that introduce a treatment or exposure to study its effect on real patients. An RCT is a planned experiment and can provide sound evidence of cause and effect. RCTs include methodologies that reduce the potential for bias and allow for comparison between the group receiving the intervention being tested (e.g., experimental group) and the group that does not (e.g., control group).
- *Cohort studies* identify a group of patients who are already undergoing a particular treatment or have an exposure, follow them forward over time, and then compare their outcomes with those of a similar group that has not been affected by the treatment or exposure being studied. Cohort studies are observational and not as reliable as RCTs because the two groups may differ in ways other than in the variable under study.
- *Case-control studies* are studies in which patients who already have a specific condition are compared with people who do not have the condition. The researcher looks back to identify factors or exposures that might be associated with the illness. These studies often rely on medical records and patient recall for data collection. These types of studies are often less reliable than RCTs and cohort studies because showing a statistical relationship does not mean that one factor necessarily caused the other.
- *Expert panels* report the professional opinion of a group of recognized experts in a particular clinical area. Although expert panels are potentially useful, the subjectivity associated with defining who the actual experts are and potential biases limit their value.

Locating Sources of Medical Evidence

Beyond understanding the types of research and the related hierarchy, NBRC exam candidates should have basic knowledge on how to find relevant research and other evidence-based resources. A variety of search engines and web-based repositories oriented toward medical research can be used by RTs and NBRC exam candidates to identify scientific evidence on a particular topic. Some of these sources are more highly specific to respiratory care and therefore are more commonly used and more relevant to NBRC credentialing exam candidates. These sources are summarized in **Table 14-1**.

Frequently Used Evidence-Based Sources in Respiratory Care

Also, there are some specific websites and repositories of research-backed guidelines that are especially relevant to the practice of respiratory care and the patients served. Among them, some such

Table 14-1 Commonly Used Search Engines and Web-Based Repositories for Respiratory Care Research

Search Engines for Medical Research*	
PubMed	www.ncbi.nlm.nih.gov/pubmed
Medline	www.nlm.nih.gov/bsd/pmresources.html
Google Scholar	scholar.google.com/
WebMD	www.webmd.com/
Organizations Sponsoring Evidence-Based Resources and Research Repositories*	
American Academy of Allergy, Asthma, and Immunology	www.aaaai.org
American Academy of Pediatrics	www.aap.org
American Academy of Sleep Medicine	www.aasmnet.org
American Association for Respiratory Care	www.aarc.org
American Cancer Society	www.cancer.org
American College of Allergy, Asthma, and Immunology	www.acaai.org
American College of Chest Physicians	www.chestnet.org
American Heart Association	www.heart.org/heartorg
American Lung Association	www.lungusa.org
American Thoracic Society	www.thoracic.org
ARDS Network	www.ardsnet.org
Centers for Disease Control and Prevention	www.cdc.gov
Cochrane Collaboration	www.cochrane.org
Committee on Accreditation for Respiratory Care	www.coarc.com
Cystic Fibrosis Foundation	www.cff.org
Global Initiative for COPD	www.goldcopd.com
National Board for Respiratory Care	www.nbrc.org
National Heart, Lung, and Blood Institute	www.nhlbi.nih.gov/health/indexpro.htm
Society for Critical Care Medicine	www.sccm.org
U.S. Surgeon General	www.surgeongeneral.gov
*Web addresses subject to change.	

Table 14-2 Suggested Incremental Fio_2/Positive End-Expiratory Pressure (PEEP) Combinations to Achieve Adequate Oxygenation

Conservative Approach (Higher Fio_2/Lower PEEP)													
Fio_2	0.3	0.4	0.4	0.5	0.5	0.6	0.7	0.7	0.7	0.8	0.9	0.9	0.9	1.0
PEEP	5	5	8	8	10	10	10	12	14	14	14	16	18	18–24
Aggressive Approach (Lower Fio_2/Higher PEEP)													
Fio_2	0.3	0.3	0.3	0.3	0.3	0.4	0.4	0.5	0.5	0.5–0.8	0.8	0.9	1.0	1.0
PEEP	5	8	10	12	14	14	16	16	18	20	22	22	22	24
NIH-NHLBI ARDS Network. Mechanical Ventilation Protocol Summary. Available from http://www.ardsnet.org/files/ventilator_protocol_2008-07.pdf													

sources have been particularly influential, including the ARDS Network (ARDSNet), the National Asthma Education and Prevention Program (NAEPP), and the Global Initiative for Chronic Obstructive Lung Disease (GOLD) guidelines. Excerpts from these three evidence-based guidelines are included in the following sections, and key elements of ARDSNet, NAEPP, and the GOLD guidelines are summarized in **Tables 14-2**, **14-3**, and **14-4**, respectively, and may appear in the NBRC examinations.

Table 14-3 Expert Panel Report 3: Guidelines for the Diagnosis and Management of Asthma (EPR-3)

Clinical Issue	Key Clinical Activities and Action Steps
Establish an asthma diagnosis	• Determine that symptoms of chronic airway obstruction such as history of cough, recurrent wheezing, recurrent difficulty breathing, frequent chest tightness are present, based on history and exam. • Symptoms that occur or worsen at night or with exercise, viral infection, exposure to allergens and irritants, changes in weather, hard laughing or crying, stress, or other factors • In all patients ≥ 5 years of age, use spirometry to determine that airway obstruction is at least partially reversible. • Consider other causes of obstruction.
Long-term asthma management	Reduce impairment by: • Prevent chronic symptoms. • Require infrequent use of short-acting β-agonist (SABA). • Maintain (near) normal lung function and normal activity levels. • Reduce risk by: • Prevent exacerbations. • Minimize the need for emergency care, hospitalization. • Prevent the loss of lung function (or, for children, prevent reduced lung growth). • Minimize adverse effects of therapy.
Assessment and monitoring	**Initial visit**: Assess asthma severity to initiate treatment. **Follow-up visits**: • Assess at each visit: asthma control, proper medication technique, written asthma action plan, patient adherence, patient concerns. • Obtain lung function measured by spirometry at least every 1–2 years; more frequently for asthma that is not well controlled. • Determine if therapy should be adjusted: Maintain treatment; step up, if needed; step down, if possible. **Schedule follow-up care:** Asthma is highly variable over time. See patients as follows: • Every 2–6 weeks while gaining control • Every 1–6 months to monitor control • Every 3 months if step-down in therapy is anticipated
Use of medications	Select medication and delivery devices that meet the patient's needs and circumstances: • Use a stepwise approach to identify appropriate treatment options. • Inhaled corticosteroids (ICSs) are the most effective long-term control therapy. • When choosing treatment, consider the domain of relevance to the patient (risk, impairment, or both), patient's history of response to the medication, and patient's willingness and ability to use the medication. • Review medications, technique, and adherence at each follow-up visit.

(continues)

Table 14-3 Expert Panel Report 3: Guidelines for the Diagnosis and Management of Asthma (EPR-3) (*continued*)

Clinical Issue	Key Clinical Activities and Action Steps

Patient education for self-management	Teach patients how to manage their asthma.
	
	• Teach and reinforce the following at each visit:
	
	  o Self-monitoring to assess the level of asthma control and recognize signs of worsening asthma (either symptom or peak-flow monitoring)
	
	  o Taking medication correctly (inhaler technique, use of devices, understanding the difference between long-term control and quick-relief medications):
	
	    ▪ *Long-term control* medications (e.g., ICSs, which reduce inflammation) prevent symptoms and should be taken daily; they will not give quick relief.
	
	    ▪ *Quick-relief medications* (SABAs) relax the airway muscles to provide fast relief of symptoms; they will not provide long-term asthma control. If used > 2 days/week (except as needed for exercise-induced asthma), the patient may need to start or increase long-term control medications.
	
	  o Avoiding environmental factors that worsen asthma
	
	• Develop a written asthma action plan in partnership with patient/family (sample plan available at www.nhlbi.nih.gov/health/public/lung/asthma/asthma_actplan.pdf):
	
	  o Agree on treatment goals.
	
	• Teach patients how to use the asthma action plan for the following:
	
	  o Taking daily actions to control asthma
	
	  o Adjusting medications in response to worsening asthma
	
	  o Seeking medical care as appropriate
	
	• Encourage adherence to the asthma action plan:
	
	  o Choose a treatment that achieves outcomes and addresses preferences important to the patient/family.
	
	  o At each visit, review any success in achieving control, any concerns about treatment, any difficulties following the plan, and any possible actions to improve adherence.
	
	  o Provide encouragement and praise, which builds patient confidence. Encourage family involvement to provide support.
	
	Integrate education into all points of care involving interactions with patients:
	
	• Include members of all healthcare disciplines (e.g., physicians, pharmacists, nurses, respiratory therapists, and asthma educators) in providing and reinforcing education at all points of care.

Control of environmental factors and comorbid conditions	Recommend ways to control exposures to allergens, irritants, and pollutants that make asthma worse: • Determine exposures, history of symptoms after exposures, and sensitivities. (In patients with persistent asthma, use skin or in vitro testing to assess sensitivity to perennial indoor allergens to which the patient is exposed.) • Recommend multifaceted approaches to control exposures to which the patient is sensitive; single steps alone are generally ineffective. • Advise all asthma patients and all pregnant women to avoid exposure to tobacco smoke. • Consider allergen immunotherapy by trained personnel for patients with persistent asthma when there is a clear connection between symptoms and exposure to an allergen to which the patient is sensitive.

Clinical Issue	Key Clinical Activities and Action Steps
	Treat comorbid conditions:
	• Consider allergic bronchopulmonary aspergillosis, gastroesophageal reflux, obesity, obstructive sleep apnea, rhinitis and sinusitis, and stress or depression. Treatment of these conditions may improve asthma control.
	• Consider inactivated flu vaccine for all patients > 6 months of age
Exercise-induced bronchospasm (EIB)	Prevent EIB:
	• Physical activity should be encouraged. For most patients, EIB should not limit participation in any activity they choose.
	• Teach patients to take treatment before exercise. SABAs will prevent EIB in most patients; leukotriene receptor antagonists (LTRAs), cromolyn, or long-acting β-agonist (LABAs) also are protective. Frequent or chronic use of LABAs to prevent EIB is discouraged because it may disguise poorly controlled persistent asthma.
	• Consider long-term control medication. EIB often is a marker of inadequate asthma control and responds well to regular anti-inflammatory therapy.
	• Encourage a warm-up period or mask or scarf over the mouth for cold-induced EIB.
Managing exacerbations—home care	Develop a written asthma action plan.
	Teach patients how to:
	• Recognize early signs, symptoms, and peak expiratory flow (PEF) measures that indicate worsening asthma.
	• Adjust medications (increase SABA and, in some cases, add oral systemic corticosteroids) and remove or withdraw from environmental factors contributing to the exacerbation.
	• Monitor response.
	• Seek medical care if there is serious deterioration or lack of response to treatment.
	Give specific instructions on whom and when to call.
Managing exacerbations—urgent or emergency care	Assess severity by lung function measures (for ages ≥ 5 years), physical examination, and signs and symptoms.
	Treat to relieve hypoxemia and airflow obstruction; reduce airway inflammation:
	• Use supplemental oxygen as appropriate to correct hypoxemia.
	• Treat with repetitive or continuous SABA, with the addition of inhaled ipratropium bromide in severe exacerbations.
	• Give oral systemic corticosteroids in moderate or severe exacerbations or for patients who fail to respond promptly and completely to SABA.
	• Consider adjunctive treatments, such as intravenous magnesium sulfate or heliox, in severe exacerbations unresponsive to treatment.
	Monitor response with repeat assessment of lung function measures, physical examination, and signs and symptoms; in the emergency department, including pulse oximetry.
	Discharge with medication and patient education:
	• Medications: SABA, oral systemic corticosteroids; consideration of starting ICS
	• Referral to follow-up care
	• Asthma discharge plan
	• Review of inhaler technique and, whenever possible, environmental control measures

The National Asthma Education and Prevention Program (NAEPP) — Expert Panel Report 3: Guidelines for the Diagnosis and Management of Asthma (EPR-3). Retrieved from: https://www.nhlbi.nih.gov/files/docs/guidelines/asthma_qrg.pdf

Table 14-4 Classifying and Pharmacologic Treatment of COPD—Global Initiative for Chronic Obstructive Lung Disease (GOLD)

COPD Patient Category	Severity of Airflow Obstruction (Post-Bronchodilator FEV₁)	Annual Exacerbations (and Hospitalizations)	COPD Assessment Test (CAT)*	mMRC Breathlessness Scale	Initial Pharmacologic Therapy
A	$\geq$ 50% Predicted	$\leq$ 1 (0 Hosp)	< 10	0-1	Any Bronchodilator
B	$\geq$ 50% Predicted	$\leq$ 1 (0 Hosp)	$\geq$ 10	> 2	Long-acting muscarinic (LAMA; aka anticholinergic) **or** long-acting β-agonist (LABA)
C	$\leq$ 49% Predicted	$\geq$ 2 (> 1 Hosp)	< 10	0-1	LAMA. *Note*: For persistent symptoms LAMA and LABA *or* LABA and inhaled steroids
D	$\leq$ 49% Predicted	$\geq$ 2 (> 1 Hosp)	$\geq$ 10	> 2	LAMA and LABA *Note*: For persistent symptoms LAMA/LABA/inhaled steroids triple combination therapy is recommended

Modified from Global Initiative for Chronic Obstructive Lung Disease (GOLD) - Global Strategy for the Diagnosis, Management and Prevention of Chronic Obstructive Pulmonary Disease - Updated 2016. Retrieved from: www.goldcopd.com.

ARDS Network Guidelines

The NBRC expects exam candidates to be familiar with selected disease-specific protocols. One of the most important of these evidence-based guidelines is the National Heart, Lung, and Blood Institute (NHLBI) ARDS Network (ARDSNet) protocol, which can be accessed in its entirety at www.ardsnet.org.

The ARDSNet protocol is based on an extensive series of research studies, including several RCTs. The use of ARDSNet guidelines has resulted in increased survival in mechanically ventilated patients with acute respiratory distress syndrome (ARDS) by maintaining adequate oxygenation and preventing or minimizing ventilator-associated lung injury. RTs and NBRC exam candidates should consider implementing this protocol for any patient who exhibits an acute onset of respiratory distress not associated with heart failure and meets the following criteria:

- P/F ratio < 300
- Bilateral diffuse infiltrates on x-ray consistent with pulmonary edema
- No clinical evidence of left atrial hypertension/left ventricular failure

Basic ventilator setup and adjustment are as follows:

1. Calculate the patient's predicted body weight (PBW).
2. Select any ventilator mode, but try to ensure an I:E $\leq$ 1:1.
3. Set initial V_T to 8 mL/kg PBW.
4. Reduce V_T by 1 mL/kg at intervals $\leq$ 2 hours until V_T = 6 mL/kg PBW.
5. Set the initial rate to approximate the baseline (generally 12 to 20) but no greater than 35/min.
6. Adjust the V_T and rate to achieve the goals for pH and plateau pressure.

To ensure adequate oxygenation, the goal is to maintain a Pao_2 between 55 and 80 torr or a Spo_2 between 88% and 95%. To achieve these targets, positive end-expiratory pressure (PEEP) levels of at least 5–8 cm H_2O should be used. Then incremental Fio_2/PEEP combinations such as those suggested in Table 14-2 can be used to achieve adequate oxygenation.

To help prevent lung injury, you should keep the plateau pressure at 30 cm H_2O or less, and measure it every 4 hours and after each change in PEEP or V_T. The following guidelines apply to adjusting P_{plat}:

- If $P_{plat} > 30$ cm H_2O, decrease V_T in 1-mL/kg steps to a minimum of 4 mL/kg.
- If $P_{plat} < 25$ cm H_2O and $V_T < 6$ mL/kg, increase V_T by 1 mL/kg until $P_{plat} > 25$ cm H_2O or $V_T = 6$ mL/kg.
- If $P_{plat} < 30$ cm H_2O and breath stacking/dyssynchrony occurs, consider increasing V_T in 1-mL/kg steps to 7–8 mL/kg if P_{plat} remains < 30 cm H_2O.

In terms of acid-base balance, the goal is to keep the pH between 7.30 and 7.45. If the pH rises above 7.45 (rare), you should decrease the ventilator rate. Otherwise, consider the following:

- If pH > 7.15 but < 7.30: increase the rate until pH > 7.30 or $Paco_2 < 25$ (maximum rate = 35/min).
- If pH < 7.15: increase the rate to 35/min.
- If rate = 35/min and pH < 7.15: increase V_T in 1-mL/kg steps until pH is greater than 7.15 (P_{plat} target may be exceeded); consider $NaHCO_3$ administration.

The NHLBI ARDS protocol follows these basic principles but uses a progressive transitioning from continuous positive airway pressure (CPAP) to pressure support (PS) to true unassisted spontaneous breathing. Details on this portion of the ARDS protocol are provided in the accompanying box (**Box 14-1**).

Box 14-1 NHLBI ARDS Protocol: Weaning Component

Criteria Indicating Readiness for a Spontaneous Breathing Trial

- $Fio_2 \leq 0.40$ and PEEP ≤ 8 cm H_2O, or $Fio_2 \leq 0.50$ and PEEP ≤ 5 cm H_2O
- PEEP and $Fio_2 \leq$ previous day's settings
- Acceptable spontaneous breathing efforts of the patient (↓vent rate by 50% for 5 minutes to detect effort)
- Systolic BP ≥ 90 mm Hg without vasopressors
- No neuromuscular blocking agents or blockade

Procedure

Initiate a spontaneous breathing trial of up to 120 minutes with $Fio_2 < 0.5$ and PEEP < 5 cm H_2O:

1. Place patient on T-piece, trach collar, or CPAP ≤ 5 cm H_2O with PS < 5 cm H_2O.
2. Assess for tolerance as follows for up to 2 hours:
   a. $Spo_2 \geq 90\%$ and $Pao_2 \geq 60$ mm Hg
   b. Spontaneous $V_T \geq 4$ mL/kg PBW
   c. Respiratory rate ≤ 35/min
   d. pH ≥ 7.30
   e. No respiratory distress (distress = 2 or more of the following)
      - HR $> 120\%$ of baseline
      - Marked accessory muscle use
      - Abdominal paradox
      - Diaphoresis
      - Marked dyspnea
3. If tolerated for at least 30 minutes, consider extubation.
4. If not tolerated, resume pre-weaning settings.

Data from National Heart, Lung, and Blood Institute, ARDS Clinical Network. Mechanical ventilation protocol summary 2008. Available at: http://www.ardsnet.org/files/ventilator_protocol_2008-07.pdf.

National Asthma Education and Prevention Program (NAEPP)

The National Asthma Education and Prevention Program (NAEPP) is a government agency that aims to address the growing problem of asthma in the United States. The NAEPP has created evidence-based guidelines to help guide the diagnosis and treatment of asthma. Because of the importance of these evidence-based guidelines, NBRC exam candidates need to be familiar with them. Extensive details on these guidelines can be accessed at https://www.nhlbi.nih.gov/health-topics/guidelines-for-diagnosis-management-of-asthma, and an excerpt from them is included in Table 14-3.

Global Initiative for Chronic Obstructive Lung Disease (GOLD) Guidelines

The Global Initiative for Chronic Obstructive Lung Disease (GOLD) was introduced in collaboration with the NHLBI, the National Institutes of Health (NIH), and the World Health Organization (WHO) to raise awareness and improve the prevention and treatment of chronic obstructive pulmonary disease (COPD) worldwide. Since its existence, GOLD has issued a series of guidelines that help shape the prevention, diagnosis, and management of COPD. Given the widespread prevalence of this disease, NBRC exam candidates should be familiar with these guidelines. The guidelines can be accessed in their entirety at www.goldcopd.com. However, it should be noted that selected criteria, including severity of airflow obstruction, exacerbations per year, COPD Assessment Test (CAT) scores (range of CAT scores from 0–40, with higher scores denoting a more severe impact of COPD on a patient's life) are used to govern the clinical management of COPD patients. Clinical management includes rehabilitation, oxygen therapy, tobacco cessation, and vaccinations, as well as pharmacologic therapy. Table 14-4 presents a key excerpt from the GOLD guidelines that shows the recommended first-line and alternative pharmacologic treatment for various categories of COPD severity.

Other Evidence-Based Sources in Respiratory Care

In addition to the sources of guidelines discussed previously, there are numerous other sources of evidence-based guidelines related to respiratory care. The most notable of these are the American Association for Respiratory Care (AARC) Clinical Practice Guidelines (CPGs), AARC Expert Panel Reference-Based Guidelines, and guidelines from similar organizations. These sources can be accessed directly at https://www.aarc.org/resources/clinical-resources/clinical-practice-guidelines/. Examples of the more recently updated and commonly used CPGs and other evidence-based guidelines available at the AARC website are listed in **Table 14-5**.

Table 14-5 Examples of Various Types of Evidence-Based Guidelines Available Through the AARC

Clinical Practice Guidelines
Effectiveness of pharmacologic airway clearance therapies in hospitalized patients (2015)
Effectiveness of nonpharmacologic airway clearance therapies in hospitalized patients (2013)
Inhaled nitric oxide for neonates with acute hypoxic respiratory failure (2010)
Expert Panel Reference-Based Guidelines
Blood gas analysis and hemoximetry (2013)
Surfactant replacement therapy (2013)
Aerosol delivery device selection for spontaneously breathing patients (2012)
Humidification during invasive and noninvasive mechanical ventilation (2012)
Guidelines from Related Organizations
American Society of Anesthesiologists (ASA) Practice Guidelines for the Management of the Difficult Airway (2013)
Cystic Fibrosis Foundation (CFF): Cystic Fibrosis Pulmonary Guidelines: Airway Clearance Therapies (2009)
Agency for Healthcare Research and Quality (AHRQ): Comparative Effectiveness Report Number 68: Noninvasive Positive-Pressure Ventilation (NPPV) for Acute Respiratory Failure (2012).

T⁴—TOP TEST-TAKING TIPS

You can improve your score in this section of the NBRC exam by following these tips:

- Remember that not all research evidence is created equally, and some types of studies support clinical practice more strongly than others.
- The strongest type of research evidence results from meta-analyses and systematic reviews, whereby the results of multiple clinical trials are combined and reported simultaneously.
- Less strong research evidence results from case-control studies, individual case studies, and expert opinion.
- Some of the more commonly used search engines for medical research include PubMed, Medline, Google Scholar, and WebMD.
- Some of the most notable and influential evidence-based guidelines include ARDSNet, the National Asthma Education and Prevention Program (NAEPP), and the GOLD COPD guidelines.
- According to ARDSNet guidelines, to help prevent lung injury, plateau pressures in mechanically ventilated patients should be kept at 30 cm H_2O or less and measured every 4 hours and after each change in PEEP or V_T.
- In accordance with ARDSNet, the criteria indicating readiness for a spontaneous breathing trial include the following: $Fio_2 \leq 0.40$ and $PEEP \leq 8$ cm H_2O, or $Fio_2 \leq 0.50$ and PEEP ≤ 5 cm H_2O; PEEP and $Fio_2 \leq$ previous day's settings; acceptable spontaneous breathing efforts; systolic $BP \geq 90$ mm Hg without vasopressors; and no neuromuscular blocking agents or blockade.
- ARDSNet guidelines indicate that if $P_{plat} > 30$ cm H_2O, decrease V_T in 1-mL/kg steps to a minimum of 4 mL/kg; if $P_{plat} < 25$ cm H_2O and $V_T < 6$ mL/kg, increase V_T by 1 mL/kg until $P_{plat} > 25$ cm H_2O or $V_T = 6$ mL/kg, and if $P_{plat} < 30$ cm H_2O and breath stacking/dyssynchrony occurs, consider increasing V_T in 1-mL/kg steps to 7–8 mL/kg if P_{plat} remains < 30 cm H_2O.
- According to the NAEPP, a stepwise approach should be used to identify appropriate medications options for asthma. As such, consider that inhaled corticosteroids (ICSs) are the most effective long-term control therapy, and each follow-up visit should include a review of medications, technique, and adherence to the prescription.
- In accordance with NAEPP recommendations, patient education for self-management should include developing a written asthma action plan, agreeing on treatment goals, and teaching patients how to use the asthma action plan.
- Quick-relief medications (e.g., SABAs) relax airway muscles to provide fast relief of symptoms. However, if used > 2 days/week (except as needed for exercise-induced asthma), the patient may need to start or increase long-term control medications.
- In concert with the Global Initiative for Chronic Obstructive Lung Disease (GOLD) Patient Category A (most stable, with $\geq$ 50% predicted spirometry and $\leq$ 1 exacerbation per year) hospitalizations), any bronchodilator can be tried as the initial inhaled medication therapy.
- For patients in GOLD Patient Category D (the least stable, with $\leq$ 49% Predicted Spirometry Classification, $\geq$ 2 exacerbations per year and at least one hospitalization, the first line of medication therapy is both a long-acting muscarinic antagonist (LAMA) and a long-acting β-agonist (LABA). However, if symptoms persist, a triple combination therapy involving a LAMA, a LABA, and inhaled steroids is recommended
- Other evidence-based guidelines include the AARC Clinical Practice Guidelines (CPGs) and AARC Expert Panel Reference-Based Guidelines.

POST-TEST

To confirm your mastery of each chapter's topical content, you should create a content post-test, available online via the Navigate Premier Access for Comprehensive Respiratory Therapy Exam Preparation Guide, which contains Navigate TestPrep (access code provided with every new text). You can create multiple topical content post-tests varying in length from 10 to 20 questions, with each attempt presenting a different set of items. You can select questions from all three major NBRC TMC sections: Patient Data, Troubleshooting and Quality Control of Devices and Infection Control, and Initiation and Modification of Interventions. A score of at least 70–80% indicates that you are adequately prepared for this section of the NBRC TMC exam. If you score below 70%, you should first carefully assess your test answers (particularly your wrong answers) and the correct answer explanations. Then return to the chapter to re-review the applicable content. Only then should you reattempt a new post-test. Repeat this process of identifying your shortcomings and reviewing the pertinent content until your test results demonstrate mastery.

CHAPTER 15

Provide Respiratory Care in High-Risk Situations (Section III-G)

Albert J. Heuer and Narciso E. Rodriguez

Respiratory therapists (RTs) play a vital role in providing timely and appropriate care in emergency settings. For this reason, the NBRC assesses your knowledge of providing emergency care on all its exams. Although only a small number of questions are involved in this area, the scope of required knowledge is extensive, demanding a significant portion of your preparation time.

OBJECTIVES

In preparing for the shared NBRC exam content (TMC/CSE), you should demonstrate the knowledge needed to provide respiratory care techniques in high-risk situations, as follows:

1. Cardiopulmonary emergencies
2. Lost or obstructed airway
3. Treating a tension pneumothorax
4. Disaster management
5. Medical emergency teams
6. Interprofessional communication
7. Patient transport
   - Intra-hospital patient transport
   - External Transport

WHAT TO EXPECT ON THIS CATEGORY OF THE NBRC EXAMS

TMC exam: 5 questions; 2 application, 3 analysis
CSE exam: indeterminate number of questions; however, section III-G knowledge is a prerequisite to succeed on the CSE, especially on Information Gathering and Decision-Making sections.

WHAT YOU NEED TO KNOW: ESSENTIAL CONTENT

Cardiopulmonary Emergencies

Basic Life Support

Basic life support (BLS) is the foundation for most emergency care. You should expect that concepts related to BLS will be included on the NBRC exams in the context of respiratory care provision. It is worth noting that the key steps in BLS now follow a **CABD** sequence, standing for *circulation–airway–breathing–defibrillation*. The NBRC exam counts on your current BLS certification to apply the knowledge needed in this area to any patient scenario requiring basic life support.

Table 15-1 outlines the key differences in BLS steps you need to be familiar with for the NBRC examinations as applied to adults, children (1 to puberty), and infants (less than one year old, excluding newborns).

Advanced Cardiac Life Support (ACLS)

In addition to know BLS, the NBRC expects that you will be able to treat cardiopulmonary collapse according to the American Heart Association (AHA) ACLS protocols.

Table 15-1 Summary of Basic Life Support (BLS)

BLS Element	Adults and Adolescents	Children (1 y/o to Puberty)	Infant (< 1 Year, Excluding Newborns)
Scene safety	Make sure the environment is safe for rescuers and victim.		
Recognition of cardiac arrest	Check for responsiveness. No breathing or only gasping (i.e., no normal breathing) No definite pulse felt within 10 seconds (Breathing and pulse check can be performed simultaneously in less than 10 seconds.)		
When to activate emergency medical services (EMS)/call a "code blue" after assessing unresponsiveness	Shout for help, activate EMS, and get a defibrillator.	*Witnessed collapse*: Follow steps for adults and adolescents on the left. *Unwitnessed collapse*: Give 2 minutes of CPR. Leave the victim to activate EMS and get an automated external defibrillator (AED). Return to the child or infant and resume CPR; use the AED as soon as it is available.	
Pulse check location	Carotid/femoral	Brachial	
Compression–ventilation ratio *without advanced airway*	*1 or 2 rescuers* 30:2	*1 rescuer* 30:2 *2 or more rescuers* 15:2	
Compression–ventilation ratio *with advanced airway*	Continuous compressions at a rate of 100–120/min		
	10 breaths/min (1 breath every 6 seconds)	12–20 breaths/min	
Compression location	2 hands on the lower half of the breastbone (sternum)	2 hands or 1 hand (optional for a very small child) on the lower half of the breastbone (sternum)	*1 rescuer* 2 fingers in the center of the chest, just below the nipple line *2 or more rescuers* 2 thumb-encircling hands in the center of the chest, just below the nipple line
Compression depth	2–2.4 inches (5–6 cm)	At least one-third the depth of chest or about 2 inches	At least one-third the depth of chest or about 1½ inches (4 cm)
Compression rate	100–120/min		
	Limit interruptions in chest compressions to less than 10 seconds.		
Chest recoil	Allow full recoil of the chest after each compression; do not lean on the chest after each compression.		
Breathing method	Lay personnel: mouth-to-mouth (barrier device if available) or hands-only CPR. Healthcare provider: bag-valve-mask ventilation and O_2 as soon as possible.	Same as adult	Same as adult

BLS Element	Adults and Adolescents	Children (1 y/o to Puberty)	Infant (< 1 Year, Excluding Newborns)
Foreign-body airway obstruction in a responsive victim	Abdominal thrusts (Heimlich maneuver)	Abdominal thrusts (Heimlich maneuver)	Alternate five back blows with five chest thrusts
Automated external defibrillator (AED) use	Yes	Yes; if child pads are not available, use adult pads.	Yes; if child pads are not available, use adult pads.
	Deliver one shock as soon as AED is available, followed immediately by 2 minutes of CPR, then reassess.		

Adult Resuscitation Protocols

The most common adult cardiopulmonary emergencies stem from one of four cardiac dysrhythmias that produce pulselessness. These rhythms include ventricular fibrillation (VF), ventricular tachycardia (VT), pulseless electrical activity (PEA), and asystole. Example electrocardiogram (ECG) tracings for VF and VT are depicted in **Figures 15-1** and **Figure 15-2**, respectively.

The ACLS algorithm for responding to adult cardiac arrest is also shown in **Figure 15-3**. For the NBRC exams, you should first be able to quickly recognize these lethal rhythms and then promptly apply the appropriate steps in the ACLS algorithm.

ACLS Drugs

ACLS also involves the use of a range of medications. NBRC exam candidates are expected to have a good general knowledge of the key emergency medications. **Table 15-2** summarizes the most

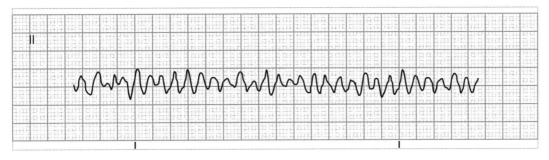

Figure 15-1 Example of Ventricular Fibrillation (VF).

Reproduced from Garcia T, Miller GT. *Arrhythmia Recognition: The Art of Interpretation.* Sudbury, MA: Jones and Bartlett Publishers; 2004.

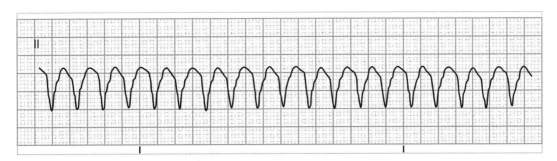

Figure 15-2 Example of Ventricular Tachycardia (VT).

Reproduced from Garcia T, Miller GT. *Arrhythmia Recognition: The Art of Interpretation.* Sudbury, MA: Jones and Bartlett Publishers; 2004.

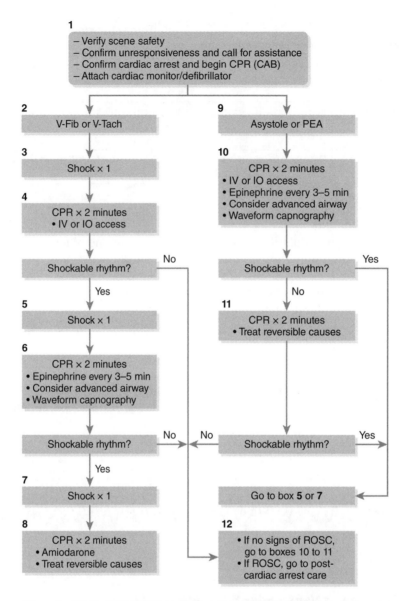

Figure 15-3 ACLS Algorithm for Adult Cardiac Arrest.

Table 15-2 ACLS Medication Summary

Medication	Initial Adult IV Dosage	Classification/Indication
Epinephrine*	1 mg every 3–5 minutes with flush	Vasoconstrictor; may improve cerebral perfusion
Atropine*	0.5 mg every 3–5 minutes, up to a maximum of 3 mg/kg	Cardiac stimulant (anticholinergic) used for selected bradycardias
Amiodarone (Cordarone)	300 mg rapid infusion followed by 150 mg in 3–5 minutes and every 10 minutes, up to 2.2 g/day	Antiarrhythmic for ventricular fibrillation (VF) and ventricular tachycardia (VT)
Lidocaine*	Initial dose of 1.0–1.5 mg/kg, with additional doses of 0.5–0.75 mg/kg every 5–10 minutes, up to 3 mg/kg	Antiarrhythmic for VF and VT, primarily as an alternative to amiodarone

*Denotes a medication that may be instilled via endotracheal tube (ETT) if IV or IO access is not established. In such cases, it is recommended that the dose be doubled and that it be followed with the instillation of 10 mL normal saline.

Table 15-3 Defibrillation Doses for Shockable Rhythms

Patient	Initial Dose*	Subsequent Doses
Adult	120–200 J or as recommended by the manufacturer	Same as initial dose (higher energy levels may be considered)
Child	2 J/kg	At least 4 J/kg (higher energy levels may be considered)
*The indicated doses are for biphasic defibrillators. For older monophasic devices, apply an initial dose of 360 J to adults and 2 J/kg to children.		

common ACLS drugs administered to adults. In the absence of intravenous (IV) or intraosseous (IO) access, some medications may be instilled through an endotracheal tube (ETT), as noted in the table.

Equipment

To succeed in this section of the NBRC exams, you should be familiar with the key equipment used in emergencies, including resuscitation devices and artificial airways. You also will be expected to know how to apply both AEDs and standard defibrillators properly. This knowledge includes selecting the initial and subsequent defibrillator energy levels or doses to apply to both adult and pediatric patients with shockable rhythms (VF and pulseless or polymorphic VT), as outlined in **Table 15-3**.

Monitoring and Assessment

You are expected to know the major ways in which a patient should be assessed during and following CPR (post-cardiac arrest care) or after return of spontaneous circulation (ROSC), as well as the quality of the ongoing resuscitation effort. This may range from assessing *chest rise* and *signs of circulation* to periodic pulse and breathing checks, generally after five cycles of CPR, to more advanced assessment methods, including electrocardiography, pulse oximetry, arterial blood gas monitoring, intra-arterial blood pressure measurement (if available), and capnography.

Candidates should note that, when available, *capnography is now recommended as a standard of care during resuscitation efforts* due to its ability to assess both the adequacy of ventilation and the effectiveness of cardiac compressions. More specifically, if the $Petco_2$ is less than 10 mm Hg (torr) and intra-arterial diastolic pressure is less than 20 mm Hg, the quality of CPR should be improved. Failure to achieve a $Petco_2$ greater than 10 mm Hg after 20 minutes of CPR can be used as an indicator to terminate resuscitative efforts.

The ongoing CPR assessment must include looking for possible reversible causes of the arrest. Some of them can be remembered as the "5 Hs" and "5 Ts" of CPR assessment, as follows:

- 5 Hs:
  - Hypovolemia
  - Hypoxia
  - Hydrogen ion (acidosis)
  - Hypo-/hyperkalemia
  - Hypothermia
- 5 Ts:
  - Tension pneumothorax
  - Tamponade (cardiac)
  - Toxins (drug overdose, anaphylactic reactions)
  - Thrombosis, pulmonary (pulmonary emboli)
  - Thrombosis, cardiac (myocardial infarction or ischemia)

Pediatric and Neonatal Emergencies

Variations of BLS techniques for children and infants are detailed in Table 15-1. When treating children, the NBRC will expect that you can follow the key pediatric advanced life support (PALS) and neonatal resuscitation protocols.

Pediatric Resuscitation

The most likely NBRC exam scenarios involving PALS are those for pulseless arrest. As depicted in **Figure 15-4**, the PALS algorithm for pulseless arrest is similar to the algorithm for adults, with the exception that the defibrillation shock and medication dosages vary by patient weight. One of the most common medical emergencies associated with pediatric patients is airway obstruction by a foreign body; consequently, you should be familiar with practices for responding to obstructed airways in both conscious and unconscious pediatric patients (see Table 15-1).

Neonatal Resuscitation

In addition to pediatric resuscitation, you must be familiar with the resuscitation protocol for neonates, as shown in **Figure 15-5** since it may be applicable to neonatal scenarios on the CSE. Babies who are flaccid, cyanotic, or apneic in the delivery room usually require stimulation and supplemental O_2. For preterm newborns < 35 weeks of gestation, low O_2 (21–30%) should be used and titrated to achieve preductal Spo_2 ranges according to **Table 15-4**. These Spo_2 ranges can also be used in the

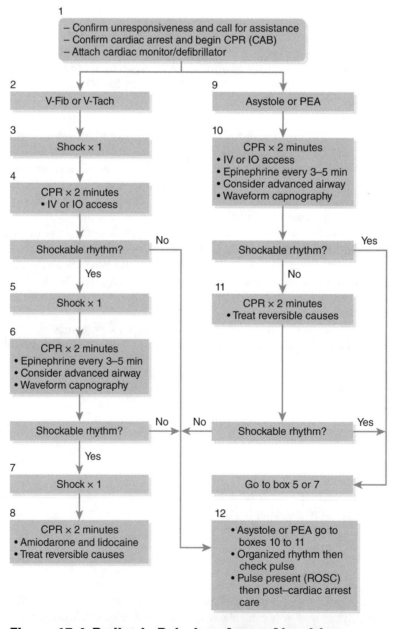

Figure 15-4 Pediatric Pulseless Arrest Algorithm.

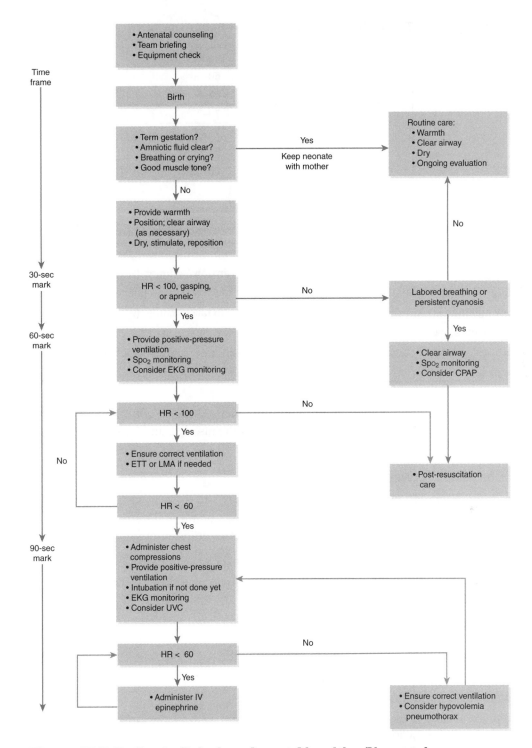

Figure 15-5 Pediatric Pulseless Arrest Algorithm/Neonatal Resuscitation Algorithm.

labor and delivery room to screen all newborns for the presence of critical congenital heart defects. A pre-/postductal Sp_{O_2} comparison must be done.

If color, heart rate, and breathing are not restored within 30 seconds after birth, you should provide manual positive-pressure ventilation (PPV) via face mask. PPV is *the most effective intervention* done in the delivery room to help improve outcomes during neonatal resuscitation. PPV can be effectively delivered with a flow-inflating bag, self-inflating bag, or T-piece resuscitator. A positive end-expiratory pressure (PEEP) of 5 cm H_2O or less is always recommended.

Table 15-4 Targeted Preductal Spo$_2$ After Birth

Time (min)	Targeted Spo$_2$
1	60–65%
2	65–70%
3	70–75%
4	75–80%
5	80–85%
10	85–95%

Table 15-5 Features of Partial and Complete Airway Obstruction

Partial Airway Obstruction	Complete Airway Obstruction
• Some air movement	• Absence of air movement/breath sounds
• Sonorous breathing, stridor, or wheezing	• Severe anxiety/agitation (while conscious)
• Choking, drooling, or gagging	• Universal choking sign (while conscious)
• Anxiety/agitation	• Inability to talk or cough (while conscious)
• Accessory muscle use	• Accessory muscle use
• Retractions/paradoxical breathing	• Retractions/paradoxical breathing
• Lethargy if persistent	• Eventual lethargy, cyanosis, unconsciousness

A heart rate of less than 60 always requires chest compressions in a neonate. If the infant does not respond to these measures, epinephrine should be administered, and intubation and mechanical ventilation considered.

Lost or Obstructed Airway

An airway emergency exists when a patent airway is lost (e.g., due to obstruction or extubation/decannulation) or attempts to provide a patent airway and assure gas exchange are difficult or fail. Airway obstruction can occur in a patient with or without an artificial tracheal airway. In either case, the obstruction can be partial or complete, with partial obstruction sometimes progressing to a complete interruption of airflow. It is essential that RTs be able to differentiate partial from complete airway obstruction and act accordingly. **Table 15-5** lists the main features that differentiate partial and complete airway obstruction.

Loss of Airway Due to Anatomic Obstruction

Table 15-6 lists the most common types of anatomic airway obstruction, their likely clinical signs, and available corrective actions.

Obstruction of Artificial Airways

Artificial tracheal airways include both oral/nasal ETTs and tracheostomy tubes. The primary causes of tracheal airway obstruction are as follows:

- Kinking of the tube
- Patient biting down on the tube (ETTs only)
- Malpositioning of the tube tip against the tracheal wall (mainly trach tubes)
- Inspissated secretions, mucus, or blood clots plugging the tube lumen
- Herniation of the cuff, causing occlusion of the tube tip (rare)
- Compression of the tube due to cuff overinflation (rare; mainly silicone ETTs)

If a patient is receiving mechanical ventilation when the obstruction occurs, the first step is always to remove the patient from the ventilator, provide manual ventilation with 100% O$_2$, and reassess the situation. If immediately available, an attempt should be made by a trained clinician to

Table 15-6 Types of Airway Obstruction, Signs, and Corrective Actions

Type of Anatomic Obstruction	Common Clinical Signs	Corrective Actions
Malpositioning of the head and neck	• Sonorous breathing • Inability to ventilate • Mask leakage with manual ventilation	• Reposition head and neck • Exaggerated jaw lift • Two-handed mask application (assistance of a second operator)
Unconsciousness/loss of upper airway muscle tone	• Sonorous breathing • Inability to ventilate • Mask leakage with manual ventilation	• Reposition head and neck • Insert pharyngeal airway • Exaggerated jaw lift • Two-handed mask application (assistance of a second operator)
Vomit, blood, or secretions in the airway	• Gurgling • Visible vomit, blood, or secretions	• Position patient sideways • Aspiration/suctioning • Empty stomach contents
Foreign-body obstruction	• Respiratory distress • Inability to ventilate • Coughing, gagging, stridor, or wheezing • Failure of the patient to make a sound • Patient making the "choking sign"	• Conscious adult or child: Heimlich maneuver • Unconscious adult or child: abdominal thrusts • Infant: Repeated cycles of five back blows and five chest compressions • Laryngoscopic/bronchoscopic removal
Laryngeal obstruction (e.g., laryngospasm, anaphylaxis, vocal cord paralysis, tumors)	• Respiratory distress • Stridor • Inability to ventilate • Increased inspiratory efforts • Paradoxical chest or abdominal movements • Hypoxemia, cyanosis	• IV steroids (e.g., prednisolone) • Epinephrine (including by aerosol) • Supplemental O_2 • Heliox therapy • Intubation • Percutaneous airway insertion • Surgery (paralysis, tumors)
Trauma (e.g., blunt trauma to larynx, mandible, burns, retropharyngeal hematoma)	• Respiratory distress • Stridor • Inability to ventilate • Increased inspiratory efforts • Hypoxemia, cyanosis	• Intubation • Tracheotomy • Therapeutic bronchoscopy • Surgery
Infection (e.g., diphtheria, epiglottitis, croup, retropharyngeal abscess)	• Respiratory distress • Stridor • Barking cough • Inability to ventilate • Labored breathing	• Supplemental O_2 • Cool mist aerosol • Intubation in a controlled environment (e.g., operating room) • Cricothyrotomy/tracheotomy • Treatment of underlying infection

insert a ventilating airway exchange catheter (tube exchanger) through the obstructed tube before removing it. This may help clear an internal obstruction and—if it can be passed into the trachea—aid in providing oxygenation and assist in reestablishing the airway. If you remove a tracheal airway without a ventilating airway exchange catheter in place, you should first try to restore ventilation and oxygenation using a bag and face mask. For trach patients, you may need to close off the stoma with a petroleum jelly gauze pad while ventilating through the upper airway.

Loss of Airway Due to Accidental Extubation (ETT) or Decannulation (Trach Tube)

Accidental extubation or decannulation can occur even with proper attention to these measures. It can be partial or complete. Because partial ETT extubation can mimic a blown cuff, the first step is to rule out a large cuff leak by quickly assessing the integrity of the balloon cuff and pilot tube and valve adaptor. If partial extubation of an ETT occurs, you should deflate the cuff, loosen the securing device, and try to reposition the tube back into the trachea. After repositioning the tube, you should check placement via auscultation, capnography, CO_2 colorimetry, and use of an esophageal detection device or endoscope, followed by a confirming chest x-ray. If this does not reestablish the airway, you will need to remove the ETT, provide bag-mask ventilation with O_2, and then consider insertion of a subglottic airway or reintubation.

If accidental extubation occurs in a patient with a trach whose trach is fresh, take the following steps:

- Call for help.
- Occlude the stoma with a sterile petroleum jelly gauze pad.
- Provide bag-mask ventilation with oxygen as needed.

In the NBRC hospital, if the stoma is well established and the patient is stable, you are expected to obtain a sterile tube of the same size or one size smaller and follow the procedure for changing trach tubes.

Difficulty in Providing a Patent Airway

A difficult airway occurs when a properly trained clinician cannot effectively ventilate a patient with a bag-valve-mask (BVM) and experiences difficulty with supraglottic airway placement or endotracheal intubation. **Table 15-7** summarizes appropriate ways of responding to a difficult airway.

Table 15-7 Responding to Difficult Airways

Difficulty With	Common Response Options
Bag-valve-mask (BVM) ventilation	• Reposition head and neck (use a neck roll if necessary) • Reposition mask • Insert pharyngeal airway • Apply exaggerated jaw lift • Have a second operator use a secure mask with two hands • Release of cricoid pressure
Supraglottic airway placement (e.g., laryngeal mask airway [LMA], King laryngeal tube [LT], Combitube)	• Assure adequate sedation • Check/confirm proper position • Check/confirm proper cuff inflation • Remove/reinsert the device (fully deflate cuff) • Place a larger/smaller device
Endotracheal intubation	• Increase head lift (lower neck flexion, head extension)* • Apply external laryngeal pressure • Use longer/shorter blade if indicated • Use tracheal tube introducer (aka "gum elastic bougie") • Use lighted stylet • Use intubating LMA ("Fastrach") • Use optical/video-assisted laryngoscopy • Use fiber-optic-guided intubation • Consider recommending rapid-sequence intubation (RSI), including premedication with moderate sedation and paralyzing agents

*Unless contraindicated (e.g., cervical spine injury).

Failed Intubation

A failed intubation occurs when the ETT cannot be inserted through the vocal cords and positioned correctly in the trachea after several attempts; *irrespective of the technique or specialized equipment used* (some sources equate failure with three unsuccessful attempts). Manifestations of a failed intubation include one or more of the following:

- Absent breath sounds
- Abdominal distention with epigastric sounds during BVM ventilation
- Lack of exhaled CO_2 (capnography or colorimetry)
- Difficulty delivering manual breaths
- Rapid decrease in SpO_2
- Deterioration in clinical status
- Stomach contents are seen on the artificial airway

It is more likely that acceptable oxygen saturation levels can be maintained if supplemental oxygen is supplied via a nasal cannula during intubation attempts. Following any failed intubation attempt, patients should be ventilated via BVM ventilation with 100% O_2. Subsequent action depends on whether or not adequate oxygenation can be maintained via BVM ventilation ($SpO_2 > 90\%$). If so, two additional attempts can be considered by the clinician who is most highly trained and experienced in intubation, and preference should be given to using the rapid sequence intubation (RSI) method. On the other hand, if the SpO_2 is $< 90\%$ and/or falling—the "cannot intubate, cannot oxygenate" (CICO) scenario should be applied, a supraglottic airway (e.g., laryngeal mask airway [LMA], King laryngeal tube [LT], Combitube) should be inserted immediately, and bag-valve ventilation reinstituted. If either pathway fails to restore satisfactory ventilation and oxygenation, the only alternative is to establish an emergency percutaneous airway (percutaneous emergency tracheostomy).

Treating a Tension Pneumothorax

A pneumothorax occurs when a tear or rupture in lung tissue permits air to escape into the pleural space, or a loss of pleural space integrity is caused by a traumatic event to the chest wall (e.g., motor vehicle accident, rib fracture, stab wound to the chest). A simple pneumothorax may occur spontaneously (e.g., during vigorous coughing) and can eventually resolve without treatment. A *tension* pneumothorax, in contrast, occurs when a large amount of air under pressure enters the pleural space. This condition is even more serious for patients receiving positive-pressure ventilation, which invariably causes a rapid buildup of pleural pressure, which compresses the heart, lungs, and great vessels, causing cardiovascular collapse. Patients experiencing a tension pneumothorax can deteriorate quite rapidly. For this reason, prompt detection and treatment are essential.

Factors that may predispose patients to a tension pneumothorax include mechanical ventilation with high airway pressures (more than 40–45 cm H_2O), chest trauma, and conditions associated with excessively high lung compliance, such as advanced emphysema (blebs, bullae). When any of these factors are coupled with a rapid decline in clinical status, you should consider the possibility of a tension pneumothorax. Although such a diagnosis is generally confirmed via a chest x-ray, you should be mindful of the following clinical manifestations:

- Rapid decline in cardiopulmonary status (hypotension, hypoxemia, increased work of breathing [WOB])
- Decreased or absent breath sounds on the affected side
- Hyperresonance to the percussion of the affected side
- Tracheal shift *away* from the affected side (severe cases)
- Rapid increase in peak and plateau pressures during volume control ventilation
- Rapid decrease in delivered volume during pressure control ventilation
- Shock or pulseless electrical activity (PEA) (severe, untreated cases)

A chest x-ray confirming the diagnosis of a tension pneumothorax will typically show hyperlucency (darkness) in the pleural space and a collapsed lung, flattening of the diaphragm, and widening of the rib spaces—all on the affected side. Also, the mediastinum typically shifts to the *opposite* side.

Box 15-1 Basic Procedure for Needle Thoracostomy

1. Place the patient in an upright position, if tolerated.
2. Locate puncture site (second intercostal space in the midclavicular line).
3. Prepare site with betadine and alcohol scrubs.
4. Insert angiocath over the top of the third rib until the catheter hub is against the chest wall.
5. Listen for a rush of air, and observe the patient's cardiorespiratory status.
6. Remove the needle, secure the angiocath, and attach a flutter valve (Heimlich valve).
7. Immediately prepare for tube thoracostomy (chest tube insertion).

Once a tension pneumothorax is confirmed, the treatment is emergency decompression of the chest via *needle thoracostomy*. As outlined in the accompanying box (**Box 15-1**), needle thoracostomy involves the insertion of a large-bore angiocath (14 gauge for adults, 18 or 20 gauge for infants) into the second intercostal space over the top of the third rib in the midclavicular line. Because needle thoracostomy converts a tension pneumothorax into a simple pneumothorax, full resolution of the problem usually requires the insertion of a conventional chest tube, as discussed in Chapter 16.

Disaster Management

NBRC exams can contain questions on the broad topic of disaster management and response. The NBRC is most likely to focus on hospital and respiratory care department preparedness for meeting the surge-capacity needs associated with mass-casualty events, as well as the implementation of triage and decontamination/isolation procedures.

In terms of preparedness, all healthcare facilities are expected to have disaster management plans in place. For most hospitals, this means being able to triple their capacity to support critically ill/injured patients for at least 10 days without external assistance. Additionally, hospitals need to plan for how the facility itself can manage direct damage or loss of resources, as might occur during natural catastrophes such as floods or earthquakes or as the result of hostile actions.

For the respiratory care department, preparedness planning involves consideration of at least the following elements:

- Estimating the number of surge patients who may require the following:
  - Ventilatory support
  - Medical gas therapy (O_2 or air)
  - Suction (vacuum)
- Assessing personnel needs and resources
  - Number of staff members needed to meet patient needs during the surge
  - Call-back procedures to obtain additional staff
  - Plan to augment staffing with nonrespiratory personnel
- Planning for equipment needs
  - Inventory and plan for using *all* available ventilators that could support the critically ill/injured (including anesthesia, transport, magnetic resonance imaging [MRI], and noninvasive positive-pressure ventilation [NPPV] ventilators)
  - Mechanism to acquire additional ventilators (e.g., from vendors, other hospitals, or the Strategic National Stockpile)
  - Plan to temporarily support and transfer patients if backup equipment unavailable (e.g., using manual resuscitators)
  - Plan to address the failure of the gas supply system, including the deployment of backup gas sources

In terms of the ventilator equipment to meet surge capacity, these devices ideally should meet the following conditions:

1. Be able to support pediatric and adult patients with either significant airflow obstruction or acute respiratory distress syndrome (ARDS);
2. Function *without* high-pressure medical gas (use low-flow O_2 to regulate Fio_2);

3. Provide adjustable volume control with V_T range of 250 to 750 mL;

4. Provide adjustable rate range of 8 to 25 per minute;

5. Provide adjustable PEEP range of 0 to 15 cm H_2O;

6. Monitor peak inspiratory pressure (PIP) and V_T;

7. Have alarms for apnea, circuit disconnect, low gas source, low battery, and high peak airway pressure; and

8. Have a battery life of at least 4 hours.

Although anesthesia, transport, MRI, and NPPV ventilators may not meet all of these expectations, they can and should be enlisted for use until more capable equipment is available.

Regarding increasing staffing, nonrespiratory personnel could be assigned to assist with selected respiratory procedures such as suctioning or vital signs/SpO_2 monitoring (e.g., emergency medical technicians [EMTs] if available) or aerosol drug therapy (e.g., physical therapists). Evidence indicates that just-in-time training for such personnel is enough to allow them to perform these duties safely.

Based on the departmental plan and likely use of facilities other than the intensive care unit (ICU) to support a patient surge, RTs should additionally be prepared to perform the following tasks:

- Transport critically ill patients within and outside the facility
- Support increased medical emergency team activity, especially on units "converted" to ICUs
- Assist in discharge/transfer of noncritically ill ICU patients
- Supervise general respiratory care provided by nonrespiratory personnel
- Obtain and put in use in-house anesthesia, transport, MRI, and NPPV ventilators
- Be prepared to receive ventilators from the Strategic National Stockpile
- Direct logistic resupply for ventilators, oxygen, and other respiratory support equipment

As outlined in **Table 15-8**, the specific role of RTs in responding to disasters also varies somewhat depending on the type of event.

Due to the large number and variable type of casualties that may present to a healthcare facility after a disaster, rapid triage is essential. Personnel assigned to triage responsibilities must evaluate each patient and quickly prioritize the various patients' management, using a scheme like that outlined in **Table 15-9**. If the disaster involves a suspected chemical, biological, radiological, or nuclear (CBRN) incident, triage takes place *outside the facility* and is conducted in conjunction with decontamination.

Table 15-8 Role of the Respiratory Therapist in Disaster Response

Category	Resulting Patient Conditions	Respiratory Therapist Roles (in Addition to Patient Monitoring)
Natural catastrophe (e.g., earthquake, flood, fire, tornado)	Trauma (chest/head), near-drowning, thermal burns, hypovolemic or septic shock, dehydration	Initial assessment/triage, infection control, cleaning, disinfection, sterilization, barrier and isolation, personal protective equipment (PPE)
Chemical (e.g., chlorine gas)	Inhalation injury, ventilatory/oxygenation respiratory failure, chemical burns, pneumonia, sepsis, acute respiratory distress syndrome (ARDS)	Prompt recognition and initial assessment, triage and decontamination, airway management, ventilation and oxygenation, common antidote therapy (e.g., atropine for nerve agents)
Biological—natural (e.g., severe acute respiratory syndrome [SARS]) or bio-terrorism (e.g., anthrax)	Inhalation injury, ventilatory/oxygenation respiratory failure, pneumonia, sepsis, ARDS	Prompt recognition and initial assessment, triage, airway management, ventilation and oxygenation, infection control, isolation techniques, antimicrobial therapy
Radiological/nuclear	Trauma, blast injuries, profound thermal burns, inhalation injury, radiation poisoning, dehydration	Prompt recognition and initial assessment, triage, and decontamination, airway management, ventilation and oxygenation, isolation and barrier techniques specific to ionizing radiation

Table 15-9 Disaster Triage Priorities

Triage Priority	Description	Action (After Decontamination if CBRN Incident)
Green/minor	Patients with minor injuries who can wait for appropriate treatment; the "walking wounded"	Move to waiting area or discharge
Yellow/delayed	Patients with potentially serious injuries, but whose status is not expected to deteriorate significantly over several hours	Move to the emergency department (ED)
Red/immediate	Patients with life-threatening but treatable injuries requiring rapid medical attention (within 60 minutes); includes compromise to the patient's airway, breathing, or circulation	Move to ED or intensive care unit (ICU) or converted tertiary care area
Black/expectant	Deceased patients or victims who are unlikely to survive given the severity of their injuries, level of available care, or both; palliative care and pain relief should be provided	Leave in receiving area or (if deceased) move to the morgue

---

Box 15-2 Criteria for Excluding Patients from Critical Care When Surge Capacity Is Exhausted (Any One)

- SOFA score indicating a mortality risk of 80% or greater
- Multiple-organ failure
- Severe acute disorder with a low probability of survival (e.g., severe trauma or burns)
- Cardiac arrest (unwitnessed or witnessed but not responsive to electrical therapy)
- Advanced untreatable neuromuscular disease
- Metastatic malignant disease
- Advanced and irreversible neurologic event or condition
- End-stage organ failure
  - New York Heart Association Class III or IV heart failure
  - Stage IV COPD (FEV1 < 30% predicted, dyspnea at rest)
- Severe baseline cognitive impairment
- Age of 85 years or older

If the surge of patients needing critical care (triage category "red/immediate") exceeds the capacity of the facility, care expectation may need to be modified. Under extreme surge conditions, critical care support may be limited to the provision of mechanical ventilation, IV fluid resuscitation, vasopressor administration, specific antidote or antimicrobial administration, and sedation and analgesia.

In addition, if the surge capacity is exhausted, some patients may need to be excluded from receiving even this basic level of critical care or even withdrawn from support. The primary criterion used to make these judgments is the patient's risk of death, with the tool most commonly employed for this purpose being the Sequential Organ Failure Assessment (SOFA) score. A patient's SOFA score combines measures of the P/F ratio, platelet count, bilirubin level, creatinine level, or urine output, severity of hypotension, and Glasgow Coma Scale score. A computed SOFA score indicating a mortality risk of 80% or greater is often the primary basis for excluding patients under extreme surge conditions from receiving critical care. Other exclusion criteria that may be considered are summarized in the accompanying box (**Box 15-2**).

For mass-casualty events, triage, decontamination, and treatment usually proceed in sequence through specific "zones," each requiring a different level of PPE for healthcare personnel. Given its potentially high risk of hazardous contamination, the initial triage area is termed the "hot zone," in which self-contained breathing apparatus (SCBA) approved by the National Institute for Occupational Safety and Health (NIOSH) should be employed. Decontamination occurs in the "warm zone," where

NIOSH-approved hooded powered air-purifying respirators (PAPRs) with FR57 filters are recommended. All respiratory therapy departments should have protocols in place for providing respiratory support to patients in the warm zone. After decontamination, patients are received in the treatment area, where standard PPE precautions are generally satisfactory.

In terms of managing large outbreaks of respiratory infections, the following considerations apply:

1. All persons with signs or symptoms of a respiratory infection (e.g., cough, labored breathing) should be instructed to maintain good respiratory hygiene/cough etiquette:
    a. Cover the nose and mouth when coughing or sneezing.
    b. Use tissues to contain respiratory secretions.
    c. Dispose of tissues in the nearest waste receptacle after use.
    d. Wash hands after contact with respiratory secretions and contaminated objects and materials.
2. Healthcare facilities should ensure that tissues, hands-free receptacles, and hand-hygiene facilities are provided to patients and visitors.
3. Healthcare facilities should offer surgical masks to persons who are coughing and encourage them to sit at least 3 feet away from others.
4. Healthcare workers should practice droplet precautions, in addition to standard precautions, when examining a patient with symptoms of a respiratory infection.
5. Once a likely infectious agent is suspected, appropriate infection control measures need to be activated:
    a. Placement of the patient in a negative-pressure isolation room (where available)
    b. Use of standard, contact, and droplet precautions
    c. Use of airborne precautions (including N95 respirators for all persons entering the room)
    d. Restriction of patient movement (and use of a surgical mask for transport)
    e. Avoiding droplet-producing procedures (e.g., nebulizers, chest physiotherapy, bronchoscopy)

Medical Emergency Teams

Today, most hospitals have established medical emergency teams (METs), also known as rapid-response teams (RRTs). Their purpose is to intervene and help stabilize patients who are rapidly deteriorating outside of the ICU setting. The team is often composed of an ICU nurse, a physician or physician assistant, and a respiratory therapist.

The MET is generally activated when a patient exhibits signs and symptoms of clinical deterioration before cardiopulmonary arrest. For adults, the specific criteria for doing so often include one or more of the following:

- Acute change in mental status or overall clinical appearance
- Heart rate < 40 or > 130, or respiratory rate < 8/min or > 30/min
- Systolic blood pressure < 90 mm Hg
- SpO_2 < 90%, especially with supplemental O_2
- Acute change in urinary output to less than 50 mL over 4 hours

The most common MET interventions performed or assisted by RTs include suctioning, adjusting the FiO_2, providing noninvasive ventilation, administering bronchodilators, arterial blood gas monitoring, and intubation. Depending on the outcome, the RT may assist during the transport of the patient to the ICU or different medical unit for further monitoring. Once the MET has responded, details of the event should be recorded in the patient's medical record.

Interprofessional Communication

One of the most effective ways to optimize patient care, especially in high-risk situations, is to ensure effective interprofessional communication. This type of communication occurs when clinicians from various disciplines, such as physicians, nurses, respiratory therapists, pharmacists, dietitians, physical therapists, and others interact, generally with the ultimate goal of enhancing patient care by minimizing hazards and risks. Interprofessional communication can occur in many forms, including the following:

- Bedside rounds
- Care planning meetings
- When executing specialized diagnostic or therapeutic interventions to reduce patient risk (e.g., pre-procedure time-out)
- Formulating and revising multidisciplinary protocols/procedures
- Interprofessional educational sessions
- Specialty consult requests

Regardless of the specific form, interprofessional communication can be most effective when it has the following features:

- Proactive—Based on a thorough and ongoing review of the patient's record, a care plan should be put in place and revised as needed based on collective input from various key disciplines.
- Documented—Though much interprofessional communication initially occurs verbally, it should be promptly and accurately documented in the patient record to be available for review by members of the patient care team.
- Secure and Confidential—Any form of oral or written communication that involves patient data should be protected so as not to breach confidentiality. This includes not mentioning patient information with bystanders nearby and ensuring written interprofessional documentation is kept away from laypersons and is maintained on a password-protected, secure electronic health record platform.
- Structured—Although some interprofessional communication occurs on an as-needed basis, communications involving patient care planning should occur at designated times, such as morning rounds, to encourage active participation by each discipline.
- Closed-Loop—When verbally communicating key information, such as observations made during a resuscitative effort, the clinician receiving such information should clearly repeat what was said back to the sender, who should then verify what was said is correct.
- Appropriate Use of Digital Communication Technology – The use of secure electronic communication platforms and approved digital devices should be considered, especially for pre-scheduled sessions (e.g., patient care planning) to maximize the number of disciplines who can actively participate.
- Fast-Track for Reporting Critical Values and Key Clinical Data – There should be one or more mechanisms for immediately flagging and reporting critical data among appropriate members of the patient care team. This includes lab results (e.g., ABG results), chest x-rays, oxygenation status, or other markers that have abruptly deteriorated or are substantially abnormal.

Patient Transport

The NBRC expects you to be competent in transporting critically ill patients, both within the hospital complex and externally via land or air transport. Related concepts covered elsewhere in this text, including airway management and O_2 cylinder duration of flow, may be included in this portion of the exams.

Intra-Hospital Patient Transport

Most transports take place within a hospital or healthcare facility. It has been determined that a disproportionate number of adverse events occur during patient transport. Most common adverse events include the following:

- Artificial airway dislodgment
- Equipment or battery failure
- Neck or spine destabilization
- Hypoxemia
- Cardiovascular instability

To help avoid some of these problems, the first step in planning for transport is to assess whether the patient is stable enough to be moved. This assessment should include vital signs, hemodynamic parameters, oxygenation, ventilation, and any other relevant clinical indicators associated with patient stability. According to the AARC, a patient should not be moved if any of the following cannot be reasonably ensured during transport:

- Provision of adequate oxygenation and ventilation
- Maintenance of acceptable hemodynamic performance
- Adequate monitoring of the patient's cardiopulmonary status
- Maintenance of airway control

In most cases, critically ill patients are transported by a team consisting of a critical care nurse and, at a minimum, either an ACLS-trained RT or a physician. The transport team should communicate in advance with the receiving team or department to confirm readiness to receive the patient, including any specialized equipment needed at the receiving site or unit. As with all patient interventions, the transport should be well documented in the record, to include the physician's order and patient status throughout the transition period.

The minimum monitoring needed during transport consists of heart and respiratory rate monitoring, ECG monitoring, pulse oximetry, and noninvasive blood pressure monitoring (all usually provided via a portable multichannel monitor). Body temperature should be monitored in those patients at risk for hypothermia. Invasive blood pressure monitoring is recommended for patients already having an arterial line in place who are under treatment with vasoactive drugs or who are hemodynamically unstable. Intracranial pressure (ICP) should continue to be monitored during transport of neurology patients with an ICP catheter in place. In addition, capnography is recommended when transporting all mechanically ventilated patients, but it is especially important in those patients for whom a specific P_{CO_2} range is being targeted, such as those with head/brain trauma.

Basic support equipment includes a drug kit (e.g., IV supplies, ACLS drugs, sedatives, analgesics), an O_2 source with sufficient duration of flow (plus a 30-minute reserve), and a fully charged battery-operated infusion pump and defibrillator (often incorporated into the portable monitor).

It should be noted that oxygen tanks must be secured appropriately in designated tank holders and should never be placed on top of stretchers and beds during transport. Additional equipment needed to transport patients with artificial airways requiring mechanical ventilation includes a transport ventilator with backup manual resuscitator with PEEP valve and mask (in case the artificial airways becomes dislodged), an intubation kit, and a battery-powered suction pump with suction supplies.

During the transport of critically ill pediatric patients, a complete kit comprising resuscitation equipment and drugs for children must accompany the patient, particularly a self-inflating bag, a face mask, and an intubation kit adapted to the age of the child, as well as an intraosseous catheterization kit. For intubated children weighing less than 15 kg (33 lb), the transport ventilator must be certified for pediatric use and be able to accurately deliver the smaller tidal volumes and higher rates required by these patients.

Ideally, the ventilator used for transport should be a high-performance portable device capable of delivering the same level and type of support as that provided to the patient in the ICU. If possible, simple single-limb circuits with a high-efficiency particulate air (HEPA) filter and heat and moisture exchanger for humidification should be used. You should determine if the patient requires a function that available portable ventilators cannot provide and look for alternative solutions *before actual transport*. Patients receiving NPPV should continue to be supported in this mode with a high-performance portable NPPV device. Whether designed for invasive or noninvasive use, the portable ventilator's interface should not allow for any accidental changes to the settings. Parameters that must be monitored include airway pressures (PIP, PEEP) and expired V_T, with mandatory alarms for high pressure, patient disconnection, interruption of the gas or electricity supply, battery status, and ventilator failure.

Basic quality assurance demands that all equipment be checked for proper operation before transport. The electrical supply and recharging capabilities of all electrically powered devices (monitor, infusion and suction pumps, ventilator) must be compatible with use at all times, with sufficient battery power for the full duration of the transport. To confirm proper operation and patient tolerance, the transport ventilator should be connected to the patient 5–10 minutes before leaving.

After confirming the equipment operation, the patient should be prepared for transport. Key aspects of patient preparation that the RT should address include the following:

- Before transport, document the patient's respiratory status and ventilator settings in the record (a transport form may be used for this purpose).
- Check and confirm all connections between the equipment and the patient before beginning transport.
- Place the patient in the same position as that maintained in the ICU.
- Verify the ETT placement and cuff pressure before (and after) transport.
- If the ETT was recently inserted, confirm proper tube position (chest x-ray) and secure appropriately before transport.
- For patients requiring strict control of $Paco_2$, obtain an arterial sample before transport and record the $Paco_2$–$Petco_2$ gradient.

During transport, each time the patient is mobilized, you should conduct a thorough verification of all equipment–patient connections. Should any problems with the patient–ventilator interface arise, you should immediately switch to manual ventilation with 100% O_2 and (if required) PEEP.

There are also special circumstances that relate to the internal transport of mechanically ventilated patients. One such situation is when the patient is being transported to receive an MRI test. In such cases, only equipment deemed "MRI safe" should be used—most notably, MRI-compatible ventilator and nonferrous metal oxygen cylinders, connections, and other respiratory equipment and supplies.

Another special situation is when transporting a mechanically ventilated patient to a hyperbaric chamber. In these situations, it is generally necessary to adjust the tidal volumes to account for the effects of Boyle's law and ensure adequate ventilation account during the hyperbaric therapy. In such situations, it is equally important to remember to return the patient to his or her original tidal volume once out of the hyperbaric chamber and for the return transport, to avoid overdistention of the lung and excessive ventilation.

External Transport

Special considerations that pertain to transporting critically ill patients outside the hospital include the following:

- Choosing the mode of transport (ground versus air)
- Managing increased patient movement and stimulation
- Accommodating the need for specialized personnel and equipment
- Addressing the effects of altitude on Pao_2 and closed air spaces (air transport)

Factors affecting the choice of transport mode include the distance to be traveled, the patient's condition, the availability of ambulance or aircraft, and the weather. **Table 15-10** summarizes the major advantages and disadvantages of transporting patients via ground, helicopter, and fixed-wing aircraft.

Once the transport mode is selected, it is important to secure the patient and all equipment to prevent unwanted movement. You also should be aware that patient overstimulation and stress will occur during transport due to vehicle movement, noise, vibration, or insufficient temperature control. These problems are particularly serious when transporting infants and children, who are most vulnerable to such stimuli. For these reasons, during external transport, all patients should be appropriately positioned and secured, with appropriate sound protection and temperature control.

In terms of monitoring, high background noise (especially in aircraft) may necessitate using an automated noninvasive system to monitor blood pressure and an amplified stethoscope to assess breath sounds. Moreover, because most alarms cannot be heard in noisy aircraft, you should depend on good patient assessment and visually monitor all alarms during the duration of the transport.

Equipment needs for air and land transport are mostly the same as those for intrahospital transport. Ideally, the transport ventilator should function using either 110-volt AC power (supplied by a

Table 15-10 Advantages and Disadvantages of Patient Transport via Ground and Air

Mode	Advantages	Disadvantages
Ground/ambulance	• Most efficient within a 100-mile distance • Often usable in inclement weather or when landing sites are not available • Provides more work area for the transport team • Less vibration and noise than a helicopter	• Generally slower than air travel • Not practical in difficult terrain
Helicopter	• Most efficient for distances between 100 and 250 miles • Faster than ground methods • May be faster for short distances in difficult terrain • Can often land near the hospital	• High noise and vibration resulting in overstimulation • May be grounded in inclement weather • Small work area • Expensive to maintain and operate • Hypobaric effects
Fixed-wing aircraft	• Fastest and most efficient for distances over 250 miles • Less vibration and noise than a helicopter • Able to travel at high altitudes, perhaps in inclement weather	• May be grounded in inclement weather • Must be landed at an airport • Small work area • Expensive to maintain and operate • Hypobaric effects

Table 15-11 Effect of Altitude on Oxygenation with $Fio_2 = 0.21$

Altitude (ft)	Pb*	Pio_2	Pao_2	Pao_2†
0	760	160	100	95
2,000	706	148	88	83
5,000	632	133	73	68
8,000	565	119	59	54
10,000	523	110	50	45

*All pressures in torr/mm Hg.

†Assumes a $P(A-a)o_2$ of 5 torr and no compensation.

generator or inverter in the ambulance or aircraft) or 12-volt DC power (the typical voltage provided by a vehicle battery/alternator). If the ventilator is to be used for air transport, ensure that its volume, pressure, and flow settings can be adjusted either manually or automatically for variations in altitude/barometric pressure. Also, include a calibrated O_2 analyzer.

For air transport, you must understand the effects of altitude on oxygenation. As the aircraft climbs to cruising altitude, atmospheric and cabin pressures decrease. As demonstrated in **Table 15-11**, in unpressurized cabins, this creates a *hypobaric* condition, which lowers the inspired, alveolar, and arterial Po_2. At altitudes greater than 5000 to 8000 feet, even a patient with normal lung function can suffer mild hypoxemia without supplemental O_2.

To compute a patient's Fio_2 needs at an altitude compared with sea level, you should apply the following formula:

$$Fio_2 \text{ at altitude} = Fio_2 \text{ at sea level} \times \frac{760}{Pb\ altitude}$$

where Pb altitude equals the barometric pressure in torr at the cruising altitude used for transport. For example, assume you are transporting a patient receiving 50% oxygen at sea level in an airplane cruising at 8000 feet (Pb = 565 torr). You would compute the needed Fio_2 as follows:

$$FiO_2 \text{ at altitude} = \frac{760}{565} = 0.67$$

Note that at 8000 ft or higher, you cannot provide a FiO_2 equivalent to 0.80 or more at sea level. For this reason, patients requiring 80% or more O_2 at sea level will likely have to either be placed on PEEP/CPAP or have their PEEP levels raised to ensure adequate oxygenation.

Some transport aircraft provide pressurized cabins. Depending on the aircraft, cabin pressures may range from that equivalent to altitudes between 5000 and 8000 feet. In these cases, you still need to compute an equivalent FiO_2, but you should substitute the known cabin pressure for the Pb at altitude. Fortunately, pulse oximetry readings are not affected by altitude and are the best way to judge the adequacy of oxygenation during transport.

In terms of cuff pressures, as altitude increases, so too does the volume of gas in the cuff (as per Boyle's law). Because the tube cuff is restricted in its ability to expand within the trachea, even small increases in volume can result in significant increases in pressure. The only right way to accommodate these changes (and those associated with descent from altitude) is to readjust the cuff pressure as the altitude changes.

In terms of ventilator function, different devices perform differently at a given altitude. For example, volume-control ventilators that use turbines or blowers will tend to deliver *lower*-than-set volumes at altitude, whereas those using differential pressure transducers to measure and regulate flow will tend to deliver *higher*-than-set volumes at altitude. One solution is to temporarily disconnect the patient (while manually providing support) and recalibrate the ventilator once you reach cruising altitude. Another solution is to follow the ventilator manufacturer's recommendation for adjusting settings at various altitudes. Alternatively, you can empirically adjust V_T or PIP according to end-tidal CO_2 levels as monitored by capnography. Unfortunately, capnometers also are affected by altitude, with the $PetCO_2$ reading being falsely low at higher altitude. This error can be overcome by recalibrating the device's high reading at the cruising altitude with a precision gas mixture (usually 5% CO_2).

Other complications are associated with "trapped" gas volume changes—that is, gas in an enclosed space that cannot equilibrate with the ambient pressure. This is a common problem in patients with a pneumothorax or excessive gas in the stomach or bowel. Such problems should be identified and managed *before transport*—for example, via insertion of a chest or nasogastric tube. In addition, in the absence of a chest tube setup, a pneumothorax that occurs in a patient being transported can be treated via an emergency decompression of the chest via needle thoracostomy, a procedure discussed earlier in this chapter.

T⁴—TOP TEST-TAKING TIPS

You can improve your score on this section of the NBRC exam by following these tips:

- Always apply the CAB sequence (circulation–airway–breathing) for CPR, and always immediately obtain or call for a defibrillator and minimize interruptions during chest compressions.
- Always provide compressions at a rate of 100–120/min with a single-rescuer compression-to-breath ratio of 30:2, regardless of the victim's age.
- When a foreign-body airway obstruction occurs in an adult, administer the Heimlich maneuver if the victim is conscious and abdominal thrusts if unconsciousness develops.
- During the resuscitation attempt of a pulseless adult patient, pharmacologic intervention should include 1 mg of epinephrine every 3–5 minutes to aid cerebral perfusion.
- For initial defibrillation of shockable heart rhythms, an initial energy level of 120–200 J should be used for biphasic defibrillators and up to 360 J for older monophasic devices.
- The compression depth for a pediatric patient (1-year-old to puberty) is one-third the depth of the chest or about 2 inches, with a rate of at least 100–120 per minute.
- Always apply chest compressions to a neonate whose heart rate is less than 60/min.
- Babies who are flaccid, cyanotic, or apneic in the delivery room usually require stimulation and supplemental O_2.

- For an unwitnessed collapse of a pediatric or neonatal patient, a single rescuer should give 2 minutes of CPR and then leave the victim to activate the emergency response system, get the AED, and then return to the child or infant and resume CPR and use the AED as soon as it is available.
- Difficulty with BVM ventilation is often rectified by repositioning the head, neck, or mask, inserting a pharyngeal airway, applying an exaggerated jaw lift, having a second clinician apply the mask with two hands, or release of cricoid pressure.
- If partial extubation of an ETT is suspected and a blown cuff is ruled out, the cuff should be deflated, the securing device should be loosened, and attempts should be made to reposition the tube back into the trachea. After repositioning the tube, placement should be checked via auscultation, capnography, CO_2 colorimetry, and use of an endoscope, followed by a confirming chest x-ray.
- A tension pneumothorax should be suspected when a patient is rapidly deteriorating and exhibits a unilateral decrease in breath sounds and chest expansion, hyperresonance to percussion on the affected side, and shift of the trachea away from the affected side.
- If a tension pneumothorax is strongly suspected or confirmed, a chest tube should be inserted immediately. If chest tube insertion equipment is not readily available, emergency decompression should be performed via needle thoracostomy.
- A needle thoracostomy involves the insertion of a large bore angiocath (14 gauge for adults, 18 or 20 gauge for infants) into the second intercostal space over the top of the third rib in the midclavicular line.
- Include a manual resuscitator and mask for backup ventilation when you are transporting a patient with an artificial airway (ETT or TT) on a transport ventilator.
- If the $Petco_2$ is less than 10 mm Hg (torr) and intra-arterial, diastolic pressure is less than 20 mm Hg, the quality of CPR should be improved.
- One of the most effective ways to optimize patient care, especially in high-risk situations, is to ensure effective interprofessional communication, which occurs when clinicians from various disciplines interact in patient care planning, formulating multidisciplinary protocols and procedures and when executing diagnostic or therapeutic interventions and treatments.
- Interprofessional communication should have the following features:
  - *Proactive*—based on a thorough and ongoing review of the patient's record.
  - *Documented*—to become a part of the patient record.
  - *Secure and confidential*—so as not to breach confidentiality.
  - *Structured* and when appropriate, occurring at designated times.
  - *Closed-loop*—whereby the clinician receiving such information should repeat what was said by the sender, who should then verify it is correct.
  - *Appropriately use digital communication technology*—to maximize the number of disciplines who can actively participate.
  - *Employ a fast-track for reporting critical values and key clinical data*—using one or more mechanisms for immediately flagging and reporting critical data which have abruptly deteriorated or are substantially abnormal.
- The minimum monitoring equipment needed when transporting mechanically ventilated patients consists of the heart and respiratory rate monitoring, ECG monitoring, pulse oximetry, and blood pressure monitoring, and capnography is recommended for those patients for whom a specific Pco_2 is being targeted, such as those with head/brain trauma.
- The best way to judge the adequacy of oxygenation during air transport is via pulse oximetry (the Spo_2 is not affected by altitude).
- Patients requiring 80% or more O_2 at sea level will likely have to either be placed on PEEP/CPAP or have their PEEP levels raised to ensure adequate oxygenation.
- Remember that during air transport, pressure changes may necessitate adjustments in Fio_2, ventilator settings, and ET cuff pressures.
- The medical emergency team (MET), also known as a rapid-response team (RRT), is generally activated when a patient's clinical status has rapidly deteriorated, but the patient is not in cardiopulmonary arrest. Their purpose is to stabilize the patient and avert a "code blue."

- For adults, the criteria for activating an MET/RRT includes but is not limited to the following: an acute decline in clinical status, a heart rate < 40 or > 130, or respiratory rate $< 8/min$ or $> 30/min$, systolic blood pressure < 90 mm Hg, and an $SpO_2 < 90\%$, especially with supplemental O_2.
- It is not necessary to wait for a physician to arrive to begin assessing a patient as part of a MET/RRT response. Given the nature of such teams, patient assessment should be done immediately by any member of the MET/RRT, including the RT, nurse, or physician assistant.

POST-TEST

To confirm your mastery of each chapter's topical content, you should create a content post-test, available online via the Navigate Premier Access for Comprehensive Respiratory Therapy Exam Preparation Guide, which contains Navigate TestPrep (access code provided with every new text). You can create multiple topical content post-tests varying in length from 10 to 20 questions, with each attempt presenting a different set of items. You can select questions from all three major NBRC TMC sections: Patient Data, Troubleshooting and Quality Control of Devices and Infection Control, and Initiation and Modification of Interventions. A score of at least 70–80% indicates that you are adequately prepared for this section of the NBRC TMC exam. If you score below 70%, you should first carefully assess your test answers (particularly your wrong answers) and the correct answer explanations. Then return to the chapter to re-review the applicable content. Only then should you reattempt a new post-test. Repeat this process of identifying your shortcomings and reviewing the pertinent content until your test results demonstrate mastery.

CHAPTER 16

Assist a Physician/Provider in Performing Procedures (Section III-H)

Albert J. Heuer

In addition to directly providing respiratory care to patients, respiratory therapists (RTs) often assist with a variety of special procedures. The NBRC expects exam candidates to be especially proficient in assisting with intubation and bronchoscopy and in having a good understanding of how to support several other interventions described in this chapter.

OBJECTIVES

In preparing for the shared NBRC exam content (TMC/CSE), you should demonstrate the knowledge needed to act as an assistant to the physician performing the following special procedures:

1. Intubation
2. Bronchoscopy (including specialized types)
3. Thoracentesis
4. Tracheostomy
5. Chest tube insertion
6. Cardioversion
7. Moderate (conscious) sedation
8. Insertion of venous or arterial catheters
9. Withdrawal of life support

WHAT TO EXPECT ON THIS CATEGORY OF THE NBRC EXAMS

TMC exam: 4 questions; 1 recall and 3 application
CSE exam: indeterminate number of questions; however, section III-H knowledge is a prerequisite to success on CSE Information Gathering and Decision-Making sections.

WHAT YOU NEED TO KNOW: ESSENTIAL CONTENT

Common Elements of Each Procedure

The procedures outlined in this chapter all have common elements that you will need to follow before, during, and after implementation. Rather than repeat these steps in the description of each procedure in this chapter, they are noted as follows:

Before Each Procedure

- Verify, interpret, and evaluate the physician's order or protocol.
- Review the medical record for contraindications, hazards, and informed consent, if appropriate.
- Wash hands, and apply standard transmission-based precautions.
- Gather all equipment.
- Identify the patient.
- Take a pre-procedure time-out, if appropriate (e.g., bronchoscopy).

During Each Procedure

- Assess and monitor the patient, and ensure that monitoring equipment is functioning correctly.
- Respond to any adverse reactions.

After Each Procedure

- Remove, properly dispose of, and process all equipment.
- Reassess the patient's clinical status.
- Respond to any adverse reactions.
- Document the procedure, the patient's tolerance of it, and any other relevant details.

Assisting with Endotracheal Intubation

Outside the operating room, endotracheal (ET) intubation generally is performed as a lifesaving measure by either properly trained RTs or physicians. Here, the focus is on your role when assisting a physician with intubation. Chapter 9 outlines the procedure as performed by RTs.

Primary indications for ET intubation include respiratory or cardiac arrest, airway compromise and protection, and invasive ventilatory support. The only absolute contraindication against intubation is a documented *do-not-resuscitate (DNR)/do-not-intubate (DNI)* order. Relative contraindications include the following:

1. Severe airway trauma or obstruction that does not permit safe passage of an endotracheal tube (ETT)
2. Head/neck injuries requiring immobilization of the cervical spine
3. Mallampati Class 4 airway or other indicators of difficult intubation

Table 16-1 summarizes the RT's role in assisting with standard bedside intubation.

Chapter 6 details the equipment and supplies needed for routine ET intubation.

Table 16-2 outlines the equipment that may be used to support difficult airway protocols. Although such protocols vary by institution, they are all meant to guide action whenever a trained professional experiences difficulty with mask ventilation or cannot quickly insert an ETT using conventional laryngoscopy in three or fewer attempts.

Table 16-1 Respiratory Therapist's Role When Assisting with Intubation

Therapist's Function	Purpose
Before the Procedure	
Confirm that no contraindications or DNR or DNI orders exist	To ensure the patient's or family's advance directives are upheld
Gather and check the operation of all equipment (Chapter 6)	To minimize delays and to ensure patient well-being
Confirm that suction (oral and tracheal) is available	To ensure secretion clearance and better visualization of the glottis
Inflate ETT cuff, check it for leaks, then fully deflate	To confirm ETT cuff integrity, prepare for insertion
Lubricate the ETT and prepare stylet (Chapter 6)	To aid tube insertion
Inspect/assess airway	To determine if difficult intubation is likely or special procedures/equipment will be needed
Remove dentures or dental appliances (e.g., bridges) if present	To facilitate laryngoscopy, avoid aspiration of appliances

During the Procedure	
Place the patient in the sniffing position, unless contraindicated (e.g., cervical spine injury)	To facilitate visualization of the glottis
Anesthetize the airway, if appropriate	To minimize the gag reflex and patient discomfort
Preoxygenate patient with Fio_2 of 100%	To prevent procedural hypoxemia
Monitor the patient's vital signs and clinical status, including response to moderate sedation, if given	To ensure patient safety and detect adverse response(s)
Assist with oral suctioning, laryngoscope insertion, application of cricoid pressure, and other measures	To help ensure a prompt and safe intubation
Inflate the cuff, manually secure ETT, ventilate and oxygenate the patient via manual resuscitator/BVM	To provide/restore ventilation and oxygenation and protect the lower airway
Assess tube placement via auscultation and CO_2 detection (Chapter 6)	To ensure tube placement and patient safety
If tube placement is in question, deflate cuff, reposition tube, and reattempt manual ventilation	To ensure patient safety
If three unsuccessful intubation attempts, recommend proceeding with the difficult airway protocol (varies by institution)	To ensure patient safety
After the Procedure	
Note and mark the ETT insertion depth and secure it in place	To ensure proper tube placement and patient safety
Ensure a chest x-ray is obtained and the tube repositioned as needed	To confirm tube placement and ensure patient safety
Reassess the patient's clinical status	To ensure patient safety
Suction patient if necessary	To maintain airway patency
Ensure appropriate humidification, ventilation, and oxygenation	To ensure patient safety
Verify that intubation and any follow-up orders (e.g., ventilator settings) have been documented in the chart	To meet legal record-keeping requirements

BVM, bag-valve-mask; DNI, do not intubate; DNR, do not resuscitate; ET, endotracheal.

Table 16-2 Equipment Commonly Used to Support Difficult Airway Protocols

Equipment or Supplies	Use
A supraglottic airway (e.g., laryngeal mask airway [LMA], Combitube, or cuffed oropharyngeal airway [COPA])	• Generally the first option in establishing an airway if ET intubation fails • It can be inserted with the patient's head/neck in a neutral position • Contraindicated if high risk of aspiration
Intubating LMA (e.g., Fastrach)	• An LMA with a large-diameter tube that allows passage of an ETT • Once the ETT is placed, the LMA is carefully removed
Fiberoptic bronchoscope	• Inserted into the ETT and used to guide intubation through the vocal cords visually • It can be performed through an intubating LMA

(continues)

Table 16-2 Equipment Commonly Used to Support Difficult Airway Protocols (*continued*)

Equipment or Supplies	Use
Standard "gum elastic Bougie" or ventilating tracheal tube introducer	• Long, narrow, flexible plastic rod with an angled tip that is inserted via laryngoscopy into the trachea • Its position is confirmed visually or via a "clicking" feel as the tip moves over tracheal rings • The ETT is inserted over the introducer, which is then withdrawn • Ventilating introducers are hollow, allowing ventilation without an ETT via either 15-mm or jet adapters
Videolaryngoscope (e.g., Glidescope, C-Mac, Airtraq)	• Laryngoscopes with either a small video screen or remote video monitor used during direct laryngoscopy to enhance visualization and tube insertion
Lighted stylet/lightwand	• Stylet with a light bulb at the tip • Inserted into ETT with a bulb at the tube bevel and the tube angled to about 120 degrees before insertion ("hockey-stick" bend) • Inserted blindly; tracheal position confirmed by midline glow below the thyroid cartilage (may require decreased room lighting)
Fiberoptic stylet (e.g., Levitan, Bonfil, Shikani, Foley)	• Equivalent in concept and use to fiberoptic bronchoscope but smaller, shorter, and typically portable (battery-powered) • It can be used with direct laryngoscopy or inserted blindly
Percutaneous cricothyrotomy kit (e.g., Nu-Trake, QuickTrach, Pertrach)	• Puncture of cricothyroid membrane and dilation of the opening until large enough to place an ETT or trach tube • Patients generally must be at least 5 years old
Jet ventilation setup (50-psi hose, adjustable regulator, jet control valve, 13- to 14-gauge angiocath or ventilating stylet)	• Manually triggered ventilation with 100% O_2 provided via either ventilating stylet inserted orally or 13- to 14-gauge angiocath inserted percutaneously into the trachea • The surgical airway of choice for children younger than 12 years due to their small tracheal diameter and the resulting hazard of cricothyrotomy
Retrograde intubation kit (syringe with angiocath needle, guidewire, introducing catheter, forceps, ventilator adapters)	• Puncture of the cricothyroid membrane using Seldinger method with a guidewire inserted toward the head • The wire is pulled from the mouth with forceps • The introducing catheter is threaded over the wire into the trachea, then the wire is removed, the ETT is inserted over the catheter, and the catheter is removed • The catheter can provide ventilation without an ETT

Positioning the Patient and Preparing the Airway

When assisting with intubation, you may need to position the patient to the head of the bed. Unless a cervical spine injury is suspected, you should then place the patient in the "sniffing" position (**Figure 16-1**). Once the patient is positioned properly, you may need to clear secretions or vomitus from the pharynx using a Yankauer suction catheter. In addition, spraying the pharynx with a local anesthetic such as 2% tetracaine (Cetacaine) aids intubation in conscious patients by blocking the gag reflex. For elective intubation, you can nebulize a 4% lidocaine solution via a small-volume nebulizer (SVN).

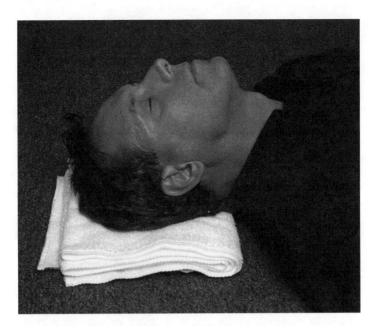

Figure 16-1 Sniffing Position for Intubation. The neck is slightly flexed, and the head is extended. Place a pillow or towels under the head and neck but not under the shoulders.

© Jones & Bartlett Learning. Courtesy of MIEMSS.

Monitoring the Patient

The patient's vital signs and SpO_2 should be monitored before, during, and immediately following intubation. In addition, heart rate and rhythm should be assessed (via electrocardiogram [ECG]) throughout the procedure. For sedated patients, special attention should be paid to adverse drug reactions, including nausea, hypotension, and respiratory depression. You should frequently communicate the patient's vital signs and clinical status to the physician who is performing the intubation, especially if any deterioration occurs.

Assisting with Tube Insertion

As an RT, you can take several measures to help the physician promptly insert the ETT. First, you should ensure the proper-size ETT is selected. For oral intubation, you also can suggest using a standard intubating stylet. Alternatively, if the patient is deemed to have a difficult airway or has suffered cervical trauma, you should suggest a fiberoptic stylet or lightwand, if available. *To prevent trauma during intubation, stylet tips must never extend beyond the ETT tip.*

During laryngoscopy, the physician may ask you to perform the Sellick maneuver. It involves the application of moderate downward pressure on the cricoid cartilage, which can help the physician better visualize the glottis and minimizes the likelihood of aspiration if the patient vomits during the procedure.

In the rare circumstance when a physician chooses the nasal route, ensure that Magill forceps are available. The ETT should also be well lubricated to aid passage through the nose. *Do not use a stylet for nasal intubation!* Once the tube tip is in the oropharynx, you may help open the mouth so that the physician can insert the laryngoscope. The physician will then use the forceps to direct the tube between the cords.

In general, each intubation attempt should not exceed 30 seconds, and you should keep the physician informed of the elapsed time. Once the ETT is positioned in the trachea, you should inflate the cuff with approximately 10 mL of air, temporarily secure the tube with your hand or tape, and then immediately begin manual ventilation with 100% O_2.

If the physician has initial difficulty with intubation, you should be prepared to perform the following tasks:

- Resume ventilating the patient with the manual resuscitator and 100% O_2.
- Suction the oral pharynx or airway.
- Have at least one smaller-size ETT readily available.

After three unsuccessful intubation attempts, you should suggest proceeding with an appropriate difficult airway option, usually defined by the institution's protocol. Typically, if the patient can be manually ventilated but not intubated using direct laryngoscopy (the "can ventilate, can't intubate" scenario), you should suggest the insertion of either a laryngeal mask airway (LMA) or an intubating LMA, followed by fiberoptic–assisted ET intubation. If it is clear that the patient cannot be manually ventilated or intubated (the "can't ventilate, can't intubate" scenario), and hypoxemia is present and worsening, you should suggest immediately proceeding with invasive airway access, via either cricothyrotomy or percutaneous jet ventilation.

Assessing Tube Placement

Immediately following intubation and manual ventilation, you should determine ETT placement via auscultation and patient observation. Additional assurance of tube placement in the trachea is provided using either a disposable colorimetric CO_2 detector or waveform capnography. You place the detector *between* the patient's ETT and manual resuscitator. If the ETT is in the trachea, the device will change color from purple (less than 0.5% CO_2) to tan/yellow (2% or more CO_2) with each exhalation. Note that during cardiac arrest—even with good tube placement and adequate ventilation—a patient's CO_2 levels may remain near zero due to poor pulmonary blood flow, yielding a false-negative result.

If waveform capnography is available, it should always be used to confirm ETT placement. A capnographic waveform will display on the monitor if the ETT is in the trachea but will be absent in the case of esophageal intubation. During cardiopulmonary arrest, waveform capnography is useful in evaluating the quality of a resuscitative effort and will generally display an abrupt increase with the return of spontaneous circulation. Unfortunately, CO_2 analysis cannot detect mainstem bronchial intubation.

After a preliminary assessment of placement and while awaiting x-ray results, you should temporarily secure the tube and record its insertion depth to the incisors using its centimeter markings. After confirming proper placement via chest x-ray, you should consider securing the tube using a commercially available device designed for this purpose.

Rapid-Sequence Intubation

Certain situations may warrant a special procedure called *rapid-sequence intubation* (RSI). RSI is the preferred method for intubating conscious patients who have not fasted and are at high risk for aspiration. As depicted in **Figure 16-2**, to facilitate intubation, the patient is immediately rendered unconscious using a short-acting anesthetic, such as etomidate, and is paralyzed using either succinylcholine or a nondepolarizing neuromuscular blocker such as rocuronium. The goal is to intubate the patient without having to provide manual ventilation immediately. Note that RSI generally is not to be used for "crash" airway management of unconscious patients. In these cases, you should proceed with or recommend immediate manual ventilation and intubation without anesthesia induction or paralysis.

Assisting with Bronchoscopy

Therapeutic indications for bronchoscopy include removal of secretions, mucus plugs, obstructing tissues, or foreign bodies. As previously discussed, fiberoptic bronchoscopy also can be used to facilitate intubation. Diagnostic use includes airway visualization to assess for injuries (e.g., smoke inhalation, tracheoesophageal [TE] fistula) or the anatomic causes of abnormalities such as hemoptysis or stridor. Also, diagnostic bronchoscopy is used to obtain fluid or tissue specimens for microbiologic or cytologic assessment via bronchial washings, brush biopsy, bronchoalveolar lavage, and endobronchial and transbronchial biopsy. Contraindications to performing fiberoptic bronchoscopy

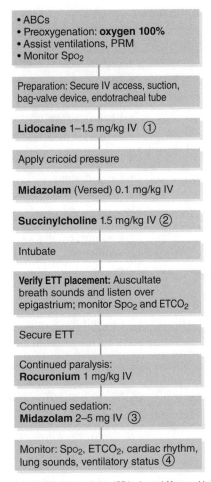

- ABCs
- Preoxygenation: **oxygen 100%**
- Assist ventilations, PRM
- Monitor Spo₂

Preparation: Secure IV access, suction, bag-valve device, endotracheal tube

Lidocaine 1–1.5 mg/kg IV ①

Apply cricoid pressure

Midazolam (Versed) 0.1 mg/kg IV

Succinylcholine 1.5 mg/kg IV ②

Intubate

Verify ETT placement: Auscultate breath sounds and listen over epigastrium; monitor Spo₂ and ETCO₂

Secure ETT

Continued paralysis:
Rocuronium 1 mg/kg IV

Continued sedation:
Midazolam 2–5 mg IV ③

Monitor: Spo₂, ETCO₂, cardiac rhythm, lung sounds, ventilatory status ④

1 **Lidocaine:** Indicated when ICP is elevated. May consider premedicating with **fentanyl** 200 mcg IV to decrease sympathetic response.
2 **Succinylcholine:** Obtain history. **Do not give succinylcholine if family history of malignant hyperthermia is noted. Succinylcholine is contraindicated in penetrating eye injury, severe burns or crush injuries that are 2–5 days old, in the presence of hyperkalemia, and in patients with chronic muscular conditions (e.g., muscular dystrophy).** The onset of **succinylcholine** is 30–60 seconds; duration is 8–10 minutes.
3 **Consider pain control measures. Neither paralytics nor sedatives provide pain control.**
4 **Keep the patient warm.** Paralyzed patients lose much of their ability to generate body heat.

Figure 16-2 Rapid-Sequence Intubation Algorithm.

Reproduced from Porter W. *Porter's Pocket Guide to Emergency and Critical Care.* Sudbury, MA: Jones and Bartlett Publishers; 2007.

are summarized in **Table 16-3**. It is imperative that all patients for whom a bronchoscopy is planned are prescreened for these contraindications.

Role of the Respiratory Therapist

Table 16-4 summarizes the potential functions you may fulfill when assisting physicians performing bronchoscopy, followed by some elaboration of the key supporting activities.

Patient Preparation

You should ensure that the patient takes nothing by mouth (NPO) at least 8 hours in advance of the procedure. Routine oral medications (especially asthma drugs) may be taken. Routine lab work, including measurement of clotting times, complete blood count (CBC), and platelet count, is essential

Table 16-3 Contraindications to Bronchoscopy

Absolute	Relative
• Absence of patient consent (except in emergencies)	• Lack of patient cooperation
• Absence of an experienced clinician to perform the procedure	• Recent myocardial infarction (MI) or unstable angina
• Lack of resources to manage complications such as cardiopulmonary arrest, pneumothorax, or bleeding	• Partial tracheal obstruction
• Inability to adequately oxygenate the patient during the procedure	• Moderate to severe hypoxemia or hypercapnia
• Coagulopathy or uncontrolled bleeding	• Uremia and pulmonary hypertension
• Severe obstructive airway disease	• Lung abscess
• Severe refractory hypoxemia	• Superior vena cava obstructions
• Unstable hemodynamic status, including dysrhythmias	• Debility, malnutrition
	• Respiratory failure requiring mechanical ventilation
	• Disorders requiring large or multiple transbronchial biopsies
	• Known or suspected pregnancy (if radiation exposure)

Table 16-4 Respiratory Therapist Role When Assisting with Bronchoscopy

Therapist's Function	Purpose
Before the Procedure	
Help to identify the potential need for a bronchoscopy, such as retained secretions or foreign-body removal	To determine which patients may benefit from the procedure to maximize clinical outcomes
Prepare and ensure proper function of equipment, including bronchoscope, light source, video monitor and recorder, medications, and specimen traps	To minimize unnecessary delay and the likelihood of patient harm from the procedure
Prepare the patient, providing patient education and premedication	To minimize untoward delays and maximize patient well-being
During the Procedure	
Monitor patient's vital signs and clinical status, including response to moderate sedation, if given	To ensure patient safety and detect adverse response(s)
Assist physician in obtaining specimens; help with medication preparation (e.g., epinephrine)	To minimize unnecessary delay and the likelihood of patient harm from the procedure
After the Procedure	
Reassess the patient's clinical status/confirm stability	To ensure patient safety
Ensure specimens are properly labeled and sent to the lab	To help ensure accurate diagnosis and treatment
Verify that the procedure and any follow-up orders have been documented in the chart	To meet legal record-keeping requirements
Clean and disinfect/sterilize equipment; ensure its proper storage (Chapter 7)	To minimize nosocomial infection risk and potential damage to equipment

to exclude a bleeding disorder—especially if a biopsy is to be performed. Pre-procedural arterial blood gases (ABGs), pulse oximetry, and spirometry may be considered to assess for risk of hypoxemia. Also, measure pulmonary reserves and document airway hyperactivity. Moderate sedation (described later in this chapter) is provided 15–30 minutes before the procedure.

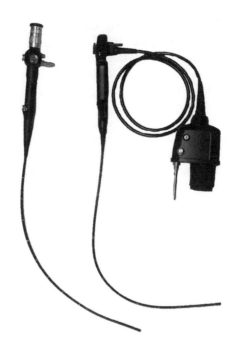

Figure 16-3 Fiberoptic Bronchoscopes.

Equipment

A fiberoptic bronchoscope (**Figure 16-3**) and light source are needed for this procedure. The bronchoscope is equipped with a thumb lever that allows angulation of the distal end of the instrument. A 2- to 2.6-mm channel runs the length of the scope. This channel is used for either therapeutic or diagnostic purposes. Injecting medications, lavaging fluids, and clearing secretions are examples of therapeutic interventions done during bronchoscopy. Diagnostic procedures include aspirating secretions and obtaining fluid or tissue samples for laboratory assessment.

It should be noted that tissue specimens are obtained using specialized instruments such as bronchial brushes and forceps.

Chapter 6 provides details on the care and maintenance of bronchoscopes, including disinfection methods.

Procedure

Bronchoscopy may be performed with the patient in a supine or sitting position. In mechanically ventilated patients, bronchoscopy is performed through the ET or tracheostomy tube using a special adaptor that allows insertion of the scope without disconnecting the ventilator. This approach provides for continued ventilation and maintenance of inspired oxygen and positive end-expiratory pressure (PEEP) levels during the procedure.

If the patient is not intubated, the upper airway should be anesthetized in the same manner as recommended for ET intubation. In addition, the bronchoscope tip is lubricated with lidocaine gel (Xylocaine 2% jelly) before passage through the nose or mouth (the latter requires a bite block). Next, 2% lidocaine liquid is injected through the bronchoscopic channel to anesthetize the vocal cords and lower airway. Once adequate anesthesia has been obtained, a detailed examination is performed. Subsequently, other procedures such as biopsies, washings, and brushings can be carried out.

Patient Monitoring, Sample Collection, and Postprocedural Care

The patient's vital signs and SpO_2 must be closely monitored before, during, and after bronchoscopy. As with ET intubation, the ECG also should be monitored, especially in high-risk patients. Patients with asthma or hyperreactive airways are prone to bronchospasm and laryngospasm, so they require especially careful preparation and monitoring. Because the Pa_{O_2} typically falls during bronchoscopy, supplemental O_2 should always be given, either via a nasal cannula (for the oral route) or a mask modified to allow passage of the scope through the nose. If the patient is intubated, the Fi_{O_2} should be increased by 10% or more during the procedure. If the Sp_{O_2} drops below 90% during bronchoscopy, immediately increase the Fi_{O_2}, or else halt the procedure and give O_2 through the bronchoscope's open channel.

When assisting with sample collection, you typically place tissue specimens in a fixing agent such as formalin. Mucus and lavage fluids are aspirated into empty sterile collection bottles for additional analysis. After proper labeling, tissue specimens and fluids are then transported to the applicable lab according to your institution's infection control protocol.

After the procedure, the patient should remain NPO for at least 2 hours or until the gag reflex is restored. Due to medication effects, outpatients should not be allowed to drive until the following day. Transient fever and mild hemoptysis may be noted for the next 24 hours, with bleeding most common after biopsy procedures.

Assisting with Specialized Bronchoscopy

In addition to a standard bronchoscopy, there are specialized variations of this procedure which are used in specific circumstances. These include endobronchial ultrasound (EBUS) and electromagnetic navigational bronchoscopy (ENB). Both of these procedures have significantly increased our ability to diagnose peripheral lung lesions and other abnormalities without substantially increasing the associated risks. EBUS combines traditional bronchoscopic technology with ultrasound to permit high-resolution imaging of lesions that would otherwise be hard to visualize. ENB uses low-frequency electromagnetic waves transmitted from a magnetic board placed below the patient's chest to allow a lesion to be visualized in three dimensions and in real time. EBUS and ENB can also be combined to further increase the diagnostic value of such systems.

While these procedures offer diagnostic advantages over a standard bronchoscopy, they also require specialized equipment and skills by the physician performing the procedure and the RT assisting them. Hence EBUS and ENB should only be done when specifically indicated, such as in those patients for whom a malignant lung tumor or other lesions in the lung periphery are suspected. While the role of the RT assisting in these procedures is very similar to that for a standard bronchoscopy as outlined in this chapter, it is crucial that the RT also receive additional training and be deemed competent in performing these specialized techniques and operating the equipment used.

Assisting with Tracheotomy

Tracheotomy is indicated to bypass partial or complete upper airway obstruction, to facilitate prolonged mechanical ventilation, or to provide access for frequent secretion clearance. There are no absolute contraindications for this procedure. However, because it can cause bleeding, elective tracheotomy should not be performed until severe coagulopathies are corrected. In addition, critically ill patients should be stabilized as much as possible beforehand.

Equipment

Bedside tracheotomy may be performed via a traditional surgical incision or by using the percutaneous dilator method. The necessary equipment is provided via a tracheotomy tray or kit. Equipment you will need to assist with this procedure includes the following:

- Personal protective equipment (PPE; gown and gloves, mask, and cap)
- Extra trach tubes (one size smaller and one size larger)
- 10-mL syringe, for adding or removing air in cuffs
- Scissors for removing tape or another securing device
- Manual resuscitator (bag-valve-mask [BVM])
- Flowmeter and O_2 source

Role of the Respiratory Therapist

In general, the physician performing the tracheotomy will often be assisted by a second clinician with surgical training. However, as outlined in **Table 16-5**, the RT also can assume a vital role, especially when the procedure is performed to replace an ETT. For details on the ongoing care of a patient with an established tracheostomy, see Chapter 9.

Potential complications include adverse reactions to sedation, tissue trauma at the incision site, airway compromise or loss of a patent airway, excessive bleeding, hypoxemia, and aspiration. Should you note or suspect any of these problems during the procedure, be sure to communicate your concern to the physician immediately.

Assisting with Thoracentesis

Thoracentesis involves inserting a needle or catheter into the pleural space to remove accumulated fluid (pleural effusion). A lateral chest x-ray can help identify the presence and amount of pleural fluid. Also, thoracic ultrasonography can help ascertain fluid location and guide needle insertion during the procedure.

Therapeutically, thoracentesis is performed whenever excessive pleural fluid interferes with lung expansion. Diagnostically, pleural fluid obtained via thoracentesis is analyzed to help determine the presence of underlying conditions such as infection, malignancy, congestive heart failure (CHF), or cirrhosis. There are no absolute contraindications for thoracentesis. Relative contraindications include the following:

- An uncooperative patient
- Severe uncorrected bleeding disorder
- Severe bullous lung disease

Table 16-5 Respiratory Therapist Role When Assisting with Tracheotomy

Therapist's Function	Purpose
Before the Procedure	
Ensure that a crash cart and intubation equipment are readily available	To enhance patient safety and address potentially life-threatening responses to this procedure
Ensure that trach tubes one size smaller and one size larger than that being inserted are available	To ensure availability of the equipment necessary to remove the old ETT, monitor the patient, and oxygenate/ventilate the patient
Patient/caregiver education	To ensure that the patient and caregiver(s) understand the procedure
During the Procedure	
Ensure adequate airway at all times	To ensure patient safety
Monitor patient's vital signs and clinical status, including response to moderate sedation, if given	To ensure patient safety and detect complications and adverse response(s)
Per the physician's instructions, deflate the ETT cuff, remove the securing device, and slowly withdraw tube (ETT should be removed just before insertion of trach tube)	To ensure an adequate airway and transition to the tracheostomy tube
Ensure proper placement of trach tube via breath sounds and CO_2 detection	To ensure patient ventilation and safety
Secure trach tube and continue ventilating through it	To ensure an adequate airway and prevent accidental decannulation
After the Procedure	
Make sure a chest x-ray is ordered	To ensure proper tube placement and lack of any major tissue trauma

Equipment

All needed equipment used for thoracentesis usually is included in a sterilized kit, with the key component being the fluid-removal device, typically consisting of an 8-Fr angiocath over a long (7.5-in) 18-gauge needle with a three-way stopcock and self-sealing valve, and a 50- to 60-mL collection syringe. For sample collection, either a large-volume sterile drainage bottle/bag (therapeutic thoracentesis) or sterile specimen or blood vials (diagnostic thoracentesis) are needed. Supplies include PPE, sterile surgical draping, chlorhexidine solution for skin asepsis, and adhesive dressings/gauze pads. Drugs include an anxiolytic and sedative (for premedication), as well as a local anesthetic (1% or 2% lidocaine) for pain. In addition to procedure-specific equipment, the RT should gather and set up the equipment needed to monitor vital signs and SpO_2 and provide supplemental O_2. It is also wise to have ready the equipment needed to insert a chest tube.

Role of the Respiratory Therapist

The RT may assist the physician before, during, and immediately following thoracentesis. Before the procedure, the assessment of the patient may indicate the presence of an effusion, by findings such as localized gravity-dependent dullness to percussion and decreased breath sounds. When such findings are combined with the presence of predisposing factors such as malignancy, CHF, or respiratory infection, you should inform the nurse and physician.

Once the decision is made to proceed with thoracentesis, the RT can assist by confirming the physician's order and signed informed consent, helping gather needed equipment, and positioning the patient. The RT may also want to recommend premedication with a cough suppressant because coughing during the procedure can cause lung or pleural trauma. Conscious patients who can be mobilized generally should be positioned sitting up and leaning slightly forward, supported in front by an adjustable bedside table. Immobile or unconscious patients should be placed with the affected side down on the very edge of the bed, slightly rotated from supine (toward the bed edge), with the arm from that side behind the head and the mid-/posterior axillary line accessible for needle insertion (elevating the head of the bed to 30 degrees may help).

During the procedure, the RT should ensure that the patient remains as still as possible and avoids coughing. In addition, you should perform the following tasks:

- Support the patient verbally and describe the steps of the procedure as needed.
- Monitor vital signs and SpO_2.
- Observe for signs of distress, such as dyspnea, pallor, and coughing.
- Provide supplemental O_2 to maintain the SpO_2 at 90% or higher.

After the procedure, the RT should ensure that all fluid specimens are appropriately labeled and processed and that the results are documented in the patient record. The RT should continue monitoring and documenting the patient's vital signs and SpO_2 and observing for changes in cough, sputum production, breathing pattern, and breath sounds, as well as the occurrence of any chest pain or hemoptysis. If dyspnea, hypotension, chest pain, or hemoptysis develops, you should immediately contact the physician. Last, where indicated or required by institutional protocol, the RT should ensure that a postprocedural imaging study (x-ray or ultrasound) is performed to rule out a pneumothorax.

Assisting with Chest Tube Insertion (Tube Thoracostomy)

Chapter 15 describes needle thoracostomy for emergency treatment of a tension pneumothorax.

For ongoing management of pneumothorax or removal of pleural fluid, blood, or pus (empyema), a chest tube needs to be inserted. As with thoracentesis, relative contraindications include an uncooperative patient and severe coagulopathy.

Equipment

When assisting the physician with chest tube insertion, one of your primary roles may be to gather the equipment. As with thoracentesis, the procedure-specific equipment is provided in a sterile kit and includes a selection of chest tubes (24- to 36-Fr), surgical instruments (scalpels, Mayo scissors, tissue forceps, Kelly clamps), a suture set, sterile draping, chlorhexidine sponges for skin asepsis, syringes, hypodermic needles, and local anesthetic. A chest tube drainage system needs to be obtained separately and set up in advance of the procedure.

After establishing access via a surgical incision, the physician inserts the tube into the pleural space. For a pneumothorax, the tube typically is placed into the fourth or fifth intercostal space at the anterior axillary line, whereas for fluid drainage, more gravity-dependent locations are used. Once secured, the tube is connected to the drainage system, to which 15–20 cm H_2O of suction is applied. Chapter 6 provides details on the setup, maintenance, and troubleshooting of chest tube drainage systems.

Role of the Respiratory Therapist

In addition to helping gather needed equipment (in some settings, including proper setup of the chest tube drainage system), your role as RT when assisting with chest tube insertion involves monitoring the patient and helping identify and respond to any adverse reactions, both during and after the procedure. Note that serious adverse responses, such as excessive bleeding or hemodynamic instability, may require special measures or even resuscitative efforts.

The chest tube is removed once the condition that led to its insertion has resolved. During the first day or two after its removal, you should help monitor the patient's status, with particular emphasis on the recurrence of the pneumothorax or underlying pathology, as well as any other adverse response. *Crepitus at the site of insertion always suggests recurrence of air leakage into the pleural space.*

Assisting with Cardioversion

Synchronized cardioversion involves the application of an electrical shock to the heart that is synchronized to occur with the R wave of an ECG. Synchronization avoids shocking the heart during its relative refractory period when a shock could cause ventricular fibrillation (VF). Cardioversion is indicated primarily to treat supraventricular tachycardia (SVT) due to atrial fibrillation and flutter. This procedure also is used to treat monomorphic ventricular tachycardia (VT) *with pulses*. It should not be used to treat multifocal atrial or junctional tachycardia. Cardioversion must never be used to treat *VF, pulseless VT, or polymorphic (irregular) VT, all of which require unsynchronized defibrillation* (Chapter 15). **Table 16-6** lists the dysrhythmias that can be treated with cardioversion, along with the recommended biphasic energy levels for adult patients. In general, immediate cardioversion is needed if the ventricular rate exceeds 150/min despite efforts to control it with appropriate drugs.

Role of the Respiratory Therapist

Your role in cardioversion primarily involves monitoring the patient and ensuring adequate oxygenation via the appropriate O_2 therapy modality. RTs with advanced cardiac life support (ACLS) training also may be responsible for applying the paddles and initiating the shock. Because in rare instances, patients receiving cardioversion may worsen and require resuscitation, you also should ensure that an intubation tray, suction equipment, and a manual resuscitator and mask (BVM) are available. Key elements in the cardioversion procedure are outlined in the accompanying box (**Box 16-1**).

Assisting with Moderate (Conscious) Sedation

Without some form of sedation, many of the procedures described in this chapter would be uncomfortable or even intolerable for the patient. For this reason, selected medications may be administered to patients to induce a state of consciousness known as *moderate or conscious sedation*.

Table 16-6 Energy Levels for Synchronized Cardioversion of Adults

Dysrhythmia	Adult Energy Levels (Joules, Biphasic)
Atrial fibrillation	120–200 J; increase in stepwise fashion if not successful
Atrial flutter	50–100 J; increase in stepwise fashion if not successful
Monomorphic VT with a pulse (if stable)	100 J; increase in stepwise fashion if not successful

Box 16-1 Key Elements of the Cardioversion Procedure

1. Ensure proper patient premedication with a sedative (e.g., midazolam [Versed]) and, optionally, analgesia (e.g., fentanyl).
2. Turn defibrillator/cardioverter on.
3. Set the device to *Sync* mode.
4. Using paddles or chest leads, confirm R-wave recognition indicating synchronization.
5. Select an appropriate energy level for the identified dysrhythmia (see Table 16-6).
6. Position conductor pads on the patient (or apply gel to paddles).
7. Position paddles on the patient.
8. Announce to team members, "Charging defibrillator—stand clear!" and then press *Charge* button.
9. Forcefully voice the final clearing command or sequence (varies by institutional protocol).
10. Apply about 25 lb of pressure on both paddles and press the *Shock* button(s).
11. Check the monitor; if tachycardia persists, increase the energy level in a stepwise fashion.
12. Be sure to reactivate *Sync* mode after each attempt.

Table 16-7 Richmond Agitation Sedation Scale (RASS)

Score	Description of Patient	Observe and/or Stimulate Patient
+4	Combative—Overtly combative, violent, immediate danger to staff	Observe patient only
+3	Very agitated—Pulls or removes tube(s) or catheter(s); aggressive	Observe patient only
+2	Agitated—Frequent, nonpurposeful movement; fights ventilator	Observe patient only
+1	Restless—Anxious, but movements not aggressive or vigorous	Observe patient only
0	Alert and calm	Observe patient only
−1	Drowsy—Not fully alert, but has sustained awakening (eye-opening/eye contact) to voice (> 10 seconds)	Verbal stimulation
−2	Light sedation—Briefly awakens with eye contact to voice (< 10 seconds)	Verbal stimulation
−3	Moderate sedation—Movement or eye opening to voice (but no eye contact)	Verbal stimulation
−4	Deep sedation—No response to voice, but movement or eye-opening to physical stimulation	Physical stimulation
−5	No response to voice or physical stimulation	Verbal and physical stimulation

When moderately sedated, the patient should be arousable, with an intact respiratory drive. Once the sedation is administered, your assessment of the patient should include vital signs, cardiopulmonary and airway status, SpO_2, and any adverse side effects from the procedure or the medications. The Richmond Agitation Sedation Scale (RASS) may be used to quantify the level of agitation or sedation of the patient. The scale assigns a score as high as +4 for a very combative patient and ranges to a –5 for one who is unarousable. An alert and calm patient would receive a score of 0, and the targeted score for moderately sedated patients is –3. The scale is summarized in **Table 16-7**.

Once the presence or absence of agitation in a patient is determined, appropriate medication and dose can be selected for moderate sedation. **Table 16-8** summarizes the most common medications used to provide moderate sedation, their major side effects, and reversing agents.

Note that there are respiratory-depressant effects of several medications used in moderate sedation. Also, the respiratory-depressant effects of propofol are potentiated by the benzodiazepines. For this reason, moderate sedation should only be used in a setting that permits continuous

Table 16-8 Moderate Sedation Medications

Drug	Classification	Key Side Effects	Reversing Agent (Antagonist)
Midazolam (Versed)	Benzodiazepine	Hypotension, sleepiness and confusion, impaired reflexes	Flumazenil (Romazicon)
Lorazepam (Ativan)	Benzodiazepine	Same as midazolam	Flumazenil (Romazicon)
Diazepam (Valium)	Benzodiazepine	Same as midazolam	Flumazenil (Romazicon)
Propofol (Diprivan)	Sedative-hypnotic/ general anesthetic	Hypotension, transient apnea, respiratory depression	None (however, a single dose lasts only minutes)
Fentanyl (Fentanyl citrate)	Opioid narcotic analgesic	Respiratory depression, confusion, nausea	Naloxone (Narcan)
Meperidine (Demerol)	Opioid narcotic analgesic	Confusion, hypotension, histamine release, nausea	Naloxone (Narcan)
Dexmedetomidine (Precedex)	Sedative, nonopioid analgesic	Hypotension, bradycardia	Atipamezole (Antisedan)
Clonidine (Catapres)	Sedative, nonopioid analgesic	Hypotension, bradycardia	None

monitoring of capnography/end-tidal CO_2, SpO_2, and vital signs and where there is available ACLS trained staff and the equipment/supplies needed to provide supplemental O_2, airway management, artificial ventilation, and cardiopulmonary resuscitation.

Assisting with Insertion of Arterial or Venous Catheters

As with most special procedures, the RT may be involved in helping monitor and support patients undergoing central venous pressure (CVP) and pulmonary artery (PA) catheterization, as well as assisting with selected components of the procedure itself. Preparation, monitoring, and patient support during CVP and PA catheterization are mostly the same as for the other special procedures discussed in this chapter—namely, equipment setup, patient premedication, vital signs/SpO_2 monitoring, and observing for adverse effects, among other tasks.

The basic equipment needed for CVP and PA catheterization is similar to that for arterial line insertion—that is, a pressurized IV system, a continuous flush device, and a pressure transducer connected to a bedside monitor displaying the pressure waveform. Because in some institutions (including the NBRC hospital) RTs may be responsible for the setup and maintenance of this equipment, you should familiarize yourself with the proper use of indwelling catheters, their troubleshooting, and the Centers for Disease Control and Prevention (CDC) central-line infection control bundle.

The procedure for inserting a CVP and PA catheter also is similar to that for an arterial line, but it is performed only by a physician or an approved physician assistant/nurse practitioner. Key differences include the catheter itself, the transducer and monitor setup, and the insertion location and method.

CVP Catheter Insertion

CVP lines most often have three ports, and because of this may be referred to as a triple-lumen catheter. The lumens are used for (1) monitoring of CVP, (2) fluid or drug administration, and (3) phlebotomy or aspiration of venous blood. CVP kits commonly include a needle for venous penetration, a stiff plastic dilator, and a guidewire coiled in a plastic sheath with a "J" tip to prevent venous wall penetration. The J tip is held straight by a small, separate sheath to accommodate entry into the hub of the insertion needle.

The most common insertion sites are the subclavian or internal jugular veins, for which the procedure is nearly identical. Usually, the head of the patient's bed is lowered, which increases venous pressure and causes the vein to swell, making it easier to penetrate and thread the guidewire. This also decreases the risk of inadvertent air embolism. The subclavian vein is entered from an insertion

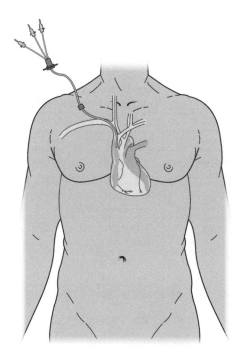

Figure 16-4 Central Venous Pressure (CVP) Catheter and Insertion Route.

Hess, Dean. *Respiratory Care: Principles and Practice, Third Edition.* Burlington, MA: Jones & Bartlett Learning, 2016.

site at the edge of the distal third of the clavicle. The internal jugular vein can be entered from the head of the clavicle or a site behind the brachial artery. A chest radiograph typically is taken after insertion to verify that the tip of the catheter is in the superior vena cava just above the right atrium.

Once inserted and secured, the CVP catheter is attached to a flushed and calibrated monitoring system like that used for pressure measurement through an arterial line. **Figure 16-4** is an illustration of a CVP catheter and insertion route. However, because central venous pressures typically are much lower than arterial pressures, two key differences in the procedure are required. First, the monitor scale for CVP measurement should be set to the low range, typically 0 to 30 mm Hg. Second, to assure accuracy in measurement and interpretation, the pressure transducer must be placed level with the patient's right atrium, identified externally at the phlebostatic axis, which is located at the intersection of the fourth intercostal space and midaxillary line. The NBRC hospital may expect the exam candidate to know that the *positioning of the transducer below the phlebostatic axis will result in erroneously high CVP readings, whereas positioning the transducer above this level will cause the reading to be lower* than the patient's actual value.

Pulmonary Artery Catheter Insertion

A typical adult pulmonary artery (PA) catheter (also known as a Swan-Ganz catheter) has at least three lumens/ports: a CVP/atrial (proximal) lumen, a distal PA lumen, and a lumen for balloon inflation (and deflation), which is used to "float" the catheter into the pulmonary artery and obtain wedge-pressure measurements. Externally, the proximal lumen port is used to aspirate blood, measure CVP, and inject drugs. The distal PA lumen port is used to measure PA wedge pressures, obtain mixed venous blood samples, and inject drugs. Other connectors may include those for a cardiac output (CO) monitor, pacemaker wires, and a Svo_2 sensor.

In terms of monitoring equipment, because PA catheters are placed in the low-pressure venous side of the circulation, the selected transducer must provide accurate measurement in the appropriate pressure range (typically 0 to 50 mm Hg), and the monitor pressure display range must be toggled to low. As with A-lines, before insertion, the transducers should be calibrated and zero balanced,

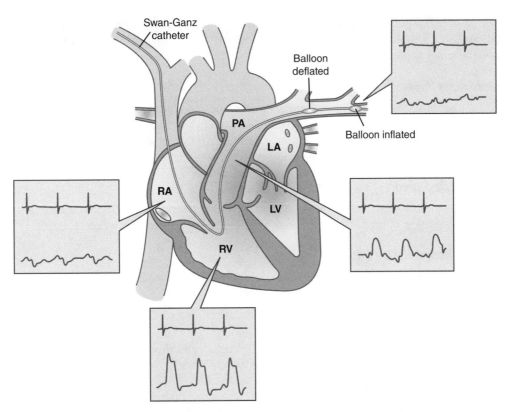

Figure 16-5 Waveforms from Various Sites on the Pulmonary Artery Catheter.

all lines and catheter ports flushed, and the balloon inflated to test for leaks (*using only the 1.0- or 1.5-mL syringe that comes with the catheter*).

PA catheters typically are introduced percutaneously via either the right internal jugular vein (the shortest and straightest path to the heart) or the left subclavian vein. When assisting with subclavian vein access, you should be on guard for a pneumothorax as a potential complication. Once the catheter is in the superior vena cava, the physician may have you inflate the balloon (again, only to the recommended 1.0- to 1.5-mL volume) to aid flotation of the catheter through the heart and into the pulmonary artery. As indicated in **Figure 16-5**, as the catheter advances, distinct pressure changes occur that indicate its position. Initially, CVP/RA (right atrial) pressure is displayed. As the catheter passes through the tricuspid valve into the right ventricle (RV), systolic pressures rise sharply due to RV contraction. As the catheter passes through the pulmonary valve into the pulmonary artery (PA), the diastolic pressures rise, and a dicrotic notch appears, corresponding to pulmonary valve closure. As the catheter eventually "wedges" into a small pulmonary artery, pulse-pressure variations disappear. This pressure is the pulmonary arterial wedge pressure (PAWP, also known as pulmonary "capillary" wedge pressure). Once the catheter is confirmed to be in the wedge position, it is slightly withdrawn until PA pressures are restored, and then the balloon is fully deflated. After that, the measurement of the PAWP is obtained by inflating the balloon, which has the same effect as actual wedging.

The physician also may ask you to obtain a mixed venous blood sample from a PA catheter, either to assess tissue oxygenation or to calculate cardiac output using the Fick method. Good guidance on properly obtaining such samples is provided in Chapter 3.

Withdrawal of Life Support

Some illnesses carry a very poor prognosis. When survival is doubtful, continuing medical care becomes futile, that is, unlikely to be of any benefit. In these cases, a collective decision to withhold or withdraw life support may be made by the patient and family, in consultation with the physician and other members of the patient care team. Although most guidelines specify that there is no ethical difference between withholding or withdrawing life support, to the RT assisting in implementing these decisions, there are some key procedural distinctions.

Withholding Life Support

For RTs, the two most common scenarios involving withholding life support are not proceeding with resuscitation and not proceeding with intubation/mechanical ventilation. Typically, the appropriate actions in these cases are governed by either a physician DNR or DNI order. Ideally, such orders derive from a patient's advance directives/living will.

Withdrawing Life Support

The two most common scenarios involving withdrawing life support that RTs will encounter are terminating a resuscitation effort and withdrawing ventilatory support to allow death.

Terminating a Resuscitation Effort

Common considerations used by physicians in deciding to terminate resuscitative efforts vary by age group and include but are not limited to the following:

For newborn infants:

- Undetectable heart rate for more than 10 minutes
- Extreme prematurity (gestational age < 23 weeks or birth weight < 400 g)
- Major chromosomal abnormality (e.g., trisomy 13)

For pediatric and adult patients:

- Presumed cause of the event/likelihood of recovery (e.g., hypothermia)
- Preexisting comorbidities
- Duration of arrest both before and after initiation of cardiopulmonary resuscitation (CPR)
- Initial and subsequent heart rhythm(s)
- Number shocks/drug dose
- Neurologic status (pupillary responses)
- End-tidal CO_2 changes

When a decision is made by the physician to terminate a resuscitation effort, the RT should cease any/all support, including bag-valve ventilation, cardiac compressions, airway management, and so forth. If an ETT has been inserted, it either should be left in place or may be removed.

Withdrawing Ventilatory Support

Once the patient, patient's family or surrogate, and members of the healthcare team agree that further aggressive medical care will not benefit a ventilator-dependent patient, consideration should be given to withdrawing such support. Both informed consent (by the patient, designated family member, or surrogate) and a physician's order are required to withdraw ventilatory support.

Three methods have been described for ventilator withdrawal: immediate extubation, withdrawal to T-tube, and terminal weaning. Based on their expertise, RTs typically assume major responsibility for implementing these procedures.

Selection of a Withdrawal Method

Although there is no evidence of any significant differences in patient comfort level or the quantity of sedating medications needed among these different approaches, some clinicians favor selecting the method based on the patient's neurologic status, as outlined in **Table 16-9**.

Ultimately, the selection of a method should be based on the patient's desire (if conscious and capable), staff familiarity and comfort with the technique, and the family's needs and expectations. Regarding staff involvement, in most institutions, clinicians who are uncomfortable with the process can remove themselves from the process.

Table 16-9 Selecting a Method

Withdrawal Method	Patient Neurologic Status	Summary Description
Immediate extubation	Brain death*	Rapid discontinuation of ventilatory support followed by immediate removal of the artificial airway
Withdrawal to T-tube	Brainstem-only injuries	Rapid withdrawal of ventilator support and placement on a T-tube with humidified O_2
Terminal weaning	Altered consciousness/conscious	Reduction in and eventual discontinuation of ventilatory support, with the artificial airway left in place during the withdrawal process
*Respiratory therapists may be asked to perform an apnea test (described elsewhere in this chapter) to help confirm brain death.		

Preparing for Withdrawal of Ventilatory Support

Before implementing ventilator withdrawal and under the direction of the attending physician, responsible healthcare team members should:

- Ensure the family understands the options, the procedure being done, and that patient comfort is paramount.
- Take measures to provide appropriate emotional support for the family (via palliative care team, pastoral care, etc.).
- Encourage the family to arrange desired support activities (e.g., playing music, praying, etc.).
- Ensure that all monitor alarms are turned off or will be overridden as needed.
- Remove patient restraints and unnecessary medical equipment (e.g., nasogastric [NG] tube).
- Maintain IV access only for analgesia/sedative administration (stop fluid loading).
- Discontinue all medications (including paralytics) that do not comfort the patient.
- Discontinue all other life-sustaining treatment (e.g., artificial nutrition/hydration, dialysis).
- Invite the family into the room and clear space for them (if the patient is an infant or young child, offer to have the parent hold the child).

Ideally, the attending physician is responsible for documenting the decision-making process, any discussions with a family/surrogate, the goals of care, and the outcome. Should the patient survive the withdrawal process, the attending physician will need to modify the patient care goals.

Sedating the Patient

Regardless of the method chosen, the key to assuring patient comfort during ventilator withdrawal is an appropriate analgesia and sedation regimen. Opioids (usually morphine) and benzodiazepines (e.g., midazolam and lorazepam) are the primary drugs used to prevent the common signs of distress that can occur during withdrawal. Some institutional protocols specify propofol (Diprivan) as the sedative instead of a benzodiazepine.

A typical protocol involves these basic steps:

1. Provide bolus dosing of opioid and benzodiazepine, followed by continuous IV infusion.
2. Titrate drug dosages to achieve adequate pain control, sedation, and relief of distress.
3. If signs of distress reoccur, provide IV push of analgesic/sedating agents until the distress is relieved.
4. Readjust infusion rates as needed to prevent reoccurrence of distress.

It should be noted that increasing drug doses beyond the levels needed to achieve adequate sedation and patient comfort to hasten death is considered euthanasia, which in most states is not an acceptable medical practice.

Table 16-10 Main Steps for Each Method of Withdrawing Ventilatory Support in Sequential Order

Immediate Extubation	Withdrawal to T-Tube	Terminal Weaning
Disconnect the ventilator circuit and turn off the ventilator.	Disconnect the ventilator circuit, and turn off the ventilator (to prevent alarming).	Set mode to IMV with normal rate (12/min for adults); remove positive end-expiratory pressure (PEEP) and pressure support.
Completely deflate the endotracheal tube (ETT) cuff.	Place the patient on a 28–35% T-tube (for comfort).	Disable apnea/backup ventilation and rate, minute ventilation, and apnea alarms.
Discretely remove the ETT.	Observe for signs of distress; recommend adjustment of sedative administration as needed.	Reconfirm patient comfort, then progressively step the IMV rate down to zero over 30 to 60 minutes.
Suction mouth if needed.	Based on family desire and concurrence of the attending physician, extubate the patient.	Observe for signs of distress; recommend adjustment of sedative administration as needed.
Place the patient on 2-L/min nasal cannula.		Disconnect the ventilator circuit, and turn off the ventilator (to prevent alarming).
Observe again for signs of distress; recommend adjustment of sedation as needed.		Complete process with either the extubation or T-tube protocol.
If signs of upper airway obstruction occur (e.g., loud breathing), reposition the patient's head and/or insert a nasopharyngeal airway.		
Stay with the patient until completion of the procedure (usually after death).		

Major Features of Each Withdrawal Method

All three methods start with the following similar steps of (1) explaining the procedure and ensuring family member questions are answered, (2) clearing the patient's airways, (3) observing for signs of distress and inadequate sedation, (4) positioning the patient with head raised as tolerated, and (5) lowering F_{IO_2} to 30%. All three methods end with removing all RT equipment and documenting the procedure. **Table 16-10** summarizes the steps unique to each method of withdrawing ventilatory support.

Apnea Test

The apnea test is one of three major components of the neurologic evaluation for brain death. This test assesses whether or not high levels of blood/brain CO_2 ($Paco_2 \geq 60$ torr) stimulate breathing. If a patient remains apneic despite a significant rise in $Paco_2$, then the results of the test would be classified as "positive"; meaning they tested *positive* for being apneic under such conditions. These results are generally associated with brain death.

T^4—TOP TEST-TAKING TIPS

You can improve your score on this section of the NBRC exam by following these tips:

- *Before* assisting with a special procedure, RTs should verify the physician's order, review the medical record, wash their hands and apply standard transmission-based precautions, gather all equipment, identify the patient, and take a pre-procedure time-out, if appropriate.

- When assisting in a special procedure, the RT should assess the patient, ensure that monitoring equipment is functioning properly, and respond to adverse reactions.
- *After* assisting with a special procedure, disposable and nondisposable equipment should be removed and disposed of or processed; the patient should be assessed; any adverse reactions should be responded to; and the procedure, the patient's response, and any other relevant details should be documented.
- The only absolute contraindication to intubation is a documented *do-not-resuscitate* (DNR)/ *do-not-intubate* (DNI) order. However, relative contraindications include severe airway trauma, head/neck injuries, and Mallampati Class 4 airway or other indicators of difficult intubation.
- To prepare a patient for intubation, the RT should gather and check the operation of all equipment; confirm that suction is available; check the ETT cuff for leaks; lubricate the ETT and prepare stylet; inspect/assess the airway and remove dentures or dental appliances.
- After tube placement is confirmed via auscultation and CO_2 detection, the RT should note the ETT insertion depth and secure it; ensure a chest x-ray is obtained; reassess the patient; suction if necessary; ensure appropriate humidification, ventilation, and oxygenation; and verify that intubation and any follow-up orders (e.g., ventilator settings) have been documented in the chart.
- If waveform capnography is immediately available, as may be the case in a hospital ICU setting, it should always be used to confirm ETT placement.
- Rapid-sequence intubation (RSI) involving the use of a short-acting anesthetic (e.g., etomidate) and a paralyzing agent (e.g., succinylcholine) is the preferred method for intubating conscious patients who are at high risk for aspiration or selected emergent intubations.
- Recommend delaying a bronchoscopy in the presence of absolute contraindications such as refractory hypoxemia, hemodynamic instability, or inability to oxygenate the patient.
- To prepare a patient for a bronchoscopy, the RT should help identify the potential need; prepare and ensure proper function of equipment, including bronchoscope, light source, video monitor and recorder, medications, and specimen traps; and provide education and ensure premedication.
- During and after the bronchoscopy, the RT should assist in obtaining and processing specimens, monitor the patient, help respond to adverse reactions (e.g., provide oxygen for hypoxemia), process the equipment, and document the procedure.
- Endobronchial ultrasound (EBUS) and electromagnetic navigational bronchoscopy (ENB) are variations of a standard bronchoscopy which have significantly increased our ability to diagnose peripheral lesions and other abnormalities without substantially increasing the risks associated with this procedure.
- To prepare a patient for a tracheostomy, the RT should ensure that an emergency crash cart and intubation equipment are readily available, verify that trach tubes one size smaller and one size larger are available, and assist with patient/caregiver education.
- When assisting with a tracheostomy, do not remove the ETT until just before insertion of the trach tube, and confirm placement via breath sounds and CO_2 detection.
- A thoracentesis is done to drain a pleural effusion. The role of the RT generally includes patient/caregiver education, preparing and positioning the patient, supporting the patient and preventing falls, monitoring vital signs and SpO_2, observing for signs of distress, and providing supplemental O_2 as needed.
- A chest tube is inserted for the ongoing management of pneumothorax or removal of pleural fluid, blood, or pus (empyema). The RT's role in such procedures involves monitoring the patient and helping identify and respond to any adverse reactions.
- Synchronized cardioversion is mainly used to treat supraventricular tachycardia (SVT) due to atrial fibrillation and flutter.
- The initial (biphasic) energy-level range for cardioverting atrial fibrillation is 120–200 J and for atrial flutter is 50–100 J.
- The Richmond Agitation Sedation Scale (RASS) is used to quantify the level of agitation or sedation of the patient. The scale ranges from +4 for a very combative patient to −5 for one who is unarousable.

- Medications that can be used in moderate sedation include benzodiazepines (e.g., midazolam, lorazepam), sedative-hypnotics (e.g., propofol), and opioid narcotics (fentanyl).
- Because moderate sedation can depress the respiratory drive, continuous monitoring of capnography/end-tidal CO_2, SpO_2, and vital signs is necessary, and ACLS-trained staff should be readily available if needed.
- CVP lines most often have three ports, and because of this may be referred to as a triple-lumen catheter. The lumens are used for (1) monitoring central venous pressure, (2) fluid or drug administration, and (3) phlebotomy or aspirating venous blood.
- A typical adult PA catheter (also known as a Swan-Ganz catheter) has at least three lumens/ports: a CVP/atrial (proximal) lumen, a distal PA lumen, and a lumen for balloon inflation (and deflation) that is used to "float" the catheter into the pulmonary artery and obtain wedge-pressure measurements.
- The three methods for withdrawing life support in mechanically ventilated patients are immediate extubation in the case of confirmed brain death, withdrawal to a T-tube as used with brainstem-function-only injuries, and terminal weaning involving an incremental reduction in ventilatory support, with the artificial airway left in place.
- An apnea test may be done with patients who have a substantial brain injury to confirm whether or not high levels of CO_2 will stimulate breathing.
- During an apnea test, the RT removes the patient from the ventilator for 10 minutes, during which time the patient receives a FiO_2 of 100%. If a rise in PCO_2 above 60 torr (confirmed via ABGs) fails to stimulate spontaneous respirations during this time, the diagnosis of brain death is supported.
- When assisting with the insertion of a CVP or PA catheter via subclavian vein access, be on guard for pneumothorax as a potential complication.
- When preparing to withdraw ventilatory support, ensure the family understands the options and that measures are taken to ensure their well-being and maximize patient comfort.

POST-TEST

To confirm your mastery of each chapter's topical content, you should create a content post-test, available online via the Navigate Premier Access for Comprehensive Respiratory Therapy Exam Preparation Guide, which contains Navigate TestPrep (access code provided with every new text). You can create multiple topical content post-tests varying in length from 10 to 20 questions, with each attempt presenting a different set of items. You can select questions from all three major NBRC TMC sections: Patient Data, Troubleshooting and Quality Control of Devices and Infection Control, and Initiation and Modification of Interventions. A score of at least 70–80% indicates that you are adequately prepared for this section of the NBRC TMC exam. If you score below 70%, you should first carefully assess your test answers (particularly your wrong answers) and the correct answer explanations. Then return to the chapter to re-review the applicable content. Only then should you reattempt a new post-test. Repeat this process of identifying your shortcomings and reviewing the pertinent content until your test results demonstrate mastery.

CHAPTER 17

Initiate and Conduct Patient and Family Education (Section III-I)

Michael J. Chaney and Albert J. Heuer

Patient and family education is an essential aspect of respiratory care. As a result, NBRC exam candidates can expect a few related test items. This chapter focuses on specific content areas that apply to patient and caregiver education.

OBJECTIVES

In preparing for the shared NBRC exams (TMC/CSE), you should demonstrate the knowledge needed to initiate and conduct patient and family education related to the following:

1. Safety and infection control
2. Home care and related equipment
3. Lifestyle changes
   a. Smoking cessation
   b. Exercise
4. Pulmonary rehabilitation
5. Disease/condition management
   a. Asthma
   b. Chronic obstructive pulmonary disease (COPD)
   c. Cystic fibrosis
   d. Tracheostomy care
   e. Ventilator dependency
   f. Sleep disorders

WHAT TO EXPECT ON THIS CATEGORY OF THE NBRC EXAMS

TMC exam: 3 questions; 1 recall, 2 application
CSE exam: indeterminate number of sections; however, section III-I knowledge is a prerequisite to succeed on the CSE, especially on Information Gathering sections. This category is a potential case management area for COPD, asthma, and sleep disorders.

WHAT YOU NEED TO KNOW: ESSENTIAL CONTENT

General Considerations in Educating the Patient, Family, and Caregivers

Regardless of the patient's disease or type of equipment used, respiratory therapists (RTs) are often involved in educating patients and caregivers on disease management as well as safe use, maintenance, basic troubleshooting, and disinfection of respiratory equipment used as part of the treatment plan. In providing this instruction, the following general principles and strategies apply:

- Proper education helps patients to manage their disease, medications, and therapies appropriately. Additionally, the ability of patients and family members to properly clean and troubleshoot equipment helps with patient safety and infection control.
- Limit educational sessions to about 1 hour or less to avoid "information overload."
- Thoroughly demonstrate all procedures and equipment; *request a return demonstration.*
- Ensure that emergency procedures, such as patient emergencies, are adequately covered.

- Remember that not all patients have the same cognitive abilities or literacy. Some patients or family members may only be able to read at the elementary level, or they may be unable to read at all.
- Leave printed "EZ read" information, with pictures if possible, about the procedures and equipment.
- Keep in mind language barriers. Use language appropriate materials or use an interpreter if available.
- Some patients have difficulties with vision. When appropriate, use materials with larger print, easy-to-distinguish font, and contrasting colors.
- For hearing-impaired patients, make sure you speak clearly and at an appropriate volume so they can hear you. Keep in mind that some patients might be reading your lips to some degree. Those with hearing aids should have them in during instruction.
- Provide directions to access web-based resources.
- Document all aspects of the education session(s) in the patient record.
- Follow up to reinforce the material, as appropriate.
- Remember that knowledge does not always change behavior. Motivation, perceived level of benefit, and removal of barriers (physical, financial, past experiences, misconceptions) are key factors in getting patients to comply with medications, therapies, or smoking cessation.

Beyond general educational strategies and principles, a variety of topics should be covered when educating patients and caregivers on disease management and the safe use of equipment involved in their care plan. They include the following:

- Safe and effective use of equipment and medications
- Basic equipment troubleshooting
- Equipment cleaning and disinfection
- Basic patient assessment
- Emergency procedures
- How to order supplies and medications
- How to contact the homecare company or healthcare facility
- Reliable sources of information about their condition and care plan

Safety

There are some basic principles that RTs need to keep in mind to help optimize patient and clinician safety and on which patients and caregivers often need education. Some of the major risk categories are those related to one or more of the following: (1) medications, (2) patient movement and ambulation, (3) electrical systems, (4) fire safety, and (5) environment and equipment considerations (**Table 17-1**). Infection control is discussed below.

Infection Control

Chapter 7 covers the main infection control principles in respiratory therapy.

The RT is responsible for educating homecare patients and caregivers regarding infection control procedures.

Specific guidance you should provide includes the following:

- Discourage patient contact from visitors with respiratory infections.
- Proper hand washing or disinfecting lotions should be applied to the hands before and after handling patients or respiratory equipment.
- Standard and transmission-based precautions should be used as appropriate.
- Wherever practical, disposable equipment (e.g., ventilator circuits) should be used.
- Sterile water should be used in nebulizers; distilled water is acceptable for humidifiers.
- Noncritical reusable items, such as blood pressure cuffs, can be cleaned with a detergent.
- Before disinfection, all reusable, semicritical objects, such as nebulizers, breathing circuits, and tracheal airway components, should be scrubbed with detergent to remove organic material, then thoroughly washed, rinsed, and allowed to air-dry.

Table 17-1 Key Healthcare Safety Risks and Strategies to Help Reduce Such Risks

Risk Category	Specific Risk	Risk Reduction Strategies
Medication	Improper dose or drug; missed medication	*Healthcare facility*: Clinician education, secure all medications, pharmacy profile for interactions, proper dose, and frequency *Home care*: Proper patient and caregiver education; ensure patient access to medication and address financial, physical, or cognitive limitations; patient follow-up for compliance; re-education as needed. Ensure that patients know what their medications do and when to take them (i.e., do they know which one is their rescue inhaler should they need it?).
Patient movement and ambulation	Back or another injury when a clinician lifts a heavy patient or object	*Caregiver*: Maintain a straight spine and lift with legs. Keep in mind your center of gravity when moving or lifting patients. Use a lift assist device (e.g., Hoyer Lift). *Patient*: exhale on exertion, for example, when going up a step. Plan your course, for example, go around obstacles rather than over them; choose a ramp instead of stairs. Stop and rest if needed. Bend at the knees instead of the waist if picking something up.
	Patient fall during ambulation	Lower bed; position lines and equipment close to the patient; account for initial patient dizziness/instability; supply oxygen as needed; use walkers and adjunctive equipment as appropriate; ensure adequate staff assistance; plan the route; start gradually; ensure patient returned to bed with rails up; monitor patient for an adverse response.
	Injury when moving a patient in bed	Ensure adequate staff assistance; log-roll patient (as a single unit); ensure bed rails are raised when done.
Electrical	Electric shock	Ensure all equipment is checked by biomedical engineering and preventative maintenance is done before use; ensure that a grounded outlet is used; remove equipment from service if electrical safety is in question.
	Electric failure	In the hospital, use only "red or emergency" outlets with a backup power supply; in home care, ensure the outlet is functioning, grounded, and that circuit amperage is adequate for equipment being used.
Fire	General	Perform periodic fire drills and competency education (RACE acronym, O_2 zone valves); ensure proper placement of fire extinguishers, smoke/fire alarms.
	Associated with supplemental O_2	Use no-smoking zones and signage; remove potential ignition sources (e.g., cigarette lighters). While cessation is preferable, for those who continue to smoke, educate them not to smoke while wearing oxygen. Do not cook over an open flame while wearing oxygen.
Environment and equipment	General healthcare environmental risks	Secure O_2 and IV tubing to avoid trips and falls; secure medications, double-verify patient and medication identification; identify patients at risk for falls or elopement; secure such patients to avoid falls or elopement.
	Risks in magnetic resonance imaging (MRI) facilities	Avoid the use of medical equipment (e.g., O_2 tanks, ventilators) or medical devices (e.g., implanted defibrillators) with ferrous metals.
	Gas cylinder accidents	Secure cylinders; store in a well-ventilated area; separate full cylinders from empty cylinders; ensure proper training and education of clinicians and, where appropriate, patients and caregivers.

- After cleaning, reusable semicritical objects should be disinfected at room temperature by immersion in either an intermediate-level disinfectant that is registered by the U.S. Environmental Protection Agency (EPA) as effective or one of the following solutions:
  - 70% isopropyl alcohol for 5 minutes
  - 3% hydrogen peroxide for 30 minutes
  - 1:50 dilution of household bleach (sodium hypochlorite) for 5 minutes
- Alternatively, once cleaned, most respiratory supplies can be disinfected at home using any one of the following techniques involving the application of heat:
  - Place in boiling water and boil for 5 minutes (if not heat sensitive).
  - Place in a microwave-safe receptacle submerged in water and microwave for 5 minutes.
  - Place in the dishwasher if the water temperature is greater than or equal to 70°C (158°F) for 30 minutes.
- Household products other than bleach (e.g., ammonia, vinegar, Borax, liquid detergents) should *not* be used to disinfect reusable semicritical equipment because they are ineffective against *Staphylococcus aureus*.
  - Cleaned and disinfected equipment should be stored in a separate "clean" area.
  - In the unlikely scenario where a reusable critical homecare item requires sterilization, use a chemical sterilant or boiling (according to the manufacturer's recommendations).

Home Care and Related Equipment

This chapter provides some key points that should be covered when educating patients, family members, and other caregivers on the use of common respiratory home-care equipment. Chapter 6 of this text provides details on the setup, maintenance, and troubleshooting of respiratory equipment used in the home and other care settings.

Home O_2 Therapy

O_2 therapy is the most common respiratory modality used at home. The following are key points for educating the home-care patient regarding oxygen therapy of any type.

- Basic care and troubleshooting of home equipment, especially how to switch to a backup system (usually a tank) should their primary system fail or there is a power outage.
- Safe use of home O_2, including the need to avoid use of oxygen near cigarettes or open flames (fireplace or stove), as well as recommendations for electrical safety (installing grounded plugs) and tank storage (location, secureness, and temperature). *A no-smoking sign should be placed on the door to the home.*
- Placement of the stationary system (concentrator). There is a limit to how much oxygen tubing can be added, so the unit must be placed as central as possible in their range of activity within the home. Other considerations for a concentrator include the heat it generates (closet or small room might not be feasible) and not placing the intake filters up against a wall or curtains. Also, warn the patient that O_2 tubing can be a trip hazard.
- Barriers to compliance. Some patients are reluctant to use O_2 because they think it is "addicting." Educating them that this is not the case is important.
- Perceived level of benefit: Educating patients that their prescribed oxygen will help them breathe easier, as well as in some cases reduce the work that their heart has to do is important as this motivates to comply with their therapy.
- Home oxygen requires a physician's order, so it is important for the RT to know the guidelines because patients will sometimes ask about getting home oxygen. Some patients think that just because they want oxygen therapy, they should be able to get it.
- To get oxygen covered by Medicare or private insurance reimbursement, certain diagnosis and blood O_2 level criteria must be met.
  - *Hypoxemia at rest* (continuous oxygen therapy to include stationary and portable systems): For patients with chronic obstructive pulmonary disease (COPD) or other chronic pulmonary disorders to qualify, their SpO_2 must be 88% or less, or their PaO_2 must be 55 torr or less, taken at rest, on room air. For hospitalized patients, this must be obtained no sooner than 48 hours before discharge.

- ○ *Coverage for sleep only* (stationary, not portable): An arterial Pao$_2$ at or below 55 mm Hg, or an arterial oxygen saturation at or below 88%, taken during sleep for a patient who demonstrates an arterial Pao$_2$ at or above 56 mm Hg, or an arterial oxygen saturation at or above 89%, while awake; or a greater-than-normal fall in oxygen level during sleep (a decrease in arterial Pao$_2$ more than 10 mm Hg, or decrease in arterial oxygen saturation more than 5%) associated with symptoms or signs reasonably attributable to hypoxemia (e.g., impairment of cognitive processes and nocturnal restlessness or insomnia).
- ○ *Hypoxemia only during exercise*: An arterial Pao$_2$ at or below 55 mm Hg or an arterial oxygen saturation at or below 88%, taken during exercise for a patient who demonstrates an arterial Pao$_2$ at or above 56 mm Hg, or an arterial oxygen saturation at or above 89%, during the day while at rest.
- ○ *Other coverage conditions*: Patients whose arterial Pao$_2$ is 56–59 mm Hg or whose arterial blood oxygen saturation is 89%, if there is evidence of dependent edema suggesting congestive heart failure; pulmonary hypertension or cor pulmonale, or erythrocythemia with a hematocrit higher than 56%.

The physician's order for home oxygen must contain a diagnosis that warrants O$_2$ therapy, the liter flow, when the therapy is needed (during sleep, just for activity, or continuous), and the anticipated length of need (6 months, 36 months, etc.). This determines what type of system the home-care company provides. Someone who only needs it for sleep would get by with just a stationary system, while someone who just needs it for activity would need a portable system. Someone who needs continuous oxygen therapy would require a stationary system with a backup, as well as a portable system.

Home O$_2$ systems include O$_2$ concentrators, liquid O$_2$ (LOX) systems, and high-pressure gaseous O$_2$ cylinders. A brief description of this equipment follows. A complete description is included in Chapter 6 of this text.

Oxygen Concentrators

An O$_2$ concentrator is an electrically powered device that physically separates the O$_2$ in room air from nitrogen. An increasingly popular variation is the portable O$_2$ concentrator (POC), which is a smaller version of the standard home concentrator, powered by household AC, 12-volt DC (available in cars, RVs, and motor homes), or batteries. To address common problems or service needs, most have indicators to warn the user of malfunction. **Table 17-2** summarizes common indicator warnings and the appropriate action the patient and caregivers should be trained to take when the indicator is activated on a POC unit.

Table 17-2 Portable O$_2$ Concentrator (POC) Warning Indicators and Corrective Actions

Indicator	Recommended Action
Low battery	• Immediately switch to AC/DC power; then charge the battery • If no alternative power is available, switch to a backup O$_2$ supply
Cannula disconnect	• Check the cannula connections • Ensure that you are breathing through your nose • If the alarm persists, switch to backup O$_2$ supply and contact the home-care provider
Capacity exceeded	• Reduce activity and switch to backup O$_2$ supply • If the alarm persists, contact the home-care provider
General malfunction	• Turn the unit off and switch to backup O$_2$ supply • Contact the home-care provider
Service needed or low O$_2$ concentration	• Contact the home-care provider to arrange for inspection and service and provision of a replacement unit.

Liquid O₂ (LOX) Systems

As described in Chapter 6, home LOX systems represent an efficient way to store large amounts of liquid oxygen, which are vaporized into a gas before being used by the patient. Though these systems are infrequently used, key points on LOX systems which should be addressed when educating on such systems are described in **Table 17-3**.

Compressed (Gaseous) O₂ Cylinders

Compressed O_2 cylinders are used in home care primarily as a backup to the concentrator, or for ambulation. For ambulation, patients typically use small aluminum cylinders, size M-6/B, M-9/C, D, or E. Because flows usually range from 0.25 to 4.0 L/min for home-care patients, a low-flow metering device should be used. Chapter 6 provides more details on the safe use of O_2 cylinders, which should be covered when educating others on this equipment.

Oxygen Appliances

The appliances of choice for home O_2 therapy are either simple low-flow devices or O_2-conserving systems. High-flow systems are used as well but primarily for bland aerosol delivery, as covered elsewhere in this text.

The low-flow device most commonly used at home is the nasal cannula. In home settings, cannulas generally are used at flows of 4 L/min or less for adults and 2 L/min or less for infants. At these flows, supplemental humidification generally is not needed. However, consideration should be given

Table 17-3 Basic Home Oxygen Troubleshooting

O₂ System	Problem	Corrective Action/Modification
Oxygen concentrator	The unit will not turn on.	Check electrical power source, including plug and circuit breaker; if the power source is working, place the patient on the gaseous backup system, as appropriate, and replace the concentrator.
	Analyzed Fio₂ is less than 85–90% of the manufacturer's specifications.	The sodium-aluminum pellets are likely exhausted. Place the patient on the gaseous backup system, as appropriate, and either replace the concentrator or send it in for maintenance.
	Low O₂ output alarm	Flowmeter is turned off, or the machine needs maintenance (see above).
	Patient on nasal cannula at 4 L/min or more complains of nasal dryness.	Add a bubble humidifier.
	General malfunction	Switch to the backup tank and contact service provider.
Liquid O₂ (LOX)	The tank is intermittently hissing.	The occasional hissing of stationary liquid O₂ systems is normal; it is likely that no action is needed, except to keep the tank upright.
	The tank is making a very loud and constant hissing sound, possibly with a steady stream of "mist" coming from the tank.	Loud and constant hissing suggests a problem; place the patient on backup O₂, and call supplier.
Gaseous oxygen tanks	O₂ regulator is turned on, but no oxygen is coming out.	Either the tank has not been turned on, or it is empty; if no flow occurs with both the tank and regulator turned on, replace the tank.
	Hissing leaking sound coming from the regulator.	Regulator is not seated properly and needs to be tightened, or the washer is missing or needs to be replaced.

to providing supplemental humidification for any patient who complains of nasal dryness or experiences related symptoms. Most portable O_2 systems incorporate a gas-conserving system to increase the duration of flow. For details on these systems, refer to Chapter 6.

Recommending, Troubleshooting, and Modifying Home O_2 Systems

Certain clinical scenarios regarding home O_2 systems commonly appear on the NBRC exams. For example, you should remember that a patient with restricted activity may need only an O_2 concentrator and a gaseous cylinder for backup. In contrast, you should always recommend a portable source (portable concentrator, LOX unit, or small cylinder) for ambulatory patients. For patients who are especially active or mobile or who need an extended duration of flow, be sure the system incorporates an O_2-conserving device. For patients who only use oxygen during sleep, a stationary system without portables will suffice.

Education should also cover basic equipment troubleshooting and modification, which may appear in some form on the NBRC exam. Table 17-3 summarizes the problems most commonly encountered with home O_2 systems, as well as the recommended corrective actions or modifications.

Bland Aerosol Therapy

Bland aerosols may be used at home to help overcome a humidity deficit (e.g., in patients with trach tubes) and as an adjunct to bronchial hygiene therapy (e.g., in patients with cystic fibrosis). The aerosol can be produced by either an ultrasonic or a jet nebulizer. If using a jet nebulizer, a 50-psi air portable compressor is required. Supplemental O_2 may be "bled in" from a concentrator or LOX system.

Aerosol Drug Administration

As in the acute-care setting, the inhalation route can be used for drug administration to home-care patients. Most inhaled drugs are available in either metered-dose inhaler (MDI) or dry-powder inhaler (DPI) form, with their effectiveness depending on proper training and use (see Chapter 6). For those who have trouble with coordination and timing of the MDI, a spacer or valved holding chamber should be used. Proper use, care, and cleaning of these devices can be found in chapter 6. If these delivery methods are not feasible, the caregiver can use a small-volume nebulizer (SVN) powered by a low-output compressor or a portable electronic (ultrasonic or mesh) nebulizer. Particular attention to issues related to longer-term use compared to short-term hospital use should be emphasized. These issues include changing or cleaning filters and changing/cleaning nebulizers, where applicable.

Airway Care and Secretion Clearance

Home-care patients with trach tubes require both daily stoma care and suctioning. Tracheostomy care can be provided by most trained caregivers, but tube changes should be performed only by a nurse, physician, or respiratory therapist who has been adequately trained in this technique.

As described in Chapter 10, tracheobronchial suctioning in the home is accomplished using a portable suction pump with collection canister and suction tubing. Although some patients can be taught to suction themselves, it is more common to train caregivers on the proper procedure. Daily maintenance and cleaning are crucial.

Airway clearance methods available for patients with intact upper airways airways are described in Chapter 10. These methods, which can be taught to home-care patients and their caregivers, include directed coughing and postural drainage, percussion, and vibration.

Lifestyle Changes

Many diseases are at least partially the result of unhealthy lifestyles. Therefore, educating and supporting patients and their family on individual lifestyle changes can have a dramatic impact on improving their health. Smoking cessation and structured exercise programs can be especially beneficial to a patient with respiratory conditions.

Smoking Cessation

Smoking is the root cause of many pulmonary and cardiovascular diseases and at least partially contributes to some of the leading causes of death in America. Hence, educating patients on smoking cessation and urging them to quit is a valuable process.

The first step in any education effort is assessing the patient's learning needs and motivation. Regarding smoking cessation, your assessment of learning needs ideally should reveal a desire to quit. Remember that knowledge does not always change behavior. Many people continue to smoke despite knowing it is bad for them, simply because they are not ready to quit. Sometimes this is due to lack of information: they know it is bad for them, but they do not know the depth or seriousness of the eventual consequences. They assume that since they do not feel bad yet, that they will not feel bad later.

Patients also might not want to quit because of negative past experiences from previous attempts. Physical and psychological withdrawal symptoms that occur when quitting, the emergence of retained secretions, or the experience of prior unsuccessful attempts can present barriers to quitting. For patients who appear hesitant to quit smoking, it may be helpful to spark motivation and remove barriers by explaining the specific health consequences of not quitting as well as the significant benefits that eventually result from quitting. For these patients, the U.S. Department of Health and Human Services recommends a strategy based on the five Rs: *relevance, risks, rewards, roadblocks,* and *repetition* (**Table 17-4**).

There is also the "Five As" approach to smoking cessation intervention. These are found in the Global Initiative for Chronic Obstructive Lung Disease [GOLD] guidelines, and they can help coach patients regarding tobacco cessation. **Table 17-5** summarizes these steps.

Table 17-4 Using the Five "Rs" to Motivate Patients to Quit Smoking (Excerpts)

Component	Description
Relevance	Encourage the patient to express why quitting is personally relevant. Motivational information has the most significant impact if it is relevant to a patient's disease status or risk, family or social situation (e.g., children in the home), health concerns, age, sex, and other important patient characteristics (e.g., prior quitting experience, personal barriers to quitting).
Risks	Ask the patient to identify the negative consequences of smoking. Suggest and highlight those consequences most relevant to the patient. Acute risks include shortness of breath, worsening of asthma, pregnancy complications, impotence, and increased CO levels. Long-term risks include heart attacks and strokes, lung cancer, and COPD, among others. Environmental risks include lung cancer and heart disease in spouses; increased risk for low-birth-weight infants; and increased risk of sudden infant death syndrome (SIDS) and asthma/respiratory infections in the children of smokers. Emphasize that smoking low-tar/low-nicotine cigarettes or use of smokeless tobacco, cigars, or pipes do not eliminate these risks.
Rewards	Ask the patient to identify potential benefits of quitting. Suggest and highlight those most relevant to the patient (e.g., quitting will improve health, sense of smell/taste, and self-esteem; home, car, clothing, and breath will smell better; quitting will set a good example for kids; quitting will result in healthier babies and children; quitting will avoid exposing others to smoke; quitting will help improve tolerance for physical activities; quitting will reduce wrinkling/aging of skin).
Roadblocks	Ask the patient to identify barriers to quitting and note elements of treatment (problem-solving, pharmacotherapy) that could address these barriers. Typical barriers might include withdrawal symptoms, fear of failure, weight gain, lack of support, depression, and enjoyment of tobacco.
Repetition	Repeat the motivational interventions as needed.

Table 17-5 Five As Approach to Smoking Cessation

Ask	Identify tobacco users by asking every patient about their tobacco use status.
Advise	Strongly urge all tobacco users to quit.
Assess	Find out if they want to quit.
Assist	Help them with their quit attempt by connecting them with the different smoking cessation resources that are available.
Arrange	Schedule a phone or face-to-face follow-up with them.

Modified from Global Initiative for Chronic Obstructive Lung Disease [GOLD] guidelines, Retrieved from https://goldcopd .org/wp-content/uploads/2018/11/GOLD-2019-v1.7-FINAL-14Nov2018-WMS.pdf

Table 17-6 Pharmacologic Treatment for Tobacco Dependence

Drug	Precautions	Side Effects	Dosage	Duration
Varenicline (Chantix) [Prescription]	Nausea	Constipation Insomnia Headache Dry mouth	Days 1–3: 0.5 mg once daily Days 4–7: 0.5 mg BID Days 8 to end: 1 mg BID	12 weeks
Bupropion (Zyban) [Prescription]	Seizure Eating disorders	Insomnia Dry mouth	150 mg each morning for 3 days, then 150 mg BID (begin treatment 1–2 weeks before quitting)	7–12 weeks post-quitting; maintenance up to 6 months
Nicotine gum (Nicorette) [OTC*]	Dependency	Mouth soreness Dyspepsia	1–24 cigarettes/day: 2-mg gum, ≤ 24/day 25+ cigarettes/day: 4-mg gum, ≤ 24/day	Up to 12 weeks
Nicotine inhaler (Nicotrol) [Prescription]	Dependency	Local irritation of mouth and throat	6–16 cartridges/day (each cartridge delivers 4 mg of nicotine)	Up to 6 months
Nicotine nasal spray (Nicotrol NS) [Prescription]	Dependency	Nasal irritation	8–40 doses/day (one dose is 1 mg of nicotine requiring 2 sprays, one in each nostril)	3–6 months
Nicotine patch (Nicoderm CQ) [OTC]	Dependency	Local skin reaction	21 mg/day 14 mg/day 7 mg/day	4 weeks, then 2 weeks, then 2 weeks

*OTC, over the counter (does not require a prescription).

Once the patient has expressed a desire to quit, you should recommend to the patient's physician implementation of a comprehensive treatment program that includes both pharmacologic support and counseling/behavioral therapies. Regarding pharmacologic therapy for smoking cessation, **Table 17-6** summarizes the commonly available medications, some of which require a physician prescription.

According to the U.S. Department of Health and Human Services, counseling, and behavioral therapies that can significantly motivate patients to stop smoking include the following measures:

- Provision of practical counseling (problem-solving/skills training)
- Provision of "intra-treatment" social support
- Obtaining "extra-treatment" social support

Table 17-7 outlines and defines the major components involved in each of these strategies and provides practical examples of discussion points or suggestions to share with the patient.

Table 17-7 Counseling and Behavioral Therapies for Smoking Cessation

Component	Discussion Points or Suggestions
Practical Counseling (Problem-Solving/Skills Training) Treatment	
Identify events, internal states, or activities that increase the risk of smoking or relapse.	• Negative mood • Being around other smokers • Drinking alcohol • Experiencing urges • Being under time pressure
Identify and practice coping or problem-solving skills. Typically, these skills are intended to cope with "danger" situations.	• Learning to anticipate and avoid the temptation • Learning cognitive strategies that will reduce negative moods • Accomplishing lifestyle changes that reduce stress, improve quality of life, or produce pleasure • Learning cognitive and behavioral activities to cope with smoking urges (e.g., distracting attention)
Provide basic information about smoking and successful quitting.	• The fact that any smoking increases the likelihood of full relapse • The peak of withdrawal symptoms (e.g., negative mood, urges to smoke, and difficulty concentrating) typically within 1–3 weeks after quitting • The addictive nature of smoking
Intra-Treatment Supportive Interventions	
Encourage the patient in the quit attempt.	• Note that effective tobacco dependence treatments are now available. • Note that half of all people who have ever smoked have now quit. • Communicate belief in the patient's ability to quit.
Communicate caring and concern.	• Ask how the patient feels about quitting. • Directly express concern and willingness to help. • Be open to the patient's expression of fears of quitting, difficulties experienced, and ambivalent feelings.
Encourage the patient to talk about the quitting process.	Ask about: • Reasons the patient wants to quit • Concerns or worries about quitting • The success the patient has achieved • Difficulties encountered while quitting
Extra-Treatment Supportive Interventions	
Train the patient to support solicitation skills.	• Show videotapes that model support skills. • Practice requesting social support from family, friends, and coworkers. • Aid the patient in establishing a smoke-free home.
Prompt support seeking.	• Help the patient identify others who are supportive. • Call the patient to remind him or her to seek support. • Inform the patient of community resources such as hotlines and helplines.
Help to arrange outside support.	• Mail/email messages to supportive others. • Call supportive others. • Invite others to cessation sessions. • Assign patients to be "buddies" for one another.

Relapse from smoking cessation is a relatively common problem that may be detected via counseling sessions, interviews, or carbon monoxide breath analysis. In the case of relapse, patients should be encouraged to continue trying and informed that smokers who are highly motivated to quit and are persistent eventually achieve their goal.

Exercise

In addition to the exercise component of pulmonary rehabilitation programs discussed in the next section of this chapter, other forms of exercise can be beneficial to patients with respiratory conditions.

In an acute-care setting, exercise can take the form of a range of motion and strengthening programs often overseen by a physical therapist. Also, many inpatients can benefit from progressive mobility therapy, which adheres to the philosophy that sitting *is better than lying down, standing is better than sitting, and assisted walking is better than being immobile.* Such a program can help shorten recovery time and reduce the length of hospital stay, even for patients receiving mechanical ventilation and other forms of respiratory care. However, great care must be taken to carefully monitor the patient to help ensure they don't become injured while performing the exercise.

For outpatients, exercise can take many forms, including aerobic training such as strength training, as well as aerobic activities such as walking, swimming, cycling, and running. Such activities can maintain the benefits achieved by a COPD patient after completing a structured pulmonary rehabilitation program or be an important part of a weight reduction/maintenance program.

Exercise programs can offer additional benefits, such as helping combat the debilitating effects of arthritis and osteoporosis. However, patients with respiratory and other serious aliments should be prescreened and cleared by a physician before beginning an exercise regimen to ensure they can tolerate the exercise. Also, such patients should be monitored during and immediately following exercise to help guard against adverse consequences.

Pulmonary Rehabilitation

Pulmonary rehabilitation is a multifaceted intervention intended to help patients with pulmonary dysfunction return to the highest level of daily functioning. Being able to perform basic activities of daily living (ADLs) restores/maintains independence, dignity, and mental well-being. Pulmonary rehabilitation also permits healthcare providers to monitor newly discharged patients to help reduce the likelihood that they will be readmitted to the hospital in the short term. This is good for the patient's quality of life and benefits hospitals by helping them avoid financial penalties for excessive short-term readmissions. Essential goals for pulmonary rehabilitation include the following:

- Improving a patient's exercise tolerance and a sense of well-being
- Reducing the severity of symptoms (e.g., dyspnea)
- Improving health-related quality of life/activities of daily living (ADLs)
- Reducing the frequency of exacerbations and hospital admissions and readmissions
- Reducing the costs of health care

Patient Selection

Candidates for pulmonary rehabilitation include patients with COPD, asthma, bronchiectasis, cystic fibrosis, and interstitial lung diseases (e.g., pulmonary fibrosis, sarcoidosis) and those for whom lung volume reduction surgery is planned or has been completed. Additional medical screening generally includes the following:

- Complete history and physical exam
- Laboratory testing (complete blood count [CBC], chem profile, α1-antitrypsin titer)
- Electrocardiogram (ECG), arterial blood gas (ABG) analysis, pulmonary function test (PFT) battery, and chest x-ray

Either a simple exercise-tolerance test (e.g., 6-minute walk test [6MWT]) or comprehensive exercise-capacity evaluation also may be prescribed. These tests are used to (1) screen patients for enrollment, (2) establish their baseline performance, (3) monitor their progress, and (4) measure improvement after program completion. Comprehensive exercise test results justifying inclusion in a rehabilitation program include a $\dot{V}O_{2max}$ that is less than 75% of the predicted value and a breathing reserve of less than 30%.

Program Components

Patient Education Topics in Pulmonary Rehabilitation

The educational topics commonly covered in pulmonary rehabilitation programs include those related to the purpose, exercise/conditioning, basic anatomy and physiology, education of the disease process and management, breathing and relaxation techniques, nutrition and diet, psychosocial support, benefit of being in a community with others who suffer from similar diseases, as well as strategies for maximizing ADLs. The rehab team is multidisciplinary to provide the patient with experts in each area listed above.

Breathing Techniques and Exercises

There are several breathing techniques used in pulmonary rehabilitation. **Table 17-8** briefly describes the rationale for these various techniques and exercises as used in pulmonary rehabilitation.

Physical Reconditioning Exercises

Exercises used in rehabilitation fall into three general categories. First, warm-up/stretch activities, conducted before other exercises. Second, aerobic activities such as walking and cycling to build up a participant's physical endurance. Last, strength-building exercises to increase a participant's ability to hold a given position and lift objects.

Monitoring

During exercise, patients' SpO_2, heart rate, respiratory rate, and blood pressure should be monitored, as well as overall appearance. Patients' targeted heart rate should be at least 60% but no higher than 75% of their predicted maximum (220 – age) to achieve the optimal cardiovascular benefit. Patients who demonstrated desaturation during activity should receive supplemental O_2 as needed. You should terminate exercise and closely monitor any patient who experiences angina, muscle cramps, severe fatigue, or excessive dyspnea or who exhibits other signs of distress. If the situation appears life-threatening, you should activate the available emergency response system.

Health (Disease) Management

Health (or disease) management programs provide care for patients with chronic disorders. These programs aim to develop patient self-management skills, improve compliance with treatment plans, reduce disease-related symptoms and hospitalizations, and enhance the quality of life. Most programs involve interdisciplinary teams with specialized expertise broadly covering all aspects of the patient's condition.

Table 17-8 Types of Breathing Techniques and Exercises for Pulmonary Rehabilitation

Breathing Exercise	Rationale
Pursed-lip breathing	Encourages a slower exhalation while creating backpressure to prevent airway collapse and air trapping
Diaphragmatic breathing	Promotes diaphragmatic excursion and effective ventilation, which reduces accessory muscle use
Inspiratory resistance breathing	Strengthens ventilatory muscles by creating an inspiratory flow or threshold resistance
Positive expiratory pressure (PEP) therapy	Improves distribution of ventilation and assists in airway clearance
Glossopharyngeal or "frog" breathing	Uses glossopharyngeal muscles to capture and swallow air, which improves spontaneous ventilation (patients with neuromuscular diseases)

Disease Management for Asthma and COPD

RTs will most often be involved as team members in programs for patients with asthma or COPD. **Table 17-9** outlines the key components and related activities common to health management programs designed for these patients.

In terms of risk reduction—especially for COPD patients—the single most crucial strategy is to quit smoking (previously covered). Other triggers that both patients with asthma and COPD should avoid include outdoor air pollution, secondhand smoke, and household dust, molds, and animal dander. It is also recommended for COPD patients to receive an annual pneumococcal vaccine, and both COPD and asthma patients should receive a flu vaccine.

Ongoing management of disease symptoms aims to reduce exacerbations and the need for hospitalization, with *self-management education* being the key. General skills that self-management education should impart to patients with chronic respiratory disease include the following:

- Knowledge about the disease
- Ability to identify and avoid exposure to environmental triggers
- Ability to assess symptoms and know when to seek medical help
- Early identification of infection/exacerbation. This can include things like fever, malaise, changes in sputum, and increased wheezing and breathlessness. If associated with CHF, look for pedal edema, fluid weight gain, dyspnea, or other signs of heart failure.
- Knowledge of how and when to use prescribed medications, and which ones are used for rescue
- Maintenance of good nutrition and physical conditioning
- Ability to effectively communicate with providers

Table 17-9 Common Components in Health Management Programs for Patients with Asthma or COPD

Component	Related Activities
Establishing a relationship with the patient/family	• Applying effective communications skills • Understanding the patient's disease experience • Assessing the patient's treatment preferences • Helping the patient and family know what to expect
Determining the severity of the disease	• Obtaining a comprehensive patient history • Evaluating the patient's pulmonary function • Assessing the patient's quality of life
Reducing further risk/slowing progression	• Identifying/avoiding triggers that worsen symptoms • Having the patient quit smoking (smoking cessation) • Ensuring the patient receives needed immunizations • Involving the patient in a rehabilitation program
Managing symptoms/reducing complications	• Setting healthy goals (personal action plans) • Providing self-management education/skill-building techniques • Involving family members in care delivery • Offering support for stress and negative emotions • Linking the patient to community resources
Providing ongoing follow-up (frequency based on disease severity)	• Retesting pulmonary function • Assessing symptom control/quality of life • Evaluating psychosocial issues such as depression • Determining the need for social/home health services

- Development of coping skills (to deal with frustration, fatigue, and other stressors)
- Breathing techniques and energy conservation methods
- Bronchial hygiene techniques and safe equipment use
- Self-management education must be tailored to the individual needs of each patient, including his or her health literacy, language, cultural beliefs, and ethnocultural practices.

Individualized educational activities should be based on *personal action plans*. An action plan is a collaborative goal-setting tool designed to help patients determine desired behavioral or lifestyle changes, plan on how to attain them, and establish follow-up mechanisms to assess progress and ensure goal achievement. The accompanying boxes (**Boxes 17-1** and **17-2**) provide an example of a simple action plan for patients with COPD and asthma, respectively.

Of course, depending on the goal and problem being addressed, you may need to refer the patient to another health professional who is better able to support the desired plan. For example,

Box 17-1 COPD Patient Action Plan

Goal plan	Begin exercising
How	Walking
Where	Around the block (about 1/3 mile)
What	Initially once around; try to increase as tolerated
When	Before lunch
Frequency	4× per week
Potential barriers	O$_2$ cylinder cart is cumbersome
Plans to overcome barriers	Get a more portable O$_2$ source Walk with someone for support and help
Follow-up	Maintain activity/distance logs (use pedometer) Discuss progress at the next office visit (3 months)

Box 17-2 Asthma Patient Action Plan

Goal plan	Reduce asthma attack frequency and severity
	• Ongoing follow-up with a pulmonologist or allergist to "step up" or "step down" treatment plan • Daily peak flow monitoring and diarizing • Strict compliance with asthma controller medications • Avoidance of known/suspected triggers • Monitoring use of short-acting adrenergic bronchodilator • Immediately contacting a physician at first signs of an exacerbation
Potential barriers	Time (monitoring, medication compliance, contacting a physician as appropriate)
Plans to overcome barriers	Document the plan, allocate time, and identify rewards (e.g., fewer sick days)
Follow-up	Review the plan with physician and revise as needed; reward compliance

if the goal involved better eating habits, you likely would refer the patient to a clinical nutritionist. Alternatively, a COPD patient experiencing secondary depression or anxiety should be referred to a mental health practitioner.

Disease Management for Cystic Fibrosis (CF)

Cystic fibrosis (CF) is a genetic disease of the exocrine glands that can affect several body systems and their functions. Most significantly, it causes problems with the pulmonary and digestive systems, but it can also cause other problems like nasal polyps, reproductive sterility, osteoporosis, and the tendency to easily bruise (from inadequate absorption of vitamins, specifically D and K, respectively). Here we will focus primarily on the educational aspect of CF disease management for the respiratory therapist. More detail on the pathophysiology, assessment, treatment, and equipment cleaning for CF can be found in Chapter 20 (*CSE Case Management Pearls*), and details on the setup, function, and troubleshooting of respiratory equipment used for CF management can be found in Chapter 6.

CF management has many aspects that are in common with COPD/asthma management. These include the following:

- Knowledge about the disease
- Ability to assess symptoms and know when to seek medical help
- Early identification of infection/exacerbation, which can include things like fever, malaise, changes in sputum, and increased wheezing and breathlessness
- Knowledge of how and when to use prescribed medications and which ones are used for rescue
- Maintenance of good nutrition (particularly a problem with CF patients due to lack of digestive enzymes and poor nutrient absorption)
- Ability to effectively communicate with providers
- Development of coping skills (to deal with frustration, fatigue, and other stressors)
- Breathing techniques
- Bronchial hygiene techniques and safe equipment use
- Self-management education tailored to the individual needs of each patient, including his or her health literacy, language, cultural beliefs, and ethnocultural practices
- Because many CF patients are minor children, education should be emphasized to meet the needs and capabilities for both the patient and the caregiver.

Pulmonary problems caused by CF include bronchospasm, airway inflammation, secretion retention, bronchiectasis, secondary infections, hypoxemia, and eventual CO_2 retention (CF is an obstructive disease). Therefore, disease management and education should focus on medication therapies (to possibly include O_2), bronchial hygiene, and infection treatment/prevention. **Table 17-10** summarizes key points for pulmonary management of CF patients.

Patients with CF have digestive problems. Pancreatic enzymes needed for breaking down proteins are not delivered, and clogged bile ducts inhibit the delivery of bile needed to break down fats. The result is poor absorption of proteins and fats (and therefore fat-soluble vitamins A, D, E, and K). This leads to poor nutrition, and for infants, difficulty in gaining weight, which can result in "failure to thrive." Treatment considerations for these problems include dietary supplements, vitamins, pancreatic enzymes, and high-calorie foods.

Disease Management for Tracheostomy Care

Patients with a tracheostomy tube are both in acute-care and home-care settings. Tracheostomy tubes are placed in the acute-care setting often because they have the advantages of being more secure, easier to suction, and better tolerated because they are more comfortable, patients can mouth words, sometimes eat, and if a PMV is applied, they can talk and cough. Trach tubes are in place for longer-term use in chronic vent-dependent patients, or in children for congenital or traumatic airway abnormalities while they await surgery or while they outgrow the anomaly. More details on tracheostomy tubes are found in the following chapters within this text:

- Chapter 16, Assisting with a tracheotomy
- Chapter 6, Indications, selection, and troubleshooting of trach tubes; PMVs

Table 17-10 Key Points for Pulmonary Disease Management of CF Patients

Problem	Medication or Therapy	Consideration(s)
Bronchospasm	Bronchodilators (b_2 agonists/anticholinergics)	• Emphasize proper inhalation technique for inhalers or nebulizer delivery. • Stress importance of adherence to ordered medication regimen, including sequencing and which meds are used for rescue.
Airway inflammation (neutrophilic)	Steroids (prednisolone) High-dose ibuprofen	Oral steroids more effective but with more side effects than inhaled corticosteroids (ICSs)
Secretion retention	Dornase alpha (Pulmozyme)	• Mucolytic developed for use in CF patients • Effectiveness is variable depending on the patient • Nebulized once or twice daily • Side effects include pharyngitis/laryngitis
	N-acetylcysteine (Mucomyst)	• Mucolytic that breaks apart mucus disulfide protein bonds • Despite widespread use, it is not very effective • Nebulize 3–5 mL of 10% or 20% solution, three or four times daily; may instill in ETT • May cause bronchospasm and rhinorrhea • Do not give if wheezing
	Hypertonic saline	• Mucokinetic that pulls water into the ciliary bed to mobilize secretions • Nebulize 2–5 mL of 3–12% solution; may instill in ETT • May cause bronchospasm; do not give if wheezing
	Vest ®	• Put on like a "vest," this percussive therapy was initially developed for mucus mobilization in CF patients • Treatment is done several times per day, usually concurrent with medication therapies • Advantages include ease of use, and therapy can be done alone without a second caregiver • Disadvantages include it is not as portable as smaller hand-held oscillatory PEP devices, and it is expensive
	Oscillatory PEP devices (see Chapter 10 for more detail on these devices)	• Hand-held devices that provide internal percussions on exhalation to mobilize secretions • Advantages are ease of use, low cost, portability, and can be used by one person, so a second caregiver is not needed
	Percussion and postural drainage (P&PD)	• Uses body positioning to promote gravitational lobe drainage, along with external percussions provided by a second caregiver either by hand or through use of an electrically or pneumatically powered percussion device • With the development of easier, more effective devices, it is not used very much anymore • It requires a second caregiver who has the technique and stamina to perform percussion. It also requires knowledge of body positioning to drain each lobe. Not all patients will tolerate some of the positions required for therapy. It is also time-consuming.

Problem	Medication or Therapy	Consideration(s)
	Other percussive devices (IPV and Metaneb®)	• Both offer adjustable pressure and percussive amplitude settings • Both have nebulization to deliver meds during percussive therapy • IPV comes in both pneumatic and electrical power. Metaneb is pneumatic. • See Chapter 10 for more detail on IPV
Hypoxemia	Oxygen therapy	• Usually not needed except in exacerbations/infections, or until significant lung involvement • Keep $SpO_2 > 90\%$ and choose a delivery system and interface that suits each patient's needs in terms of flow, length of use, and portability.
Infection treatment/ prevention	Annual flu vaccine	
	Infection control/hygiene practices	• Hand hygiene • Equipment care and cleaning (see Chapter 20 CF section) • Avoidance of infection sources
	Antibiotics (to treat *Pseudomonas aeruginosa*)	
	Inhaled Tobramycin (Tobi)	• Nebulized in a Pari Neb bid for 28 days alternating months • Also available in DPI podhaler • For all antibiotics, because of the potential for resistance, stress the importance of closely following the prescribed regimen. • Advantage of inhaled over oral is the potential for high-dose delivery to the airways with minimal systemic effects
	Aztreonam (Cayston)	• Nebulized in an Altera Neb bid for 28 days alternating months
	Colistimethate (Colistin)	• Nebulized in a Pari Neb bid
	Ciprofloxacin	• Oral antibiotic, but because resistance builds quickly (3–4 weeks), it is not recommended

- Chapter 9, Provide tracheotomy care (cleaning and changing tubes, cuff leaks)
- Chapter 10, Suctioning via a tracheal airway

Educational considerations not covered elsewhere in this text include:

- Emphasize the importance of infection control to include handwashing, sterile technique during cleaning and changing equipment, and during suctioning, as well as proper storage of equipment.
- Ensure caregivers are familiarized and competent with care, cleaning, changing, and troubleshooting trach tubes and associated equipment.
- Caregivers must recognize an abnormal stoma site and when to contact the physician. This includes redness, swelling, abnormal drainage of pus or blood, or granuloma tissue.
- Caregivers must be knowledgeable about how to handle trach emergencies:
  - Blocked tube—suction and remove inner cannula to clear the blockage
  - Accidental decannulation—reinsert trach tube or half-size smaller tube according to insertion procedure guidelines

- Mask ventilate or orally intubate if a trach tube cannot be reinserted
- Difficult airway—use an airway-exchange cannula; have second caregiver present; recommend bronchoscopic/fiberoptic exchange
- In severe cases where oxygenation and ventilation cannot be maintained, and a secure airway cannot be obtained, call a code or the emergency services (e.g., 911)

Home Mechanical Ventilation and Related Caregiver Education

Although most patients are weaned from mechanical ventilation in an acute-care facility, some ventilator-dependent patients are discharged to the home setting. Many of these patients have underlying cardiopulmonary conditions such as COPD, whereas others may have been diagnosed with neuromuscular diseases (e.g., ALS) or have spinal cord trauma.

Patients being considered for discharge to the home with mechanical ventilation should meet the following criteria:

- Be clinically stable for at least two weeks and have the desire to go home
- Have been on continuous ventilation for at least 30 days without successful weaning
- Not require cardiac monitoring
- Have a tracheostomy tube in place (unless using noninvasive ventilation)
- Demonstrate control of any seizure activity with the prescribed medication protocol
- Not require acute-care IV medications such as vasodilators
- Have family members and caregivers willing and capable of taking on responsibilities
- Have undergone a complete medical and financial assessment by the case manager

In general, patients should *not* be considered for home ventilatory support in these circumstances:

- They require more than 40% O_2 or more than 10 cm H_2O positive end-expiratory pressure (PEEP).
- They need continuous invasive monitoring.
- The home physical environment is deemed, inaccessible (may need access ramp), unsafe, or caregivers inadequate.

Ideally, the patient should be placed on the ventilator that will be used in the home setting *before discharge*. When this approach is used, caregivers can be further oriented to the equipment and their role and responsibilities in a well-controlled setting with full medical support.

The key patient factor in ventilator selection is the type of airway—that is, tracheostomy versus intact upper airway. For patients with trach tubes requiring continuous support, the common choice is an electrically powered, volume-controlled ventilator using a single-limb circuit (Chapter 6). For patients with an intact upper airway who need only intermittent support (e.g., at night), electrically powered, pressure-limited ventilators with noninvasive interfaces are popular choices. Patients who would otherwise be suited for noninvasive positive-pressure ventilation (NPPV) but object to mask or mouthpiece interfaces may be considered candidates for negative-pressure ventilation, usually via a chest cuirass or "pneumosuit."

Key considerations for home-care ventilation include the following:

- A backup ventilator should be available for patients who:
  ○ Cannot maintain spontaneous ventilation for four or more hours
  ○ Live in an area where a replacement ventilator cannot be provided within two hours
- Caring for a ventilator-dependent patient in the home is labor-intensive and involves extensive education and training for the family and caregivers, including infection control measures.
- Additional equipment needed may include a hospital bed, wheelchair with ventilator transport deck and O_2 tank carrier, supplemental O_2, suction equipment, feeding pump, and all related supplies that accompany these pieces of equipment.
- Arrangements must be in place for emergencies, including power outages.

The NBRC also expects exam candidates to be able to educate caregivers on the safe use and basic troubleshooting of home mechanical ventilation systems. Aspects of ventilator troubleshooting

Table 17-11 Home Ventilator Troubleshooting

Problem	Corrective Action/Modification
The unit will not turn on.	Ensure adequate patient ventilation, and use a backup ventilator or manual resuscitator, as appropriate; then check power sources, such as the plug and circuit breaker.
The ventilator-dependent patient lives in a rural area that experiences frequent power outages.	Ensure that the utility company is notified in writing of the patient's needs and that a backup power source such as a generator is in place.
A caregiver cannot immediately fix an alarm, and the patient appears to be in distress.	Remove patient from ventilator, use a backup ventilator or manual resuscitator as needed, and call 911; consider cardiopulmonary resuscitation (CPR) as appropriate.
Patient with a trach tube is in distress; when off the ventilator, extreme resistance is felt when bagging.	Call 911, attempt to pass a suction catheter, and then resume manual ventilation with 100% Fio_2; consider CPR as appropriate.
Patient on pressure-limited ventilation objects to the discomfort of the nasal mask.	Consider a different interface, such as nasal pillows, or recommend a negative-pressure ventilator.

are covered elsewhere in this text, but the most common problems and corrective actions or modifications specific to home mechanical ventilation are summarized in **Table 17-11**.

Sleep Disorder Management

Sleep-disordered breathing and apnea-hypopnea syndrome are disorders characterized by either complete cessation of breathing (apnea) or notable reduction in ventilation (hypopnea) during sleep. Physiologic causes include airway obstruction due to relaxation or collapse of the upper airway tissues (obstructive sleep apnea [OSA]) or a failure of the respiratory center to activate the respiratory muscles (central sleep apnea [CSA]). Diagnosis of sleep disorders, including the use of the polysomnography exam (PSG), is discussed in Chapter 1.

Disease management begins once the sleep disorder is diagnosed, usually via a sleep study. Typically, a sleep specialist first reviews the findings of the sleep study and related tests with the patient. Following diagnosis, patient education should begin.

Patient Education for Sleep Disorders

Ideally, patient education activities should be included as a component of a comprehensive disease management program, delivered by a multidisciplinary team that consists of a sleep specialist, the patient's primary care doctor, and allied healthcare providers, including RTs. Educational topics should include the following:

- Nature of the disorder
  - Basic pathophysiology
  - The natural course of the disease
  - Associated disorders (e.g., hypertension)
- Treatment
  - Treatment options and goals
  - What to expect from the treatment
  - Patient's role in the treatment
  - Consequences of untreated disease, such as the following:
    - Decreased quality of life
    - High blood pressure
    - Heart disease, heart attack, stroke
    - Fatigue-related motor vehicle and work accidents

- Counseling
  - Risk/exacerbating factor identification and modification
  - Complementary behavioral strategies
  - Sleep hygiene
  - Drowsy driving/sleepiness
  - Genetic counseling*
- Follow-up and evaluation
  - Need to monitor goals, side effects, and complications
  - Involvement of the patient in quality assessment and feedback

There are several treatment options for both OSA and CSA, which are described in **Table 17-12.** They can be used alone or in some cases in conjunction with one another. Generally, the patient's physician will prescribe one or more of these treatment options. If these treatment options are adopted as part of the care plan, the RT will often be responsible for further educating the patient and caregiver on them.

Table 17-12 Treatments for Obstructive and Central Sleep Apnea

Obstructive Sleep Apnea (OSA)	Central Sleep Apnea (CSA)
Weight reduction—applicable to obese patients with OSA; seldom successful if the sole therapy	*Treatment of the underlying disorder*—for example, if CSA due to heart failure causing *Cheyne-Stokes breathing* (CSB), optimize cardiac function
Avoidance of alcohol and drugs that depress the central nervous system (e.g., sedatives or hypnotics)	*Continuous positive airway pressure (CPAP)*—may improve cardiac function in patients with congestive heart failure and CSB-type apnea
Alteration in sleep posture—avoiding the supine position (with positional devices as needed) and instead of sleeping in either a side-lying or head-up position	*Bilevel positive airway pressure (BiPAP)*—effective for treating patients with *hypercapnic CSA* (hypoventilation syndrome)
CPAP—generally most effective treatment for OSA; CPAP levels set by titration; poor compliance is a concern	*Adaptive servo-ventilation* (ASV)—treatment for most forms of CSA, especially CSB-related; should be prescribed based on PSG exam
Oral appliances—oral devices that position the tongue/mandible; best used in patients with mild to moderate OSA associated with overbites or temporomandibular joint (TMJ) problems	*Nocturnal O_2 therapy*—for CSA secondary to heart failure; improves left ventricular ejection fraction and decreases the apnea-hypopnea index (AHI); used in conjunction with positive airway pressure (PAP) therapies
Uvulopalatopharyngoplasty—surgery that removes portions of the soft palate, uvula, and tonsils; not always effective in resolving OSA	*Acetazolamide (Diamox)*—increases excretion of HCO_3^-, causing metabolic acidosis, which can lower the $Paco_2$ apneic threshold; most effective in CSB with heart failure
Tracheostomy—a last resort for patients with severe OSA who do not benefit from the more common medical or surgical interventions	*Theophylline*—a phosphodiesterase inhibitor with respiratory stimulant properties that is effective in CSB patients with heart failure
Modafinil (Provigil)—a brain-stimulating agent used to treat narcolepsy; also, may help patients with OSA who continue to experience daytime sleepiness despite CPAP therapy	*Sedative-hypnotics* (e.g., temazepam [Restoril] and zolpidem [Ambien])—may minimize ventilatory instability with sleep-wake transitions (non-hypercapnic CSA only)
Upper airway stimulation therapy—applies electrical impulses to upper airway muscles to maintain the tone and airway patency	

---

* Strong evidence is emerging of a genetic link to certain sleep disorders, including narcolepsy, restless legs syndrome, and OSA (e.g., Marfan syndrome–associated OSA).

Despite some recent advances related to upper airway stimulation therapy, nasal continuous positive airway pressure (CPAP) remains the most widely used home treatment for OSA. A CPAP setup consists of a flow generator, breathing circuit, patient interface (e.g., nasal mask, nasal pillows), and headgear. Most systems provide pressures up to 20–30 cm H_2O. The optimal CPAP pressure is typically determined by a titration study, which is conducted either in conjunction with a polysomnography exam in the sleep lab or at home using an auto-titrating device. Many units now have a ramp feature that gradually raises the pressure to the prescribed level over a time interval. This gradual elevation helps some patients fall asleep and may increase therapy compliance.

Whereas CPAP applies a constant airway pressure, the separate inspiratory and expiratory pressure settings available with bilevel positive airway pressure (BiPAP) systems make this mode a better choice to support patients needing enhanced ventilation, such as those with CSA or neuromuscular weakness. BiPAP also may increase patient comfort and therefore improve patient compliance, even among those patients with OSA.

Although CPAP is an effective treatment for sleep apnea, several problems associated with this therapy may warrant corrective action or modification, as summarized in **Table 17-13.**

Compliance/Adherence to Therapy

As indicated earlier, successful treatment of sleep apnea depends on patient compliance with the prescribed therapy. Unfortunately, between 20% and 40% of sleep apnea patients do not comply with their treatment.

Generally, good CPAP adherence is defined as use of the device for a minimum of four hours per night at least five nights per week. When combined with patients' subjective reporting of compliance issues, objective compliance data provided from the PAP device's memory can help identify and rectify problems with adherence to therapy. Given that the initial weeks of therapy are crucial in assuring subsequent patient compliance, it is essential that identified problems be corrected as soon as possible after treatment begins. In addition to assessing equipment or interface alternatives for patients receiving PAP therapy, interventions that can help improve compliance include (1) in-person individual or group teaching/learning sessions provided at the sleep clinic, (2) in-person individual reinforcement provided in the home by a nurse or RT, (3) provision of selected media (e.g., videos, DVDs, written brochures/handouts, or Internet-based resources) combined with frequent phone calls from a management team member during the early period of use, or (4) participation in a telemedicine program.

Documentation

Regardless of the clinical intervention and the setting in which it has occurred, the accompanying education related to safety, equipment use, smoking cessation, pulmonary rehabilitation, and disease management must be documented in the patient record. This is often done in the progress notes and care plan, but it is becoming common for documentation systems to now have a separate section for each clinical discipline to document patient education efforts.

Table 17-13 Problems Associated with CPAP and Corrective Action

Problem	Corrective Action/Modification
Patient complaints of overall discomfort from excessive flow and noise	Use the ramp feature to build up to prescribed pressure gradually.
Skin irritation or facial soreness from excessive mask pressure	Use different interface (e.g., nasal pillows), add supplemental cushioning, adjust straps on headgear, and ensure proper cleaning of the interface.
Conjunctivitis	Adjust the interface to eliminate leak around eyes.
Epistaxis (nosebleed) or excessive nasal dryness	Add a circuit humidifier or ensure adequate household humidity.
Inability to maintain adequate pressure	Check circuit connections for the leak, use a chin strap to prevent pressure loss through the mouth, or use a different interface.

T⁴—TOP TEST-TAKING TIPS

You can improve your score on this section of the NBRC exam by following these tips:

- Avoid using technical or "textbook" terms when educating patients and caregivers.
- Basic principles for educating patients and caregivers include limiting educational sessions to about 1 hour; thoroughly demonstrating all procedures/equipment; requesting a return demonstration; leaving printed "EZ read" information and directions to access web-based resources; documenting all aspects of the education process and following up.
- Strategies to enhance medication safety within a healthcare facility include ensuring clinician education; securing all medications; pharmacy profiling for interactions; and ensuring proper dose and frequency.
- Strategies to maximize medication safety within a home-care setting include providing proper patient and caregiver education, ensuring patient access to medication and addressing financial or cognitive limitations, monitoring patient compliance through follow-up, and providing re-education as needed.
- Measures to ensure electrical safety within a hospital setting include ensuring all equipment is checked by biomedical engineering and that preventative maintenance is done, ensuring that a grounded outlet is used, removing equipment from service if electrical safety is in question, and using only "red or emergency" outlets with a backup power supply.
- Electrical safety measures at home include ensuring outlet is functioning and grounded and that circuit amperage is adequate for the equipment being used.
- Measures to ensure fire safety within a general hospital setting include periodic fire drills and competency education (RACE acronym, O_2 zone valves) and proper placement of fire extinguishers and smoke/fire alarms.
- Strategies to minimize fire risks in hyperbaric conditions include following strict hyperbaric protocol, including the use of special fabrics, and avoiding static electricity and other sparks.
- Risks in magnetic resonance imaging (MRI) facilities can be reduced by *avoiding* the use of medical equipment (e.g., O_2 tanks, ventilators) or medical devices (e.g., implanted defibrillators) with ferrous metals.
- Adequate equipment disinfection can be achieved in a home-care setting by using any of the following: 70% isopropyl alcohol for 5 minutes, 3% hydrogen peroxide for 30 minutes, or 1:50 dilution of household bleach (sodium hypochlorite) for 5 minutes.
- Household products other than bleach (e.g., ammonia, vinegar, Borax, liquid detergents) should *not* be used to disinfect reusable semi-critical equipment because they are ineffective against *Staphylococcus aureus*.
- Patients with a SpO_2 of less than 88% or a PaO_2 of less than 55 torr on room air will generally qualify for home O_2 therapy reimbursement through Medicare and most other health payers.
- When experiencing a problem with a home oxygen concentrator system, the patient or caregiver should be instructed to turn the unit off, switch to backup O_2 supply, and contact the home-care provider.
- When an oxygen concentrator will not turn on, the RT troubleshooting the problem should first check the electrical power source, including the plug and circuit.
- If the FiO_2 measured from the outlet of an oxygen concentrator is less than 85–90% of the manufacturer's specifications, the sodium-aluminum pellets are likely exhausted, and the concentrator should be replaced or sent in for maintenance.
- It's generally best to recommend a portable oxygen system such as a portable oxygen concentrator for active oxygen-dependent patients.
- Assessing the patient's readiness to quit, medications, counseling, and accounting for the potential of relapses are all major components of a smoking cessation program.
- Pharmacologic treatment for nicotine dependence includes varenicline (Chantix), bupropion (Zyban), and nicotine replacement (Nicorette Gum).
- The five "Rs" in motivating patients to quit smoking are as follows: emphasizing the *Relevance* that quitting has to them, identifying the health *Risks* that will be reduced, focusing on the

Rewards of quitting, noting the potential *Roadblocks* to quitting and strategies to overcome them, and providing *Repetition* of interventions for trying to quit or remain tobacco-free.

- The five "As" for smoking cessation intervention are: *Ask* every patient about their tobacco use status, *Advise* all tobacco users to quit, *Assess* whether they want to quit, *Assist* them with their quit attempt by connecting them with the different smoking cessation resources, and *Arrange* a phone or face-to-face follow-up with them.
- Many inpatients can benefit from progressive mobility therapy, which adheres to the philosophy that *sitting is better than lying down, standing is better than sitting, and assisted walking is better than being immobile*. Such programs can help shorten recovery time and reduce the length of hospital stay.
- Patients with respiratory and other serious ailments should be prescreened and cleared by a physician before beginning an exercise to ensure they can tolerate the exercise; Also, such patients should be monitored during and immediately following exercise to help guard against adverse consequences.
- Always recommend that rehabilitation patients who smoke, enroll in a smoking cessation program as a condition of participation.
- Essential goals for pulmonary rehabilitation include improving a patient's exercise tolerance and sense of well-being, reducing the severity of symptoms, improving health-related quality of life/activities of daily living (ADLs), reducing the frequency of exacerbations and hospital admissions/readmissions, and reducing healthcare costs.
- Primary components of a pulmonary rehabilitation program include exercise/conditioning, basic anatomy and physiology, education of the disease process and management, breathing and relaxation techniques, nutrition and diet, psychosocial support, the benefit of being in a community with others who suffer from similar diseases, as well as strategies for maximizing ADLs.
- Common elements of disease management programs for patients with COPD and asthma include the following: establishing a relationship with the patient/family; determining the severity of disease; reducing further risk/slowing progression; managing symptoms/reducing complications; providing ongoing follow-up.
- General self-management education should impart to patients with chronic respiratory disease: knowledge about the disease, identifying and avoiding triggers, ability to assess symptoms and knowing when to seek medical help, early identification of infection/exacerbation, knowledge of how and when to use prescribed medications, and which ones are used for rescue, good nutrition and physical conditioning, effective communication with providers, coping skills, breathing techniques and energy conservation methods, bronchial hygiene techniques, and safe equipment use.
- Self-management education must be tailored to the individual needs of each patient, including his or her health literacy, language, cultural beliefs, and ethnocultural practices.
- Individualized educational activities should be based on personal action plans.
- Key components of CF management are to mobilize secretions and prevent/treat *Pseudomonas aeruginosa* infection.
- Inhaled antibiotics for CF are tobramycin, Colistin, or Cayston.
- When choosing a secretion mobilization device, considerations should include effectiveness, cost, portability, and ease of use.
- When dealing with a trached patient, strict adherence to infection control guidelines is crucial to prevent infection.
- Caregivers must recognize an abnormal stoma site, which includes redness, swelling, abnormal drainage of pus or blood, or granuloma tissue.
- Caregivers must be knowledgeable about how to handle trach emergencies. These include a blocked tube, accidental decannulation, and difficult airway.
- In severe cases where oxygenation and ventilation cannot be maintained, and a secure airway cannot be obtained, activate the emergency response system (call a code or 911).
- In general, patients should not be considered for home ventilatory support if they require more than 40% O_2 or more than 10 cm H_2O PEEP, if they need continuous invasive

monitoring, if the home physical environment is deemed unsafe, or if caregiver support is inadequate.

- For home-care ventilation, a backup ventilator should be available for patients who cannot maintain spontaneous ventilation for 4 or more hours or live in an area where a replacement ventilator cannot be provided within 2 hours.
- If a caregiver cannot immediately fix a home ventilator alarm and the patient appears to be in distress, the caregiver should be instructed to remove the patient from the ventilator, use a backup ventilator or manual resuscitator as needed, call 911, and consider CPR, as appropriate.
- Always recommend a polysomnography study for a patient suspected of having a sleep disorder; if a diagnosis of OSA is confirmed, recommend CPAP or BiPAP therapy.
- Treatment options for OSA include weight reduction, avoidance of alcohol, sleeping in either a side-lying or head-up position, CPAP, oral appliances, uvulopalatopharyngoplasty surgery, tracheostomy (a last resort), and upper airway stimulation therapy (newer therapy that applies electrical impulses to maintain the tone and airway patency).
- Skin irritation or facial soreness from excessive CPAP mask pressure can be addressed by using a different interface (e.g., nasal pillows), adding supplemental cushioning, adjusting straps on headgear, and ensuring proper cleaning of the interface.

POST-TEST

To confirm your mastery of each chapter's topical content, you should create a content post-test, available online via the Navigate Premier Access for Comprehensive Respiratory Therapy Exam Preparation Guide, which contains Navigate TestPrep (access code provided with every new text). You can create multiple topical content post-tests varying in length from 10 to 20 questions, with each attempt presenting a different set of items. You can select questions from all three major NBRC TMC sections: Patient Data, Troubleshooting and Quality Control of Devices and Infection Control, and Initiation and Modification of Interventions. A score of at least 70–80% indicates that you are adequately prepared for this section of the NBRC TMC exam. If you score below 70%, you should first carefully assess your test answers (particularly your wrong answers) and the correct answer explanations. Then return to the chapter to re-review the applicable content. Only then should you reattempt a new post-test. Repeat this process of identifying your shortcomings and reviewing the pertinent content until your test results demonstrate mastery.

SECTION II

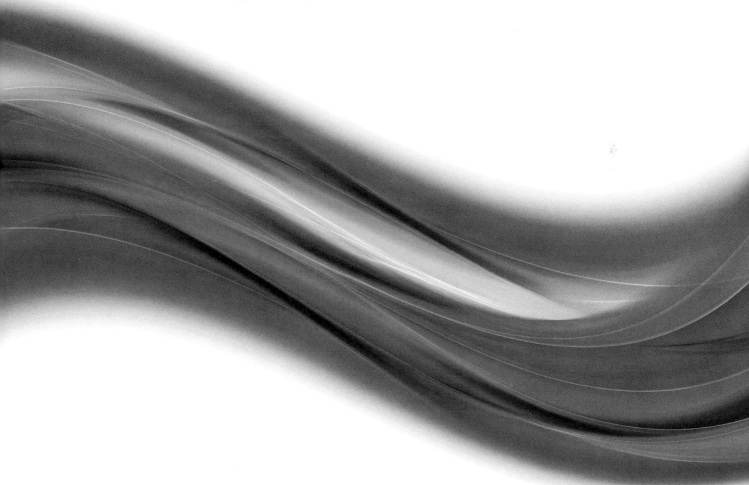

Clinical Simulation Exam (CSE)

CHAPTER 18

Preparing for the Clinical Simulation Exam

Narciso E. Rodriguez

Your path to registry requires taking and passing the NBRC Clinical Simulation Exam (CSE) after scoring above the high cut score in the TMC exam. Besides being the most expensive exam in that pathway ($200 per each new and repeat attempt), it is also the most difficult and the longest (four hours in duration). First-time pass rates for the CSE have historically averaged between 50% and 60%, the lowest of any NBRC exam. Thus, if you want to avoid the high reapplication fee and achieve the Registered Respiratory Therapist (RRT) credential on your first attempt, you will want to be well prepared for this unique exam.

In our experience, the "difficulty" of the CSE and the resultant high failure rate experienced by RRT candidates are more often due to poor or ill-informed preparation than to the level or complexity of the test itself. Yes, the CSE has a unique structure, and yes, correctly navigating through a problem's sections requires skill in application and analysis. However, knowing these simple facts should guide you to take a different approach when preparing for the CSE.

To properly prepare for the CSE, we recommend that you become thoroughly familiar with both the content and structure of the CSE and recognize how that knowledge can help guide your exam preparation.

Lastly, it is important to mention that if you do not earn the RRT credential within the time limit allowed by the NBRC (three years after achieving the high cut score in the TMC), you will be required to retake and pass the TMC exam at the high cut score to regain eligibility. Any previous passing performance on the TMC and CSE are nullified. After passing the TMC exam at the high cut score, you will have another three years to earn the RRT credential. We strongly recommend that you attempt your CSE examination as soon as possible after achieving your high cut score in the TMC exam but allow at least 3 to 4 weeks for proper preparation.

CSE CONTENT

Whereas the TMC exam is organized exclusively by topical content, the NBRC organizes the CSE by both topical content and disease category. With this knowledge in hand, you should then prepare for the exam by focusing on both the exam's topical coverage and disease management.

CSE Topical Coverage

As with the NBRC TMC exam, you must know exactly which topics are covered on the CSE. Most of this information is provided to you via the CSE detailed content outline in the current NBRC candidate handbook (www.nbrc.org).

First and foremost, the CSE covers the same topical content as that on the TMC exam. Knowing that the simulation exam content spans the same topical content included on TMC means that if you recently took and *passed* the TMC at the RRT level cut score, you are already reasonably well prepared for the CSE's topical content.

Second, a topical content review for the CSE should include a review of all previous chapters in this text. All NBRC topical content is covered in Chapters 1–17 of this text, corresponding to the 17 major NBRC exam topics.

However, to better focus your topical review for the CSE, we recommend that you first carefully assess your TMC exam score report and use that information to prioritize your CSE topic-oriented preparation time. To do so, review your three major TMC section scores (i.e., Patient Data Evaluation,

Troubleshooting and Quality Control of Devices and Infection Control, and Initiation and Modification of Interventions). Then flag any section on which you scored less than 75%. You should then focus your attention on these flagged sections and their corresponding book chapters in preparing for the CSE topical content.

CSE Content by Disease Category

What most candidates miss—and, in our opinion, why many fail the CSE—is that this exam's content is also organized by disease category. Currently, the CSE includes 20 cases or problems (plus two not graded test cases for a total of 22 problems), selected from seven disease management categories. **Table 18-1** outlines these categories, the number of cases that are on the current CSE, and some example cases for each category.

We recommend that you spend the majority of your CSE prep time focusing on disease management by case. Specifically, your preparation for the CSE should include a review of assessment and problem identification, procedures, skills, and treatment plans/protocols related to these seven disease management categories and the example cases identified by the NBRC.

Table 18-1 Disease Management Categories and Cases Likely to Appear on the CSE

Category		Likely # of Cases	Examples of Cases That May Appear
Adult Chronic Airways Disease	Intubation and mechanical ventilation	2	Mechanical ventilation (invasive and noninvasive)
	Noninvasive management	2	Preoperative/postoperative evaluation, pulmonary function test (PFT) evaluation, home care/rehabilitation, infection control
	Outpatient management of COPD	1	
	Outpatient management of asthma	1	
	COPD diagnosis	1	
Adult Trauma		1	Chest/head/skeletal injury, burns, smoke inhalation, hypothermia
Adult Cardiovascular	Heart failure	1	Congestive heart failure, coronary artery disease, valvular heart disease, cardiac surgery
	Other: e.g., arrhythmia, pulmonary hypertension, myocardial ischemia/infarction, pulmonary embolism	1	
Adult Neurological or Neuromuscular		1	Myasthenia gravis, Guillain-Barré syndrome, tetanus, muscular dystrophy, drug overdose
Adult Medical or Surgical	Cystic fibrosis or non-cystic fibrosis bronchiectasis	1	Thoracic surgery, head and neck surgery, carbon monoxide poisoning, obesity–hypoventilation syndrome, AIDS
	Infectious disease	1	
	Acute respiratory distress syndrome	1	
	Other: e.g., immunocompromised, shock, bariatric, psychiatric	2	
Pediatric	Acute asthma	1	Epiglottitis, croup, bronchiolitis, asthma, foreign-body aspiration, toxic substance ingestion, bronchopulmonary dysplasia
	Other: e.g., infectious disease, bronchiolitis, chronic lung disease of prematurity, congenital defects	1	
Neonatal	Respiratory distress syndrome	1	Delivery room management, resuscitation, infant apnea, meconium aspiration, respiratory distress syndrome.
	Resuscitation	1	
Total		**20**	

Preparation by Case Is the Key to CSE Success!

How should you prepare for disease management by case? Differently! Topical content is relatively easy to specify and is well covered here and in many comprehensive respiratory care textbooks. However, disease management by case is not as well defined, so it requires a different preparatory approach. In our experience, the best strategy is to use appropriate resource materials to review the pathophysiology and the medical, surgical, and respiratory management of each of the common disorders identified by the NBRC in Table 18-1.

What are the appropriate resource materials? We recommend that you access whatever textbook resources were used in your respiratory or cardiopulmonary pathophysiology course(s) in school. These materials may include focused pathophysiology and disease management texts written for respiratory therapists or relevant disease-oriented chapters in more comprehensive texts. However, because pathophysiology-focused texts are organized by disease category and emphasize both diagnosis and management, they are a better choice for CSE preparation than most comprehensive texts.

Either way, you should extract and summarize in writing at least the following basic information about each of the common disorders identified by the NBRC:

- Definition and causes (etiology)
- Pathophysiology (how the disorder alters structure or function)
- Clinical manifestations (signs and symptoms)
- Test results used to confirm the diagnosis (e.g., lab results, PFT, imaging studies)
- Differential diagnosis (including which findings distinguish this condition)
- General medical/surgical treatment
- Respiratory management (therapy and assessment)
- Common complications and their management

Figure 18-1 provides an example of a good summary extraction for bronchiolitis, as it might appear on an index card. Because many RT programs require it, you may already have a collection of

RSV bronchiolitis	
Etiology	A clinical syndrome that occurs in children <2 years of age and is characterized by upper respiratory symptoms (e.g., rhinorrhea) followed by lower respiratory infection with inflammation which results in wheezing and crackles (rales).
Pathophysiology	Occurs when viruses infect the terminal bronchiolar epithelial cells causing direct damage and inflammation in the small bronchi and bronchioles. Edema, excessive mucus, and sloughed epithelial cells lead to obstruction of small airways and atelectasis. Pathologic changes begin 18 to 24 hours after infection and include bronchiolar cell necrosis, ciliary disruption, and peribronchiolar lymphocytic infiltration.
Clinical S&S	Occurs primarily in children <2 years of age and generally presents with fever, cough, and respiratory distress (e.g., increased respiratory rate, retractions, wheezing, crackles). It is preceded by a one- to three-day history of URT symptoms (e.g., nasal congestion and discharge). Respiratory distress, increased work of breathing, respiratory rate, and oxygenation all can change rapidly with crying, coughing, and agitation. Oxygen desaturation can occur under all these circumstances as well as during sleep when chest wall muscles relax. Further narrowing intrathoracic airways.
DX tests	It is diagnosed clinically. Features include an early viral upper respiratory infection followed by increased respiratory effort and wheezing and crackles Chest x-rays and lab studies are not necessary to make the diagnosis and should not be routinely performed. However, they may be necessary to evaluate the possibility of secondary or comorbid bacterial infection, complications, or other conditions in the differential diagnosis.
Differential Dx	The differential diagnosis includes a variety of acute and chronic conditions that affect the respiratory tract, including recurrent viral-triggered wheezing or asthma, pneumonia, chronic pulmonary disease, foreign body aspiration, aspiration pneumonia, congenital heart disease, heart failure, and vascular ring.
General Med Surg Rx	Severe bronchiolitis usually requires treatment in the emergency department or inpatient setting. Supportive care includes maintenance of adequate hydration, respiratory support, and monitoring for disease progression.
Respiratory Mgmt.	Nasal suctioning, supplemental O_2 to maintain SpO_2 >90 to 92%. If worsens, a trial of heated humidified high-flow nasal cannula (HFNC) therapy and CPAP can be done before endotracheal intubation. Trial of inhaled bronchodilator and nebulized hypertonic saline can also be done, but their routine use is not recommended.

Figure 18-1 Example Disease Management Case Summary: Bronchiolitis.

index cards or page forms like this one covering most of the common disorders you need to review for the CSE exam. To facilitate your CSE review, we have encapsulated much of this information for you in Chapter 20 as "Clinical Simulation Exam Case Management Pearls."

We also recommend that you copy the clinical manifestations and the test results used to confirm the diagnosis to the back of each summary card or sheet. In this manner, you turn each summary into a "flashcard" that you can use to assess and enhance your diagnostic skills—for example, given these findings, what is the most likely disorder? The importance of building your diagnostic skills in preparing for the CSE is discussed in more detail subsequently.

In addition to these resources, you should gather and review selected clinical practice guidelines covering the conditions listed in Table 18-1. A good place to start is with the American Association for Respiratory Care (AARC) Clinical Practice Guidelines (CPG), other guidelines and clinical resources, which are available online at the AARC site (http://www.aarc.org). The AARC guidelines are an invaluable source of information with which all therapists should be familiar and from which the NBRC draws essential content.

Although the AARC guidelines provide excellent procedural guidance (especially regarding assessing respiratory care interventions), you need to supplement this knowledge with current disease management guidelines, as provided mainly by professional medical organizations. Disease management guidelines covering most of the cases likely to appear on the CSE are readily available online and easily found using the U.S. Department of Health and Human Services' National Guideline Clearinghouse (http://guideline.gov). **Figure 18-2** provides a partial screenshot of a search for bronchiolitis guidelines on this site. Here, as in many cases, multiple guidelines were retrieved on the prevention, diagnosis, and treatment of this disorder. In such cases, the National Guideline Clearinghouse often provides very useful short syntheses of the available guidelines. Knowing that the NBRC cases selected for inclusion on the CSE generally abide by professional organization guidelines should provide enough motivation to obtain and review them when preparing for this exam.

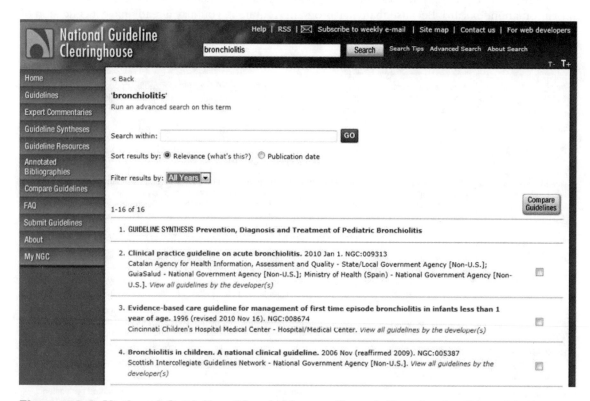

Figure 18-2 National Guideline Clearinghouse Search Results for Bronchiolitis Guidelines.

CSE STRUCTURE

In addition to understanding its unique content, as part of your preparation for your upcoming CSE, you need to consider the exam's unique structure, which differs substantially from other NBRC written exams. Your success on the CSE requires that you fully understand this structure and know how to apply this information when preparing for this exam.

Overall Structure and Sections

As previously discussed, rather than using single-concept, multiple-choice items, the CSE takes you through a set of clinical cases or patient management problems. Each case consists of a variable number of sections (averaging four to eight sections on the current CSE) in which you assess the patient's status and recommend or take appropriate actions as the situation evolves. Sections in which you collect and evaluate information are termed Information Gathering (IG) sections, whereas sections in which you recommend or implement interventions are called Decision-Making (DM) sections.

Figure 18-3 provides an example "flow chart" showing the structure of a hypothetical simulation of a case involving an immunocompromised cancer patient. This problem includes five sections, two IG sections, and three DM sections, with no "branching" (with the shorter problem format introduced in 2015, branching is less common than it was with the older, longer problems). Branching occurs when a selected answer triggers you to an alternate pathway (a branch) in the simulation. If present, branching may allow you to correct a wrong decision (a corrective branch). Branching also may allow for equivalent decisions—for example, initiating full ventilatory support with assist-control (A/C) ventilation or normal-rate synchronized intermittent mandatory ventilation (SIMV).

For every section of an NBRC simulation, content experts set both a maximum score (sum of all correct choice score values) and a minimum pass score. For example, an IG section may have a maximum score of 22 (IG Max) and a minimum pass score of 17 (IG Min), meaning that for that section, you would ideally get a score of at least 17 out of 22 or about 77% "correct." Although these minimum pass scores vary by problem, they typically range between 77% and 81% for IG and 60% and 70% for DM. To determine the CSE pass/fail, the NBRC set a cut score equal to the total minimum pass scores for every problem's IG and DM sections.

What does this scoring method mean for you, the candidate? Very simply, it means that the CSE IG and DM scores are essentially "averaged." Thus, a low score in one area (say, DM) can be offset by a high score in the other area (in this case, IG). As an example, we have seen cases where DM scores in the 30–40% correct range have been offset by IG scores above 90%, with the result being "Pass" and congratulations, RRT! Of course, the best way to assure passing the CSE is to do well on both IG and DM sections.

Relationship Between Information Gathering and Decision Making

Section 1 in Figure 18-3 is an example of an IG section in which a proper assessment would reveal that the patient is on 40 L/min and 70% O_2 with a Pao_2 of 58 torr. Vitals are HR = 133/min and RR = 26/min with evidence of respiratory distress. Breath sounds reveal diffuse coarse crackles that correspond with bilateral infiltrates on chest x-ray. The patient has a fever and is positive for a *Pseudomonas* infection.

Section 2 is an example of a DM section, in which the correct initial action (one among many choices) is to recommend/initiate invasive mechanical ventilation using the ARDSNet protocol. Note that this correct action or decision (like all actions in a CSE case) depends on the prior collection and proper evaluation of the relevant information—in this case, the evidence indicating that the problem is acute respiratory distress syndrome (ARDS) (P/F < 100 with bilateral infiltrates not due to a cardiac problem).

Understanding this linkage between the IG and DM sections is critical to your CSE preparation. Key pointers related to this understanding include the following:

1. You need to know which information to gather.
2. You need to know what the information means.
3. Your decisions always must be made in context.
4. The context usually involves a presumptive diagnosis.

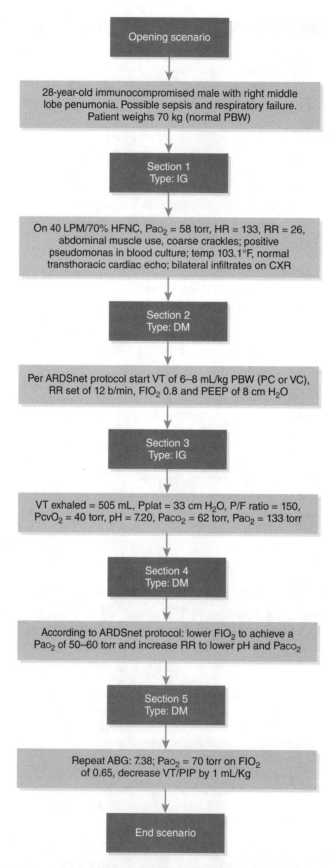

Figure 18-3 Flow Chart of Hypothetical Simulation for an Immunocompromised Oncology Patient.

Relationship Between NBRC Topics and CSE Skills

The good news is that your topical preparation for the CSE (and for the TMC exam) will help you address these important points. Simulation exam IG sections assess knowledge and skills like those emphasized in Section I of the topical content outlines (that is, which information you need to know and what it means). Likewise, the skills required to do well on CSE DM sections correspond mainly to the Section III topics. Knowing these parallels in coverage and emphasis can be extremely helpful in planning your preparation.

Disease Management and Diagnostic Reasoning

Given these close parallels between topical content and CSE skills, disease management preparation is essential to succeed in the CSE. Your decision making always must be made in context (pointer 3 mentioned above), and that context usually involves making a diagnosis (pointer 4 mentioned above). In our example problem (see Figure 18-3), it is never stated that the patient has developed or is developing ARDS. Instead, you must presume this to be the case—that is, you make a presumptive diagnosis. To make a presumptive diagnosis, you must carefully interpret the information you selected in the Information Gathering sections. Only by knowing or having a good idea of the problem you are dealing with can you make good management decisions. Thus, making correct decisions requires making a correct presumptive diagnosis.

However, you are not a physician, and disease diagnosis is not specified in the NBRC exam topical outlines, right? Well, yes and no. You are *not* a physician, but some essential themes embedded in major topic III-F of the NBRC topical outline (Utilize Evidence-Based Medicine Principles) are the following three skills:

- Determine the patient's pathophysiological state.
- Recommend changes in a therapeutic plan when indicated.
- Apply evidence-based or clinical practice guidelines.

This is precisely what is meant by making your decisions in context. First, determining the pathophysiological state means determining a presumptive diagnosis. Second, recommending the appropriate therapy and goals for the pathophysiologic state means taking actions or making recommendations with good knowledge of what is wrong with the patient at the time the decision must be made. Moreover, as in our example, the actions you recommend should be based on current practice guidelines whenever possible.

Based on our experience, it is in these areas that candidates have the most difficulty on the CSE, which explains why low DM scores are the most common reason for exam failure. To overcome this problem, we recommend you apply a technique called *reciprocal reasoning*. Reciprocal reasoning simply means that instead of thinking from disease or disorder to clinical findings (a common approach when studying for pathophysiology exams), you reverse this reasoning and think from clinical findings back to likely disorder (the process used by physicians in making diagnoses). For example:

Instead of Asking	Ask
What are the clinical findings that a patient suffering from ARDS would exhibit?	What is the likely problem in an immunocompromised man who exhibits respiratory distress, severe hypoxemia, and bilateral infiltrates on x-ray?

Of course, many disorders share at least some clinical findings. In our example (Figure 18-3), the initial information is also at least partially consistent with acute pulmonary edema due to heart failure. This, of course, is why we recommend that your disease management preparation should include identifying the common differential diagnoses for each condition and understanding what distinguishes the given diagnosis from those with similar findings. Returning to our example, the correct selection of the echocardiogram with its normal findings (along with the likelihood of *Pseudomonas aeruginosa* pneumonia) would rule out congestive heart failure (CHF)/pulmonary edema as the cause of the patient's problem. The bottom line is that you should not link a diagnosis to findings without consideration of other possible causes; instead, you should become familiar with common differential diagnoses and know what distinguishes each from the others.

SUMMARY OF CSE PREPARATION DO'S AND DON'TS

In review, some strategies used to prepare for the CSE are like those used to study for the TMC exam. At the same time, the unique content and structure of this exam demand a different approach. The following "Do's and Don'ts" summarize the approach we recommend to maximize your chances of passing the CSE.

Do's

- Do take the exam as soon as possible after achieving the high cut score in the TMC examination but allow 3 to 4 weeks for proper preparation.
- Do set aside approximately 3 to 4 weeks during which you can dedicate ample quality time for preparation for the CSE.
- Do focus on both the exam's topical coverage and disease management.
- Do prioritize your topical content review by assessing your TMC scores.
- For your topical review, do emphasize major NBRC topical content Section I (Chapters 1–5 in this text) and Section III (Chapters 9–17).
- Do spend the majority of your CSE preparation on disease management by case.
- Do use pathophysiology-focused texts for CSE disease management preparation.
- Do access and review current clinical practice and disease management guidelines.
- Do prepare written summaries covering the basic information about each common disorder you are likely to see on the CSE.
- Do be familiar with common differential diagnoses for a given disorder and know what distinguishes each from the others.
- Do use practice exam questions and simulation to get accustomed to the exam format and content.

Don'ts

- Don't prepare for the CSE by focusing solely on topical content.
- Don't prepare for the CSE by thinking from disorder to clinical findings; instead, reverse this reasoning, and think from clinical findings back to likely disorder.
- Don't link a diagnosis to findings without considering other possible causes (e.g., differential diagnoses).
- Don't underestimate the amount of quality time needed to adequately prepare for the exam.

CHAPTER 19

Taking the Clinical Simulation Exam

Narciso E. Rodriguez

To pass the NBRC Clinical Simulation Exam (CSE), you need to master the relevant content. However, your success on the CSE also requires that you fully understand its structure and format and use this information to become more proficient in taking this unique exam. Specifically, the CSE requires a different set of skills from those needed to succeed on multiple-choice exams (the *Test-Taking Tips* covered in the Navigate 2 companion website). This chapter intends to provide you with those skills, thereby increasing your likelihood of passing this portion of your boards.

CSE COMPUTER TESTING FORMAT AND OPTION SCORING

Rather than asking many single-concept, multiple-choice questions, the NBRC CSE has you progress through a set of short patient cases. Currently, the CSE includes 20 cases plus two that are being "pre-tested" and are not graded. Because the ungraded cases are not identified, you need to treat all problems as counting toward your CSE scores. You have 4 hours to complete all 22 cases.

Each case involves, on average, four to six sections. In the *Information Gathering (IG) sections*, you gather and assess the patient's status and/or response to interventions; in *Decision-Making (DM) sections*, you take actions or make recommendations.

As depicted in **Figure 19-1**, the computer presents each section of the case in three scrolling windows: the scenario window, the options window, and the history window. The scenario window provides current information about the patient or the evolving situation. The options window contains all the choices available to you in each section. The history window displays the options you chose and their results for the current and previously completed sections. A button allows you to "toggle" back and forth between these two different information views. A digital clock to help track elapsed time also can be toggled on/off, and a help screen can be activated anytime during the exam.

Section scenarios also direct you to either "CHOOSE ONLY ONE" or "SELECT AS MANY" for the responses provided in the options window. For IG sections, you always can select as many items as you consider necessary to assess the patient's current status according to the given scenario. In most DM sections, you are directed to select the single *best* action or recommendation according to the data gathered previously. Occasionally, DM sections permit the selection of multiple actions.

This response format differs significantly from the TMC format in several respects. First, some CSE sections allow you to select multiple options. Second, *once you choose a CSE option, you cannot change your response*. Third, each CSE response is graded on a multiple-point scale, rather than as merely right or wrong. Finally, every answer you select provides feedback.

We provide guidance on selecting multiple options later in this chapter. Regarding not being able to change responses, you want to be as confident as possible about choosing an option before checking it. However, due to the unique way options are scored and the allowance for corrective action, only infrequently will a given choice cause serious or permanent "damage" from which you cannot recover.

Part of the reason that a "wrong" choice may not seriously affect your overall CSE grade is that your responses are scored on a variable scale, like that depicted in **Table 19-1**. What this example scale makes clear is that some responses are "less wrong" than others—and some "more right" than others. Thus, if you must make an error in responding, you want it to be a minor error (–1) as opposed to a serious one (–2 to –3).

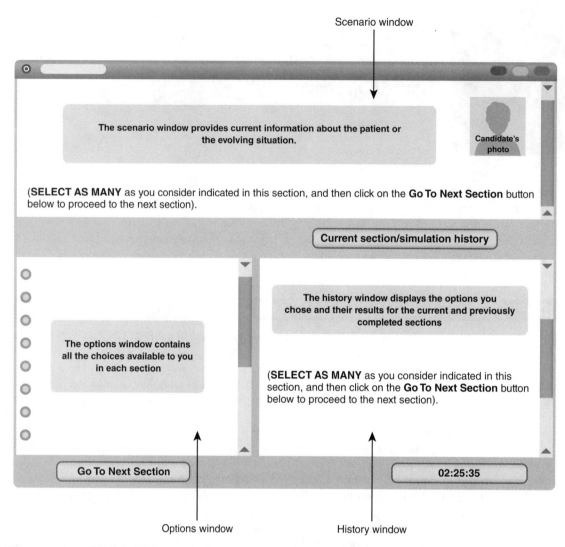

Scenario window

The scenario window provides current information about the patient or the evolving situation.

Candidate's photo

(**SELECT AS MANY** as you consider indicated in this section, and then click on the **Go To Next Section** button below to proceed to the next section).

Current section/simulation history

The history window displays the options you chose and their results for the current and previously completed sections

The options window contains all the choices available to you in each section

(**SELECT AS MANY** as you consider indicated in this section, and then click on the **Go To Next Section** button below to proceed to the next section).

Go To Next Section

02:25:35

Options window

History window

Figure 19-1 NBRC Clinical Simulation Exam Testing Format.

NBRC Candidate Handbook & Application, Figure 4 (p. 14). Copyright © 2016. The National Board for Respiratory Care, Inc. Reproduced with permission from the National Board for Respiratory Care, Inc.

Table 19-1 Illustrative CSE Options Scoring Scale*

Score	General Meaning
+3[†]	Critically necessary in identifying or resolving the problem
+2	Strongly facilitative in identifying or resolving the problem
+1	Somewhat facilitative in identifying or resolving the problem
−1	Uninformative or potentially harmful in identifying or resolving the problem
−2	Wastes critical time in identifying the problem or causes some patient harm
−3[†]	Unnecessarily invasive, gravely harmful, or illegal action

*Not official NBRC scaling.
[†]+3 or −3 scoring is rare; most options are scored in the +2 to −2 range.

However, how do you know if a given choice is an error, or how serious the error might be? Technically, you do not know. However, every option in a CSE case provides feedback. For IG options, this typically includes either the requested patient data or feedback such as "Results pending" or "Sample sent to the laboratory" or "Not performed" or "Physician disagrees." Likewise, for DM sections, feedback may include new patient status information or "Done" or "Ordered" or "Not done—make another selection in this section" or "Physician disagrees—make another selection in this section." Although none of this feedback definitively indicates that a right or wrong choice has been made, when considered in context, you usually can infer the impact and take appropriate corrective action.

For IG sections, feedback such as "Not performed" or "Physician disagrees" suggests that your choice may be wasting time, may cause harm to the patient, or may be unnecessarily invasive. If you receive this type of feedback and remaining unselected options could provide equivalent information but are quicker, easier to obtain, less harmful, or less invasive, be sure to select them. In this manner, you will likely be able to "cancel out" a negatively weighted response with a positive one.

For DM sections, the "Not done" or "Physician disagrees" feedback that directs you to make another selection may or may not indicate an error. In some cases, this feedback is used to force a choice (without penalty) that guides you to the next programmed section of the case. However, the same type of feedback may indicate that you have made an error. This is usually apparent if after making a decision, you are directed to a section indicating a worsening of the patient's status. If so, do not fret over what may have been an incorrect action or recommendation. Instead, realize that likely you are being allowed to correct your initial error. Such "corrective branches" in a case never allow you to recoup any lost points completely, but they do allow you to lessen the impact of a wrong prior decision. For example, if a DM choice scored as –2 provides a corrective branch, likely the best remedial action will be scored +1, with the net result still being negative *but less so*. In these situations, the key is to use the feedback provided in the case to recognize the potential error and correct it immediately.

SCENARIO GUIDANCE

Typically, the opening scenario describes the setting, your role, and basic patient information. As the case evolves, subsequent scenarios provide additional patient information, including response to therapy. **Table 19-2** provides our general guidance regarding CSE scenarios as a series of basic "*Do's and Don'ts*."

If the scenario indicates an emergency:

- Gather only essential or quick-to-obtain information; do not waste time performing or recommending complex or lengthy assessment procedures.
- Once the problem at hand is clear, immediately proceed with the appropriate emergency protocol or action.

Also, from the opening scenario onward, you should be building your list of potential problems and figuring out how to distinguish among those with common signs and symptoms—that is, performing a *differential diagnosis*. **Table 19-3** lists examples of differential diagnoses that often

Table 19-2 Scenario Do's and Don'ts

Do's	Don'ts
Do decide if the situation is an emergency and begin "differential diagnosis" early on.	**Don't** make assumptions about the scenario—consider only the facts presented to you.
Do identify and assess all key patient data (objective/subjective), including any information indicating changes in patient status.	**Don't** worry if the setting (e.g., pulmonary function test [PFT] lab or patient's home) or situation is unfamiliar to you. Your basic knowledge of respiratory care will always apply, regardless of setting or situation.

Table 19-3 Examples of Clinical Simulation Exam Differential Diagnoses

Example Differential Diagnoses	Key Information to Seek
Adult	
Reversible obstruction (asthma) versus irreversible (Emphysema)	Pre-/post-bronchodilator results
Myasthenia gravis versus Guillain-Barré syndrome	Tensilon test, AChR, CSF fluid tests
Congestive heart failure (CHF) versus ARDS	History; pulmonary artery wedge pressure or echocardiogram
Carbon monoxide (CO) poisoning versus alcohol/drug overdose	History (CO exposure), HbCO
Pediatric/Neonatal	
Epiglottitis versus laryngotracheobronchitis (croup)	Symptoms + neck x-rays (AP and lateral)
Childhood asthma versus foreign body aspiration	History, physical (e.g., unilateral wheezing), response to β-agonist therapy, chest/neck x-rays
Newborn pulmonary hypertension versus RDS	Pre-postductal SpO_2, chest x-ray
Transient tachypnea of the newborn (TTN) versus RDS	History, disease progression, chest x-ray

Table 19-4 Information Gathering Do's and Don'ts

Do's	Don'ts
Do review and consider all options first.	**Don't** be too curious about unfamiliar options—if you have never heard of it, it likely is there to distract you.
Do prioritize options yielding data that can identify the problem or resolve the situation at hand.	**Don't** skimp on choices—trying to figure out the problem with the least amount of data is a mistake that will cost you points.
Do select options in a logical order, from basic to advanced choices.	**Don't** select all options—usually at least some of the choices carry a penalty.

show up on the CSE, along with some of the diagnostic tools that can help distinguish between them. This is important because *depending on the diagnosis/problem at hand, treatments can be very different.*

INFORMATION GATHERING (IG) GUIDANCE

Do's and Don'ts

You determine the diagnosis or problem at hand as well as the patient's response to therapy primarily via the IG sections of the case. As with CSE scenarios, important Do's and Don'ts apply to selecting options in IG sections, as outlined in **Table 19-4**.

Regarding reviewing and considering all IG options, it is important to note that the CSE options window usually *must be scrolled down to reveal all choices.* Don't miss out on possible good choices by failing to reveal all the options available to you on that section!

The most important criterion to consider in selecting available IG options is their *relevance*—that is, *will the information help identify the problem or resolve the situation at hand?* For example, if the patient likely has a progressive neuromuscular disorder or is being considered for weaning from ventilatory support, a vital capacity measurement may be relevant, and therefore would be indicated.

However, the same measure would not provide useful information (and would waste time) when caring for a patient with acute myocardial infarction in the emergency department (ED).

We also recommend selecting IG options in a logical order, from *basic to advanced*. For example, if the patient's pulse is irregular or arrhythmias are suspected, consider selecting the ECG, if available, for the additional information it may provide. In this manner, the selection of one option may indicate the need to choose another.

Selection of one option can also sometimes rule out the selection of other options. For example, when assessing a newborn infant in respiratory distress, if inspection and breath sounds indicate bilateral lung expansion, you would not select an option to perform transillumination (to diagnose a pneumothorax).

"Always Select" Choices

Although you probably have been taught that there are few, if any, absolutes in patient management, when taking the CSE, a few generally do apply. Typically, this information is vital, harmless to the patient, quick to obtain, and almost always helpful in identifying the problem at hand or the patient's response to therapy. Information in the "Always Select" category includes the following:

- General appearance (e.g., color)
- Vital signs
  - Respiratory rate—always
  - Heart rate—always
  - Pulse oximetry Sp_{O_2} (*obtain Sa_{O_2} via CO-oximetry if the patient has experienced smoke inhalation*)
  - Blood pressure—if the patient has a cardiovascular problem
  - Body temperature—if infection/hypothermia is likely
- Level of consciousness
  - *Basic*: sensorium assessment (e.g., "oriented × 3")
  - *Advanced*: Glasgow Coma Scale score (e.g., for patients who are unconscious or brain-injured)
- Breath sounds
- History of present illness (if readily available)

Selecting Respiratory-Related Information

As described in **Table 19-5**, additional respiratory-related information that you may want to consider will depend on the situation at hand. For example, an arterial blood gas is needed only if knowledge of the patient's acid-base balance, ventilation, or oxygenation is required to identify the problem or to make a decision. Likewise, other common respiratory-related information will be relevant in some situations but not in others.

Table 19-5 Selecting Respiratory-Related Information

Information	Select To
Arterial blood gas	Assess acid-base balance, ventilation, or oxygenation
Tracheal position	Identify pneumothorax (shift away) or atelectasis (shift toward)
Percussion	Identify pneumothorax (hyperresonant note) or consolidation/pneumonia (dull note)
MIP/NIF	Assess respiratory muscle strength (neuromuscular disorders, weaning)
Vital capacity (VC)	Assess inspiratory/expiratory muscle function (neuromuscular disorders, weaning)
$\dot{V}_E$, RR, RSBI	Evaluate the adequacy of ventilation (need for ventilatory support/weaning)
Sputum production	Assess for infection or secretion clearance problems

Selecting Pulmonary Function and Exercise Test Information

Similarly, you should be sensible in seeking pulmonary function test (PFT) or exercise test information. For example, not every patient situation calls for a diffusing capacity study or comprehensive exercise evaluation. You can help eliminate some of these unnecessary choices by asking yourself a simple question: *"If I had this information in this situation, what would I do with it?"* **Table 19-6** provides additional guidance on selecting PFT or exercise test data in CSE IG sections.

Of course, PFT information also serves as a good illustration of testing that should be deferred in emergencies. For example, you would *not* recommend obtaining bedside spirometry data for a patient in the ED who is currently being treated for a severe exacerbation of asthma or chronic obstructive pulmonary disease (COPD).

Selecting Laboratory Tests

Laboratory tests also appear as common options in IG sections of the CSE exam. **Table 19-7** lists the lab tests that most frequently appear on the CSE exam, along with their common use. As with PFTs, selection of lab data is situation specific. For example, although cardiac enzymes would be a good choice when assessing an adult patient with acute chest pain, they would not be needed to evaluate a child with metabolic acidosis due to renal failure.

Table 19-6 Selecting Pulmonary Function and Exercise Test Information

Test	Select To
Spirometry (FEV)	Assess surgical risk; detect obstruction/reversibility
Functional residual capacity (FRC), residual volume (RV), total lung capacity (TLC)	Differentiate between obstructive and restrictive conditions
Bronchoprovocation	Assess for airway hyperresponsiveness and inflammation
Diffusing capacity (DLco)	Identify the cause of restrictive disorders; assess the feasibility of lung reduction surgery
Exercise testing	Evaluate tolerance for exertion (e.g., for pulmonary rehabilitation), diagnose coronary artery disease, differentiate cardiac versus pulmonary limits to exercise capacity

Table 19-7 Selecting Laboratory Tests

Information	Select to:
Hemoglobin (Hb), hematocrit (Hct), red blood cells (RBCs)	Evaluate O_2 carrying capacity; assess for anemia, hemodilution, hemoconcentration, or bleeding
White blood cells (WBCs), differential	Assess for presence of bacterial/viral infections
Platelets, INR, prothrombin time (PT)	Evaluate blood clotting and bleeding abnormalities (especially if ordering/performing an ABG)
Electrolytes	Determine the type of metabolic acid-base imbalance (anion gap); identify causes of selected cardiac arrhythmias and neuromuscular abnormalities
Blood urea nitrogen (BUN), creatinine	Assess renal function and metabolic acid-base imbalances
Lactate/lactic acid	Determine the presence of tissue hypoxia (e.g., shock, ARDS, cyanide poisoning), sepsis
Total protein, albumin	Assess for malnutrition, weaning difficulties, or liver disease
Cardiac enzymes (CK, troponin, BNP)	Assess for myocardial damage (e.g., myocardial infarction) or congestive heart failure

Table 19-8 Selecting Imaging Studies

Information	Select to:
Chest x-ray	Assess for atelectasis, consolidation, pneumothorax, and tube and catheter positions
Neck x-ray	Differentiate causes of stridor (croup versus epiglottitis); to help detect foreign-body aspiration (only for radiopaque objects)
CT/MRI	Thoracic: Detect tumors, aortic aneurysm, effusions, and chest trauma Head/neck: Evaluate for traumatic brain, neck, or spine injury
CT angiography	Identify the presence and extent of pulmonary embolism
Thoracic ultrasound	Detect fluid in thorax, pneumothorax, or chest trauma; guide thoracentesis
V/Q perfusion scan	Help diagnose or rule out a pulmonary embolism
PET scan	Identify malignant tumors

Selecting Imaging Studies

The other common diagnostic procedures that often appear in IG sections are various imaging modalities. As with lab tests, not all imaging tests apply to all situations. As outlined in **Table 19-8**, you should select the test only if it is indicated and can provide the information needed to identify or resolve the problem at hand. In terms of emergencies, you should note that chest and neck x-rays, computed tomography (CT) scans, and thoracic ultrasounds are all standard tools in emergency medicine and may be indicated in selected situations, especially head or chest trauma.

ANALYSIS: THE MISSING LINK BETWEEN INFORMATION GATHERING AND DECISION MAKING

In our experience, many candidates who fail the CSE do so not because they select the wrong information, but rather because they do not apply the information to the situation at hand. This problem is usually evident when the candidate has a high IG score but a low DM score.

The problem in these cases is failing to understand that information gathering involves not one but two key steps:

1. You must select the right information.
2. Once the information is in hand, you need to *analyze what it means.*

Based on our prior guidance, selecting the right information should not be overly difficult. The more challenging task is analyzing what the selected information means and what to do with it. As indicated in **Figure 19-2**, *analysis* represents the missing link between gathering the needed information and making the correct decisions.

Of course, to correctly analyze patient information, you first must know what constitutes "normal" for every data element. Tables of normal values and reference ranges are provided for all essential patient data throughout Section I of this text (Chapters 1–17).

However, beyond "knowing your normal," you need to recognize what an abnormal result means, in terms of both altered function *and* treatment options. A simple example would be a fall in SpO_2 from 93% to 88% in an adult on 2 L/min nasal O_2 who recently underwent upper abdominal surgery. You would rightfully conclude that this result is below normal and requires an increase in FIO_2 or O_2 flow. However, you should also consider that this finding may indicate developing atelectasis, which could require some form of lung expansion or airway clearance therapy. As previously discussed, this simple finding should also provoke consideration of other, more advanced information, such as the patient's most recent chest x-ray.

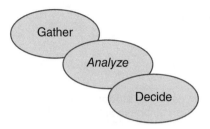

**Figure 19-2 Analysis:
The Critical Link Between
Information Gathering
and Decision Making.**

DECISION-MAKING GUIDANCE

Most simulation problems include at least one or two DM sections. However, the possibility exists of having a case in which the majority (if not all) of the sections are DM sections. These sections typically provide you with options for managing the problem, usually in the form of taking an action or making a recommendation.

Do's and Don'ts

As with IG sections and as delineated in **Table 19-9**, there are "Do's and Don'ts" that apply to selecting options in DM sections.

The first "Do" is the most critical—that is, selecting the *best* action based on your analysis of the information you have gathered. Although there are hundreds of different patient situations that you might encounter, only a limited number of decision-making actions apply to the most common clinical findings seen on the simulation exam.

Decision Making Based on Physical Assessment Findings

As shown in **Table 19-10**, several common physical findings can help you identify the most likely problem and, therefore, the most appropriate action. For example, if you hear wheezing on auscultation in an adult, the most likely problems are bronchospasm and congestive heart failure. If other data (e.g., the patient's history) indicate bronchospasm, the most appropriate action would be bronchodilator administration. Conversely, if the problem appears to be congestive heart failure, diuresis, and administration of a positive inotropic agent should be recommended. Wheezing in a child also could be due to bronchospasm, but may indicate foreign-body aspiration, in which case bronchoscopic removal would be indicated.

Decision Making Based on Problems with Secretions and/or Airway Clearance

Similar guidance applies if the information given indicates potential problems with secretions or airway clearance (**Table 19-11**). Again, the findings suggest the problem, and the problem (in the context of the clinical scenario) establishes the action or actions needed to resolve it. This is the basic sequence of reasoning that must guide you in linking information and action.

Decision Making Based on Problems Involving Acid-Base Imbalances

Because a substantial number of CSE cases usually involve disturbances in acid-base balance, you need to be proficient both in blood gas interpretation and in the management of these disturbances. **Table 19-12** provides a basic summary of the problems and appropriate actions indicated for the

Table 19-9 Decision-Making Do's and Don'ts

Do's	Don'ts
Do select the best action based on your analysis of the prior information.	**Don't** worry if your favorite action is missing.
Do think about your choice before making a selection.	**Don't** select more than one choice unless directed to do so.
Do read all responses carefully (e.g., "Physician disagrees," "Action taken").	**Don't** select unfamiliar actions.

Table 19-10 Basic Decision Making Based on Physical Assessment Findings

Information Gathering	Analysis (Likely Problems)	Decision Making/Action
Wheezing	Bronchospasm	Bronchodilator therapy
	CHF	Diuretics, positive inotropes*
	Foreign body (child)	Bronchoscopy
Stridor	Laryngeal edema	Cool mist/racemic epinephrine
	Foreign body (child)	Laryngoscopy*
	Tumor/mass	Bronchoscopy*
Rhonchi/tactile fremitus	Secretions in large airways	Bronchial hygiene therapy, suctioning
Dull percussion note, bronchial breath sounds	Infiltrates, atelectasis, consolidation	Lung expansion therapy, O_2 therapy
Opacity on chest x-ray	Infiltrates, atelectasis, consolidation	Lung expansion therapy, O_2 therapy
Hyperresonant percussion	Pneumothorax	Evacuate air*/lung expansion therapy
Dull percussion	Pleural effusion	Evacuate fluid*/lung expansion therapy

*Actions you would recommend.

Table 19-11 Basic Decision Making for Problems with Secretions or Airway Clearance

Information Gathering	Analysis (Likely Problems)	Decision Making/Action
Weak cough	Poor secretion clearance	Bronchial hygiene therapy, suctioning
Amount: more than 30 mL/day	Excessive secretions	Bronchial hygiene therapy, suctioning
Yellow/opaque sputum	Acute airway infection	Treat the underlying cause, antibiotic therapy*
Watery, frothy secretions	Pulmonary edema	Treat underlying cause (CHF*), PAP therapy (CPAP/BiPAP), O_2 therapy

*Actions you would recommend.

most common acid-base imbalances you will see on the CSE. For example, besides identifying the presence of an acute metabolic acidosis in a patient with shock-like symptoms, you would need to know that this condition likely is lactic acidosis and that measures to improve tissue oxygenation need to be implemented, including providing a high F_{IO_2} and improving cardiac output.

Table 19-12 Basic Decision Making for Acid-Base Imbalance

Information Gathering	Analysis (Likely Problems)	Decision Making/Action
$\downarrow pH = \dfrac{HCO_3}{\uparrow Paco_2}$	Acute ventilatory failure (acute respiratory acidosis)	Mechanical ventilation*
$\leftrightarrow pH = \dfrac{\uparrow\uparrow HCO_3}{\uparrow Paco_2}$	Chronic ventilatory failure (compensated respiratory acidosis, as in COPD)	Low-flow O_2, bronchial hygiene therapy; if worsens $\Rightarrow$ NPPV*; HFNC, avoid intubation if possible
$\uparrow pH = \dfrac{\uparrow HCO_3}{Paco_2}$	Acute metabolic alkalosis	Hypokalemia $\Rightarrow$ give potassium* Hypochloremia $\Rightarrow$ give chloride*
$\downarrow pH = \dfrac{\downarrow HCO_3}{Paco_2}$	Acute metabolic acidosis	Increase ventilation (temporary); if lactic acidosis $\Rightarrow$ give O_2 and restore perfusion; treat underlying cause*

$\uparrow$, increased; $\downarrow$, decreased; $\leftrightarrow$, normal/unchanged; $\uparrow\uparrow$, compensation.
*Actions you would recommend.

Table 19-13 Basic Decision Making for Oxygenation Disturbances

Information Gathering	Analysis (Likely Problems)	Decision Making/Action
$Pao_2 > 60$ torr $Fio_2 < 0.60$	Moderate hypoxemia (V/Q imbalance)	O_2 therapy Treat underlying cause*
$Pao_2 < 60$ torr $Fio_2 > 0.60$	Severe hypoxemia (pulmonary shunting)	O_2 therapy, PEEP/CPAP Treat underlying cause*

*Actions you would recommend.

Decision Making Based on Problems Involving Disturbances of Oxygenation

When responding to blood gas data, we strongly recommend that you assess oxygenation separately from acid-base balance and ventilation. In this regard, recognizing the presence of hypoxemia represents only part of the needed task in a CSE case. You must then identify the basic pathophysiologic cause of the low Po_2 or saturation and treat it accordingly, as outlined in **Table 19-13**. To that end, we teach the 60/60 rule: If the Pao_2 is greater than 60 torr on less than 60% O_2, the likely problem is a V/Q imbalance, which usually responds well to simple O_2 therapy.

In contrast, if the arterial Po_2 is less than 60 torr on more than 60% O_2, the likely problem is a severe shunting (likely due to ARDS), which in addition to supplemental O_2 will require either positive end-expiratory pressure (PEEP) or continuous positive airway pressure (CPAP). Note that a similar rule uses 50% O_2 and a Po_2 of 50 torr. Because both cutoffs (60/60; 50/50) represent a P/F ratio of 100, they are equivalent.

PACING YOURSELF WHEN TAKING THE CSE

Our last suggestion is the simplest: You need to pace yourself to ensure that you can complete all CSE cases in the available time. In our experience, candidates who do not complete all CSE problems are destined to fail. Based on the number of problems currently included on the CSE (20 graded plus two being pre-tested) and the exam time limit of 4 hours, you should spend, on average, no more than 10 minutes on each problem. However, because problems vary in complexity, our best advice for the current CSE is to ensure completion of at least five problems every hour.

SUMMARY GUIDANCE AND NEXT STEPS

To succeed on the NBRC CSE exam, you need to be proficient in the management of a wide variety of cases that respiratory therapists (RTs) can encounter in clinical practice. In addition to good knowledge of disease management, you need to apply a consistent reasoning process as you progress through each section of your CSE problems:

GATHER → ANALYZE → DECIDE

1. *Gather* the information most consistent with the situation at hand.
2. *Analyze* the information to identify the likely problem and current patient status.
3. *Decide* on the action(s) most likely to resolve the identified problem.

Consistent application of this process will help boost both your scores, increasing your likelihood of passing the CSE, and obtaining your Registered Respiratory Therapist (RRT) credential.

Your next steps? Apply what you have learned here by completing the practice problems available online at the accompanying Jones & Bartlett Navigate 2 companion website. These practice problems are designed to give you experience with the CSE format and to help you apply the case management and CSE test-taking skills reviewed here. If you score poorly on any individual practice problem or consistently have difficulty with either information gathering or decision making, we recommend you review this chapter's guidance and the corresponding disease management "pearls" provided in Chapter 20.

Clinical Simulation Exam Case Management Pearls

Narciso E. Rodriguez and Albert J. Heuer

As emphasized in Chapters 18 and 19, success on the NBRC Clinical Simulation Examination (CSE) requires proficiency in case management. In the NBRC "hospital," respiratory therapists (RTs) are expected to be broadly experienced in managing a large variety of disorders, including those affecting various organ systems and patient age categories, as well as different levels of acuity.

Although it is impossible to cover every disorder that RTs might encounter on the CSE, this chapter aims to assist candidates in reviewing the management of the problems most likely to appear in each category of the CSE. We do so by using the basic NBRC CSE disease categories as the organizing principle. For each disorder, we then provide "pearls" or valuable pointers covering both the essential elements of assessment and information gathering needed to evaluate the typical case and the currently recommended treatments or decisions required to achieve successful outcomes.

A careful review of these management pearls, in combination with the available online resources accompanying this book, will provide a strong foundation for your success on the CSE.

ADULT CHRONIC AIRWAY DISEASE

Number of Simulations in the CSE: 7 Cases

This is probably the most critical section of the CSE, having the largest number of cases. A significant amount of time must be spent in this area to be successful in this examination.

Chronic airway diseases encompass several disease entities (emphysema, chronic bronchitis, cystic fibrosis, asthma, and bronchiectasis), all characterized by chronic, progressive airway obstruction that (in most cases) is not *fully* reversible with treatment. This set of conditions are commonly referred to as chronic obstructive pulmonary diseases or COPD. In the case of emphysema and chronic bronchitis, airway obstruction is mostly caused by inflammation due to long-term inhalation of noxious particles or gases, especially tobacco smoke.

Asthma is a chronic inflammatory disease characterized by airway inflammation, intermittent and *reversible* airflow obstruction, and bronchial hyperresponsiveness. Since asthma can affect most age groups but is more prevalent in children and young adults, it will be discussed in the pediatric section. Bronchiectasis and cystic fibrosis are discussed somewhere else in this chapter. In this section, we will only focus on emphysema and chronic bronchitis.

The NBRC CSE exam now differentiates between outpatient and in-hospital/critical care management of the COPD patient. To assist candidates in preparing for this disease management category, we cover each separately.

COPD: Outpatient Management

Assessment/Information Gathering

The primary disease entities categorized as COPD are emphysema and chronic bronchitis. *Emphysema* is defined in pathologic terms as irreversible destruction of the alveolar and airway walls causing enlargement of the distal air spaces, the collapse of the small airways, air trapping, and hyperinflation. *Chronic bronchitis* is defined by its symptoms—that is, productive cough for at least 3 months per year for at least 2 years. Although most patients with COPD exhibit elements of both disorders, some key characteristics differentiate patients with a primary diagnosis of emphysema from those suffering mainly from chronic bronchitis (**Table 20-1**).

Table 20-1 Emphysema Versus Chronic Bronchitis

Characteristic	Emphysema	Chronic Bronchitis
Age	More than 50 years old	More than 35 years old
Cough	Late; scanty sputum	Early; copious mucopurulent sputum
Dyspnea	Severe, early	Mild, late
Appearance	Thin and cachectic; barrel chest (elevated ribs), accessory muscle use at rest	Normal weight or obese; cyanotic, peripheral edema, jugular venous distention
Chest exam	↓ Breath sounds, hyperresonant to percussion, ↓ diaphragm excursion, barrel chest	Rhonchi, wheezing
X-ray	Hyperinflation, small heart, flattened diaphragm, ↑ A-P diameter on a lateral film	Prominent vessels, large heart (↑ CT ratio)
Spirometry	FEV_1/FVC ($FEV_1\%$) < 70% after bronchodilator therapy	FEV_1/FVC ($FEV_1\%$) < 70% after bronchodilator therapy
Lung volumes	Increased RV, TLC	Increased RV
Airway resistance	Increased (small airways)	Increased (large airways)
Compliance	Increased	Normal
DLco	Decreased	Normal
Arterial blood gases	Mild hypoxemia; may have normal Pa_{CO_2}	Chronic respiratory acidosis with moderate hypoxemia
Other lab tests	Decreased α_1-antitrypsin*	Polycythemia

*Evident in less than 1% of COPD patients; should be assessed if emphysema appears at a young age (45 years or younger) or without a history of smoking.

FEV, forced expiratory volume; FVC, forced vital capacity; RV, residual volume; TLC, total lung capacity.

Treatment/Decision Making

Treatment of stable COPD aims to increase patients' life expectancy and quality of life while also decreasing complications and exacerbations requiring hospitalization. Comprehensive care should include:

- Smoking cessation
- Disease management education
- Pulmonary rehabilitation
- Avoidance of triggers
- Dietary counseling
- Prevention of recurrent infections via immunization against influenza and pneumococcal pneumonia
- Antibiotics only for those patients who are most likely to have a bacterial infection or are most ill

As indicated in **Table 20-2**, additional treatment is "stepped up" according to the stage of disease progression and the severity of symptoms. Note that neither mucolytics nor the routine use of antibiotics is recommended to manage stable COPD, even in its advanced stages.

Disease management should be implemented for all COPD patients, with the following management goals:

- Slow disease progression/reduce mortality
- Improve health status/quality of life
- Increase tolerance for activities of daily living
- Relieve life-altering symptoms
- Prevent or minimize hospital admissions

Table 20-2 Chronic Obstructive Pulmonary Disease (COPD) Treatment Approaches by Severity Stage

Stage I: Mild	Stage II: Moderate	Stage III: Severe	Stage IV: Very Severe
Diagnostic/Prognostic Criteria			
• $FEV_1/FVC < 70\%$ • $FEV_1 \geq 80\%$ predicted	• $FEV_1/FVC < 70\%$ • $FEV_1 = 50–79\%$ predicted • SOB on exertion	• $FEV_1/FVC < 70\%$ • $FEV_1 = 30–49\%$ predicted • SOB on exertion • Frequent exacerbations	• $FEV_1/FVC < 70\%$ • $FEV_1 < 30\%$ predicted or • $FEV_1 < 50\%$ predicted + chronic respiratory failure
"Stepped" Treatment Approaches *(All stages should include disease management education, smoking cessation, pulmonary rehabilitation, and influenza and pneumococcal vaccination.)*			
• SABA or inhaled anticholinergic (e.g., tiotropium) PRN	• Regular use of LABA • Consider combined LABA + long-acting anticholinergic	• Add inhaled steroids if frequent exacerbations • Consider combining steroid + LABA (e.g., fluticasone + salmeterol)	• Add long-term O_2 therapy if justified • Consider lung volume reduction surgery (emphysema only)
FEV, forced expiratory volume; FVC, forced vital capacity; LABA, long-acting β-agonist; RV, residual volume; SABA, short-acting β-agonist; SOB, shortness of breath; TLC, total lung capacity.			

Key elements in COPD disease management include the following:

- Smoking cessation and avoidance of other triggers/risk factors
- Preventive care (healthy lifestyle, flu + pneumococcal vaccinations, exercise)
- "Stepped" treatment to control/reduce symptoms (described previously)
- Patient education appropriate to the disease stage and patient/caregiver health literacy
- Dietary management
- Self-management "action" plans to deal with exacerbations and minimize hospital readmissions
- Prophylactic use of antibiotics for infection prevention
- Pulmonary rehabilitation, ideally with community support
- Psychological counseling as needed
- Ongoing monitoring and follow-up (at least twice per year) to maximize compliance with the care plan

COPD—In-Hospital, Critical Care Management

The need for acute care of patients with COPD typically occurs due to an exacerbation of the condition, causing worsening of symptoms and overall deterioration of respiratory status.

Assessment/Information Gathering

Signs and symptoms of an acute exacerbation of COPD may include any of the following:

- Increased dyspnea
- Increased heart and respiratory rate
- Increased cough and sputum production
- Change in sputum color or character
- Use of accessory muscles of respiration
- Peripheral edema
- Development or increase in wheezing and chest tightness
- Change in mental status

- Fatigue
- Fever
- A decrease in FEV_1 or peak expiratory flow
- Hypoxemia

Change in mental status or a combination of two or more of the following new symptoms indicates a severe acute exacerbation:

- Dyspnea at rest
- Cyanosis
- Respiratory rate > 25/min
- Heart rate > 110/min
- Use of accessory muscles of respiration

When a patient with known COPD presents with a moderate to severe exacerbation, the following should be considered:

- History:
  - Baseline respiratory status
  - Present treatment regimen and recent medication use
  - Signs of airway infection (e.g., fever and change in volume and color of sputum)
  - Duration of worsening symptoms
  - Limitation of activities (e.g., decreased ability to walk, eat, or sleep due to dyspnea)
  - History of previous exacerbations
  - Increased cough
  - A decrease in exercise tolerance/increase in dyspnea
  - Chest tightness
  - Change in alertness
  - Other nonspecific symptoms, including malaise, difficulty sleeping, and fatigue
  - Symptoms associated with comorbid acute and chronic conditions
- Physical Examination:
  - Measurement of vital signs (T, P, R, + BP)
  - Measurement of SpO_2
  - Respiratory distress
  - Accessory respiratory muscle use
  - Increased pulmonary findings (e.g., wheezing, decreased air entry, prolonged expiratory phase)
  - Peripheral edema
  - Somnolence and hyperactivity
  - Acute comorbid conditions
- Laboratory/Imaging:
  - Chest radiograph to exclude an alternative diagnosis
  - Arterial blood gas (in patients with a SpO_2 < 88%, history of hypercapnia, somnolence, or other evidence of impending respiratory failure [e.g., tachypnea, accessory muscle use])
  - Theophylline level (if theophylline is being utilized)
  - Sputum culture and sensitivity if exacerbation likely due to infection (e.g., fever and change in volume and color of sputum)
  - Brain natriuretic peptide (BNP) to help rule out left ventricular failure (congestive heart failure [CHF]) as the cause of dyspnea

Note that in patients with an acute COPD exacerbation, spirometry is of little value. For that reason, oximetry and arterial blood gases (ABGs) should be monitored. Likewise, unless the diagnosis is unclear or the need exists to evaluate comorbidities, there is little evidence supporting the routine ordering of electrocardiography or echocardiography for these patients.

Treatment/Decision Making

Basic Management

Basic management of the patient requiring treatment for an acute exacerbation of COPD includes the following:

- Provide supplemental O_2 to maintain PaO_2 of 60–65 torr/SpO_2 of 88–92%
- Recommend increasing the β-agonist dose and frequency
- Recommend adding inhaled anticholinergic (if not already prescribed)
- Recommend systemic steroids (in addition to inhaled steroids)
- Recommend antibiotic and antiviral therapy if secretions are copious and purulent
- Provide nutritional support
- Discuss palliative care or end-of-life options with patients and family members for those with end-stage disease

Assessing Patient Response

Evidence indicating a positive response to treatment of an acute exacerbation of COPD includes the following: decreased work of breathing and improved oxygenation; decrease in cough, sputum production, fever, or dyspnea; decrease in respiratory and heart rate; decrease in accessory muscle use.

Patients who fail to respond to treatment of an acute exacerbation normally should be admitted to the hospital. Indicators of treatment failure include the following:

- A marked increase in the intensity of symptoms
- The onset of new physical signs indicating deterioration (e.g., cyanosis, peripheral edema, cardiac arrhythmias)
- Increasing hypoxemia despite supplemental O_2
- New or worsening CO_2 retention or pH < 7.25–7.30
- Newly occurring cardiac arrhythmias
- Decreased level of consciousness

Ventilatory Support

Patients suffering an acute exacerbation of COPD who fail to respond to initial basic management and develop worsening respiratory acidosis, fatigue, and a decreased level of consciousness usually will require ventilatory support. Due to the many complications associated with invasive ventilation and the fact that intubated COPD patients can be very difficult to wean unless contraindicated, non-invasive positive-pressure ventilation (NPPV) is the preferred approach.

- Good initial NPPV settings are as follows:
  - Inspiratory positive airway pressure (IPAP) = 10 cm H_2O, expiratory positive airway pressure (EPAP) = 5 cm H_2O. Readjust as needed according to exhaled tidal volume.
  - Backup rate = 10/min
  - Enough expiratory time to allow complete exhalation (I:E ratio of 1:3 or lower)
  - FiO_2 to assure $SpO_2 \geq$ 88–95%
- Adjust to relieve tachypnea and reduce accessory muscle use
- Always aim for a normal pH, not necessarily a normal PCO_2
- To increase tidal volume and ventilation during NPPV, increase the IPAP pressure
- If air trapping/auto-PEEP occurs during NPPV and the PCO_2/pH are adequate, raise EPAP and IPAP equally (this raises EPAP but keeps ΔP constant)

Weaning from NPPV is best accomplished by progressively decreasing the time off the ventilator during the day; many patients will still require at least some nocturnal support. Intubation and invasive ventilation may be required if contraindications against using NPPV are present (**Table 20-3**).

Table 20-3 Contraindications Against Using Noninvasive Positive-Pressure Ventilation (NPPV)

Contraindications Against Using NPPV	
Respiratory	**Non-Respiratory**
Respiratory arrest	Cardiac arrest/hemodynamic instability
Upper airway obstruction	Mental status changes (i.e., obtundation)
Unable to protect the airway	Active upper gastrointestinal bleeding
Unable to clear respiratory secretions	Facial surgery or trauma
High risk for aspiration	Facial deformity
	Nonfitting mask (i.e., significant air leaks)
	Nausea or vomiting

Intubation and invasive ventilation also may be required in the presence of:

- NPPV failure, for example:
  - Worsening of ABGs in first 1 to 2 hours
  - Lack of improvement in ABGs after 4 hours
- Severe acidosis (pH < 7.25) and hypercapnia ($Paco_2$ > 60 torr)
- Severe hypoxemia (P/F ratio < 200)
- Severe tachypnea (> 35 breaths/min)
- Other complications (e.g., metabolic abnormalities, sepsis, pneumonia, pulmonary embolism, barotrauma, massive pleural effusion)

ADULT TRAUMA

Number of Simulations in the CSE: 1 Case

Regardless of the specific injury, all trauma management begins with efforts to secure the airway and restore and maintain adequate perfusion, ventilation, and oxygenation using the appropriate basic and advanced life support protocols. All trauma patients initially should receive 100% O_2 via a non-rebreathing mask, bag-valve-mask (BVM), or advanced airway. Simultaneous rapid assessment of the victim should quickly reveal the specific type of injuries sustained and direct the additional management needed beyond the initial resuscitation stage.

Chest Trauma

Chest trauma may result from either a penetrating or a blunt injury. Penetrating chest trauma most commonly is due to knife, gunshot wounds, industrial accidents, or lacerations from broken bones. In penetrating trauma, injury can occur to *any* thoracic structure. In addition to specific structural damage, bleeding can cause hemothorax or hemopericardium, and air leakage can result in pneumothorax or pneumopericardium.

"Sucking" chest wounds result from penetration through the chest wall and lung. They get their name from the sound they often make when the patient inhales, and air taking the path-of-least-resistance is sucked in through the wound. These injuries initially should be covered with an occlusive dressing (e.g., Vaseline gauze pad) to permit adequate ventilation and help prevent a tension pneumothorax. Definitive treatment of penetrating chest trauma always involves surgical repair.

Most blunt chest trauma occurs in motor vehicle accidents (MVAs). Other causes of blunt chest trauma include falls, sports injuries, crush injuries, and explosions. The injuries seen in blunt chest trauma are caused primarily by the rapid deceleration that occurs with a direct impact or direct blow to the thorax. **Table 20-4** summarizes the various rib cage, pulmonary, and cardiac injuries that can occur with blunt chest trauma, their key clinical findings, main diagnostic tests, and basic treatment options.

As outlined in Table 20-4, the general management of blunt chest trauma varies according to the type of injury. Respiratory management pearls follow.

Table 20-4 Summary of Blunt Chest Trauma Injuries

Injury	Clinical Findings	Diagnosis	Treatment
Rib Cage Injuries			
Fractured ribs, sternum	Pain, tenderness, and crepitus at fracture sites; inspiratory pain	CXR	Epidural analgesia
Flail chest (flail segment, one or more ribs broken in two or more places)	Fracture site/inspiratory pain, paradoxical chest motion (*in* with inhalation/*out* with exhalation); dyspnea, tachypnea	CXR	Epidural analgesia, surgical fixation
Airway/Pulmonary Injuries			
Laryngeal or tracheal crush injury/fractures	Severe respiratory distress with stridor, inability to speak	Bronchoscopy, CT scan	Cricothyrotomy, tracheotomy, surgical repair
Pulmonary contusion	Dyspnea, tachypnea, tachycardia, crackles, hypoxemia (may be delayed)	CXR, CT scan	Supplemental O_2, PEEP/CPAP, mechanical ventilation
Pneumothorax	Dyspnea, inspiratory pain If tension: cyanosis, tachypnea, tachycardia, hypotension, pulsus paradoxus, ↓ breath sounds, and hyperresonance on affected side; a mediastinal shift away from the affected side	Clinical findings, CXR, thoracic ultrasound, CT scan (imaging to follow treatment if tension pneumothorax)	Needle decompression, tube thoracostomy (chest tubes)
Hemothorax	↓ Breath sounds and dullness to percussion on affected side; signs of shock	CXR, thoracic ultrasound	Tube thoracostomy (chest tubes)
Cardiac Injuries			
Myocardial contusion	Dysrhythmias (e.g., tachycardia); accumulation of pericardial fluid (pericardial tamponade)	CXR, 12-lead ECG, serum troponin, cardiac echo	Antiarrhythmic agents, pericardial drainage, surgery
Pericardial tamponade	Hypotension, ↓ heart sounds, distended jugular veins, tachycardia	CXR, 12-lead ECG, serum troponin, cardiac echo, thoracic ultrasound	Pericardiocentesis, IV fluids, inotropic agents; avoid positive-pressure ventilation
Commotio cordis	Sudden cardiac arrest due to blow to the precordial region	History	Early CPR and rapid defibrillation

CPAP, continuous positive airway pressure; CT, computed tomography; CXR, chest x-ray; ECG, electrocardiogram; PEEP, positive end-expiratory pressure.

Assessment/Information Gathering

- Because the full effects of pulmonary contusion may not be apparent for 24–48 hours, patients should be admitted and closely monitored, primarily for worsening hypoxemia and development of acute respiratory distress syndrome (ARDS).
- Recommend diagnostic tests according to the type of trauma (see Table 20-4); also, recommend complete blood count (CBC), hemoglobin, hematocrit (to assess for blood loss or hemodilution), coagulation tests, and ABGs.
- *Do not* recommend an initial chest x-ray or CT scan if there are clear signs of a tension pneumothorax; instead, recommend immediate treatment via needle decompression or tube thoracostomy. Then and only then should the patient undergo imaging studies.
- Fractures of the lower "floating" ribs (11–12) may be associated with diaphragmatic tears and trauma to the liver or spleen; recommend an abdominal ultrasound (for hemoperitoneum) and computed tomography (CT) scan (to assess organ damage).

Treatment/Decision Making

- Indications for endotracheal (ET) intubation in chest trauma patients include apnea, profound shock, inadequate ventilation, and compromised airway.
- Recommend epidural analgesia for rib cage fracture pain; epidurals allow painless deep breathing and coughing without depressing respiration.
- Adjunctive measures to recommend in the care of patients with chest trauma include early mobilization and aggressive bronchial hygiene therapy (to prevent pneumonia).
- *Do not* recommend steroids for treatment of pulmonary contusion.
- Unless contraindicated as with a pneumothorax, consider lung expansion therapy such as incentive spirometry (IS), positive expiratory pressure (PEP), or percussive ventilation for a patient unable to adequately perform IS.
- Only recommend mechanical ventilation to correct abnormal gas exchange (with pulmonary contusion)—*not to* treat chest wall instability (flail chest).
  - Intubation and assist-control (A/C) modes (VC, PCV, PRVC, or bilevel ventilation) with positive end-expiratory pressure (PEEP) is the standard approach.
  - Recommend a trial of mask continuous positive airway pressure (CPAP) or bilevel positive airway pressure (BiPAP) for the alert, compliant patient with marginal respiratory status.
  - Apply the National Heart, Lung, and Blood Institute (NHLBI) ARDS protocol if ARDS develops.
  - Recommend independent lung ventilation for patients with severe unilateral contusion if (1) severe shunting persists or (2) "cross-over" bleeding is affecting the good lung.
  - Consider ECMO as a short-term approach for patients with reversible conditions and profound respiratory failure.

Head Trauma (Traumatic Brain Injury)

Trauma to the brain causes hemorrhage and edema. In a "closed head" traumatic brain injury (TBI), tissue swelling, and blood pooling increase intracranial pressure (ICP). When the ICP rises above 15 to 20 mm Hg, cerebral blood flow can decrease to a critical level, resulting in secondary ischemia. Prolonged cerebral ischemia causes worsening brain injury or brain death. Therefore, the general goal of managing head trauma is to avoid secondary injury by preserving cerebral blood flow. Respiratory management pearls follow.

Assessment/Information Gathering

- The initial assessment should include airway patency, SpO_2, level of consciousness, ability to communicate, and pupil size and reactivity.
- Continuous capnography (expired CO_2) monitoring should be implemented if available to help avoid hypercapnia.
- Use the Glasgow Coma Scale (Chapter 2) to help categorize the severity of the injury as mild (score 14 or 15), moderate (9 to 13), or severe (8 or less).
- Assess for other related injuries (see the sections on the chest and spinal cord injuries) and hemodynamic stability/shock.
- Note that Cheyne-Stokes breathing and slow/irregular respirations are common in TBI.
- Recognize the signs of a potentially life-threatening hematoma: hemiparesis or aphasia, unequal and sluggish pupillary responses, progressive decline in mental status, and coma.

Treatment/Decision Making

- Initial emergency management:
  - Recommend that a cervical collar be kept in place until the patient is evaluated for spinal cord damage.
  - Initially provide 100% O_2 via a nonrebreathing mask, BVM, or advanced airway to keep SpO_2 above 95%, *while maintaining the patient's head and neck in a neutral position.*
  - If providing ventilation, initially aim to keep the $PaCO_2$ between 35 and 40 torr (normocapnia).

- Recommend fluid resuscitation and vasopressors to keep mean arterial pressure (MAP) greater than 75 mm Hg.
- Recommend IV mannitol or hypertonic saline if the patient exhibits posturing and unequal or nonreactive pupils.
- If the Glasgow Coma Scale score is 8 or less, or if the patient is unable to protect the airway, recommend rapid-sequence intubation; if oral/nasal intubation is not possible due to airway trauma, recommend cricothyrotomy or tracheotomy.
- If a life-threatening hematoma is likely, recommend its surgical removal.
  - Ongoing management/monitoring:
    - Recommend continuous monitoring of arterial blood pressure (BP or A-line), ICP, and SpO_2; the goal is to keep ICP less than 20 mm Hg and cerebral perfusion pressure (CPP) at 60 mm Hg or higher (CPP = MAP – ICP) to avoid cerebral hypoxia.
    - Recommend vasopressors (e.g., norepinephrine) to maintain MAP/CPP as needed.
    - To help lower ICP, recommend the following:
      - Elevating the head of the bed 30–40 degrees
      - Sedating the patient with a benzodiazepine or propofol
      - Initiating osmotherapy (mannitol/hypertonic saline) or ventricular drainage to decrease ICP
      - Prescribing an anticonvulsant (e.g., phenytoin) if seizures are a problem
      - Neuromuscular blockade, high-dose barbiturate coma, or decompressive craniectomy if ICP remains high
      - Judicious suctioning or any other intervention which is likely to stimulate the patient and raise ICP.
    - *Do not* recommend high-dose steroids (they do not improve survival).
  - If mechanical ventilation is required:
    - Aim to achieve $PaCO_2$ of 35–40 torr, PIP ≤ 30 cm H_2O, SpO_2 > 95%, and good patient–ventilator synchrony.
    - Avoid hypercapnia (causes cerebral vasodilation and increases ICP).
    - Avoid high levels of PEEP (can decrease MAP, increase ICP, and decrease CPP).
    - Avoid prophylactic/routine hyperventilation (lowers ICP but can cause cerebral ischemia). Consider only in the following circumstances:
      - To lessen ICP increases before procedures such as suctioning
      - In the presence of confirmed cerebral herniation
      - As salvage therapy when high ICP does not respond to standard treatment
    - If neuromuscular blockade has been implemented, implement a strict management protocol to ensure support should ventilator disconnection or failure occur.

Spinal Cord Injuries

Spinal cord injury (SCI) is seen most often in motor vehicle accidents, falls, gunshot wounds, and sporting accidents. Cord neurons may suffer destruction from direct trauma; compression by bone fragments, disc material, edema, or hematoma; or ischemia from interruption of blood flow.

There are two broad classes of SCI: tetraplegia and paraplegia. Tetraplegia involves injury to the cord's cervical segments (C1–C7) and partial or complete loss of muscle function in all four extremities. Injuries resulting in paraplegia occur lower in the cord (thoracic, lumbar, or sacral segments), causing loss of motor and sensory function in the lower limbs and trunk. Tetraplegia and paraplegia can be further classified as being complete (no sensory or motor function below the injury) or incomplete (preservation of some sensory or motor function).

In general, the higher the level of injury, the greater its effect on respiration. Patients with injuries above the C3 level suffer damage to the nerves innervating the respiratory muscles and, therefore, typically require some form of artificial ventilatory support. Mid-cervical injuries (C3–C5) may leave some nerves intact and allow the patient to breathe without ventilatory support, at least some of the time. Patients suffering injuries below the C5 level may be able to breathe on their own but can experience a reduced vital capacity and inability to effectively cough and clear secretions. Cervical cord injuries also can cause loss of autonomic function, resulting in *neurogenic shock* and the accompanying signs of hypotension, vasodilation, bradycardia, and hypothermia.

The full impact of an SCI may not be immediately apparent. After the initial insult, edema, bleeding, or ischemia can gradually cause worsening of the injury, in some cases progressing in severity from incomplete to complete.

As with all trauma management, initial efforts require rapid stabilization of the patient with concurrent assessment for the specific type and extent of the injury. Additional respiratory management pearls follow.

Assessment/Information Gathering

- Conduct assessment only when the patient's head, neck, and spine are immobilized and maintained in a neutral position.
- Continuous pulse oximetry *and* end-tidal CO_2 (capnometry) monitoring should be implemented for all patients with severe SCI.
- Carefully evaluate airway patency, respiratory rate, chest and abdominal movement, and the presence of chest-wall or head injuries (approximately one in four patients with SCI also has head trauma). *If apnea is present, assume complete high cervical injury and immediately initiate manual ventilation.*
- Determine by recent history and observation if the patient was under the influence of drugs or intoxicated with alcohol (can mimic SCI or mask some neurologic findings).
- Recommend measurement of pulse, blood pressure, and core temperature to detect hypotension and differentiate among causes of shock:
  - Shock is likely *neurogenic* if the patient has an injury above T6 with bradycardia and hypothermia (the patient's skin may also be flushed, warm, and dry due to vasodilation).
  - Shock is likely *hemorrhagic* if the patient has an injury at or below T6 with tachycardia and normal core temperature (extremities may be cold and clammy with pallor or acrocyanosis evident).
- Recommend ABG, CBC, hemoglobin and hematocrit (for blood loss); chemistry panel, coagulation profile, blood lactate, and base deficit (to assess for shock); and toxicology screen (to differentiate drug-related CNS effects).
- For any patient with cervical pain or neurologic deficit (and in all elderly patients admitted with a suspected neck injury), recommend CT scan or standard anteroposterior (AP), lateral, and *odontoid* neck x-rays (the odontoid beam is directed through the open mouth to assess the C1 area).
- Recommend magnetic resonance imaging (MRI) (1) if CT/x-ray is negative, but the clinical picture supports cord damage, or (2) to assess for soft tissue "non-osseous" injuries such as hemorrhage and hematoma.
- Recommend bladder catheterization and input/output (I/O) monitoring to help assess the patient's circulatory status and relieve the complications of urinary retention (often seen in neurogenic shock).
- After any needed resuscitation, recommend evaluation of the patient's sensory response (to touch + pinprick) and motor strength (limb flexor/extensor muscles) using a standardized assessment tool.
- After stabilization, if the patient is conscious and exhibits spontaneous respirations, recommend assessment of respiratory muscle function via measurement of vital capacity (Vc) and maximum inspiratory pressure/negative inspiratory force (MIP/NIF).

Treatment/Decision Making

Treatment of SCI involves at least two phases: the immediate acute postinjury phase (typically in the emergency department [ED] and intensive care unit [ICU]) and a subsequent chronic phase of lifelong care.

Acute Phase Recommendations

- The patient initially should be immobilized and treated in the supine position; if repositioning is needed (e.g., to avoid aspiration), the patient should be carefully "log-rolled" so that the head, neck, and torso are turned as a unit.

- To further help avoid aspiration, recommend insertion of a nasogastric (NG) tube.
- Initially provide 100% O_2 via a nonrebreathing mask or manual resuscitator to keep Spo_2 above 95%, *while maintaining the patient's head and neck in a neutral position.*
- If the patient is agitated, combative, or fighting against restraints, recommend either a short-acting sedative/hypnotic (e.g., midazolam) or an antipsychotic (e.g., haloperidol or droperidol).
- Airway management:
  - Always maintain the cervical spine in neutral alignment.
  - To maintain airway patency and prevent aspiration, keep the oropharynx clear of secretions; however, avoid vigorous suctioning that could cause gagging, retching, or bradycardia.
  - If ET intubation is indicated, recommend either fiberoptic intubation or rapid sequence orotracheal intubation with manual in-line neck stabilization.
  - Be prepared for severe bradycardia from vagal stimulation during intubation; preoxygenation and IV atropine or topical lidocaine spray can minimize this response.
  - If the patient is likely to remain ventilator-dependent, recommend a tracheotomy early in the hospitalization period.
  - Because patients with SCI are at high risk for aspiration and pneumonia, initiate rigorous ventilator-associated pneumonia (VAP) protocol for those receiving mechanical ventilation.
- Management of shock:
  - Recommend fluid resuscitation and vasopressors, with the goal being a systolic BP higher than 85–90 mm Hg with a normal heart rate (60–100/min) and rhythm.
  - Recommend atropine to treat significant bradycardia.
  - For a patient in neurogenic shock, recommend vasopressors that include β-stimulation such as dopamine or norepinephrine (pure α-adrenergic agents such as phenylephrine can worsen bradycardia).
- Recommend external rewarming or warm, humidified O_2 to treat hypothermia.
- In some SCI protocols, administration of high doses of methylprednisolone within 8 hours of the initial injury is considered an option; if this choice is offered as a recommendation on the CSE, select it.

Chronic Phase

In the chronic phase of SCI management, the goals are to prevent atelectasis and pneumonia, liberate the patient from full-time ventilatory support (if feasible), and enhance the quality of life. The following chronic phase guidelines apply mainly to those patients who retain some respiratory muscle function:

- Ensure that a comprehensive discharge plan addresses needed home modifications, caregiver training, medical equipment, and assistive technologies, emergency provisions (e.g., backup generator), transportation needs, vocational and recreational activities, and supportive community resources.
- For ventilator-dependent SCI patients, recommend large tidal volumes (up to 1.0 L) to relieve the common sensation of dyspnea that these patients experience.
- To facilitate speech for a ventilator-dependent patient with a trach who has good secretion control, deflate the cuff and either attach a one-way speaking valve (Chapter 9) or increase the tidal volume.
- For patients likely to require long-term ventilatory support, recommend a trial of noninvasive ventilation (positive or negative pressure) or diaphragmatic pacing.
- To help avoid atelectasis and promote at least part-time liberation from mechanical ventilation, implement inspiratory muscle training (see Chapter 10).
- Recommend an abdominal binder to improve diaphragmatic function (properly positioned binders facilitate chest expansion by compressing the abdominal contents to increase intra-abdominal pressure, and thus elevating the diaphragm into a more optimal position for breathing).
- Teach patients with an intact upper airway glossopharyngeal or "frog" breathing (breathing by repetitive swallowing of mouthfuls of air).

- To facilitate coughing and secretion removal, implement or teach caregivers to apply the "quad cough" technique, or use a mechanical insufflation–exsufflation device.
- Because sleep-disordered breathing is a common complication of SCI, recommend either an in-home or laboratory polysomnography exam for symptomatic patients.

Burns/Smoke Inhalation

Burns are among the most devastating and complex forms of trauma. Most burns are due to flame exposure, with burns due to hot liquids (scalding) being the next most common, followed by inhalation injuries. Less common are burns caused by electrical current and chemicals.

The severity of a burn and the patient's likelihood of survival are determined by the percentage of body surface area (BSA) affected and the burn depth. Percent BSA is estimated using either the standardized Lund and Browder chart or the "rule of nines" (adult head 9%, each arm 9%, each leg 18%, front and rear torso 18% each). Burn depth can be either partial thickness (not extending through all skin layers) or full thickness (extending through all skin layers into the subcutaneous tissues).

In general, a severe burn is one extending into or through the dermis and covering more than 25–30% BSA. In patients who experience such burns, the release of cytokines and other inflammatory mediators from the burn site can cause body-wide/systemic effects. Cardiovascular changes include increased capillary permeability, with massive loss of both fluid and protein into the interstitial space. Vasoconstriction occurs in both the peripheral circulation and the gut, along with a decrease in heart contractility. If not immediately treated, these changes can result in "burn shock" and multiple-organ failure.

Compounding this problem are *direct* inhalation injuries, which occur in as many as one-third of all serious burns. Inhalation injuries can include one or more of the following: (1) direct thermal damage to the upper airway from inhaling hot gases (thermal injury below the larynx is rare), (2) chemical injury to the lungs due to inhalation of toxic by-products of combustion found in smoke, and (3) damage to O_2 delivery and cellular O_2 utilization through exposure to carbon monoxide or hydrogen cyanide gas. Inhalation injuries significantly increase mortality over that predicted from cutaneous burns alone. Indeed, some estimates suggest that as many as three out of four deaths following major burns are due to inhalation injury.

Management of major burns proceeds through several phases, here referred to as the "four Rs": *R*esuscitation, *R*esurfacing, *R*ehabilitation, and *R*econstruction. Typically, the full range of needed support throughout these four phases is provided in specialized burn centers. Most respiratory management occurs during the resuscitation phase, in which essential support is provided to vital organ systems to help ensure patient survival. Key management pearls during this phase follow.

Assessment/Information Gathering

- Recommend CBC, electrolytes, lactate, ABG, CO-oximetry (to assess for carboxyhemoglobin concentration), and a coagulation profile.
- Assess the sensorium and coma level (Glasgow Coma Scale) if the patient is unresponsive.
- Recommend chest x-ray (may be negative early on).
- Monitor SpO_2 and watch for signs and symptoms of hypoxemia.
- Assess for signs of inhalation injury: facial/neck burns, singed nasal hairs, sooty sputum, dyspnea, cyanosis, hoarseness, coughing, and stridor (closed-space fire victims are most prone to inhalation injuries).
- Assess for signs and symptoms of cyanide (CN) poisoning: headache; confusion, seizures or coma, chest tightness, nausea/vomiting, mydriasis; dyspnea, tachypnea, hyperpnea, and either hypertension (early) or hypotension (late). Note also that blood lactate is typically high (≥ 8 mmol/L), indicating tissue hypoxia/anaerobic metabolism.
- Reevaluate the patient's airway and oxygenation status frequently (inhalation injuries may take several hours to develop).
- Because chest x-rays may not detect inhalation injuries, recommend fiberoptic bronchoscopy to assess airway damage.

Treatment/Decision Making

- Recommend covering the patient to prevent heat and fluid loss.
- Immediately administer as high an O_2 concentration as possible (via a nonrebreathing mask or high-flow cannula) to all patients suspected of inhalation injury; after that, titrate the oxygen level to maintain the SpO_2 above 90%.
- Recommend immediate IV access and fluid and electrolyte replacement therapy (a 70-kg patient may need 8–10 L or more over the first 24 hours following injury).
- Recommend urinary catheterization to help monitor fluid balance (the output goal is approximately 1.0 mL/kg/h).
- Recommend morphine analgesia for severe pain; be on guard for respiratory depression.
- If the patient has electrical burns, recommend a 12-lead ECG and cardiac biomarkers.
- Circumferential full-thickness burns of the thorax significantly reduce chest-wall compliance; recommend prompt escharotomy (incision/removal of the charred, dead tissue) to allow for adequate ventilation.
- Patients with smoke inhalation should be admitted if they are hypoxemic ($PaO_2 < 60$ torr), have an HbCO greater than 15%, have metabolic acidosis, or are experiencing bronchospasm and painful or difficulty swallowing.
- If %HbCO is greater than 25% with signs of neurologic or cardiac impairment, recommend hyperbaric oxygenation (at 3 ATA) treatment if available.
- If cyanide poisoning is suspected (e.g., combustion of certain plastics), recommend immediate treatment with either hydroxocobalamin (also known as vitamin B_{12a} or "cyanokit") or sulfanegen TEA.
- If bronchospasm is present, recommend aerosolized bronchodilators, *N*-acetylcysteine (Mucomyst), and heparin (to prevent plugging from fibrin clots and cellular debris); accompany aerosol therapy with bronchial hygiene/airway clearance therapy appropriate to the patient's condition.
- Do *not* recommend prophylactic steroids or antibiotics for inhalation injuries (antibiotics should be used only when respiratory tract infection is suspected or confirmed).
- Patients should be referred to a burn center in the following circumstances:
  - Partial-thickness burns exceeding 10% BSA, full-thickness burns exceeding 5% BSA, or circumferential burns
  - Burns with associated inhalation injury
- Airway management:
  - If airway injury is confirmed, recommend ET intubation; if the vocal cords are damaged or the patient is likely to require mechanical ventilation for more than 10–12 days, recommend tracheotomy.
  - In patients with neck/facial burns and airway edema, reintubation after accidental extubation can be very difficult. To avoid this problem:
    - Recommend adequate patient sedation to prevent self-extubation.
    - Properly secure the ET tube (ETT), which may require stapling the tape to the patient's skin.
    - Be prepared with backup methods to secure the airway (e.g., laryngeal mask airway [LMA], cricothyrotomy).
  - To prevent acute ETT obstruction from endobronchial debris, provide proper humidification, and implement a rigorous bronchial hygiene/airway clearance protocol.
- Mechanical ventilation:
  - Consider an initial trial of noninvasive ventilation for the burn patient with mild to moderate respiratory distress but no significant inhalation injury or facial burns.
  - Apply active humidification (*not* a heat and moisture exchanger [HME]) to minimize insensible water loss and prevent tube occlusion.
  - Use high minute volumes to accommodate high metabolic rates (best achieved via high rates as opposed to high V_T); accept mild to moderate respiratory acidosis to prevent compounding the pulmonary injury.

- If acute hypoxemic respiratory failure develops (P/F ratio < 300 and bilateral diffuse infiltrates on x-ray consistent with pulmonary edema), apply the NHLBI ARDS protocol for ventilator management.
      - Rigorously apply the VAP protocol to minimize the likelihood of pneumonia (acute bacterial invasion peaks at 2–3 days after inhalation injury).
- Weaning/extubation:
      - Recognize that staged excisions and skin grafting procedures can delay weaning for days or weeks.
      - Recommend inhaled racemic epinephrine for patients who develop mild stridor after extubation; if stridor is more severe, consider noninvasive ventilation or heliox therapy.

CARDIOVASCULAR DISEASE

Number of Simulations in the CSE: 2 Cases

The NBRC expects candidates to be proficient in the management of common cardiovascular disorders, including congestive heart failure (CHF), coronary artery disease (CAD), and pulmonary embolism. Because some of these conditions often involve surgical intervention, you also need to understand the perioperative management of patients undergoing valve repair/replacement and coronary artery bypass grafting (CABG).

Congestive Heart Failure (CHF)

Heart failure occurs when the heart's ability to pump blood is not adequate to meet the body's metabolic needs. The most common cause is impaired contractility of the left ventricle (LV), due to coronary artery disease (CAD), myocardial infarction (MI), dilated cardiomyopathy, valvular heart disease, or hypertension. Right ventricular (RV) failure also can occur, most commonly due to LV failure, RV infarction, pulmonary hypertension, pulmonary emboli, or tricuspid regurgitation.

Signs and symptoms vary according to the severity and progression of the disease. Patients with advanced disease typically exhibit signs and symptoms of fluid retention and pulmonary congestion (thus the term *congestive heart failure*), including dyspnea, orthopnea, and paroxysmal nocturnal dyspnea. Additional findings may include fatigue, chest pain or pressure, and palpitations. If the RV is involved, jugular venous distention, peripheral edema, hepatomegaly, and ascites are common findings. Auscultation may reveal a gallop rhythm (with an S_3 sound and often an S_4 sound) and, in valvular disease, heart murmurs.

As indicated in **Table 20-5**, functional impairment in patients with heart failure is categorized by the level of dyspnea they experience.

With proper disease management, even patients with New York Heart Association (NYHA) Class III/IV heart failure can remain relatively stable most of the time. However, patients with heart failure can quickly decompensate and develop acute dysfunction, most typically resulting in pulmonary edema or hypotension/shock. The following pearls address the basics in the management of stable heart failure and acute decompensation.

Table 20-5 New York Heart Association (NYHA) Heart Failure Symptom Classification

NYHA Class	Level of Impairment
I	No symptom limitation with ordinary physical activity
II	Ordinary physical activity somewhat limited by dyspnea (e.g., long-distance walking, climbing two flights of stairs)
III	Exercise limited by dyspnea with moderate workload (e.g., short-distance walking, climbing one flight of stairs)
IV	Dyspnea at rest or with minimal exertion

Assessment/Information Gathering

To identify or manage stable CHF:

- Assess for the signs and symptoms previously noted.
- Recommend testing of serum electrolytes (fluid balance, sodium levels), blood urea nitrogen (BUN) and creatinine (renal function), as well as brain natriuretic peptide (BNP—a hormone useful in diagnosing CHF and its response to treatment).
- Recommend a chest x-ray; look for cardiomegaly, pulmonary vascular congestion, Kerley B lines (horizontal lines in lower lung zones representing edematous interlobular septa), and pleural effusion.
- Recommend 12-lead ECG; look for indicators suggesting LV or RV hypertrophy or ischemia/CAD (discussed subsequently).
- If the ECG indicates ischemia/CAD, recommend a stress test, cardiac catheterization, or coronary computed tomographic angiography (CTA) to confirm or exclude CAD as the cause (see the subsequent section on CAD).
- Recommend an echocardiogram to assess for systolic and diastolic function, hypertrophy, chamber size, and valve abnormalities (discussed subsequently).

To assess for decompensation/pulmonary edema:

- Assess for signs of acute decompensation (e.g., sudden onset of restlessness, confusion, diaphoresis, dyspnea, increased work of breathing, tachypnea, tachycardia).
- Assess peripheral perfusion; look for cold, pale, cyanotic, or mottled skin and slow capillary refill.
- Assess cough and sputum production; look for frothy or pinkish/blood-tinged sputum.
- Assess breath sounds (marked bilateral crackles and wheezing indicate acute decompensation).
- Assess for chest pain (its presence suggests acute myocardial ischemia/infarction).
- Initiate SpO_2 monitoring, and obtain an ABG (which typically shows hypoxemia with respiratory alkalosis).
- Recommend an immediate chest x-ray (which typically reveals bilateral fluffy infiltrates).
- Recommend cardiac biomarkers (troponin, CK, and CK-MB) to assess for MI.
- Recommend an echocardiogram (to help determine possible mechanical causes such as cardiac tamponade or valve problems).
- Do *not* recommend pulmonary artery (PA) catheter insertion unless the patient's diagnosis cannot be confirmed without it, or there are unexpected responses to therapy.

Treatment/Decision Making

To manage stable CHF:

- Recommend disease management education, with an emphasis on sodium and fluid restriction, smoking cessation, daily monitoring of BP, weight control, and moderate aerobic exercise.
- Recommend the following medications for all CHF patients:
  - An angiotensin-converting enzyme (ACE) inhibitor (e.g., captopril) or angiotensin receptor blocker (e.g., valsartan)
  - A β-blocker (e.g., carvedilol)
  - Depending on the severity of symptoms, additional medications may include digoxin (especially with atrial fibrillation), a diuretic (preferably a loop diuretic such as furosemide or the potassium-sparing torsemide), and an aldosterone antagonist such as spironolactone.

To manage decompensation/pulmonary edema:

- Initiate O_2 therapy with the highest FiO_2 possible (via nonrebreathing mask at 12–15 L/min or high-flow cannula at 30–40 L/min) to obtain a SpO_2 above 90%.
- Recommend CPAP or BiPAP with 100% O_2 (improves gas exchange and decreases venous return and ventricular preload).

- Recommend morphine or a benzodiazepine such as lorazepam to reduce anxiety (morphine also may decrease preload via venous dilation).
- Recommend the appropriate ACLS protocol for any associated arrhythmia or MI.
- Recommend the following medications (these recommendations assume the patient is *not* hypotensive):
  - A vasodilator such as nitroglycerin, sodium nitroprusside, or nesiritide (to decrease preload and afterload)
  - A rapid-acting loop diuretic such as furosemide or torsemide
  - If the patient is hypotensive, recommend an inotropic agent such as dobutamine to maintain a mean arterial pressure of at least 70–75 mm Hg.
- Recommend intubation and invasive ventilation if the patient develops severe dyspnea or respiratory acidosis on CPAP/BiPAP.
- In the patient with persistent hypotension and pulmonary edema due to an acute MI, recommend intra-aortic balloon pumping (if available) until angioplasty or cardiac surgery can be performed.

Coronary Artery Disease (CAD) and Acute Coronary Syndrome (ACS)

CAD is a pathologic process affecting the coronary arteries, most commonly due to atherosclerosis. The buildup of atherosclerotic plaque narrows the arteries and reduces blood flow to the myocardium, eventually causing ischemia, angina, and infarction. Risk factors include hyperlipidemia (especially elevated low-density lipoprotein [LDL]), diabetes, hypertension, smoking, sedentary lifestyle and obesity, and a family history of CAD.

The primary symptom of CAD is *angina pectoris*. Angina can vary in severity from that occurring only with strenuous exercise to constant pain at rest. Angina is *stable* if the pattern of discomfort remains unchanged over time; it is *unstable* when abrupt changes occur in the frequency, intensity, or duration of the pain or its precipitating factors.

When CAD progresses to cause partial or complete blockage of a coronary artery resulting in unstable angina or MI, the condition is known as an *acute coronary syndrome* (ACS). As indicated in **Table 20-6**, the two categories of ACS are defined primarily by the ECG: the ST-segment elevation myocardial infarction (STEMI) type and the non-ST-segment elevation myocardial infarction (NSTEMI)/unstable angina type. Because STEMI-type MI involves complete obstruction of a coronary artery, it is the more serious event and the one generally requiring the most rapid and aggressive response. The following management pearls address both stable CAD and ACS.

Assessment/Information Gathering

To identify or assess CAD with stable angina:

- Assess vital signs, including *all peripheral pulses*.
- Auscultate the carotid arteries, listening for bruits (indicating atherosclerosis).
- Obtain patient history, to include current symptoms, risk factors, and family history; assess for chest pain and palpitations, shortness of breath, fatigue, and limited tolerance for exertion.
- Recommend a 12-lead ECG to identify the presence and severity of myocardial ischemia; *note that a normal ECG does not exclude CAD.*
- Recommend the following lab tests: electrolytes, fasting glucose (to assess for diabetes/diabetes control), lipid panel (total cholesterol, high-density lipoprotein [HDL], LDL, and triglycerides), and C-reactive protein (an inflammatory marker that increases in atherosclerotic disease).

Table 20-6 Basic Classification of Acute Coronary Syndrome

Classification	Recognition	Presumed Cause
STEMI or new left bundle branch block (LBBB)	ST-segment elevation in two or more contiguous chest leads (V1–V6)	Complete coronary artery occlusion
NSTEMI/unstable angina	Ischemic ST-segment depression or dynamic T-wave inversion with pain	Partial or intermittent occlusion

- Recommend a chest x-ray.
- Recommend stress echocardiography or radionuclide stress testing (imaging with thallium-201 or technetium-99m) to identify the presence and magnitude of ischemia and MI.
- Recommend either coronary arteriography/cardiac catheterization (the gold standard for diagnosing CAD) or minimally invasive CT angiography to help identify the exact location and extent of coronary artery blockage.

To identify or assess for ACS:

- Assess for centralized chest pain, pressure, fullness, or "squeezing" sensation; pain may radiate to the jaw, shoulder, arm, and back. *Note that some patients with MI may be asymptomatic.*
- Measure SpO_2 and vital signs, and assess for hypotension and the potential for cardiogenic shock.
- Assess for dyspnea, diaphoresis, nausea, lightheadedness, confusion, and syncope.
- Auscultate the lungs, and listen for crackles (indicating CHF/pulmonary edema).
- Recommend 12-lead ECG; look for ST-segment deviation (± 1 mm or higher) or T-wave inversion in multiple chest leads.
- Recommend electrolytes, coagulation panel, and *serial measurement* of cardiac biomarkers whose levels increase with MI. These include creatine phosphokinase (CK), CK-MB, and troponin. *However, do not delay treatment to wait for lab results because these markers can take several hours to show up in blood tests!*
- Recommend a chest x-ray.

Treatment/Decision Making

The nature and urgency of treatment provided to patients with CAD vary according to the severity of their disease process. In general, patients with stable angina are managed conservatively using a comprehensive disease management protocol, whereas those presenting with acute coronary syndrome receive more urgent care.

Management of CAD with Stable Angina (Including Post-MI)

- Recommend participation in a cardiac rehabilitation program that provides smoking cessation (see Chapter 17), encourages regular exercise (30 min/day of moderate activity), and assists with weight control and healthy dieting (low saturated fat, high fiber).
- If the patient has diabetes, recommend careful blood glucose control via hemoglobin A_{1C} monitoring.
- Recommend pharmacologic therapy:
  - An antiplatelet drug (e.g., low-dose aspirin, warfarin, clopidogrel)
  - An antianginal drug (e.g., nitroglycerin—sublingual, tab, spray) for relief and a β-blocker (e.g., metoprolol), a calcium-channel blocker (e.g., nifedipine), a long-acting nitrate (e.g., isosorbide extended-release), or ranolazine for control
  - For patients with CAD and high LDL levels, recommend a statin (e.g., atorvastatin [Lipitor]).
- For patients with stable angina but significant limitations to activity (NYHA Class III/IV heart failure), recommend either elective percutaneous coronary angioplasty or coronary artery bypass grafting (CABG)

Management of Acute Coronary Syndrome/MI

- Support the ABCs (airway, breathing, circulation) as needed; be prepared to implement the applicable ACLS protocol.
- Initially, recommend that all patients with suspected ACS (STEMI or NSTEMI) receive the following ("MONA" + β-blocker):
  - *M*orphine for pain
  - *O₂* to maintain SpO_2 above 90%

- ○ <u>N</u>itroglycerin, unless contraindicated (hypotension [systolic BP < 90 mm Hg] or evidence of RV infarction)
- ○ <u>A</u>spirin (or clopidogrel if aspirin is contraindicated)
- ○ A β-blocker such as metoprolol, unless contraindicated (hypotension, shock, bradycardia, uncompensated CHF, asthma)
- Recommend a chest x-ray.
- For STEMI, new left bundle branch block (LBBB), or likely MI with cardiogenic shock:
  - ○ If available, recommend emergency revascularization via either percutaneous coronary angioplasty (PCA) or CABG within 90 minutes;
  - ○ If not possible, recommend immediate fibrinolytic/thrombolytic therapy using a tissue plasminogen activator (t-PA) such as alteplase or reteplase.
- For initially responsive NSTEMI: recommend conservative management with antianginal therapy, antiplatelet therapy, and antithrombin therapy (heparin, either unfractionated or low molecular weight)—*not* fibrinolytic therapy—followed by a stress test and, if needed, diagnostic angiography.
- For worsening NSTEMI (rising CK/troponin, new ECG changes, refractory angina, severe arrhythmias, hemodynamic instability, onset of heart failure): recommend urgent revascularization via either PCA or CABG.

Valvular Heart Disease

Valvular heart disease—especially that affecting the aortic and mitral valves—can cause significant disability that usually requires surgical correction. Regarding assessment and information gathering, note that the clinical findings in valvular heart disease are often similar to those in CHF. For this reason, echocardiography should be recommended in all patients exhibiting signs and symptoms of heart failure. Specifically, both two-dimensional (2D) and Doppler echocardiogram are indicated if a valve problem is suspected. Two-dimensional echocardiography provides real-time analysis of chamber and valve mechanical function, whereas the Doppler method allows measurement of actual blood flow.

In terms of treatment and decision making, note that with minor exceptions, cardiac valve disorders require surgical intervention to repair or replace the damaged tissue. Consequently, as an RT, valvular heart disease involvement most often will occur in the perioperative and postoperative settings.

Cardiac Surgery

Cardiac surgery is associated with significant pulmonary complications, even among patients with healthy lungs. Typically, a diminished postoperative functional residual capacity (FRC) increases the likelihood of atelectasis, whereas the reduced vital capacity and impaired airway clearance due to pain and analgesia make the patient prone to secretion retention and pneumonia. Moreover, fluid imbalances and the general inflammatory response to the surgery often increase capillary leakage and lung water, further aggravating V/Q inequalities and worsening hypoxemia.

Initial postoperative respiratory care aims to restore the FRC and maintain adequate gas exchange via mechanical ventilation with PEEP to help avoid or minimize these problems. Subsequent efforts involve weaning and extubation, followed by rigorous bronchial hygiene therapy.

With the advent of new anesthesia strategies and minimally invasive techniques, including "off-pump," transcatheter aortic valve replacement (TAVR) and robotically assisted cardiac surgery, there has been a dramatic decrease in the frequency of postoperative pulmonary complications as well as the need for lengthy ventilatory support. Both achievements depend in part on the integral role that RTs play in managing cardiac surgery patients, as summarized in the following management pearls.

Assessment/Information Gathering

Ideally, patient assessment should occur before surgery and subsequently upon admission to the postoperative unit, with continuous monitoring taking place while the patient is receiving care.

- Via chart review and patient interview, assess the patient preoperatively for the following postoperative risk factors (all likely to increase complications/ICU length of stay):
    - *Demographics*: advanced age (75 years or older), female gender
    - *Degree of cardiac dysfunction*: NYHA Class III or IV, low ejection fraction (EF < 40%), prior CABG or current valve disorder, previous MI, need for preoperative intra-aortic balloon pump
    - *Comorbidities*: COPD, CHF, diabetes, hypertension, cerebrovascular disease, renal impairment, drug abuse, obesity, smoking history
    - *Operative factors*: emergency (nonelective) procedure, cardiopulmonary bypass (versus "off-pump"), left main coronary artery graft, multiple vessel grafts, valve repair/replacement, expected lengthy procedure. Recommend bedside spirometry for any patient with a history of lung disease or smoking; measure forced vital capacity (FVC), slow vital capacity (SVC), and inspiratory capacity (IC).
- To help reduce postoperative complications, provide *preoperative* patient education, to include discussion of airway and ventilator management, as well as training in the selected lung expansion and airway clearance methods.
- After surgery, on admission to the postsurgical unit or placement on a ventilator:
    - Initiate continuous pulse oximetry and capnography.
    - After the patient has been on the ventilator for 20 minutes, obtain a blood gas analysis and compute the $P(A-a)o_2$ and P/F ratio.
    - Recommend 5-lead ECG telemetry monitoring (including leads II and V5 for detecting ischemia), ideally with computerized ST-segment analysis.
    - Recommend hemodynamic monitoring, ideally to include direct radial arterial pressures (use the right side for aortic surgery) and CVP (do *not* recommend routine use of a PA catheter).
    - Recommend careful monitoring of fluid output via a urinary catheter, chest tube drainage, and NG tube.
    - Recommend a postsurgical chest x-ray to assess for ETT position and vascular line placement and to evaluate the patient's lung fields for lung expansion/atelectasis, infiltrates, pneumothorax, bleeding, pleural effusion, or pulmonary edema.
    - Where feasible, recommend blood-sparing sampling and point-of-care ABG testing (to minimize blood loss).
    - Recommend anti-embolism stockings (reduces the risk of deep vein thrombosis [DVT] and pulmonary embolism).

Treatment/Decision Making

Most patients who undergo cardiac surgery are provided with ventilatory support immediately after transfer from the operating room (OR). Initial ventilator settings vary by institutional protocol but generally include the following elements:

- *Mode*: full ventilatory support (pressure or volume control A/C)
- *Tidal volume*: 8–10 mL/kg (to treat/prevent post-op atelectasis) with plateau pressure of 30 cm H_2O or less
- *Rate*: to provide $Petco_2$ (capnography) of 30–40 torr, normalize pH
- *Fio_2*: match the operating room %O_2 or initially provide 100% O_2 to obtain $P(A-a)o_2$; immediately titrate down to maintain the Spo_2 above 90% with PEEP
- *PEEP*: initially 5–10 cm H_2O

Ideally, these patients should be weaned from ventilatory support and extubated within 2 to 6 hours after leaving the OR—a strategy known as the *fast-track* approach. Early extubation and spontaneous breathing decrease intrapleural pressure, which in most patients increases LV end-diastolic volume, EF, and cardiac output. Of course, not all patients can or should be fast-tracked. Thus, the first step is deciding who is ready to wean, followed by implementation of a rapid weaning and extubation protocol.

Assess the patient to determine if he or she is ready to fast-track. Example criteria in fast-track protocols include the following:

- The patient meets respiratory and acid-base criteria:
  - The patient is spontaneously breathing with $\dot{V}e$ 5–12 L/min
  - $Fio_2 \leq 0.50$ and PEEP $\leq$ 8 cm H_2O with $Spo_2 \geq 90\%$
  - pH 7.35–7.50 with arterial $HCO_3^- > 21$ mmol/L
- The patient meets neurologic criteria:
  - Can move all extremities/lift head and legs off the bed on command
  - Nods appropriately to questions
  - Has intact cough reflex
- The patient meets hemodynamic criteria:
  - Blood pressure is within an acceptable range (e.g., mean arterial pressure [MAP] > 75 mm Hg or systolic BP 100–120 mm Hg) without vasoactive drug support
  - No evidence of major bleeding; chest tubes drainage < 50–100 mL/h
  - Heart rate < 120/min with no significant arrhythmias
  - Cardiac index > 2.0 $L/min/m^2$; EF > 40%
  - CVP < 17 mm Hg
- For patients meeting fast-track criteria for whom sedation has been discontinued, follow a standard spontaneous breathing trial protocol (see Chapter 11) using CPAP or CPAP + pressure support (to maintain FRC):
  - Judge weaning to be successful if the patient remains hemodynamically stable with an acceptable pattern of breathing (e.g., rapid shallow breathing index [RSBI] < 100) and no signs of distress.
  - If the weaning attempt is unsuccessful, try again every 30–60 minutes until the patient can maintain adequate oxygenation and ventilation without hemodynamic compromise for at least 30 minutes with pressure support of 5 cm H_2O or less.
  - Recommend extubation or (if the protocol allows) extubate the patient if the patient is stable for at least 30 minutes without signs of distress.
  - Be prepared for reintubation or provision of noninvasive ventilation should the patient deteriorate after ETT removal.
- As soon as possible after successful extubation:
  - Recommend that the patient sit up in a chair and begin to ambulate.
  - Recommend initiation of appropriate airway clearance therapy, to include at least deep breathing and directed coughing, and lung expansion therapy if needed; helping patients with median sternotomies splint their incisions (using a "cough pillow") can facilitate effective coughing.
  - Continue to monitor the patient for signs of atelectasis or pneumonia (progressive hypoxemia, dyspnea, decreased breath sounds, dull percussion note, fever, tracheal deviation towards the affected side), even after transfer to a step-down unit.

Pulmonary Arterial Hypertension (PAH)

Pulmonary arterial hypertension is a clinical finding, not a single disease. It is associated with a diverse number of conditions characterized by a mean pulmonary artery pressure (mPAP) > 25 mm Hg at rest or > 30 mm Hg with exercise. As indicated in **Table 20-7**, these various conditions fall into one of five groups.

Assessment/Information Gathering

Symptoms

- You should suspect pulmonary hypertension in any patient with *unexplained* dyspnea, especially on exertion. Dyspnea is unexplained either if it occurs in patients with no signs of specific heart or lung disease; or signs of lung or heart disease, but it is more severe than the underlying condition would suggest.
- Other potential symptoms include fatigue, chest pain/angina, and dizziness/syncope (may only occur with physical activity)

Table 20-7 Pulmonary Hypertension Groupings and Associated Conditions

Group	Associated Conditions

I	• Pulmonary arterial hypertension (PAH):
	  ○ Idiopathic
	  ○ Inherited (familial)
	• Drug and toxin-induced
	• Congenital heart disease
	• Persistent pulmonary hypertension of the newborn (PPHN)

II	• Pulmonary hypertension associated with left heart disease:
	  ○ Left ventricular failure (LVF)
	  ○ Left-sided valve disorders (e.g., mitral stenosis)

III	• Pulmonary hypertension associated with lung disease:
	  ○ COPD
	  ○ Interstitial lung disease
	  ○ Sleep-disordered breathing
	  ○ Hypoxemic vasoconstriction (e.g., ARDS)

IV	• Pulmonary hypertension caused by thrombi/emboli

V	• Miscellaneous causes:
	  ○ Thrombocythemia
	  ○ Connective tissue diseases (e.g., sarcoidosis)
	  ○ Sickle cell disease
	  ○ Chronic renal failure
	  ○ Liver cirrhosis ("portopulmonary hypertension")
	  ○ HIV
	  ○ Vasculitis
	  ○ Pulmonary vessel compression (e.g., adenopathy, tumor)

Table 20-8 Functional Classes of Pulmonary Hypertension

Class	Description
I	Patients in whom regular physical activity does not cause undue dyspnea or fatigue, chest pain, or near syncope.
II	Patients who are comfortable at rest but for whom ordinary physical activity causes undue dyspnea or fatigue, chest pain, or near syncope.
III	Patients who are comfortable at rest, but even minimal activity causes undue dyspnea or fatigue, chest pain, or near syncope.
IV	Patients may have dyspnea and fatigue even at rest, typically manifest signs of right-heart failure, and are unable to carry out any physical activity without symptoms.

Based on the severity of symptoms relative to the level of physical activity, the World Health Organization (WHO) has established four functional classes of pulmonary hypertension. As depicted in **Table 20-8**, these classes are similar to the NYHA Functional Classification of heart failure.

Physical Signs

- Vital signs/SpO$_2$
- Tachycardia at rest
- Reduced pulse pressure (the difference between systemic systolic and diastolic)

- Desaturation (> 3–4%) with exertion
- Heart sounds:
  - Loud pulmonary component of the second heart sound (P2)
  - Pansystolic murmur indicating tricuspid regurgitation
  - Diastolic murmur indicating pulmonic insufficiency
- Lung sounds:
  - Unremarkable unless there is associated left heart (Group II) or pulmonary disease (Group III) processes
- Inspection (signs of right heart failure in advanced disease):
  - Jugular vein distention
  - Hepatomegaly
  - Peripheral edema
  - Ascites
  - Cool extremities
  - Central cyanosis

Recommending Diagnostic Tests

- Pulmonary artery (PA) catheterization (***the gold standard for diagnosis***)
  - Confirms presence of hypertension (mPAP > 25 mm Hg at rest) and its severity (mild: < 35 mm Hg; moderate: 35–45 mm Hg; severe > 45 mm Hg)
  - Can differentiate pulmonary arterial hypertension (PAH; Group I) from other causes such as left ventricular failure (LVF), for example:
    - PAH: normal pulmonary artery wedge pressure (PAWP; < 15 mm Hg), high pulmonary vascular resistance (PVR; > 3 mm Hg/L/min or > 240 dynes-sec/cm^5)
    - LVF: high PAWP (> 15 mm Hg), normal PVR (< 3 mm Hg/L/min or < 240 dynes-sec/cm^5)
    - Can identify patients with PAH who can be treated with oral calcium-channel blockers (the *vasodilator test*)
- IV/inhaled prostacyclins or inhaled nitric oxide:
  - Positive response: mPAP decrease ≥ 10 mm Hg, to < 40 mm Hg
- Imaging tests:
  - Echocardiography (for screening *and* diagnosis); findings can include:
    - Right ventricular systolic pressure ≥ 40 mm Hg (equivalent to PA systolic if no outflow obstruction)
    - Enlarged, "D-shaped" RV, septal bowing into the LV during systole
    - Tricuspid regurgitation
    - Dilated RA and vena cava
    - Pericardial effusion
  - Chest CT:
    - Enlarged main pulmonary artery (diameter > 29 mm)
    - May identify thrombi within the pulmonary arteries (Group IV)
  - Chest x-ray:
    - Not especially helpful in identifying early-stage PAH
    - Can help identify left heart failure (Group II), pulmonary disease (Group III) or some miscellaneous (Group V) processes
    - In advanced disease: enlargement of the central pulmonary arteries, cardiomegaly
- Electrocardiogram (findings usually seen late in the disease process; can help exclude other diagnoses)
  - Right-ventricular hypertrophy/right-axis deviation
  - Right atrial enlargement
  - Right bundle branch block
- Pulmonary function tests and sleep studies—mainly to identify or rule out Group III conditions as causes:
  - Exercise tests (see Chapters 3 and 4)
  - 6-minute walk test (6MWT)
  - 6MWT < 330 meters associated with higher mortality in PAH patients.

- ○ It helps monitor patient progress and evaluate response to therapy.
- ○ Cardiopulmonary exercise test:
  - It can be difficult for patients to perform (due to debilitating dyspnea).
  - $\dot{V}o_{2max} < 10$ mL/kg/min predicts survival.
- Laboratory tests:
  - ○ Serum troponin (associated with RV overdistention and ischemia)
  - ○ BNP (correlates with PVR, cardiac output, and functional class of patients with PAH)
  - ○ Other tests specific to suspected conditions (e.g., D-dimer for pulmonary embolism)

Treatment/Decision Making

Treatment for pulmonary hypertension *varies by condition grouping and by the severity of patient symptoms* (World Health Organization [WHO] functional classification). **Table 20-9** outlines the different treatment strategies according to condition grouping. The remainder of this pearl focuses on treatment/decision making for PAH (Group I)

For patients with PAH, recommend:

- Pulmonary vasodilator therapy (see **Table 20-10**)
- Diuretics as appropriate (to reduce symptoms of right ventricular failure)
- Oral thrombolytic therapy (e.g., warfarin) if PAH is idiopathic
- O_2 therapy for hypoxemia
- Influenza and pneumococcal vaccination
- Lifestyle modifications (e.g., aerobic exercise, sodium-restricted diet)

In terms of pulmonary vasodilator therapy, Table 20-10 summarizes the current categories and available preparations approved for use. Preparations include those for oral, parenteral (IV and SQ), and inhalation administration via nebulizer (currently the prostacyclins include: epoprostenol, treprostinil, and iloprost).

Recommend:

- An *oral agent* for patients with WHO functional Class II or III symptoms (*Note*: Calcium-channel blockers are indicated to treat PAH *if and only if* the patient has a positive response to the vasodilator test; *these agents are contraindicated in patients with right heart failure or those who are hemodynamically unstable.*)
- *Combination therapy* using oral or oral and inhaled agents with differing mechanisms of actions for patients whose symptoms persist when receiving a single drug

Table 20-9 Common Treatment Strategies for Pulmonary Hypertension

Group	Common Treatment Approaches
I (PAH, CHD, PPHN)	• Pulmonary vasodilators • Atrial septostomy • Lung/heart-lung transplantation
II (Left heart failure)	• LVF: Diuretics, β-blockers, ACE inhibitors • Valve disease: repair/replace
III (Lung disease)	• COPD/ILD: O_2 therapy • Sleep disorders: CPAP/BiPAP
IV (Thrombo-embolic disorders)	• Anticoagulants/thrombolytics • Pulmonary thromboendarterectomy
V (Miscellaneous)	• Treatment by a specific cause

ACE, angiotensin-converting enzyme; BiPAP, bilevel positive airway pressure; CHD, congenital heart disease; COPD, chronic obstructive pulmonary disease; CPAP, continuous positive airway pressure; ILD, interstitial lung disease; LVF, left ventricular failure; PAH, pulmonary arterial hypertension; PPHN, persistent pulmonary hypertension of the newborn.

Table 20-10 Categories and Drugs Used to Treat Pulmonary Hypertension

Category/Agent	Available Routes
Calcium-Channel Blockers	
Diltiazem (Cardizem)	Oral
Nifedipine (Procardia)	Oral
Prostacyclins	
Epoprostenol (Flolan)	IV, Inhalation (off-label)
Treprostinil (Remodulin)	IV, SQ (continuous)
Treprostinil (Tyvaso) solution	Inhalation
Treprostinil (Orenitram) tabs	Oral
Iloprost (Ventavis)	Inhalation
Phosphodiesterase-5 (PDE-5) Inhibitors	
Sildenafil (Viagra, Revatio)	Oral
Tadalafil (Adcirca)	Oral
Vardenafil (Levitra)	Oral
Endothelin Receptor Antagonist (ERAs)	
Bosentan (Tracleer)	Oral
Ambrisentan (Letairis)	Oral
Macitentan (Opsumit)	Oral
Guanylate Cyclase (sGC) Stimulators	
Riociguat (Adempas)	Oral

- ○ The combination of ambrisentan (an endothelin receptor antagonist [ERA]) and tadalafil (a PDE-5 inhibitor) is recommended as first-line therapy for newly diagnosed patients with group I PAH and WHO Class II or III symptoms.
- ○ The U.S. Food and Drug Administration (FDA) warns *against* combining phosphodiesterase-5 (PDE-5) inhibitors and guanylate cyclase (sGC) stimulators due to an unfavorable safety profile.
- *Continuous parenteral prostacyclin therapy* (i.e., Flolan, Remodulin) for patients with severe symptoms (WHO functional Class IV) or those with WHO Class III disease that progresses despite treatment with oral/inhaled agents

What about nitric oxide? Inhaled nitric oxide (INO) is appropriate for use only in the acute care setting, with very limited indications. *It is not used to manage patients with chronic pulmonary hypertension.* Currently, INO is approved only for the treatment of term and near-term neonates ($\geq$ 34 weeks) with hypoxemic respiratory failure ($Pao_2 < 100$ torr on $Fio_2 = 1.0$ or an oxygenation index > 25) associated with persistent pulmonary hypertension of the newborn (PPHN). Common "off-label" uses of INO (for which evidence of effectiveness is lacking or inconclusive) include the following:

- Prevention of bronchopulmonary dysplasia/chronic lung disease in infants
- Management of pulmonary hypertension after cardiac surgery in infants and children with congenital heart disease
- Treatment of pulmonary hypertension associated with ARDS in children and adults
- Treatment of pulmonary arterial hypertension/acute right ventricular failure in adults
- Treatment of sickle cell crisis

Pulmonary Embolism (PE)

Acute pulmonary embolism (PE) is a cardiovascular condition that is common and sometimes fatal. A PE refers to obstruction of the pulmonary artery or one of its branches by a thrombus (most common), tumor, air, or fat that originates elsewhere in the body. A PE can lead to pulmonary

Table 20-11 Pulmonary Emboli Acuity Classification

Classification	Description
Acute	Patients with acute PE typically develop symptoms and signs immediately after obstruction of pulmonary vessels. It can be fatal.
Subacute	Some patients with PE may also present subacutely within days or weeks following the initial event.
Chronic	Patients with chronic PE slowly develop symptoms of pulmonary hypertension over many years (i.e., chronic thromboembolic pulmonary hypertension; heart failure).

Table 20-12 Common Pulmonary Emboli Risk Factors

Category	Risk Factors
Hypercoagulation disorders	• Oral contraceptives • Polycythemia • Multiple myeloma
Trauma/surgery	• Bone fractures, especially long bones • Large soft tissue injury • Postoperative states: Major abdominal/pelvic surgery, hip/knee joint replacement, postoperative intensive care • Obstetrics: Late pregnancy, cesarian section, puerperium
Venous stasis	• Limited mobility: hospitalization, geriatric care • History of previous venous thromboembolism • Prolonged sitting (e.g., car or plane travel) • Congestive heart failure • Varicose vein, thrombophlebitis
Others	• Cardiovascular: congenital heart disease, hypertension, superficial venous thrombosis, central venous catheter • Humoral: estrogen use: oral contraception, hormone replacement therapy • Miscellaneous: chronic obstructive lung disease, neurologic impairment, latent malignancy, thrombotic defects, obesity

hypertension and right heart failure in the long term. The evaluation of patients with a suspected PE should be efficient so that patients can be diagnosed, and therapy administered quickly to reduce the morbidity and mortality associated with this condition.

Assessment/Information Gathering

The clinical presentation of PE is variable and often nonspecific, making the diagnosis challenging. Patients with PE can present acutely, subacutely, or chronically. See **Table 20-11** for presentation classification.

The initial patient assessment must include assessing for predisposing factors that will make the diagnosis of a PE more likely. **Table 20-12** list some of the factors predisposing a patient to pulmonary emboli.

A PE presentation can range from no symptoms at all for a small clot to shock or sudden death in the case of large blockages. The most common presenting symptom is *dyspnea,* followed by *chest pain* (classically pleuritic in nature), *cough,* and signs of *deep venous thrombosis.* Additional symptoms include orthopnea, wheezing, and hemoptysis. The onset of dyspnea is frequently rapid, usually within seconds or minutes.

Additional common presenting signs on examination include:

- Tachypnea
- Calf or thigh swelling, erythema, edema, tenderness, palpable cords
- Tachycardia
- Rales
- Decreased breath sounds
- An accentuated pulmonic component of the second heart sound
- Jugular venous distention
- Fever, mimicking pneumonia
- Hypoxemia and respiratory alkalosis in the ABG results

Recommending Diagnostic Tests

During a PE, laboratory tests are not diagnostic but rather confirm or rule out the presence of alternative diagnoses and provide prognostic information if PE is diagnosed:

- *Complete blood count and serum chemistries*: Laboratory findings include leukocytosis and elevated serum lactate dehydrogenase (LDH) and aspartate aminotransferase (AST).
- *Arterial blood gas (ABG)*:
  - Unexplained hypoxemia in the setting of a normal chest radiograph should raise the clinical suspicion for PE and prompt further evaluation.
  - Respiratory alkalosis and hypocapnia can also be present.
  - Hypercapnia, respiratory, and lactic acidosis are uncommon but can be seen in patients with massive PE associated with obstructive shock and respiratory arrest.
- *Troponin*: Serum troponin I and T levels are useful prognostically but not diagnostically.
- *D-dimer*: An elevated D-dimer alone is insufficient to make a diagnosis of PE but can be useful to rule out PE. D-dimer testing is best used in conjunction with clinical probability assessment to determine further testing.
  - Due to their high sensitivity, and the fact that accurate results are available quickly, a "sensitive D-dimer" testing that uses quantitative or semiquantitative rapid enzyme-linked immunosorbent assays (ELISA) is preferred. However, D-dimer testing will often be falsely positive for patients with recent surgery or trauma, so testing in such instances may be contraindicated.
  - For D-dimer assays, a level ≥500 ng/mL is usually considered positive, and <500 ng/mL is deemed to be negative.
- *Electrocardiography*: The most common findings are tachycardia and nonspecific ST-segment and T-wave changes.
- *Chest radiograph*: It helps to rule out for an alternative cause of the patient's symptoms. It is also performed to determine eligibility for ventilation-perfusion (V/Q) scanning.
- *Computed tomography pulmonary angiography* (CTPA): For most patients with suspected PE, CTPA, also called chest CT angiogram with contrast, is the first-choice diagnostic imaging modality because it is sensitive and specific for the diagnosis of PE.
  - CTPA is widely available, and, in most settings, it can be performed on an urgent or emergent basis.
- *Ventilation-perfusion scan*:
  - V/Q scanning is mostly reserved for patients in who CTPA is contraindicated or inconclusive, or when additional testing is needed.
  - V/Q scans results are reported as normal, low-probability, intermediate-probability, and high-probability.
- *Pulmonary angiography*:
  - Pulmonary angiography, in which contrast is injected under fluoroscopy via a catheter introduced into the right heart, was the historical gold standard for the diagnosis of PE.
  - With the widespread emergence of CTPA, this procedure is infrequently used and reserved for rare circumstances for patients with a high clinical probability of PE, in whom CTPA or V/Q scanning is nondiagnostic and in whom a diagnosis determines an important clinical decision.

Treatment/Decision Making

The initial approach to patients with suspected pulmonary embolism (PE) should focus upon stabilizing the patient while clinical evaluation and definitive diagnostic testing are ongoing.

The following actions are recommended:

- Respiratory support:
  - Supplemental oxygen should be administered to target oxygen saturation of ≥ 90%.
  - Severe hypoxemia, hemodynamic collapse, or respiratory failure should prompt consideration of intubation and mechanical ventilation.
- Intravenous fluids to treat hypotension if present.
- Vasopressors to provide adequate perfusion if not restored with IV fluids.
- Anticoagulation therapy
- Thrombolytic therapy: Thrombolysis and catheter-based therapies may be considered on a case-by-case basis when the benefits are assessed by the clinician to outweigh the risk of hemorrhage.
- Embolectomy is indicated in patients with hemodynamically unstable PE in whom thrombolytic therapy is contraindicated. This relatively high-risk procedure is also a therapeutic option in those who fail thrombolysis. Emboli can be removed surgically or using a catheter.
- Inferior vena cava (IVC) filter is indicated for most patients with PE in whom anticoagulation is contraindicated or patients in whom the risk of bleeding is unacceptably high.
- Patients with PE should always receive supportive care with analgesia to treat the pleuritic pain and chest discomfort, intravenous fluids, and oxygen, as clinically indicated.
- Early ambulation does not promote embolization and, when feasible, should be encouraged in most patients with acute PE, once the patient is definitively treated.

The prognosis from pulmonary embolism (PE) is variable. A patient with a single, small, subsegmental pulmonary embolism may be asymptomatic, but one with a massive PE and shock generally has a poor prognosis. In general, if left untreated, a diagnosis of PE is associated with an overall mortality of up to 30% compared with 2–11% in those treated with anticoagulation.

NEUROMUSCULAR DISORDERS

Number of Simulations in the CSE: 1 Case

Neuromuscular disorders commonly encountered by RTs include those for which acute muscle weakness/paralysis is the major presenting symptom (such as myasthenia gravis [MG] and Guillain-Barré syndrome [GBS]) and chronic disorders in which a slow but progressive decline in muscle function eventually results in respiratory insufficiency and failure (such as muscular dystrophy [MD] and amyotrophic lateral sclerosis [ALS]). Also, tetanus (included in this section for completeness) is rarely encountered by RTs, but it is another neuromuscular disorder that may appear in the CSE.

In neuromuscular cases, assessing a patient's level of consciousness is an "Always Select" option, with obtaining the Glasgow Coma Scale score being important if the patient is unconscious. The gag reflex and ability to swallow are both important, as is assessing upper airway protection, whereas more sophisticated tests such as electroencephalograms (EEGs) and intracranial pressure (ICP) measurements have narrower indications. **Table 20-13** summarizes our guidance on selecting information in managing these cases.

Neuromuscular Disorders with Acute Manifestations (Guillain-Barré Syndrome and Myasthenia Gravis)

Guillain-Barré syndrome (GBS) is an acute, inflammatory neuropathy affecting the spinal root and peripheral nerves. Inflammation destroys the myelin sheaths surrounding the nerves, causing severe muscle weakness and diminished reflexes. GBS often occurs following viral or bacterial infections, especially *Campylobacter jejuni* (diarrhea) and cytomegalovirus (CMV) upper respiratory infections. GBS also has been reported to develop after certain immunizations.

Myasthenia gravis (MG) is an autoimmune disease in which excessive anti-acetylcholine receptor (anti-AchR) antibody blocks the acetylcholine receptors at the myoneural junction, causing a characteristic progressive loss of muscle strength with repeated use (*fatigability*). Once diagnosed, the condition typically is recurrent, with fluctuating episodes of weakness followed by periods of remission. A severe episode of weakness, termed a *myasthenic crisis*, can involve life-threatening respiratory muscle weakness. Myasthenic crises commonly are triggered by viral infections, surgery, childbirth, or drug-related issues.

Because one of these acutely presenting neuromuscular conditions often appears on the CSE and because candidates frequently confuse the two, we have summarized our case management pearls in the form of a comparative table (**Table 20-14**).

Treatment/Decision Making

Respiratory Management to Implement/Recommend for Both Diseases (GB+MG)

- Implement Vc, NIF monitoring every 4 to 8 hours
- Provide O_2 therapy as needed to keep $SpO_2 > 90\%$

Table 20-13 Selecting Neurologic or Neuromuscular-Related Information

Information	Select To
Muscle tone	Differentiate lower motor neuron disorders (hypotonia) from upper neuron disorders (hypertonia)
Deep tendon reflex	Assess for peripheral neuropathy, polymyositis, muscular dystrophy, or paralysis
Gag reflex	Assess the level of consciousness/anesthesia or upper airway control
Ability to swallow	Assess upper airway control/aspiration risk
Glasgow Coma Scale score	Determine the level/depth of coma and mortality risk
Babinski reflex	Assess for brain damage
EEG	Stage sleep or confirm brain death
EMG/nerve conduction	Test neuromuscular function in disorders such as ALS, myasthenia gravis, and muscular dystrophy
ICP	Monitor patients with traumatic brain injury

Table 20-14 Guillain-Barré Syndrome Versus Myasthenia Gravis

Guillain-Barré Syndrome	Myasthenia Gravis
Assessment/Information Gathering	
History and Clinical Signs and Symptoms	
• History of recent febrile illness • Rapidly progressing *ascending* symmetrical muscle weakness/paralysis • Sensory dysesthesias (pain or discomfort to touch) • Decreased or absent deep tendon reflexes • Dysautonomia (rapid, wide fluctuations in BP, frequent cardiac arrhythmias) • Dysphagia (indicating bulbar muscle involvement), loss of gag reflex • Dyspnea, often progressing to respiratory insufficiency	• History of painless muscle weakness that worsens with repeated use • *Descending* and often episodic muscle weakness/paralysis • Ptosis (drooping eyelids) • Ophthalmoplegia/diplopia (weakness of eye muscles, double vision) • Dysphagia (indicating bulbar muscle involvement), loss of gag reflex • Normal deep tendon reflexes • Respiratory distress (advanced/untreated)

Table 20-14 Guillain-Barré Syndrome Versus Myasthenia Gravis (*continued*)

Assessment/Information Gathering	
Diagnostic Tests to Recommend and Characteristic Findings	
• Lumbar puncture to gather cerebral spinal fluid: increased protein content, low WBC	• Antibody tests: ↑ anti-acetylcholine receptor (anti-AchR) antibody
• Electromyography (EMG) and nerve conduction studies (NCS): slowing or blockage of nerve conduction	• EMG/NCS: decreased amplitude of muscle action potential with repeated stimulation
• Antibody tests: ↑ antiganglioside antibodies	• Positive tensilon (edrophonium) test: dramatic improvement in muscle strength within 1 minute of administration*
• Liver enzymes: ↑AST, ALT	• CT or MRI scan: may show the presence of a thymoma (thymus gland tumor)
• Serology—positive for *C. jejuni* or CMV	
• Breath sounds—normal unless aspiration and pneumonia due to loss of upper airway reflexes (indicated by basilar crackles and wheezes)	• Breath sounds: normal unless aspiration or pneumonia due to loss of upper airway reflexes (indicated by basilar crackles and wheezes)
• Spirometry: ↓Vc, ↓ MIP/NIF, ↓ MEP	• Spirometry: ↓Vc, ↓ MIP/NIF, ↓ MEP
• Blood gases: if respiratory involvement, acute respiratory acidosis; hypoxemia only if aspiration and pneumonia	• Blood gases: if respiratory involvement, acute respiratory acidosis; hypoxemia only if aspiration or pneumonia due to loss of upper airway reflexes
• Chest x-ray: normal unless aspiration and/or pneumonia	• Chest x-ray: normal unless aspiration and/or pneumonia
Treatment/Decision Making	
General Medical/Surgical Treatment to Recommend	
• Vital signs, SpO_2, and ECG monitoring (dysautonomia requires continuous HR, BP, and arrhythmia monitoring)	• Vital signs and SpO_2 monitoring; close observation during a myasthenic crisis
• Plasmapheresis (plasma exchange)	• Acetylcholinesterase inhibitor therapy, such as pyridostigmine (Mestinon)
• IV immunoglobulin therapy	• Immunosuppressant therapy, such as hydrocortisone or azathioprine (Imuran)
• Analgesics for dysesthesia (NSAIDs, opioids)	• Plasmapheresis (plasma exchange)
• Fluids/Trendelenburg positioning for severe hypotension (for patients who are sensitive to vasoactive medications)	• IV immunoglobulin therapy
	• Thymectomy (especially if a thymoma is present)
• Deep vein thrombosis (DVT) prophylaxis for immobility	• DVT prophylaxis for immobility
• Physical rehabilitation during the recovery stage	• Physical rehabilitation during the recovery stage

↑, increased; ↓, decreased; ALT, alanine aminotransferase; AST, aspartate aminotransferase; BP, blood pressure; CMV, cytomegalovirus; EMG/NCS, electromyogram and nerve conduction studies; HR, heart rate; MEP, maximum expiratory pressure; MIP, maximum inspiratory pressure; NIF, negative inspiratory force; NSAID, nonsteroidal anti-inflammatory drug; Vc, vital capacity.

*A patient who improves when given tensilon is said to be in a *myasthenia crisis*, while one who worsens when given tensilon likely is having a *cholinergic crisis* (due to excessive acetylcholine at the myoneural junction). Other symptoms include diaphoresis, bronchorrhea, bronchospasm, and miosis. Atropine is the treatment.

- Recommend intubation and mechanical ventilation if:
  - Vc < 1.0 L or < 15 mL/kg (or rapidly declining to such levels)
  - MIP/NIF < –25 cm H_2O, MEP < 40 cm H_2O (or rapidly declining)
  - Inability to cough, swallow, and protect the airway
  - ABG evidence of respiratory failure
  - Aspiration pneumonia with severe hypoxemia
- Recommend trach if:
  - Severe weakness, especially if bulbar involvement
  - Likely need for mechanical ventilation > 10 days
- Implement rigorous infection control/VAP protocol

Muscular Dystrophy

Muscular dystrophies constitute a group of more than 30 inherited diseases that cause progressive muscle weakness and loss, eventually resulting in the inability to walk, swallowing difficulty, respiratory muscle insufficiency, and respiratory failure. The most common variant is Duchenne-type muscular dystrophy (DMD), an X-linked recessive trait disorder that occurs almost exclusively in males. Diagnosis of DMD is based on patient history and physical findings and is confirmed by genetic testing or protein analysis of muscle tissue, which will demonstrate an absence of the dystrophin protein.

Assuming an early diagnosis, DMD typically progresses through four stages: (1) normal respiratory function, (2) adequate ventilation but ineffective cough, (3) adequate daytime ventilation but inadequate nighttime ventilation, and (4) inadequate daytime and nighttime ventilation. During each stage, the role of the RT varies according to the functional limitations experienced by the patient. For this reason, the DMD management pearls presented here follow this four-stage progression. Note that other chronic neuromuscular diseases such as amyotrophic lateral sclerosis (ALS) follow a pattern like DMD and, therefore, require similar treatment and decision making.

Assessment/Information Gathering

- Stage 1: Normal respiratory function
  - Recommend annual visits to a physician and routine immunizations (pneumococcal vaccination at 2 years old, yearly influenza vaccine beginning at 6 months of age).
  - Establish baseline respiratory function (i.e., SpO_2, FVC, FEV_1, peak cough flow, MIP, and MEP); *reassess at every subsequent visit (over the patient's entire lifetime).*
- Stage 2: Adequate ventilation, ineffective cough
  - Recommend biannual visits to a pulmonologist after age 12, after confinement to a wheelchair, or after the patient's Vc drops below 80% predicted; follow up on respiratory function measures.
  - Recommend annual polysomnography for sleep-disordered breathing.
  - Recommend assessment for dysphagia.
  - Recommend annual chest x-ray.
- Stage 3: Adequate daytime ventilation, inadequate nighttime ventilation
  - Recommend quarterly visits to the pulmonologist; follow up on respiratory function measures and dysphagia.
  - Measure awake $PetCO_2$.
- Stage 4: Inadequate daytime and nighttime ventilation
  - Recommend quarterly visits to the pulmonologist; follow up on respiratory function measures and dysphagia.
  - Implement continuous monitoring of SpO_2 with regular assessment of $PetCO_2$.

Treatment/Decision Making

- Stage 1: Normal respiratory function
  - Begin patient/caregiver education in disease management, with emphasis on preventive care (e.g., immunizations, regular visits to the doctor), airway clearance strategies, and monitoring of respiratory function.
- Stage 2: Adequate ventilation, ineffective cough
  - Train and have caregivers implement an airway clearance regimen such as manually assisted coughing or mechanical insufflation–exsufflation once peak cough flow is less than 270 L/min (4.5 L/sec), or MEP is less than 60 cm H_2O.
  - Train and have caregivers incorporate volume recruitment/deep lung inflation (e.g., inexsufflation) into the airway clearance regimen when FVC is less than 40% predicted or less than 1.25 L (in adults); avoid incentive spirometry, which generally is not effective in patients with respiratory muscle weakness.
- Stage 3: Adequate daytime ventilation, inadequate nighttime ventilation
  - Recommend/initiate nocturnal noninvasive positive-pressure ventilation (NPPV) for respiratory insufficiency or sleep-disordered breathing. Criteria include the following:

- Signs and symptoms of hypoventilation (fatigue, dyspnea, headache, lack of concentration, hypersomnolence)
- SpO_2 < 95% (air) or $PetCO_2$ > 45 torr while awake
- Apnea-hypopnea index > 10/h or at least four O_2 desaturation events/h (oxygen desaturation index [ODI] ≥ 4)
    - Avoid simple CPAP because it does not overcome hypoventilation, and *do not* recommend negative-pressure ventilation because it can cause upper airway obstruction in these patients.
    - Provide the patient and caregivers with the training needed to manage ventilatory support in the home.
- Stage 4: Inadequate daytime and nighttime ventilation
    - Recommend/initiate daytime NPPV when the patient's $PetCO_2$ is more than 50 torr, when the SpO_2 remains below 92% while the patient is awake, or when ventilatory support is required to relieve persistent dyspnea.
    - Use oral/mouthpiece interfaces for daytime NPPV; some patients with DMD also can use a mouthpiece while sleeping.
    - Recommend invasive ventilation via tracheostomy if NPPV is contraindicated, if it is not feasible due to paralysis/weakness of the muscles controlling swallowing (bulbar weakness), or if the patient/caregivers express a preference for the invasive route.
    - Provide the patient and caregivers with the training needed to manage continuous ventilatory support in the home.

Hypoxemia can occur in patients with DMD. When this condition is due to hypoventilation, the appropriate treatment is to lower the PCO_2 (which raises the PO_2) via assisted ventilation, not via administering O_2. Likewise, if the hypoxemia is due to mucus plugging or atelectasis, O_2 therapy will merely mask the underlying problem. In these cases, the best management approach is the rigorous application of the selected airway clearance regimen, with the goal being the restoration of a SpO_2 of 92% or higher.

Tetanus

Tetanus is a neuromuscular disorder caused by wound exposure to a toxin produced by *Clostridium tetani*, an anaerobic bacterium often found in the soil. The tetanus toxin blocks the inhibitory motor and autonomic neurons in the spinal cord, resulting in intense muscle spasms/rigidity as well as sympathetic overactivity. The toxin does not affect sensory neurons, so patients remain fully aware and typically experience severe pain associated with the muscle spasms.

Fortunately, tetanus is rare in developed countries due to widespread immunization. However, because you might encounter cases of tetanus among those individuals who have not been immunized, the following pearls should help guide management should a patient with this condition present to your hospital.

Assessment/Information Gathering

- Look for a recent history (typically 4 days to 2 weeks) of either a contaminated penetrating wound (including unsterile needle punctures by illicit drug users) or a necrotic or anaerobic infection (e.g., infected umbilical stumps, septic abortions, anaerobic periodontal infections, chronic diabetic ulcers).
- Assess for the following symptoms:
    - *Trismus* (intense spasms of the masseter muscle, commonly called "lockjaw")
    - Dysphagia and abnormal gag reflex (insertion of a tongue blade causes the patient to bite down instead of gagging)
    - Spasms of the facial muscles, causing unnatural expressions such as an odd grin (called *risus sardonicus*)
    - Neck stiffness progressing to *opisthotonus* (severe spasm in which the head and heels arch or "bow" backward in extreme hyperextension)
    - Rigid abdominal wall

- Sympathetic overactivity—for example, irritability, restlessness, sweating, tachycardia, and reflex spasms in response to minimal external stimuli such as noise, light, or touch
  - Electromyography (EMG)—continuous discharge of motor units
- No laboratory or imaging tests can confirm the diagnosis; however, the presence of serum antitoxin levels greater than 0.01 U/mL can help rule out a diagnosis of tetanus.
- Recommend a toxicology screen for drug-induced dystonias or strychnine poisoning and a neurology assessment for other causes of seizures.

Treatment/Decision Making

- Upon diagnosis, recommend immediate IM administration of tetanus immunoglobulin.
- If the wound is contaminated, recommend that it be cleaned and debrided.
- Recommend an antibiotic such as metronidazole (Flagyl) to control further *C. tetani* growth.
- If ventilation and upper airway function are compromised, recommend intubation, mechanical ventilation, and intensive care.
- Because intubation may cause severe reflex laryngospasm, recommend rapid-sequence intubation with succinylcholine choline.
- Recommend IV administration of a benzodiazepine (e.g., midazolam) to provide sedation and control spasms.
- If benzodiazepine administration fails to control spasms, recommend a nondepolarizing neuromuscular blocking agent such as vecuronium or pancuronium (with ventilatory support); magnesium sulfate also can be recommended to reduce spasms and autonomic overactivity.

ADULT MEDICAL OR SURGICAL

Number of Simulations in the CSE: 5 Cases

This section is one of the most important and challenging of the CSE. Besides having the second largest number of cases, you also need to prepare for a large variety of medical or surgical conditions that can appear in this section of the CSE. Below we focus on the most common disorders you may be expected to help manage in this category of the exam (as listed in the NBRC CSE detailed content outline).

Cystic Fibrosis

Cystic fibrosis (CF) is a genetically inherited autosomal recessive disease that is more common in white persons than in individuals of other ethnic backgrounds. CF affects the exocrine glands, causing chronic respiratory infections and gastrointestinal dysfunction, including pancreatic enzyme insufficiency. End-stage lung disease is the principal cause of death in persons with CF. Definitive diagnosis is based on genetic testing.

Assessment/Information Gathering

For the patient *not* already confirmed by genetic testing to have CF:

- Obtain patient history, looking for the following findings:
  - Chronic cough with sputum production
  - Recurring respiratory infections
  - History of sinusitis
  - History of bowel obstruction or steatorrhea (fatty stool)
  - Failure to thrive/retarded growth
- Conduct or review a physical examination, looking for the following findings:
  - Abnormal breath sounds (e.g., wheezes, crackles, rhonchi)
  - Failure to thrive/retarded growth:
    - Body weight below the lower limit of normal
    - Body mass index (BMI) < 19

- Presence of nasal polyps
- Digital clubbing
- Signs of pancreatic insufficiency:
  - Steatorrhea (fatty stool)
  - Abdominal distention and flatulence
  - Weight loss/fatigue
- Recommend a sweat chloride test (considered positive for CF if > 60 mmol/L).
- Recommend a chest x-ray, looking for the following findings:
  - Hyperinflation (due to air trapping)
  - Peribronchial thickening
  - Infiltrates with or without lobar atelectasis
  - Right ventricular hypertrophy (advanced cases)
  - Bronchiectasis (best confirmed via high-resolution CT scan)
- Recommend spirometry and lung volume measurements (to make the diagnosis and to establish a patient baseline for assessing disease progression), looking for the following findings:
  - Decreased FEV_1 and FEV_1/FVC (obstruction)
  - Increased RV/TLC ratio (air trapping)
  - Decreased TLC and Vc (late stage only, indicating lung scarring/fibrosis)
- Recommend sputum Gram stain as well as culture and sensitivity, looking for the following pathogens:
  - *Pseudomonas aeruginosa, Haemophilus influenzae, Staphylococcus aureus, Burkholderia cepacia, Escherichia coli,* or *Klebsiella pneumoniae.*
  - The presence of *P. aeruginosa* supports a diagnosis of CF.

If the patient is being seen in the clinic or ED for acute respiratory distress, obtain the following information:

- Recent history:
  - Development of fever
  - Increase in productive cough with purulent sputum
  - Increased fatigue, weakness, or poor appetite/weight loss
  - New-onset or increased hemoptysis
- Physical assessment:
  - Labored breathing with intercostal retractions and use of accessory muscles
  - Severe wheezing, rhonchi, or rhonchial fremitus
- Diagnostic tests:
  - New infiltrate on chest x-ray
  - Labs: leukocytosis; low Na^+, Cl^-, and K^+; hypochloremic metabolic acidosis
  - ABG/pulse oximetry: moderate hypoxemia, SpO_2 < 90% on room air

Treatment/Decision Making

For the immediate treatment of the CF patient in respiratory distress:

- Minimize the patient's contact with other CF patients and apply applicable transmission-based precautions.
- Provide supplemental O_2 to maintain a SpO_2 above 90%.
- To relieve airway obstruction, implement or recommend a combined aerosol drug and airway clearance regimen that includes the following elements:
- An aerosolized bronchodilator (e.g., albuterol), followed by
- Aerosolized dornase alfa (Pulmozyme), hypertonic saline (HyperSal), or *N*-acetylcysteine (Mucomyst), followed by:
  - Appropriate airway clearance therapy (to include directed coughing), followed by
  - If *P. aeruginosa* colonization or infection is confirmed, an aerosolized antibiotic:
    - Tobramycin (TOBI): via breath-enhanced nebulizer (e.g., Pari LC) or DPI (TOBI Podhaler)
    - Polymyxin E (Colistin): via breath-enhanced nebulizer (e.g., Pari LC)
    - Aztreonam (Cayston): via mesh nebulizer (e.g., Altera)

- Assess the effectiveness of this regimen by noting the patient's subjective response plus changes in SpO_2, sputum production, breath sounds (may clear or increase due to the movement of secretions into the larger airways), spirometry (FEV_1), and chest x-ray.
- Recommend oral, IV, or inhaled antibiotics (as described previously) specific to the colonizing organism(s).

Once the patient is stabilized, and the diagnosis confirmed, recommend implementation of a comprehensive disease management program:

- Annual influenza immunizations
- A high-energy/high-fat diet with increased salt intake, pancreatic enzyme replacement, and vitamin supplements
- Regular exercise activity (improves airway clearance and reduces exacerbations)
- Patient education:
  ○ Medication usage, including proper sequencing and inhaler technique(s)
  ○ Airway clearance techniques (including adjustments to fit the patient's lifestyle)
  ○ Use of action plans to respond to worsening signs and symptoms
  ○ Infection control, including proper hand hygiene, containment of respiratory secretions, avoidance of direct contact with other patients with CF, and proper cleaning and disinfection of reusable home care equipment, especially reusable nebulizers (see accompanying box [**Box 20-1**])
- Clinic visits every 2–3 months:
  ○ Assessment of growth and development, nutritional status, and BMI
  ○ Lung function (FEV_1 and SpO_2)
  ○ Collection of sputum sample for Gram stain as well as culture and sensitivity
  ○ Assessment of therapy effectiveness in retarding disease progression
  ○ Counseling regarding psychosocial issues
  ○ PA and lateral chest x-ray every 2–4 years

Non-Cystic Fibrosis Bronchiectasis

Bronchiectasis is an acquired and irreversible disorder of the major bronchi and bronchioles that is characterized by permanent abnormal dilatation and destruction of the bronchial walls. Bronchiectasis shares many clinical features with COPD, including inflamed and easily collapsible (high compliance) airways, obstruction to airflow, and frequent office visits and hospitalizations due to exacerbations.

Box 20-1 Home Cleaning and Disinfecting of Drug Nebulizers for Patient with CF

- Clean the nebulizer parts with dish detergent soap and water.
- Disinfect the nebulizer parts using one of the following methods:
  ○ Heat methods:
    - Place in boiling water, and boil for 5 minutes.
    - Place in a microwave-safe receptacle submerged in water, and microwave for 5 minutes.
    - Use a dishwasher (temp ≥ 70°C or 158°F) for 30 minutes.
    - Use an electrical steam sterilizer.
  ○ Cold methods:
    - Soak in 70% isopropyl alcohol for 5 minutes.
    - Soak in 3% hydrogen peroxide for 30 minutes.
- Do not disinfect with acetic acid, bleach, or benzalkonium chloride.
- Rinse with sterile or filtered (≤ 0.2-micron filter) water.
- Air-dry parts before storage

The diagnosis is established clinically based on cough on most days with tenacious sputum production, often one or more exacerbations/year, and radiographically by the presence of bronchial wall thickening and airway dilatation on chest CT scans.

Assessment/Information Gathering

The classic clinical manifestations of bronchiectasis are cough and the daily production of mucopurulent and tenacious sputum lasting months to years.

Additional clinical findings include:

- Less specific complaints include dyspnea, wheezing, and pleuritic chest pain
- Patients often report frequent bouts of "bronchitis" requiring therapy with repeated courses of antibiotics.
- History of repeated respiratory tract infections over several years, although a single episode of severe pulmonary infection can be the cause.
- Additional symptoms include cough, daily sputum production, dyspnea, rhinosinusitis, hemoptysis, and recurrent pleurisy.
- Crackles and wheezing are common, with digital clubbing occurring in a small number of patients.
- Laboratory tests:
  - A complete blood count with differential
  - Sweat chloride and mutation analysis of the cystic fibrosis transmembrane conductance regulator (CFTR) gene to rule out CF
  - Sputum smear and culture for bacteria, mycobacteria, and fungi
- The chest radiograph may show linear atelectasis, dilated and thickened airways, and irregular peripheral opacities.
- High-resolution computed tomography (HRCT) and multidetector computed tomography (MDCT) of the chest are the *diagnostic standard* for bronchiectasis.
- Characteristic features of bronchiectasis on HRCT and MDCT include airway dilatation, lack of airway tapering, bronchial thickening, and cysts. Also, mucopurulent plugs or debris accompanied by postobstructive air trapping may be observed.
- Pulmonary function testing is used for functional assessment of impairment due to bronchiectasis. Obstructive impairment (i.e., reduced or normal FVC, low FEV_1, and low FEV_1/FVC) is the most frequent finding.

Treatment/Decision Making

Treatment of bronchiectasis is aimed at controlling infection, reducing inflammation, and improving bronchial hygiene. Antibiotics and bronchopulmonary hygiene are the mainstays of bronchiectasis management.

For most causes of bronchiectasis, treatment of the underlying disease is not possible, as the bronchiectasis is most often a manifestation of scarring that resulted from a prior injury or pulmonary infection. However, some disease processes can be controlled to prevent further scarring of the lung tissue.

Treatment of Acute Exacerbations

Recommend:

- Oral, intravenous, and inhaled antibiotic medications: Inhaled antibiotics (e.g., tobramycin, aztreonam, colistin) can be used during acute exacerbations.
- Mucolytic agents and airway hydration: Nebulized hypertonic saline solution, mannitol, and mucolytic agents can be used to manage secretion clearance during exacerbations.
- Airway clearance therapy: Help to improve cough and help patients to expectorate the tenacious secretions and mucous plugs that frequently complicate bronchiectasis.
- Bronchodilators: Aerosol bronchodilator therapy, as used in asthma and COPD, may be appropriate if indicated.

- Anti-inflammatory medications: Since inflammation plays a significant role in bronchiectasis, recommending anti-inflammatory agents such as oral or inhaled glucocorticoids, nonsteroidal anti-inflammatory agents (NSAIDs), and statins might be beneficial.

For the long-term management of bronchiectasis, follow the recommendations for the long-term management of adult chronic airway disease found at the beginning of this chapter.

Pneumonia

Pneumonia is a bacterial, viral, or other microbial infection of one or both lungs that causes the alveoli to fill up with fluid or pus. If the infection is overwhelming, the alveoli become filled with fluid, RBCs, leukocytes, and macrophages, and that section of the lungs is said to be *consolidated*. Symptoms can be mild or severe and may include cough, sputum production, fever, chills, and difficulty breathing.

Many factors affect how severe pneumonia is, such as the type of organism causing the lung infection, age, and overall individual health. Pneumonia tends to be more serious for children under the age of five, adults over the age of 65, people with certain conditions such as heart failure, diabetes, or COPD, or people who have weak immune systems due to HIV/AIDS, chemotherapy (a treatment for cancer), or organ or blood and marrow stem cell transplant procedures.

Pneumonia can be classified according to the place of acquisition as the following:

- Nursing home–acquired pneumonia
- Community-acquired pneumonia (CAP)
- Hospital-acquired pneumonia (HAP)
  - Ventilator-associated pneumonia (VAP)

In addition to *where* the pneumonia process begins, the *type of organism* causing the infection can also vary. **Table 20-15** lists the most common causes of pneumonia and their classification.

Assessment/Information Gathering

Common pneumonia symptoms can vary from mild to so severe that hospitalization, intubation, and mechanical ventilation may be required. Common signs and symptoms of bacterial or viral pneumonia include:

- Cough, which may produce greenish, yellow, or even bloody sputum
- Fever, sweating, and chills
- Shortness of breath, tachypnea, and shallow breathing
- Pleuritic chest pain that gets worse when taking a deep breath or coughing
- Loss of appetite, low energy, and fatigue
- Confusion and lethargy, especially in the elderly

Viral pneumonia may start with flu-like symptoms, such as wheezing and generalized malaise; a high fever may occur after 12–36 hours. Bacterial pneumonia may cause a temperature as high as 105°F along with profuse sweating, cyanosis, and confusion.

Community-Acquired Pneumonia (CAP)

Community-acquired pneumonia (CAP) is defined as an acute infection of the pulmonary parenchyma in a patient who has acquired the infection in the community, as distinguished from hospital-acquired (nosocomial) pneumonia (HAP). CAP is most commonly caused by a bacterial agent (> 50%), but up to 40% can also be caused by viruses, especially during the winter season. The most common cause of CAP is *Streptococcus pneumoniae*.

CAP assessment includes the following:

- Clinical features are cough, fever, pleuritic chest pain, dyspnea, and purulent sputum production.
  - Mucopurulent sputum is most frequently associated with bacterial pneumonia.
  - Scant or watery sputum is more suggestive of an atypical pathogen.
- On physical examination, approximately 80% are febrile.
- Other features are GI symptoms such as nausea, vomiting, diarrhea.

Table 20-15 Pneumonia Classification According to Causing Agent

Classification	Causing Organism

Bacterial pneumonia	• Gram-positive:
	  ○ *Streptococcus*
	  ○ *Staphylococcus*

	• Gram-negative:
	  ○ *Haemophilus influenzae*
	  ○ *Klebsiella*
	  ○ *Pseudomonas aeruginosa*
	  ○ *Moraxella catarrhalis*
	  ○ *Escherichia coli*
	  ○ *Serratia* species
	  ○ *Enterobacter* species

	• Atypical organisms:
	  ○ *Mycoplasma pneumoniae*
	  ○ *Legionella pneumophila*
	  ○ *Chlamydia psittaci*
	  ○ *Chlamydia pneumoniae*

Viral pneumonia	• Influenza infection
	  ○ Respiratory syncytial virus (RSV)
	  ○ Parainfluenza virus
	  ○ Adenovirus
	  ○ Coronavirus (SARS)

Pneumonias by other organisms	• Aspiration • *Pneumocystis jiroveci* • Fungal infections • Tuberculosis • Cytomegalovirus

- Mental status changes are possible in the most severe presentation.
- Leukocytosis, typically between 15,000 and 30,000 per mm^3 with a leftward shift is commonly noted.
- Leukopenia can also occur and generally predicts a poor prognosis.
- Chest x-ray assessment:
  - *The presence of infiltrates on a chest radiograph is considered the gold standard for diagnosing pneumonia* when clinical and microbiologic findings are supportive.
  - The radiographic appearance of CAP depends on the causing agent and severity.
  - Depending on the severity of the pneumonia, the chest radiograph may show lobar consolidation, interstitial infiltrates, and cavitation.
  - Right middle lobe infiltrates and consolidation are commonly associated with aspiration pneumonia.
- CT scanning is not generally recommended for routine use in CAP since the cost is high, and there is no evidence that it improves outcome.
- Microbiology assessment:
  - For outpatients with CAP, routine diagnostic tests are recommended and performed according to suspected etiology.

- Hospitalized patients with CAP should have blood cultures, and sputum Gram stain performed if possible.
  - Sputum samples should be from a deep cough specimen obtained before antibiotics are given.
  - *A "good" sputum sample is one with polymorphonuclear leukocytes (PMNs) but few (or no) squamous epithelial cells (SECs) on Gram stain.*
- Patients with CAP admitted to the intensive care unit should, in addition to blood cultures, have *Legionella* and *Pneumococcus* urinary antigen tests and sputum culture (either expectorated or endotracheal aspirate) performed.
- Newer tests include polymerase chain reaction (PCR) for detecting *Chlamydia pneumoniae* and *Mycoplasma pneumoniae* as well as 14 other respiratory tract viruses. These tests are rapid, sensitive, and specific.

Ventilator-Associated Pneumonia (VAP)

Ventilator-associated pneumonia (VAP) is a type of hospital-acquired pneumonia (nosocomial pneumonia) or healthcare-associated pneumonia (HCAP) that develops after more than 48 hours of mechanical ventilation. Patients with severe nosocomial pneumonia who require mechanical ventilation *after* the onset of infection *do not* meet the definition of VAP.

VAP is associated with an increased risk of death in the ICU. Accurate diagnosis is important so that appropriate treatment can be instituted early while simultaneously avoiding antibiotic overuse and consequently, the development of multidrug resistant organisms (MDROs).

VAP assessment and information gathering include the following:

- VAP should be suspected in mechanically ventilated patients with new or progressive pulmonary infiltrates on imaging that presents with clinical findings of infection (e.g., fever, mucopurulent secretions, leukocytosis).
- VAP patients present with a gradual or sudden onset of the following:
  - Dyspnea and respiratory distress.
  - Fever, tachypnea, increased or purulent secretions, hemoptysis, rhonchi, crackles, reduced breath sounds, bronchospasm, and hypoxemia.
  - Reduced tidal volume during mechanical ventilation, increased inspiratory pressures, decreased lung compliance, increased plateau pressures are common findings.
  - Worsening hypoxemia in the ABG, leukocytosis, positive cultures (bronchoscopic or tracheal aspirates).
  - New or progressive infiltrates on chest radiograph or computed tomography (CT).
- Respiratory samples should be obtained before the initiation of antibiotics or change of antibiotic therapy.
- VAP diagnosis is confirmed when lower respiratory tract aspirates identify a pathogen.
  - Invasive methods for respiratory sampling generally involve nonbronchoscopic methods (e.g., mini-BAL) or bronchoscopic methods (e.g., bronchoscopic bronchoalveolar lavage [BAL] or protected specimen brush [PSB]).
  - Noninvasive sampling (i.e., endotracheal aspirates) is the alternative approach if invasive methods are not available. The sample is directly aspirated into a sterile specimen trap that can be sent for microbiologic analysis.

Treatment/Decision Making

For both CAP and VAP, the following recommendations apply:

- Antibiotic selection for each patient should be based on a careful assessment of the possible causing organism(s), the clinical disease course, and the risk factors for developing MDROs.
- O_2 therapy should be used to treat hypoxemia and decreased work of breathing.
- Aggressive bronchopulmonary toilet and hyperinflation therapy protocols are recommended to help manage secretions and offset alveolar consolidation and atelectasis.
- High-flow nasal cannula, bilevel noninvasive therapy, and CPAP should be used as indicated in the nonintubated patient in the presence of hypoxia and hypercapnia caused by alveolar consolidation and atelectasis.

- If hypercapnic or hypoxic respiratory failure occurs, intubation and mechanical ventilation must be implemented to support the patient.
- Ventilatory management of the intubated patient with pneumonia should follow established guidelines of lung-protective strategies for hypoxic and hypercapnic respiratory failure.
- Extracorporeal membrane oxygenation (ECMO), if available, should be recommended for those with profound hypoxemic failure.
- If the etiology of the pneumonia has been identified using reliable microbiologic methods, antimicrobial therapy should be directed at that pathogen.

For VAP prevention, a ventilator bundle can be recommended consisting of:

- Elevation of the head of the bed to 30 to 45 degrees
- Daily awakening trials and assessment of readiness for weaning/extubation
- Peptic ulcer disease prophylaxis
- Deep venous thrombosis prophylaxis
- Regular oral care with chlorhexidine

Prevention for both CAP and VAP continue to be the best treatment approach. Always recommend immunizing high-risk populations against influenza (flu shot) and *S. pneumoniae* (pneumococcal vaccine). Immunization is especially important for the very young, the immunocompromised, individuals older than 60 years, and those with chronic heart and lung diseases (e.g., COPD).

Acute Respiratory Distress Syndrome

Acute respiratory distress syndrome (ARDS) is a rapidly progressive form of acute respiratory failure characterized by *noncardiogenic* pulmonary edema, causing severe hypoxemia that is refractory to usual oxygen therapy. The pulmonary edema results from an increase in the permeability of the alveolar-capillary membrane due to a variety of injuries. In combination, these injuries cause a decrease in aerated lung tissue, impaired gas exchange (due to shunting), decreased lung compliance, and increased pulmonary vascular resistance and pulmonary arterial pressures.

Common conditions causing lung injury and associated with the onset of ARDS include the following:

- Pulmonary:
  - Pneumonia
  - Pulmonary contusion
  - Aspiration of gastric contents
- Extrapulmonary disorders:
  - Sepsis
  - Shock/trauma
  - Burns (inhalation injuries)
  - Pancreatitis

The primary differential diagnosis for ARDS is cardiogenic pulmonary edema, *which needs to be excluded as a cause in making treatment decisions.* Currently, ARDS is defined by its major clinical features as follows (the "Berlin Definition"):

- Acute onset (within one week of a known clinical insult or new/worsening respiratory symptoms)
- Bilateral infiltrates/opacities consistent with pulmonary edema on chest radiograph or CT
- Pulmonary edema *not* due to cardiac failure or fluid overload; if no clear-cut cause (e.g., aspiration), objective data such as echocardiography needed to rule out hydrostatic edema
- Refractory hypoxemia with a P/F ratio < 300 on PEEP/CPAP = 5 cm H_2O

Assessment/Information Gathering

- Assess for the history of abrupt onset of new/worsening respiratory symptoms.
- Assess for signs of respiratory distress (i.e., tachypnea, use of accessory muscles of respiration, thoracoabdominal paradox, diaphoresis).

Table 20-16 ARDS Classification Based on P/F Ratio*

Severity	P/F ratio
Mild	201–300
Moderate	101–200
Severe	P/F < 100
*Note that the American Thoracic Society uses a definition which classifies P/F Ratios of 200–300 as Acute Lung Injury (ALI) and ARDS as a P/F Ratio < 200.	

- Assess for diffuse crackles on auscultation (based on the underlying cause, other adventitious sounds may occur, e.g., wheezing with aspiration pneumonia).
- Evaluate for presence of severe hypoxemia: tachycardia, central cyanosis, SpO_2 < 90% on FiO_2 > 30%, P/F ratio < 300.
- Based on the P/F ratio, ARDS is further classified according to the Berlin definition as being mild, moderate, or severe (see **Table 20-16**).
- Confirm *absence* of findings suggesting cardiac failure or fluid overload (e.g., no S_3 or S_4 gallop, no jugular venous distention, no cardiomegaly or pleural effusions on chest x-ray).
- Recommend ABG (for objective assessment of PaO_2, P/F ratio, acid-base balance).
- Recommend chest radiograph or CT scan (looking for characteristic bilateral infiltrates/opacities).
- Recommend plasma BNP to help rule out CHF/cardiogenic pulmonary edema.
- Recommend echocardiography to rule out cardiogenic pulmonary edema.
- Recommend CVP to help rule out overhydration, adjust the fluid balance, and assess $ScvO_2$.
- Recommend additional evaluation relevant to suspected cause(s) (e.g., if sepsis is suspected cause, assess for fever, hypotension, and related lab data such as the presence of bacteria [in blood, lungs], CBC [leukocytosis], and blood lactate [tissue hypoxia]).

Treatment/Decision Making

If ARDS is diagnosed, implement a lung-protective ventilation protocol, such as the following (slightly modified from the ARDSNet protocol):

- Start in any ventilator mode with initial V_T of 8 mL/kg predicted body weight (PBW).
  - To calculate PBW use the following formulas:
    - Male: PBW (kg) = 50 + 2.3 [height (in.) – 60]
    - Female: PBW (kg) = 45.5 + 2.3 [height (in.) – 60]
- Aim to keep the plateau pressure (P_{plat}) at or below 30 cm H_2O.
- Set an initial respiratory rate sufficient to the patient's minute ventilation requirements (generally 7–9 L/min for adults).
- Set an initial I:E ratio of 1:2 or 1:3.
- Titrate PEEP and FiO_2 to maintain a SaO_2 of 88–95% or PaO_2 of 55–80 torr.
- Aim to get the FiO_2 below 60% as soon as possible; use higher PEEP to keep FiO_2 in a safe range.
- Over the first 4 hours, reduce V_Ts in steps to 7 mL/kg, then to 6 mL/kg.
- If P_{plat} cannot be kept at or below 30 cm H_2O with V_T 6 mL/kg, consider alternative strategies, such as the following:
  - Further, reduce V_T to as low as 4 mL/kg in 1-mL/kg steps (allows rates of 30–35/min to maintain pH/$PaCO_2$).
  - Unless contraindicated (e.g., high ICP) and as long as the pH can be kept at or above 7.20, allow the $PaCO_2$ to rise ("permissive hypercapnia").
  - Sedate/paralyze the patient to minimize dyssynchrony or allow permissive hypercapnia.
  - As a last resort, consider eliminating patient effort, dyssynchrony, and the opposing force of muscle tone using a neuromuscular blocking agent such as cisatracurium (Nimbex).

Proven Adjunctive Therapies to Recommend

- Fluid-conservative therapy using diuretics to maintain neutral fluid balance/prevent fluid overload (contraindicated in patient with signs of tissue hypoperfusion or those in shock)
- Patient positioning:
  - Elevate the head of the bed 30–45° to prevent ventilator-associated pneumonia.
  - Place the patient in the prone position for a majority of the day (at least 16 hours daily).

"Rescue" Therapies to Consider

Rescue therapies are interventions that may have short-term positive outcomes, such as improved oxygenation, but on average, do not affect patient mortality. Rescue therapies to recommend for patients with life-threatening hypoxemia that does not respond to the previously described protocol and adjunctive therapies include the following:

- Inhaled nitric oxide (INO) therapy (doses of 5 to 20 ppm).
- Extracorporeal membrane oxygenation (ECMO) to treat the profound hypoxemic failure while allowing the lung to heal under a more aggressive lung protecting settings.

Ineffective Therapies (Do Not Recommend)

- Corticosteroids
- Surfactant therapy
- Beta-agonists
- *N*-acetylcysteine
- Use of a PA catheter for routine management of ARDS patients also is *not* recommended. Fluid balance usually can be adjusted by monitoring the CVP and other volume indicators. The CVP line can also provide an indication of cerebral perfusion and O_2 uptake via its O_2 parameters ($Pcvo_2$ and $Scvo_2$).

Drug Overdose and Poisonings

Harmful accidental or intentional abusive exposure to various drugs or chemicals is a common occurrence that often requires supportive respiratory care. With so many different harmful agents potentially involved, it is impossible to cover all the responses needed to deal with every specific substance. Instead, we focus on the general aspects of drug overdose and poisoning management.

Assessment/Information Gathering

Symptoms of a drug overdose and poisoning vary according to the specific substance involved and the route by which it enters the body. Given this enormous variability in presentation, resuscitation and stabilization of the patient come first, with in-depth symptom assessment and identification of the specific offending substance of secondary importance (see the discussion of treatment and decision making).

Nonetheless, general knowledge of the diagnostic process in cases of suspected drug overdose or poisonings can help direct therapy, especially when considering antidote treatment. To that end, the following guidelines apply when assessing a patient for harmful exposure to drugs or chemicals:

- If available, try to determine what the patient ingested, injected, or was exposed to, including when and how much.
- Quickly assess the patient's level of consciousness and vital signs, looking for key clusters of symptoms (called toxidromes) that might indicate the offending agent's general category or classification (**Table 20-17**).
- Obtain an ABG to assess for hypoxemia, hypercapnia, and acid-base imbalances.
- Recommend or conduct CO-oximetry to measure HbCO levels (carbon monoxide poisoning).
- Recommend serum electrolytes and calculation of the anion gap (look for high-anion-gap metabolic acidosis in salicylate, methanol, and ethylene glycol poisoning).
- Recommend urinalysis to identify the presence of offending drugs or drug by-products.

Table 20-17 Categories of Drugs or Poisons and Their Typical Symptoms

Drug Category	Example Agents
Narcotic	Opiate analgesics (morphine, heroin, fentanyl, oxycodone)
Sedative-hypnotic	Barbiturates, benzodiazepines
Adrenergic/sympathomimetic	Ecstasy, amphetamines, methamphetamines
Cholinergic/parasympathomimetic	Neostigmine, organophosphates (insecticides), chemical warfare nerve agents (e.g., sarin)
Anticholinergic	Atropine, anticholinergic bronchodilators (e.g., tiotropium), diphenhydramine (Benadryl), bupropion (Zyban)

Table 20-18 Reversing Agents or Antidotes for Selected Drugs and Chemicals

Category or Drug	Reversing Agent
Opioid narcotics	Naloxone (Narcan)
Acetaminophen	*N*-acetylcysteine
Benzodiazepines	Flumazenil (Romazicon)
β-adrenergic blockers	Glucagon
Calcium-channel blockers	Calcium chloride, glucagon
Carbon monoxide	100% O_2, hyperbaric O_2
Cyanide	Nitrites, hydroxocobalamin, sulfanegen TEA
Organophosphates	Atropine, pralidoxime

- Recommend a quantitative toxicology screen to measure serum levels of common agents such as acetaminophen, salicylates, ethanol/methanol, barbiturates, and cyclic antidepressants.
- Recommend an ECG if the patient is unstable or is suspected of having ingested any drugs with potential cardiac toxicity (e.g., digoxin).

Treatment/Decision Making

- Always prioritize the ABCs (airway, breathing, circulation) in managing drug overdoses or poisonings.
- Recommend intubation for any overdose/poisoning patient who is obtunded or any patient for whom upper airway control is suspect or aspiration is a concern.
- Provide supplemental O_2 as needed to maintain the SpO_2 above 90% (administer 100% O_2 for suspected carbon monoxide poisoning).
- Unless there is evidence of cardiac depression, recommend fluids to treat hypotension.
- If the patient is obtunded and exhibits miosis and respiratory depression, *assume* opioid overdose and recommend naloxone (Narcan) administration.
- For patients suspected of orally ingesting an overdose of drugs, recommend gastric lavage or activated charcoal administration (*both require airway protection*).
- In cases of salicylate or barbiturate overdose, recommend alkaline diuresis via bicarbonate administration.
- Recommend hemodialysis for *life-threatening* ingestions of alcohols, amphetamines, salicylates, barbiturates, and lithium.
- Once the drug or chemical agent is identified, recommend the appropriate reversing agent or antidote (**Table 20-18**), and notify the Poison Control Center.

Sleep Disorders

Sleep disorders or *dyssomnias* represent a variety of conditions in which individuals have difficulty initiating and maintaining normal sleep.

Assessment/Information Gathering

The primary symptom associated with sleep disorders is excessive daytime sleepiness.
Predisposing/associated factors (to assess via the patient history) include insomnia, snoring/cessation of breathing, frequent awakenings, morning headaches, hypertension, obesity/increased neck circumference, male gender, and age > 50.

Various scales, questionnaires, and interview mnemonics are used to help screen patients for the presence of sleep disorders and the need for further testing, such as the following:

- *Epworth Sleepiness Scale*: Asks patients to rate their chances of falling asleep during certain activities. If score ≥ 10, recommend polysomnography (PSG) exam.
- *STOP-BANG* questionnaire: *S*nore, *T*ired, *O*bserved (sleep apnea), *P*ressure (blood), *B*MI, *A*ge, *N*eck circumference, *G*ender (male); any three positive findings indicate a high risk of OSA.
- *I SNORED* mnemonic: *I*nsomnia, *S*noring, *N*octurnal awakenings/not breathing, *O*besity, *R*estorative sleep (need to nap), *E*xcessive daytime somnolence, *D*rug or alcohol use; a positive finding on any six of the seven indicates a high risk of OSA.

Recommend further testing if any multiple predisposing factors are present, or the applicable scale or questionnaire threshold score is reached or exceeded. Additional testing may involve the following:

- Laboratory-based attended PSG exam—*the gold standard for diagnosis; recommend if available.*
- Full overnight 7–10+ channel PSG (includes sleep staging), usually requiring a second full night to assess/adjust treatment.
- A "split-night" study—baseline PSG followed by CPAP or BiPAP titration on the same night (decision to titrate may be based on initial 2- to 3-h PSG results).
- Portable limited channel monitoring (e.g., Type 3 device measuring airflow, respiratory effort, heart rate, and SpO_2 [no sleep staging]—recommend if full PSG not available. *Do not recommend for patients with significant comorbidities (e.g., CHF).*
- Overnight oximetry (if PSG and portable monitoring not available); measures desaturation events (SpO_2 drop of at least 3–4%)—*recommend when a cause cannot be identified* (e.g., obstructive vs central sleep apnea).
- Attended PSG/portable monitoring basic interpretation is as follows:
  - Abnormal respiratory events detected by lab PSG or portable monitoring include obstructive, central, and mixed apneas (cessation of airflow ≥ 10 sec); hypopneas; respiratory effort–related arousals (RERAs); Cheyne-Stokes breathing; and O_2 desaturations.
  - Sleep apnea is confirmed if the number of abnormal events exceeds 5 per hour; 5–15 events/h = mild; 15–30 events/h = moderate; > 30 events/h = severe.

The condition is *obstructive* (OSA) if most events involve continued effort to breathe and *central* (CSA) if most events do not involve an effort to breathe; if the inspiratory effort is initially absent during the event but resumes later, it is characterized as a *mixed* apnea.

Overnight oximetry interpretation is as follows:

- Oxygen desaturation index (ODI) = average # desaturations/hours of sleep.
- ODI ≥ 15 indicates the presence of sleep apnea-hypopnea syndrome (SAHS); may obviate the need for PSG.
- CT90 $< 5\%$ helps rule out SAHS (CT90 = cumulative percentage of overall sleep time with $SpO_2 < 90\%$).

Treatment/Decision Making

If OSA is the primary problem, treatment and decision-making considerations are as follows:

- The decision regarding treatment usually is made by the patient in collaboration with the sleep specialist and primary care provider.
- Positive airway pressure/PAP (CPAP or BiPAP) is the treatment of choice for OSA and should be an option available to all patients with OSA.

- Always recommend titration (PSG or auto) of the CPAP/BiPAP pressure levels; after the optimum pressure level(s) are determined, you should assist the patient in selecting an acceptable interface and learning how to use and manage the equipment properly.
- If a patient refuses or rejects CPAP, you should recommend and assess equipment or interface alternatives to improve tolerance (e.g., various mask options, added humidification, ramp feature, auto-titration, pressure relief [aka C-flex, EPR], BiPAP or adaptive servo-ventilation [ASV]; *auto-titration generally should be avoided in patients with significant comorbidities*, e.g., those with CHF, COPD, hypoventilation syndromes).
- For OSA patients (1) who decline PAP as the initial treatment, (2) who subsequently cannot tolerate PAP, or (3) for whom PAP on follow-up is judged ineffective, alternative treatment approaches are available, as summarized in **Table 20-19**.

If central sleep apnea (CSA) is the primary problem, treatment options to consider or recommend are the following:

- The decision regarding treatment usually made by the patient in collaboration with the sleep specialist and primary care provider.
- Treatment of the underlying disorder (e.g., if CSA is due to heart failure causing *Cheyne-Stokes breathing* [CSB], recommend optimizing cardiac function)

Table 20-19 Treatment Options Other Than PAP for Obstructive Sleep Apnea (OSA)

Treatment	Description	Comments
Behavioral strategies	Weight loss for obese patients*	Goal is body mass index (BMI) ≤ 25 kg/m^2
	Aerobic exercise (e.g., walking, biking)	1–1½ hours, 3 days/week suggested
	Good sleep habits (sleep hygiene)	See **Box 20-2**
Positional therapy	Pillow, backpack, tennis ball, commercial device or alarm†	To avoid supine positioning
Oral appliances	Mandibular repositioning appliances	To hold the mandible forward
	Tongue retaining devices	To hold the tongue forward
Upper airway nerve stimulation	An implanted system that senses breathing patterns and electrically stimulates the hypoglossal nerve to maintain airway patency	For patients ≥ 22 years old with moderate to severe OSA (AHI 20–65), < 25% central apneas and no complete soft palate collapse
Surgical management	Reconstruction of mandible, uvula, or other facets of the upper airway	Generally, not first choice; best for obstruction readily correctable by surgery.

*Although weight loss as modest as 10% of body weight can often alleviate symptoms, dietary approaches have a low long-term success rate.

†Correction of OSA by positional therapy should be documented via polysomnography before initiating this treatment as a primary treatment.

Box 20-2 Counseling Patients on Good Sleep Habits

- Establish a regular sleep time.
- Create a proper sleep environment.
- Make the bedroom for sleeping only.
- Do not worry or stress while in bed.
- Avoid alcohol, caffeine, and tobacco.
- Exercising 20 to 30 minutes three or four times a week enhances the ability to sleep. However, exercising vigorously within three hours of bedtime is not recommended because of the possibility of becoming too aroused to sleep.

Modified from *Edlin's Health and Wellness*, 12th edition. Burlington, MA: Jones & Bartlett Learning; 2016.

- Positive airway pressure:
  - CPAP—may improve cardiac function in patients with congestive heart failure and Cheyne-Stokes breathing type apnea.
  - BiPAP—effective for treating patients with *hypercapnic CSA* (hypoventilation syndrome).
  - ASV—treatment for most forms of CSA, especially Cheyne-Stokes breathing-related; should be prescribed based on PSG exam.
- Nocturnal O_2 therapy—for CSA secondary to heart failure; improves LVEF and decreases apnea-hypopnea index (AHI); usually used in conjunction with positive airway pressure therapy.
- Pharmacologic therapy:
  - Acetazolamide (Diamox): $\uparrow$ HCO_3^- excretion $\rightarrow$ metabolic acidosis $\rightarrow$ lower $Paco_2$ apneic threshold; most effective in Cheyne-Stokes breathing with heart failure.
  - Theophylline: a phosphodiesterase inhibitor with respiratory stimulant properties that is effective in Cheyne-Stokes breathing patients with heart failure.
  - Sedative-hypnotics (e.g., temazepam [Restoril] and zolpidem [Ambien]: may minimize ventilatory instability with sleep-wake transitions.

Bariatric Surgery

Obesity, defined as a body mass index (BMI) $\geq$30 kg/m^2, is a chronic illness identified in children, adolescents, and adults. There are several well-established health hazards linked to obesity, including type 2 diabetes, heart disease, stroke, cancers, osteoarthritis, liver disease, obstructive sleep apnea, and depression. The risk of developing cardiopulmonary complications rises with increasing body mass, while weight loss can reduce the risk and improve medical conditions, such as hypertension and diabetes.

As required by the American Society of Metabolic and Bariatric Surgery (ASMBS), bariatric surgery centers encourage (or require) patients to participate in lifestyle changes prior to surgery to demonstrate their commitment to their health. Bariatric surgery should be performed in conjunction with a comprehensive preoperative assessment and a follow-up plan consisting of nutritional, behavioral, and medical programs led by an interdisciplinary team.

Assessment/Information Gathering

- Assess indications for surgery as listed below:
  - Adults with a BMI $\geq$ 40 kg/m^2 without any additional comorbidities.
  - Adults with a BMI 35.0 to 39.9 kg/m^2 with at least one serious comorbidity (e.g., type 2 diabetes, obstructive sleep apnea [OSA], hypertension, obesity-hypoventilation syndrome [OHS], Pickwickian syndrome (combination of OSA and OHS), asthma, impaired quality of life, and disqualification from other surgeries as a result of obesity, among others).
  - Adults with a BMI between 30.0 to 34.9 kg/m^2 *and* one of the following comorbid conditions: uncontrollable type 2 diabetes and metabolic syndrome.
- Assess for contraindications for surgery:
  - Bariatric procedures *should not* be performed for glycemic or lipid control or for cardiovascular risk reduction independent of the body mass index (BMI) parameters.
  - Other medical or psychiatric conditions that preclude a bariatric surgical procedure include:
    - Untreated major depression or psychosis
    - Uncontrolled and untreated eating disorders (e.g., bulimia)
    - Current drug and alcohol abuse during the preceding two years
    - Severe cardiac disease with prohibitive anesthetic risks
    - Severe coagulopathy
    - Inability to comply with nutritional requirements, including lifelong vitamin replacement
- *The preoperative assessment* includes the following:
  - A presurgical psychological assessment to include behavioral, cognitive/emotional, current life situation, motivations, and expectations
  - Nutritional assessment (by a registered dietitian) to make sure patients make nutritional plans for prior to, around the time of, and after bariatric surgery

- Medical assessment to include a complete history and physical examination to assess for comorbid illnesses and appropriateness as a surgical candidate
- Anesthetic and airway risk assessment due to the risks of general anesthetics causing respiratory and cardiovascular changes that impact the delivery of perioperative analgesia and the predisposition to a difficult airway during intubation

Treatment/Decision Making

A detailed discussion of surgical procedures involved in bariatric surgery is beyond this text. However, since you may encounter the name of some of these procedures on your examination, below is the list of the procedures endorsed by ASMBS to perform this surgery:

- Adjustable gastric banding
- Sleeve gastrectomy
- Roux-en-Y gastric bypass
- BPD/duodenal switch
- Bariatric re-operative procedures
- Intragastric balloons

Perioperative and Postoperative Management of the Bariatric Patient

The following management methods are recommended in bariatric patients:

- ET intubation remains the preferred airway to secure the airway in obese patients. ETT size has an impact on micro-aspiration and postoperative complications.
- Position the patient in a "beach chair" and "leg flexion position" to facilitate ventilation during surgery.
- Postoperatively, keep the patient in a semi-Fowler's position. After bariatric surgery, respiratory function is compromised since obesity induces severe restrictive syndrome when lying flat and can induce atelectasis.
- Mechanical and pharmacologic measures with low molecular weight heparins for thromboprophylaxis. Dosage and duration of treatment should be individualized.
- Protein intake should be monitored in the early postoperative period. Iron, vitamin B_{12}, and calcium supplementation are mandatory.
- Glycemic and lipid control must be strict in the postop period for patients with diabetes.
- If the patient has OSA as a comorbidity, treatments such as CPAP should be employed if warranted.

Shock

Shock is a life-threatening condition of circulatory failure. Shock is defined as a state of cellular and tissue hypoxia due to reduced oxygen delivery and increased oxygen consumption or inadequate oxygen utilization. Shock is initially reversible but must be recognized and treated immediately to prevent progression to irreversible multiorgan failure (MOF) and death.

"Undifferentiated shock" refers to the situation where shock is recognized, but the cause is unclear. When a patient presents with undifferentiated shock, it is important that the healthcare provider immediately initiate therapy while rapidly identifying the etiology so that therapy can be administered to reverse shock and prevent MOF and death.

Four general types of shock are recognized: distributive, cardiogenic, hypovolemic, and obstructive (see **Table 20-20**):

- Distributive shock is characterized by severe peripheral vasodilatation.
- Cardiogenic shock is due to intracardiac causes of cardiac pump failure that result in reduced cardiac output (CO).
- Hypovolemic shock is due to reduced intravascular volume, which, in turn, reduces CO.
- Obstructive shock is mostly due to extracardiac causes of cardiac pump failure and often associated with reduced right ventricle output.

Table 20-20 Classification of Shock and Possible Causes

Classification	Type	Definition	Causes
Distributive	Septic shock (sepsis)	Life-threatening organ dysfunction resulting from dysregulated host response to infection with severe circulatory, cellular, and metabolic abnormalities. Results in tissue hypoperfusion and hypotension requiring vasopressor therapy and elevated lactate levels (more than 2 mmol/L)	Most common pathogens associated with sepsis and septic shock are gram-positive bacteria, including *Streptococcus pneumoniae* and *Enterococcus* sp.
	Systemic inflammatory response syndrome (SIRS)	SIRS is a clinical syndrome of a strong inflammatory response caused by either infectious or noninfectious causes.	• Infectious causes include gram-positive (most common) and gram-negative bacteria, fungi, viral infections, parasitic, and rickettsial infections. • Noninfectious causes include, among others, pancreatitis, burns, fat embolism, air embolism, and amniotic fluid embolism.
	Anaphylactic shock	A clinical syndrome of severe hypersensitivity reaction mediated by immunoglobulin E (Ig-E), resulting in cardiovascular collapse and respiratory distress due to bronchospasm	Common allergens include drugs (e.g., antibiotics, NSAIDs), food, insect stings, and latex.
	Neurogenic shock	Occur in the setting of trauma to the spinal cord or the brain	Caused by the disruption of the autonomic pathway resulting in decreased vascular resistance and changes in vagal tone.
	Endocrine shock	Due to underlying endocrine etiologies	• Adrenal failure (addisonian crisis) • Myxedema
Cardiogenic	Cardiomyopathic	Due to heart muscle failure leading to decreased cardiac output and systemic hypoperfusion	• MI (involving >40% of the LV or with extensive ischemia) • RV infarction • CHF exacerbation due to dilated cardiomyopathy • Stunned myocardium from prolonged ischemia (e.g., cardiac arrest, hypotension, cardiopulmonary bypass) • Advanced septic shock • Myocarditis • Myocardial contusion • Drug-induced (e.g., β-blockers)
	Arrhythmogenic	Due to cardiac arrhythmias leading to decreased cardiac output and systemic hypoperfusion	• Tachyarrhythmia: Atrial tachycardias (fibrillation, flutter, reentrant tachycardia), ventricular tachycardia and fibrillation • Bradyarrhythmia: Complete heart block, Mobitz type II second degree heart block
	Mechanical	Due to structural anomalies of the heart leading to decreased cardiac output and systemic hypoperfusion	Severe valvular insufficiency, acute valvular rupture, critical valvular stenosis, acute or severe ventricular septal wall defect, ruptured ventricular wall aneurysm, atrial myxoma

Classification	Type	Definition	Causes
Hypovolemic	Hemorrhagic	Decreased intravascular volume and increased systemic venous assistance cause by a sudden loss of intravascular volume (bleeding)	• Bleeding due to trauma • Vascular etiologies (e.g., aortoenteric fistula, ruptured abdominal aortic aneurysm, tumor eroding into a major blood vessel) • Spontaneous bleeding due to anticoagulant use
	Non-hemorrhagic	Decreased intravascular volume due to the shifting of intravascular fluid	• GI losses: vomiting, diarrhea, NG suction or drains • Renal losses: medication-induced diuresis, endocrine disorders such as hypoaldosteronism • Skin losses/insensible losses: burns, Stevens-Johnson syndrome, toxic epidermal necrolysis, heatstroke, pyrexia • Third-space loss: pancreatitis, cirrhosis, intestinal obstruction, trauma
Obstructive	Pulmonary vascular	Caused by impaired blood flow from the right heart to the left heart	Hemodynamically significant PE, severe pulmonary hypertension, severe or acute obstruction of the pulmonic or tricuspid valve, venous air embolus
	Mechanical	Impaired filling of right heart or due to decreased venous return to the right heart due to extrinsic compression	Tension pneumothorax or hemothorax, pericardial tamponade, constrictive pericarditis, restrictive cardiomyopathy, severe dynamic hyperinflation caused by elevated intrinsic/extrinsic PEEP, left or right ventricular outflow tract obstruction
Mixed/unknown		Circulatory failure caused by other causes or a combination of the above	• Endocrine (e.g., adrenal insufficiency, thyrotoxicosis, myxedema coma) • Metabolic (e.g., acidosis, hypothermia) • Other: trauma with more than one shock category, acute shock etiology with pre-existing cardiac disease, late under-resuscitated shock, miscellaneous poisonings

Assessment/Information Gathering

The clinical findings associated with undifferentiated shock vary according to the etiology and stage of presentation (pre-shock, shock, end-organ dysfunction). The evaluation should include a thorough history and assessment of sensorium, mucous membranes, lips and tongue, neck veins, lungs, heart, and abdomen, as well as skin and joints.

Hypotension, oliguria, mental status changes, and cool, clammy skin are sentinel clinical findings that should raise the suspicion of shock and prompt immediate treatment with intravenous fluids and further evaluation with laboratory studies and relevant imaging.

The most common clinical findings in all four types of shock are explained below:

- Hypotension may be *absolute* (e.g., systolic blood pressure < 90 mm Hg; mean arterial pressure < 65 mm Hg), *relative* (e.g., a drop in systolic blood pressure > 40 mm Hg), *orthostatic* (> 20 mm Hg fall in systolic pressure or > 10 mm Hg fall in diastolic pressure with standing), or *profound* (e.g., vasopressor-dependent).
  - Note: hypotension *does not have to be present* for the diagnosis. Patients in the early stages of shock can be normotensive or hypertensive.

- *Tachycardia* is an early compensatory mechanism in patients with shock.
- *Oliguria* in shock is caused by the shunting of renal blood flow to other vital organs, direct injury to the kidney (e.g., aminoglycoside toxicity), or due to intravascular volume depletion (e.g., from vomiting, diarrhea, or hemorrhage).
- *The altered sensorium* in shock is usually due to poor cerebral perfusion or metabolic encephalopathy.
- *Cool, clammy skin* is caused by compensatory peripheral vasoconstriction that redirects blood centrally, to maintain vital organ perfusion.
- A cyanotic, mottled appearance is a late and worrisome feature of shock.
- Bedside telemetry or ECG should be performed in patients with undifferentiated hypotension and shock.
  - ECG may reveal an arrhythmia or ST-segment changes consistent with ischemia or pericarditis.
  - A low-voltage ECG may be suggestive of pericardial effusion.

Laboratory tests should be performed early in the evaluation of patients with undifferentiated hypotension/shock to identify the cause of shock and early organ failure. Recommend the following tests:

- Serum lactate
- Renal and liver function tests
- Cardiac enzymes and natriuretic peptides
- Complete blood count and differential
- Coagulation studies and D-dimer level
- Blood gas analysis
  - A high anion gap metabolic acidosis should always raise the clinical suspicion for the presence of shock.
- Elevated serum lactate levels (>2 mmol/L), have traditionally been used as surrogates for the presence of hypoperfusion and tissue hypoxia.
- The presence of an elevated serum lactate level (>4 mmol/L) has been associated with adverse outcomes, including the development of shock and increased mortality.
- A chest x-ray is recommended in most patients with suspected shock to detect common causes (e.g., pneumonia) or complications of shock (e.g., ARDS).
- A chest x-ray may be clear in hypovolemic shock or obstructive shock from a PE.
- When the diagnosis or the type of shock remains undetermined or mixed, hemodynamic measurements obtained by pulmonary artery catheter (PAC) can be helpful.
- Adequacy of cardiac output can be evaluated by measurement of $ScvO_2$ or SvO_2, in addition to signs of tissue perfusion.

Treatment/Decision Making

Treatment for shock is usually specific to the type of shock affecting the patient. However, there are three common interventions to all patients that you can recommend in your exams:

- Identify the type of shock
- Provide oxygenation support
- Blood pressure management

Treatment/Decision Making for Hypovolemic Shock

For hypovolemic shock recommend the following:

- Identify and treat the underlying cause.
- Treat electrolyte and acid-base disturbances.
- Treat the volume deficit through fluid resuscitation. The preclinical and clinical treatment of hypovolemic shock consists of immediate intravascular volume replacement with balanced crystalloids.

- The choice of replacement fluid depends in part upon the type of fluid that has been lost. For patients with hypovolemic shock, three major classes of replacement fluids are commonly used:
    - Crystalloid solutions (saline solutions, lactated Ringer's, Plasma-Lyte, bicarbonate buffered 0.45% saline)
    - Colloid-containing solutions (albumin solutions, hyperoncotic starch, dextran, gelatin)
    - Blood products or blood substitutes (packed red blood cells, plasma)
- The rate of fluid repletion should be individualized depending on the underlying cause and rate of fluid loss, estimated total body deficit, underlying electrolyte abnormalities, and predicted future losses.
- Monitor fluid administration response to prevent irreversible shock and to prevent over-resuscitation and iatrogenic hypervolemia.
- Recommend measuring laboratory parameters, including chemistries and lactate level within 6 hours and urinary sodium within 24 hours of fluid resuscitation.
- Do *not* recommend vasopressors unless profound hypotension unresponsive to the fluid infusion is present. Vasopressors, in the absence of adequate resuscitation, tend to further reduce tissue perfusion since they *do not* correct the primary problem.

Treatment/Decision Making of Cardiogenic Shock

For cardiogenic shock, recommend the following:

- Ventilatory support to:
    - Protect the airway and maintain oxygen supply in patients with a deterioration in consciousness or cardiac arrest.
    - Treat acute respiratory failure, most often due to cardiogenic pulmonary edema
    - Help to raise the arterial pH in metabolic acidosis.
- Prompt management of hypotension and hypoperfusion to provide circulatory support.
- To reverse hypotension, maintain vital organ perfusion, and maintain coronary perfusion pressures recommend pharmacologic (norepinephrine, dopamine) and nonpharmacologic methods.
- Hemodynamic monitoring for patients with refractory shock despite revascularization.
- Do *not* delay reperfusion therapy to insert a balloon-tipped pulmonary artery catheter.
- Careful monitoring of volume status since too much fluid in patients with extensive left ventricular infarction will result in pulmonary edema and should be avoided.
- Patients with volume overload and cardiogenic pulmonary edema without hypotension may require therapy with diuretics, morphine, supplemental oxygen, and vasodilators.
- Do *not* routinely recommend an intra-aortic balloon pump (IABP).
- IABP may only be beneficial in patients with mechanical defects and selected other patients who are rapidly deteriorating.
- Temporary mechanical circulatory support devices are increasingly being recommended in patients with severe cardiogenic shock (left ventricular and biventricular assist devices, durable left ventricular assist device [LVAD], Impella RP System, ECMO).
- Recommend early reperfusion/revascularization if indicated.
    - Some patients will require only percutaneous coronary intervention (PCI) of the infarct-related artery; others may require immediate coronary artery bypass surgery (CABG). Some patients may need both.

The short-term prognosis of cardiogenic shock is directly related to the severity of the initial hemodynamic disorder. In general, patients most commonly succumb to multiorgan dysfunction due to organ hypoperfusion. In-hospital mortality continues to be high despite technological and pharmacologic advances.

Treatment/Decision Making for Obstructive Shock

Patients with obstructive shock have hypotension with reduced cardiac output due to an extracardiac cause of pump failure. The final treatment approach will depend on the main cause of the mechanical obstruction (pericardial tamponade, tension pneumothorax or hemothorax, air, fat, or thrombus embolism). The following recommendations apply:

- A rapid examination of the heart, chest, abdomen, major arteries, and veins using point-of-care ultrasonography in the preoperative area or operating room may confirm the cause(s) of shock.
- Recommend decompression or specific surgical interventions to relieve the obstruction.
- Recommend an intra-arterial catheter to continuously monitor arterial blood pressure (BP), pulse pressure (PP), and respiratory variations in the pressure waveform as a dynamic parameter to determine fluid responsiveness.
- Recommend a central venous catheter for infusion of vasoactive drugs, venous access for fluid and blood administration, measurements of central mixed venous oxygen saturation ($Scvo_2$), and additional data to manage intravascular volume status.
- Administration of fluids and vasopressors *do not* correct the cause of obstructive shock but may provide temporary hemodynamic stability to allow definitive surgical treatment.
- Use anesthetic induction and maintenance agents with minimal hemodynamic effects in surgical patients in shock. Doses are usually reduced to avoid exacerbation of hypotension.

Treatment/Decision Making of Distributive Shock: Septic Shock (Sepsis)

Sepsis is characterized by systemic inflammation due to infection. There is a continuum of severity ranging from sepsis to septic shock. Securing the airway (if indicated), correcting hypoxemia, and establishing venous access for the early administration of fluids and antibiotics are priorities in the management of patients with sepsis and septic shock

The following recommendations apply for the management of septic shock:

- Oxygen should be administered to all patients with sepsis, and oxygenation should be monitored continuously with pulse oximetry.
- Intubation and mechanical ventilation may be necessary to support the increased work of breathing that typically accompanies sepsis.
- Intubation is also indicated for airway protection since encephalopathy and a depressed level of consciousness frequently complicate sepsis.
- Treatment to support the circulation by the infusion of balanced crystalloid solutions, administration of vasopressors (norepinephrine, vasopressin if needed), in some cases also inotropic drugs (e.g., dobutamine), and organ replacement therapy.
- Venous access should be established as soon as possible in patients with suspected sepsis. Most of these patients will require central venous access at some point during their course to facilitate fluid resuscitation.
  - Note: the insertion of a central line should *not* delay the administration of resuscitative fluids and antibiotics.

The following tests are recommended:

- Complete blood counts with differential, chemistries, liver function tests, and coagulation studies, including D-dimer level.
- Elevated serum lactate may indicate the severity of sepsis and is used to follow the therapeutic response.
- ABGs to assess for acidosis, hypoxemia, or hypercapnia.
- Peripheral blood cultures (aerobic and anaerobic cultures from at least two different sites), urinalysis, and microbiologic cultures from suspected sources (e.g., sputum, urine, intravascular catheter, wound or surgical site, body fluids) from readily accessible sites.
- Imaging targeted at the suspected site of infection is warranted (e.g., chest radiography, computed tomography of the chest and abdomen).
- While the diagnostic value of procalcitonin in patients with sepsis is poorly supported by evidence, its importance in deescalating antibiotic therapy is well established in populations other than those with sepsis, those with CAP and respiratory tracts infections.

Treatment/Decision Making for Distributive Shock: Anaphylactic Shock

Anaphylaxis is an acute systemic reaction usually mediated by IgE-dependent hypersensitivity reactions. The diagnosis of anaphylaxis is based primarily upon clinical symptoms and signs, as well as a detailed description of the acute episode, including antecedent activities and events occurring within the preceding minutes to hours.

Patients with severe anaphylactic reactions require constant monitoring, as late reactions including arrhythmias, myocardial ischemia, and respiratory failure may manifest as late as 12 hours after the initial event.

The following recommendations apply for the initial management of septic shock:

- Call for help (summon the medical emergency team in a hospital setting or call 911 in a community setting).
- Removal of the trigger cause, if promptly identified (e.g., stop the infusion of a suspect medication).
- Intramuscular (IM) injection of epinephrine as soon as possible, followed by additional epinephrine by IM or intravenous (IV) injection.
- Placement of the patient in the supine position with the lower extremities elevated.
- Provide supplemental oxygen as needed.
- Establish access, and provide volume resuscitation with IV fluids as soon as possible.
- Recommend continuous monitoring of blood pressure (BP), heart rate, and respiratory rate, as well as monitoring of oxygen saturation by pulse oximetry for the duration of the episode.
- Intubation should be performed immediately if marked stridor or respiratory arrest is present.
  - The early presence of upper airway edema represents rapidly developing airway compromise, requiring prompt action.
  - Recommend an emergency cricothyroidotomy to secure the airway if upper airway edema prevents access to the glottic aperture.
- Agents that may be given as adjunctive therapies to epinephrine in the treatment of anaphylaxis include H_1 antihistamines, H_2 antihistamines, bronchodilators, and glucocorticoids.
- Recommend inhaled bronchodilators for the treatment of bronchospasm not responsive to epinephrine, to be administered by a mouthpiece (or facemask for those whose age or condition requires) and a nebulizer, as needed.

All patients who have experienced anaphylaxis should be sent home with the following:

- An anaphylaxis emergency action plan
- A prescription for more than one epinephrine autoinjector
- Printed information about anaphylaxis and its treatment
- Documented advice to follow up to an allergist, with a referral if possible

The Immunocompromised Patient

In this category, the NBRC may present you with several disorders in which their hallmark is the *patient's susceptibility to infection* with organisms of low natural virulence for otherwise immunologically healthy patients. Pulmonary infection (pneumonia) remains the most common form of tissue-invasive infection in the immunocompromised patient. In particular, the incidence of pulmonary fungal infection is high in immunocompromised individuals despite advances in antifungal prophylaxis and therapy.

The spectrum of potential pathogens known to cause pulmonary infections in immunocompromised individuals has grown as a result of intensified immunosuppression, prolonged patient survival, the emergence of antimicrobial-resistant pathogens, and improved diagnostic assays. **Table 20-21** lists the most common pathogens likely to cause pulmonary infections on these patients.

A few general considerations apply in the immunocompromised patient with suspected pulmonary infection:

- Multiple simultaneous infectious processes are common.
- Early imaging (CT scan) and specific microbiologic diagnoses are essential to the care of immunocompromised patients.

Table 20-21 Classification of Pathogens Causing Pulmonary Infections in the Immunocompromised Patient

Classification	Pathogen
Bacteria	• *S. pneumoniae* • *H. influenzae* • *Mycoplasma* • *Legionella* • *Chlamydia* • *Neisseria meningitidis*
Fungi	• *Pneumocystis jiroveci* • *Aspergillus* • *Cryptococcus* species • *Candida albicans* • Agents of mucormycosis (*Rhizopus*, *Mucor*, and *Lichtheimia* spp)
Viruses	• Cytomegalovirus (CMV) • Community-acquired respiratory viruses (influenza, parainfluenza, respiratory syncytial virus [RSV], metapneumovirus, and adenovirus) • Herpes simplex and varicella zoster viruses
Parasites	• *Strongyloides* • Toxoplasmosis (*Toxoplasma gondii*)

- Invasive procedures (biopsies and bronchoscopy) are often necessary to establish a microbiologic diagnosis.
- Microbicidal therapy must be started as soon as possible.
- Laboratory assay results must be interpreted cautiously and must take into account the clinical context of each patient.

Assessment/Information Gathering

Early diagnosis and specific therapy of opportunistic infections are the cornerstone of successful management of these patients. Below are some important points to consider for the assessment and information gathering of these patients:

- Suspect the possibility of an immunocompromised disorder if:
  - *Neutropenia* is present. Neutropenia is the most common risk factor for pulmonary infection in immunocompromised patients.
  - *Glucocorticoids* have been given for a long period of time. Glucocorticoids cause depression of phagocytic function of alveolar macrophages and neutrophils, alterations in antigen presentation and lymphocyte mobilization and decrease mobilization of inflammatory cells into areas of infection.
  - *HIV infection* is confirmed.
  - *Transplantation* of solid organs and hematopoietic cells has occurred.
  - *Autoimmune and inflammatory* conditions are present (e.g., lupus, rheumatoid arthritis, scleroderma).
  - *Biologic and T cell suppression and lymphocyte depletion* agents are being used to treat certain malignancies.
- Fever and pulmonary infiltrates are the most common signs of a pulmonary infection in the immunocompromised.
- Three types of pulmonary infiltrates are common:
  - Consolidation, with a substantial replacement of alveolar air by tissue density material, typically with air bronchograms and a peripheral location of the abnormality.

- Peribronchovascular (or interstitial) distribution, in which the infiltrate is predominantly oriented along with the peribronchial or perivascular bundles.
- Nodular, space-occupying, nonanatomic lesions with well-defined, rounded edges surrounded by aerated lung.
- Features useful in making a preliminary diagnosis:
  - Travel and occupation
  - Prolonged duration of neutropenia
  - Potential or witnessed aspiration
  - Presence of potential pulmonary pathogens in prior cultures
  - History of frequent antimicrobial exposure
  - Cardiac abnormalities (endocarditis), indwelling catheters, or an intravascular clot (bacteremic seeding of the lungs)
  - Metastatic tumors, particularly intrathoracic malignancies
  - Diabetes mellitus with sinopulmonary infection (mucormycosis)

Treatment/Decision Making

Recommend the following actions:

- Oxygen should be administered to all patients with suspected hypoxemia, and oxygenation should be monitored continuously with pulse oximetry.
- Intubation and mechanical ventilation may be necessary to support the increased work of breathing caused by the infection and the underlying immune disease of the host.
- CT scan should be performed, since the pattern of involvement can be helpful in establishing the etiology of the process. A chest CT frequently reveals abnormalities even when the chest radiograph is negative or has only subtle findings.
- Chest x-ray should be performed. The initial findings and progression of the chest radiograph provide important clues to both the differential diagnosis of pulmonary infection and the appropriate diagnostic evaluation.
- Immediate empiric antibiotic therapy is recommended while awaiting diagnostic studies results.
- Once the causative agent(s) are identified, begin establishing specific antibiotic therapy.
- A reduction of the overall level of immune suppression (if possible) may be as important as antimicrobial therapy in the ultimate success of treatment.

Survival of the immunocompromised patient has improved with the availability of newer antimicrobial agents, including azole antifungals, macrolides, antivirals, and antiretroviral drugs. Despite these advances, pulmonary infection remains the most common form of documented tissue invasive infection observed in these patients increasing their morbidity and mortality in the hospital setting.

PEDIATRIC PROBLEMS

Number of Simulations in the CSE: 2 Cases

In the "NBRC hospital," RTs must be able to help manage a variety of acute and chronic childhood disorders. These include asthma, croup (laryngotracheobronchitis), epiglottitis, bronchiolitis, congenital defects, and foreign-body aspiration (FBA), among others.

Croup (Laryngotracheobronchitis) and Epiglottitis

Croup is a *viral* infection of the upper airway that occurs most commonly in children 6 months to 3 years of age. It is most often caused by the parainfluenza virus, adenovirus, respiratory syncytial virus (RSV), or influenza A and B. Infection causes inflammation and swelling of *subglottic* tissue, including the larynx, trachea, and larger bronchi.

Epiglottitis is a *bacterial* infection of the upper airway that occurs most commonly among children 2 to 8 years old. Before immunizations against *Haemophilus influenzae*, this organism was the most common cause. Today, *Staphylococcus aureus* and group A *Streptococcus*–associated epiglottitis is more commonplace. The infection causes acute inflammation and swelling of the epiglottis, aryepiglottic folds, and arytenoids, which if not treated, can progress to airway obstruction and death within hours.

Because one of these acutely presenting pediatric airway disorders often appears on the CSE and because candidates frequently confuse the two, we have summarized our case management pearls in the form of a comparative table (**Table 20-22**).

Table 20-22 Croup Versus Epiglottitis

Croup	Epiglottitis
Assessment/Information Gathering: History and Clinical Signs and Symptoms	
• Age: infant/toddler	• Age: toddler to school-age
• Initial cold-like symptoms with a possible low-grade fever that progresses to more severe symptoms (often at night), including hoarseness, barking cough, and inspiratory stridor (with severe stridor, intercostal retractions may appear)	• Abrupt onset of acute illness with high fever (typically up to 40°C [104°F]), and sore throat/difficulty swallowing (often with drooling), accompanied by stridor (with possible retractions) and labored breathing
• Confirm physical findings as above plus assess for agitation; in more severe cases, look for significant tachypnea and tachycardia; lethargy, hypotonia, and cyanosis are late signs	• Confirm physical findings as above plus assess for restlessness, irritability, and extreme anxiety; the child also may prefer sitting upright and leaning forward; as obstruction worsens, breath sounds may decrease; as with croup, lethargy, hypotonia, and cyanosis are late signs of impending respiratory failure
	• Determine immunization status (*H. influenzae*)
Assessment/Information Gathering: Diagnostic Tests to Recommend	
• Diagnosis based mainly on typical age, history, and physical exam findings	• Diagnosis based primarily on typical age, history, and physical exam findings
• Recommend lateral neck x-ray, looking for characteristic subglottic "steeple sign"	• Recommend lateral neck x-ray, looking for characteristic "thumb sign" indicating a swollen epiglottis
	• To confirm the diagnosis, recommend visualizing the inflamed epiglottis via nasal fiberoptic laryngoscopy (a skilled operator is essential!)
	• To help substantiate the presence of a bacterial infection, recommend a complete blood count (CBC) and differential, looking for elevated WBC, with left shift ($\uparrow$ bands)
Treatment/Decision Making: General Medical/Surgical Treatment to Recommend	
• Recommend close respiratory and cardiac monitoring, including SpO_2	• Recommend close respiratory and cardiac monitoring, including SpO_2
• Recommend adequate hydration	• Minimize procedures that could precipitate airway compromise, such as venipuncture and upper airway manipulation
• Recommend an antipyretic for fever	• Recommend an antipyretic for fever
• Recommend systemic corticosteroids (oral or IM); aerosolized budesonide is an option	• Recommend mild sedation for comfort and to reduce anxiety
• Do *not* recommend antibiotics or viral serology; lab tests are of limited value	• Recommend a broad-spectrum antibiotic (after the airway is secure) such as a cephalosporin, with treatment to continue for 7–10 days
• If the patient is admitted to the hospital, recommend droplet precautions	

Treatment/Decision Making: Respiratory Management to Implement/Recommend	
• Initiate supplemental O_2 therapy as needed to keep $Spo_2 > 90\%$	• Initiate supplemental O_2 therapy as needed to keep $Spo_2 > 90\%$
• Recommend or administer aerosolized racemic epinephrine (0.25–0.50 mL 2.25% solution with 3.0 mL saline), repeated up to three times as needed	• If acute respiratory arrest occurs, ventilate the child with 100% O_2 via manual resuscitator and call for intubation
• If repeat racemic epinephrine treatments fail to relieve symptoms, recommend heliox via a high-flow cannula or nonrebreathing mask	• Recommend fiberoptic–assisted nasotracheal intubation under controlled conditions (e.g., rapid-sequence intubation)
• If symptoms persist for more than 4 hours after initial treatment, recommend hospital admission with close monitoring of the respiratory status	• If intubation cannot be accomplished and airway obstruction persists or worsens, recommend crico-thyroidotomy or emergency tracheotomy
• In the rare situation where obstruction worsens, consciousness decreases, or respiratory acidosis develops, recommend intubation and mechanical ventilation	

Bronchiolitis

Bronchiolitis is a viral respiratory tract infection, primarily affecting infants younger than two years old. RSV causes most bronchiolitis infections, with the parainfluenza virus and adenoviruses also being responsible for some cases. Inflammation in the bronchioles causes edema and excessive mucus production, which can lead to airway obstruction, air trapping, and atelectasis. Most cases are self-limiting and treated on an outpatient basis. More severe cases may require hospitalization and mechanical ventilation.

Assessment/Information Gathering

- Assess for age-related diagnosis (younger than 24 months) and seasonal occurrence (predominantly November to March).
- Look for an immediate prior history (1 to 3 days) of cold-like upper respiratory tract symptoms (e.g., nasal congestion, mild cough), followed by worsening respiratory distress.
- Assess for signs of lower respiratory tract infection, including cough, wheezing, crackles, tachypnea (respiratory rate greater than 60–70/min), grunting, nasal flaring, intercostal retractions, mild fever, and possible cyanosis.
- Assess for risk factors indicating the likelihood of severe disease or need for hospitalization, including age younger than 12 weeks, a history of prematurity, underlying chronic lung disease, congenital heart disease, or an immune deficiency syndrome.
- Assess Spo_2.
- Because the diagnosis typically is based on history and physical findings alone, do *not* routinely recommend imaging studies, lab work, or PFTs; a chest x-ray *may* be considered if a hospitalized infant does not improve after standard treatment.

Treatment/Decision Making

- Recommend hospitalization if the patient meets the following criteria:
  - Exhibits persistent/worsening respiratory distress (tachypnea, nasal flaring, retractions, grunting) or episodes of apnea with cyanosis or bradycardia
  - Needs supplemental O_2 to maintain $Spo_2 > 90\%$
  - Requires continuous maintenance of airway clearance (using bulb suctioning)
  - Exhibits significant restlessness or lethargy
  - Is dehydrated and unable to maintain oral feedings enough to prevent dehydration

- Recommend the hospitalized infant be placed under contact and respiratory (droplet) isolation precautions.
- Initiate supplemental O_2 to maintain the SpO_2 above 90%.
- Recommend nasal suctioning as needed, before feedings, and before aerosol therapy.
- Recommend repeated clinical assessment to detect deteriorating respiratory status.
- For patients with more severe disease or those with reported episodes of apnea with cyanosis and bradycardia, recommend continuous cardiac and respiratory rate monitoring.
- Do *not* recommend routine bronchodilator therapy (most wheezing is due to edema, not bronchospasm); if wheezing and respiratory distress persist, recommend a trial of inhaled racemic epinephrine or albuterol and continue the therapy only if there is objective evidence of a positive response.
- Do *not* recommend corticosteroids.
- Do *not* recommend ribavirin.
- Do *not* recommend antibiotics unless a coexisting bacterial infection is confirmed.
- Recommend hospital discharge when the infant meets the following criteria:
  ◦ Is breathing at a rate less than 60–70/min with no signs of distress
  ◦ Has a SpO_2 of 92% or higher on room air
  ◦ Is taking oral feedings and is adequately hydrated
- Recommend family education to help prevent recurrent respiratory infections includes the following:
  ◦ Avoid infant/child exposure to secondhand smoke.
  ◦ Limit infant/child exposure to sick siblings and settings likely to spread infections (e.g., daycare programs).
  ◦ Implement proper hand decontamination, respiratory hygiene, and cough etiquette.
- Recommend the monoclonal antibody palivizumab (Synagis) for prophylaxis against RSV for *high-risk infants*—that is, those born prematurely and those with either chronic lung disease or congenital heart disease.

Asthma

Asthma is a chronic inflammatory disease characterized by airway inflammation, intermittent airflow obstruction, and bronchial hyperresponsiveness. Asthma can affect most age groups but is more prevalent in children and young adults.

Diagnosis requires documenting recurrent episodes of airflow obstruction that are at least partially reversible. Also, other causes of airflow obstruction with similar symptoms need to be excluded before a definitive diagnosis can be made. These differential diagnoses include allergic rhinitis, foreign body aspiration, vocal cord dysfunction, bronchiolitis, bronchiectasis, bronchopulmonary dysplasia, cystic fibrosis, and gastroesophageal reflux.

The NBRC expects candidates to be familiar with two types of asthma treatment: long-term outpatient management and management of acute exacerbations requiring ED or hospital admission.

Assessment/Information Gathering (Long-Term Management)

The goal of asthma outpatient management is control of the disease, to include preventing recurrent symptoms and minimizing medication use. Achieving this goal requires careful assessment of disease control, regular monitoring of symptoms, and a step-based approach to treatment.

Table 20-23 summarizes the National Asthma Education and Prevention Program (NAEPP) guidelines for assessing asthma control in children 5–11 years old. **Table 20-24** summarizes the NAEPP guidelines for assessing asthma control in youth > 12 years of age and adults.

Key management pearls in assessing for asthma include the following:

- Recommend or obtain a family history with a focus on close relatives having asthma, allergic disorders, sinusitis, eczema, or nasal polyps.
- Look for a history of recurrent episodes of wheezing, coughing (usually unproductive), and shortness of breath, commonly occurring at night.

Table 20-23 Classification of Asthma Control in Children 5–11 Years Old

Components of Control	Well Controlled	Not Well Controlled	Very Poorly Controlled
Symptoms	≤ 2 days/week but not multiple times per day	> 2 days/week or multiple times on ≤ 2 days/week	Throughout the day
Nighttime awakenings	≤ 1/month	≥ 2/month	≥ 2/week
SABA use for symptom control	≤ 2 days/week	> 2 days/week	Several times per day
Interference with normal activity	None	Some limitation	Extremely limited
Lung function	FEV$_1$ or PF > 80% predicted* FEV$_1$% > 80%	FEV$_1$ or PF 60–80% predicted* FEV$_1$% 75–80%	FEV$_1$ or PF < 60% predicted* FEV$_1$% < 75%

FEV$_1$, forced expiratory volume in 1 second; FEV$_1$%, ratio of FEV$_1$/FVC; PF, peak expiratory flow; SABA, short-acting β-agonist.

*Predicted normal or personal best.

Data from the National Asthma Education and Prevention Program. *Expert Panel Report 3 (EPR3): Guidelines for the Diagnosis and Management of Asthma.* Bethesda, MD: U.S. Department of Health and Human Services; 2007. Note that the control elements/definitions vary somewhat for children younger than 5 years old. See the complete report for details.

Table 20-24 Classification of Asthma Control in Youth > 12 Years Old and Adults

Components of Control	Well Controlled	Not Well Controlled	Very Poorly Controlled
Symptoms	≤ 2 days/week	> 2 days/week	Throughout the day
Nighttime awakenings	≤ 2/month	1–3/week	≥ 4/week
SABA use for symptom control	≤ 2 days/week	> 2 days/week	Several times per day
Interference with normal activity	None	Some limitation	Extremely limited
Lung function	FEV$_1$ or PF > 80% predicted* FEV$_1$% > 80%	FEV$_1$ or PF 60–80% predicted* FEV$_1$% 75–80%	FEV$_1$ or PF < 60% predicted* FEV$_1$% < 75%

FEV$_1$, forced expiratory volume in 1 second; FEV$_1$%, ratio of FEV$_1$/FVC; PF, peak expiratory flow; SABA, short-acting β-agonist.

*Predicted normal or personal best.

Data from the National Asthma Education and Prevention Program. *Expert Panel Report 3 (EPR3): Guidelines for the Diagnosis and Management of Asthma.* Bethesda, MD: U.S. Department of Health and Human Services; 2007. Note that the control elements/definitions vary somewhat for children younger than 5 years old. See the complete report for details.

- Assess the onset, duration, and pattern of symptoms, as well as any aggravating factors such as exercise, cold air, or smoke exposure.
- Recommend assessment for conditions presenting with similar symptoms, such as bronchiolitis, foreign-body aspiration (infants and children), and vocal cord paralysis.
- Recommend a chest x-ray (to help rule out conditions with similar symptoms).
- Recommend spirometry (FEV$_1$, FEV$_1$/FVC, peak flow) to establish baseline values and "personal bests."
- Recommend eosinophil counts and IgE levels (to assess for ectopic asthma).
- In the young adult for whom a diagnosis is in doubt, recommend bronchial provocation testing or expired nitric oxide analysis.

Treatment/Decision Making (Long-Term Management)

Recommend or implement a comprehensive disease management program involving both the child and key family members (Chapter 17), as follows:

- Identification and management of environmental triggers and control of coexisting conditions that can aggravate asthma (e.g., sinusitis, gastroesophageal reflux)
- Regular monitoring of symptoms
- Use of action plans to deal with acute exacerbations
- Careful selection and implementation of drugs and delivery approaches
- Step-based drug treatment consistent with the level of disease control

Table 20-25 summarizes the step-based drug treatment regimen for childhood asthma recommended by the NAEPP. Step 1 is the norm for well-controlled asthma with intermittent symptoms. Higher steps may be required for persistent asthma to maintain good control. Step-ups are considered whenever the patient's asthma becomes inadequately controlled. **Table 20-26** summarizes the steps for youth older than 12 years and adults.

Table 20-25 Step-Based Approach to Drug Therapy for Childhood Asthma

Step	Preferred Drug Regimen
1	Short-acting β-agonist as needed (dosages vary for children)
2	Add a low-dose inhaled corticosteroid (dosages vary for children)
3	Add LABA, LTRA, or theophylline to the low-dose inhaled corticosteroid or step up to a medium-dose inhaled corticosteroid
4	Medium-dose inhaled corticosteroid + LABA
5	High-dose inhaled corticosteroid + LABA
6	High-dose inhaled corticosteroid + LABA + oral systemic corticosteroid

LABA, long-acting β-agonist (e.g., salmeterol or formoterol); LTRA, leukotriene receptor antagonist (e.g., montelukast or zafirlukast).

Data from the National Asthma Education and Prevention Program. *Expert Panel Report 3 (EPR3): Guidelines for the Diagnosis and Management of Asthma*. Bethesda, MD: U.S. Department of Health and Human Services; 2007. Note that the treatments by step vary somewhat for children younger than 5 years old. See the complete report for details.

Table 20-26 Step-Based Approach to Drug Therapy for Youth Older Than 12 Years of Age and Adults

Step	Preferred Drug Regimen
1	Short-acting β-agonist (SABA) as needed
2	Add a low-dose inhaled corticosteroid
3	Add LABA, LTRA, theophylline, or zileuton to the low-dose inhaled corticosteroid or step up to a medium-dose inhaled corticosteroid
4	Medium-dose inhaled corticosteroid + LABA, or medium-dose inhaled corticosteroid + LTRA, theophylline, or zileuton
5	High-dose inhaled corticosteroid + LABA (consider omalizumab for patients with allergies)
6	High-dose inhaled corticosteroid + LABA + oral systemic corticosteroid (consider omalizumab for patients with allergies)

LABA, long-acting β-agonist (e.g., salmeterol or formoterol); LTRA, leukotriene receptor antagonist (e.g., montelukast or zafirlukast).

Data from the National Asthma Education and Prevention Program. *Expert Panel Report 3 (EPR3): Guidelines for the Diagnosis and Management of Asthma*. Bethesda, MD: U.S. Department of Health and Human Services; 2007. Note that the treatments by step vary somewhat for children younger than 5 years old. See the complete report for details.

Note that *a short-acting β-agonist should always be available as needed to relieve symptoms.* Patients can take up to three doses at 20-minute intervals. However, use more often than two days per week indicates inadequate control and the need for a step-up in treatment.

Decision making in long-term outpatient asthma management is based on assessing the patient's level of control

- If the patient's asthma is well controlled (see Tables 20-23 and 20-24):
  - Recommend maintaining the current drug regimen/step and having the patient follow up with the doctor in 1 to 6 months.
  - If the patient's asthma remains well controlled for 3 months or longer, recommend a step *down* in the drug regimen.
- If the patient's asthma becomes not well controlled:
  - Assess the patient's compliance with the drug regimen, inhaler technique, and control of environmental factors and coexisting conditions.
  - If the patient's compliance is confirmed and environmental factors and coexisting conditions are under control, recommend a step-up in the drug regimen and reevaluation by the doctor in 2−6 weeks.
- If the patient's asthma becomes very poorly controlled:
  - Assess the patient's compliance with the drug regimen, inhaler technique, and control of environmental factors and coexisting conditions.
  - If the patient's compliance is confirmed and environmental factors and coexisting conditions under control:
    - Recommend a short course of oral systemic corticosteroids.
    - Recommend a step-up in the drug regimen and reevaluation by the doctor in 2 weeks.

Assessment/Information Gathering (Acute Exacerbation)

Acute exacerbations of asthma can vary substantially in terms of their severity. Because the severity of the exacerbation determines the initial treatment approach, RTs must be able to assess the patient on several clinical indicators quickly. **Table 20-27** applies these measures to categorize asthma exacerbations by the level of severity.

In assessing the severity of the patient's exacerbation, two important points should be emphasized:

- Early on, the patient's arterial blood gas typically reveals respiratory alkalosis with mild to moderate hypoxemia; *normalization of the pH ("the cross-over point") usually indicates a rising $Paco_2$ and progression toward respiratory acidosis and failure.*
- The progression to life-threatening respiratory failure is marked by a rapid decline in status; typically manifested by the development of drowsiness, bradypnea, bradycardia, decreased breath sounds, and fatigue.

Treatment/Decision Making (Acute Exacerbation)

Once the severity of the exacerbation is determined, the appropriate management begins. **Table 20-28** outlines the recommended initial treatment regimens for patients presenting to the ED suffering an acute worsening of asthma symptoms, according to their severity.

After initial management, you reassess the patient and implement or recommend further action based on the response to therapy. For the patient being managed for moderate or severe symptoms, the following guidelines apply:

- Recommend discharge from the ED to home if:
  - The patient's symptoms are relieved by treatment.
  - The FEV_1 or PEF is restored ($\geq$ 70% predicted/personal best).
  - The response is sustained for at least 1 hour without further intervention.
- Recommend hospital admission to a medical unit if:
  - Mild to moderate symptoms continue despite appropriate treatment.
  - The FEV_1 or PEF is not adequately restored (40–69% predicted/personal best).

Table 20-27 Assessing the Severity of Asthma Exacerbation

Assessment	Severity		
	Moderate	Severe	Life-Threatening
Breathlessness	Dyspnea at rest; talks in phrases	Dyspnea at rest; talks in words	Limited effort indicating fatigue
Sensorium/behavior	Alert/may be agitated	Alert/usually agitated	Drowsy or confused
Respiratory rate	Tachypnea	Tachypnea	Bradypnea possible
Work of breathing/ respiratory distress	May show accessory muscle use with retractions	Usually shows accessory muscle use with retractions	May exhibit thoracoabdominal paradox
Heart rate/pulse	Tachycardia with pulsus paradoxus	Tachycardia with pulsus paradoxus	Bradycardia (indicating fatigue)
Breath sounds	Prominent expiratory wheezing	Prominent inspiratory + expiratory wheezes	Absence of wheezing ("silent chest")
FEV_1 or PF (% predicted)	≥ 40%	25–40%	< 25% (if able to perform)
Pao_2/Sao_2 (room air)	≥ 60 torr/90%	< 60 torr/90%	< 60 torr/90%
$Paco_2$/pH	< 35–40 torr/↑ pH	> 40 torr/N or ↓ pH	> 45–50 torr/↓ pH

FEV_1, forced expiratory volume in 1 second; N, normal; PF, peak expiratory flow.

Data from the National Asthma Education and Prevention Program. *Expert Panel Report 3 (EPR3): Guidelines for the Diagnosis and Management of Asthma.* Bethesda, MD: U.S. Department of Health and Human Services; 2007.

Table 20-28 Initial Emergency Management of Asthma Exacerbations

Moderate	Severe	Life-Threatening
• O_2 to achieve Sao_2 ≥ 90% • SABA by SVN or MDI + valved holding chamber; up to 3 doses in the first hour • If no immediate response, recommend oral steroids	• O_2 to achieve Sao_2 ≥ 90%; consider heliox if available • High-dose SABA plus ipratropium by SVN or MDI + valved holding chamber, every 20 minutes or CBT for 1 hour • Oral steroids • Trial application of NPPV*	• Intubation and mechanical ventilation with 100% O_2 • Inhaled SABA + ipratropium • IV steroids • IV magnesium sulfate ($MgSO_4$)

CBT, continuous bronchodilator therapy; MDI, metered-dose inhaler; NPPV, noninvasive positive-pressure ventilation; SABA, short-acting β-agonist; SVN, small-volume nebulizer.

*In the patient with severe symptoms whose $Paco_2$ is rising, a trial of NPPV may forestall further deterioration. Successful application requires that the patient be conscious and cooperative and not have any contraindications. If the patient has already progressed to life-threatening respiratory failure, application of NPPV may merely delay needed intubation and invasive support.

- Recommend admission to the ICU if:
  - Severe symptoms continue despite appropriate treatment.
  - The patient is drowsy or confused.
  - The FEV_1 or PEF remains below 40% predicted.
  - The $Paco_2$ indicates hypercapnia.

Should the patient require intubation and mechanical ventilation, the following guidelines apply:

- Initially, use control mode ventilation (*no patient triggering*). Sedate the patient as necessary.
- Ensure adequate oxygenation.
  - Set the initial Fio_2 to 1.0 (100% O_2).
  - Titrate Fio_2 down to maintain Spo_2 > 90%.
- Avoid further air trapping/hyperinflation.
- Apply a low minute volume.

- Set the rate at the *low end* of the age-appropriate range (about 15/min for school-age children).
- Set V_T to 6–8 mL/kg (predicted body weight).
- Keep the plateau pressure $\leq$ 30 cm H_2O.
- Accept a high $Paco_2$ as long as the pH $>$ 7.2 (permissive hypercapnia).
- Provide an I:E ratio of 1:4 or 1:5.
- Maintain an age-appropriate low rate.
- Use high flows during volume control ventilation to shorten the inspiratory time.
- Use of external PEEP to treat air trapping in asthma is controversial and should not routinely be recommended; consider it only if auto-PEEP can be accurately measured, is contributing to hyperinflation, and is not alleviated using the low-Ve and low-I:E-ratio strategies.
- Controlled ventilation with low rates, volumes, and I:E ratios, together with permissive hypercapnia, typically requires neuromuscular blockade (which also will facilitate intubation) and heavy sedation (always used in combination with pharmacologic paralysis).

For patients being discharged from the ED or hospital, it is essential to provide the patient and family with guidance on how to prevent relapses. To that end, the patient and family should be educated as follows:

- Referred to seek follow-up asthma care within a month
- Provided with instructions for all prescribed medications
- Assessed for the proper technique using the prescribed inhaler(s)
- Trained to follow an action plan if symptoms worsen

Foreign-Body Aspiration

Foreign-body aspiration (FBA) is a common medical emergency and the leading cause of accidental deaths in infants and toddlers. Most events occur in those $<$ 3 years old (peaking at 1–2 years of age).

About two-thirds of aspirated foreign bodies in children consist of organic material/foodstuff, such as seeds and nuts (peanuts being most common in the United States). Because most organic foreign bodies are at least somewhat radiolucent, they may not be detected via standard chest x-ray. Many organic foreign bodies also tend to absorb moisture and swell, thus worsening any initial obstruction. Moreover, some organic foreign bodies can cause severe airway inflammation.

Inorganic foreign bodies commonly include teeth, coins, pins, crayons, and small plastic objects, such as small toy parts. Many of these are radiopaque and thus easily visible on x-ray. However, most plastic objects may escape detection on a standard chest radiograph.

Most aspirated foreign bodies end up in the bronchial tree, with the remainder lodging in the larynx or trachea. Although the mainstem bronchi separate at nearly equal angles in small children, foreign bodies are still more likely to lodge in the right mainstem bronchus or its segmental bronchi.

Key pointers in the assessment and treatment of patients with FBA are discussed below.

Assessment/Information Gathering

- Most children with FBA will have a recent history of a witnessed choking event (i.e., sudden onset of cough and dyspnea or cyanosis in a previously healthy child).
- A child suffering from FBA causing complete airway obstruction will typically be in acute respiratory distress without air exchange (and unable to cough or make sounds) or be unconscious, cyanotic, and in respiratory arrest; *immediate action is required* (see Treatment/Decision Making).
- Partial airway obstruction is the more common finding in a child suffering from FBA. Signs and symptoms vary according to location and time elapsed since aspiration:
  - *Larynx/trachea*: Acute respiratory distress with stridor, diffuse wheezing, dyspnea, hoarseness, aphonia with possible retractions and cyanosis (must be addressed immediately)
  - *Large bronchi*: Choking, persistent coughing, dyspnea, tachypnea, regional decrease in breath sounds with localized/unilateral wheezing (later may include signs and symptoms of pneumonia or atelectasis)

- *Lower airways*: An initial choking episode that may be followed by a lack of any remarkable signs or symptoms until late-phase complications develop (e.g., pneumonia, atelectasis, abscess).
- Signs and symptoms typical of late-phase FBA include unilateral decreased breath sounds with course rhonchi, persistent cough and unilateral wheezing, and recurrent or non-resolving pneumonia.
- Signs and symptoms of FBA can mimic other respiratory problems, such as asthma, bronchitis, croup, and bronchiolitis (presence of unilateral wheezing is a key distinguishing feature).
- You should be highly suspicious of FBA in any child exhibiting these signs and symptoms, or one with an asthma-like condition or respiratory tract infection that is unresponsive to the usual therapy.
- If the child has a fever and FBA is suspected, either the object is causing chemical inflammation, or the child has developed late-phase obstructive pneumonia or possible a lung abscess.
- Recommend a chest x-ray, which may appear normal in many patients. Common abnormal findings are unilateral air trapping/hyperinflation/obstructive emphysema (best viewed on an expiratory film) or atelectasis with/without mediastinal shift; actual visualization of a radiopaque object is uncommon. Late-phase findings include lobar pneumonia, consolidation, bronchiectasis, or lung abscess.
- Left and right lateral decubitus x-rays can be helpful if an expiratory film cannot be obtained (the side with the foreign body usually will not deflate when placed in the dependent position).
- If signs and symptoms suggest an object in the larynx or trachea and the child is in no immediate danger, recommend PA + lateral neck x-rays (even if the object is radiolucent, subglottic density or swelling may be apparent).
- If x-ray findings reveal no firm evidence of a foreign body in a child with a history of sudden choking and persistent coughing who is clinically stable, recommend further assessment via diagnostic fiberoptic bronchoscopy (proceeding to rigid bronchoscopy for removal if necessary).
- If signs and symptoms suggest FBA, but bronchoscopy for a foreign body is negative, recommend a CT scan.

Treatment/Decision Making

- Aspirated foreign bodies should be removed as soon as possible; delayed extraction is associated with increased morbidity and mortality.
- If the obstruction is complete, first attempt to manually dislodge the object (back blows/chest thrusts on infants; Heimlich maneuver if > 1 year of age); avoid these methods if the child can speak or cough because they may worsen the obstruction.
- If the obstruction persists after back blows/Heimlich maneuver and a laryngeal object is suspected, recommend immediate laryngoscopy/retrieval with McGill forceps; do not "blindly" sweep pharynx.
- If laryngoscopy cannot remove a foreign laryngeal body and complete obstruction/asphyxia persists, recommend emergency cricothyroidotomy.
- For a confirmed radiopaque object that appears below the larynx and is causing a severe obstruction or if x-rays reveal significant air trapping with a mediastinal shift, recommend rigid bronchoscopy under general anesthesia.
- For patients with persistent symptoms of partial obstruction below the larynx (cough, wheezing, dyspnea, localized decrease in breath sounds/wheezing) or those suspected of FBA but without major symptoms, recommend fiberoptic bronchoscopy to identify the cause and location of the obstruction.
- If a small/solid object is visualized via fiberoptic bronchoscopy, an experienced operator may be able to remove it via special (urologic) tools that can fit through a pediatric scope's 1.2-mm working channel; otherwise, rigid bronchoscopy will be necessary.

- Following successful foreign-body removal, the patient should be admitted for observation; recommend short-term treatment with inhaled corticosteroids and bronchodilators if coughing and wheezing persist (usually due to transient bronchial hyperresponsiveness); if increased secretions/bronchorrhea occur, recommend appropriate airway clearance therapy; do not recommend antibiotics unless there is evidence of infection (e.g., fever, purulent secretions, increased white blood cells [WBCs]).
- All caregivers should be provided with instruction to help prevent FBA, including the following:
  ○ Avoid feeding hard or round foods to children younger than 4 years of age.
  ○ Provide adult supervision whenever solid foods are fed to infants/young children.
  ○ Always feed infants in an upright sitting position.
  ○ Teach children to chew their food well and avoid vocalizing or playing while eating.
  ○ Avoid chewable medications until at least 3 years of age.
  ○ Follow age recommendations on toy packages, avoiding any toys with small parts, and specifically keeping marbles, small rubber balls, and latex balloons away from children (the leading non-food cause of fatal FBA).
  ○ Be aware of interactions with older children, who may share dangerous objects.
  ○ Take a course in basic life support and choking first aid.

Bronchopulmonary Dysplasia

Bronchopulmonary dysplasia (BPD) is a syndrome defined primarily by the long-term need for supplemental O_2 among premature infants (less than 32 weeks' gestation) for at least 28 days after birth. Within this broad definition, three levels of BPD are recognized, all based on assessing the infant's status at 36 weeks' postconceptual age:

- *Mild*: infant can maintain satisfactory oxygenation breathing room air.
- *Moderate*: infant needs supplemental O_2, but no more than 30%, to maintain satisfactory oxygenation.
- *Severe*: infant needs more than 30% O_2 to maintain satisfactory oxygenation.

BPD is associated with prolonged treatment with O_2 and positive-pressure ventilation (PPV), especially in premature or low-birth-weight ($\leq$ 1250 g) infants and those being managed for infant respiratory distress syndrome (IRDS). Pathologic changes are complex and include airway inflammation, bronchial smooth muscle and arteriole hypertrophy, bronchomalacia, interstitial edema, alveolar hypoplasia, capillary obliteration, and pulmonary fibrosis.

Assessment/Information Gathering

- Evaluate for the presence and severity of BPD using the 36-week assessment guidelines described previously.
- Assess for risk factors: prematurity, low birth weight, IRDS, mechanical ventilation, high Fio_2 needs or maintenance of SpO_2 more than 95%, sepsis, and patent ductus arteriosus.
- Conduct or review a physical examination, looking for tachypnea, retractions, crackles, and expiratory wheezing.
- Recommend or review a chest x-ray, which will typically show decreased lung volumes with diffuse areas of both atelectasis and hyperinflation, with possible evidence of fibrosis or pulmonary interstitial emphysema.
- Obtain an arterial blood gas analysis, which typically indicates respiratory acidosis with hypoxemia.
- Recommend an echocardiogram to detect pulmonary hypertension and cor pulmonale (due to pulmonary vasoconstriction, arteriole hypertrophy, and capillary obliteration).

Treatment/Decision Making

The best way to reduce the impact of BPD is to prevent it. To help prevent BPD, recommend or implement the following measures for high-risk infants:

- Provide the lowest level of supplemental O_2 needed to maintain a SpO_2 in the 88–92% range, with slightly higher levels acceptable for infants who are 33 weeks or more postconceptual age.
- Administer prophylactic surfactant treatment using the "intubation–surfactant–extubation" approach described for IRDS.
- Consider prophylactic vitamin A administration (decreases the risk of BPD development in extremely low-birth-weight infants).
- Consider early (before the infant is a few days old) prophylactic caffeine administration (decreases the incidence of BPD and the duration of PPV).

If the infant is already intubated and receiving PPV with O_2, recommend the following measures:

- Select volume-control (VC) ventilation, not pressure-control (PC) ventilation.
- Implement permissive hypercapnia to avoid volutrauma by using low tidal/minute volumes; this requires letting the $Paco_2$ rise as long as the pH remains higher than 7.20.
- Wean the infant to nasal CPAP as soon as possible, accepting $Paco_2$ levels as high as 60–65 torr as long as they remain stable and the pH can be kept at or above 7.3.
- Do *not* recommend inhaled nitric oxide unless persistent pulmonary hypertension of the newborn is a coexisting diagnosis.
- Do *not* recommend high-frequency ventilation (it does not offer any benefit over conventional modes).

Other recommendations include the following:

- Ensure adequate calorie intake (infants with BPD have higher-than-normal calorie needs).
- Restricting fluids and providing diuresis (using hydrochlorothiazide and spironolactone, not furosemide) may provide some benefit.
- Administer a β_2 bronchodilator such as albuterol to help alleviate episodic bronchospasm, should it occur.
- Perform a tracheotomy on infants likely to need continued ventilator support beyond 48 weeks' postconceptual age.

Corticosteroids were once a mainstay of therapy for BPD. However, due to their severe side effects in premature infants (including the development of cerebral palsy), their routine use is no longer recommended. Some neonatologists will still consider corticosteroids in the most severe cases, with current evidence favoring the use of hydrocortisone over dexamethasone.

Most infants with BPD improve gradually over time. Complete weaning off supplemental O_2 can take weeks to months, often is conducted in the home, and may require a calibrated low-flow meter (capable of accuracy to ± 0.25 L/min).

Critical Congenital Heart Defects

A critical congenital heart defect (CCHD) is a structural abnormality in the circulatory system of an infant that is apparent at birth, causes *right-to-left* shunting with cyanosis and hypoxemia, and normally requires surgical correction early in life. CCHDs include the classic "five Ts"—tetralogy of Fallot (TOF), total anomalous pulmonary venous return (TAPVR), transposition of the great arteries (TGA), tricuspid atresia, and truncus arteriosus—as well as hypoplastic left heart syndrome (HLHS) and pulmonary atresia with intact septum.

In several of these defects, survival depends on the maintenance of pulmonary blood flow through an *open* or *patent* ductus arteriosus (PDA). As long as the ductus arteriosus remains patent in these patients, major symptoms may not always be apparent. Unfortunately, if CCHD is not recognized and corrected before discharge, infants with these "ductal-dependent" defects can develop life-threatening cardiogenic shock when the ductus closes. For this reason, early detection of these defects is essential.

Assessment/Information Gathering

- Recommend and perform pulse oximetry screening for CCHDs on all infants 24 hours after birth (see **Figure 20-1** for the screening protocol).
- Conduct or review the physical examination, looking for the following findings:

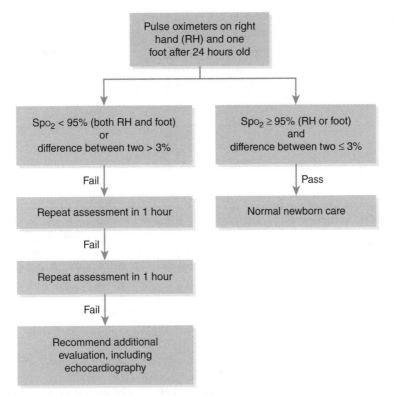

Figure 20-1 Basic Pulse Oximetry Screening Protocol for CCHD.
Screening should be performed after 24 hours of life or as late as
possible if an early discharge is planned. The infant *passes* the screen if
while breathing room air *both* the right hand and the foot SpO_2 are 95%
or greater, with the difference between them being 3% or less. The infant
fails the screen if *any* SpO_2 is less than 90% on initial assessment or if two
additional measurements (for a total of three) confirm either a low SpO_2
at both measurement sites or more than a 3% difference between them.
Infants failing the screen should undergo further assessment to confirm
CCHD, including echocardiography.

- ○ Presence of central cyanosis or persistent pallor (Note that cyanosis generally requires
  a SpO_2 less than 80%; however, even at these levels, cyanosis may not be apparent in
  dark-skinned infants or those with anemia.)
- ○ Abnormal cardiovascular findings, including abnormal heart rate, precordial activity, and
  sounds; pathologic murmurs; weak or absent peripheral pulses; and a large difference
  between upper and lower extremity blood pressure
- ○ Abnormal respiratory findings, including tachypnea, labored breathing at rest, coughing,
  wheezing, and increased distress when feeding
- • For cyanotic infants, assess the PaO_2 after 10 minutes of breathing 100% O_2 (the hyperoxia
  test):
  - ○ $PaO_2 < 150$ torr on 100% O_2: *intracardiac,* R to L shunt/CCHD likely
  - ○ $PaO_2 > 150$ torr but < 200 torr: inconclusive results
  - ○ $PaO_2 > 200$ torr: *pulmonary,* R to L shunt likely (e.g., RDS, PPHN)
- • Recommend a chest x-ray, which may reveal a telltale heart shape:
  - ○ "Snowman" with total anomalous pulmonary venous return
  - ○ "Boot" with pulmonary atresia, tetralogy of Fallot, and tricuspid atresia
  - ○ "Egg on string" with transposition of the great arteries
- • Recommend an ECG to detect axis deviation:
  - ○ Right-axis deviation indicating right ventricular hypertrophy: transposition of great
    arteries, total anomalous pulmonary venous return, tetralogy of Fallot

Table 20-29 Effect of Ventilator Settings on Pulmonary Resistance and Blood Flow

Ventilator Setting	Increases PVR/Decreases Blood Flow
Minute ventilation	Low ($\uparrow$ $Paco_2$, $\downarrow$ pH)
Inspired O_2 concentration	Low (e.g., 18% by adding N_2)
Peak/mean airway pressure	High
PEEP	High
I:E ratio	High

- ○ Left-axis deviation indicating left ventricular or biventricular hypertrophy: truncus arteriosus, transposition of great arteries, tricuspid atresia
- If available, recommend neonatal 2D and Doppler echocardiography for infants who test positive for CCHD in the pulse-oximetry screening or hyperoxia test; these imaging modalities provide definitive detection of CCHD and other cardiac anomalies.

Treatment/Decision Making

- Recommend surgical correction for any infant with a confirmed CCHD.
- If an infant with a suspected or confirmed CCHD presents with or develops cardiogenic shock, treat according to the neonatal resuscitation protocol (Chapter 15).
- If an infant with a confirmed ductal-dependent defect exhibits severe cyanosis with evidence of heart failure and pulmonary edema, recommend IV prostaglandin E_1 (PGE_1 or alprostadil) to dilate the ductus arteriosus; be prepared for apnea and hypotension as possible side effects.
- If the infant in heart failure exhibits systemic hypotension or low cardiac output, recommend an inotropic agent such as dopamine.
- For infants requiring mechanical ventilation, the neonatologist may request changes in ventilator settings to alter vascular resistance and blood flow through the pulmonary circulation; **Table 20-29** summarizes how key ventilator settings can affect pulmonary vascular resistance and blood flow.

NEONATAL PROBLEMS

Number of Simulations in the CSE: 2 Cases

In the NBRC hospital, all RTs are expected to be familiar with perinatal care, including the care delivered in the delivery room and the neonatal intensive care unit (NICU). To ensure success on CSE problems in this area, in this section we cover delivery room management including, newborn resuscitation, meconium aspiration syndrome (MAS), apnea of prematurity, and IRDS.

Delivery Room Management and Resuscitation

Typically, RTs will be called to the delivery room to assist with neonatal management after high-risk deliveries, especially those involving births occurring before 35 weeks' gestation. The focus in these cases is on rapid assessment and protocol-based resuscitation and stabilization.

Assessment/Information Gathering

- Immediately after birth, assess the neonate's heart rate, respiratory rate, muscle tone, reflexes, and color—that is, the basic parameters included in the 1-minute Apgar score; also assess for meconium staining.
- Repeat the Apgar score at 5 minutes; if it is less than 7, repeat the assessment every 5 minutes for up to 20 minutes (never delay action to perform the Apgar score for an infant needing immediate support).

Table 20-30 Silverman-Anderson Index for Assessing Respiratory Distress

Feature	Score		
	0	1	2
Chest/abdominal movement	Synchronized	Lag on inspiration	Seesaw movement
Intercostal retractions	None	Just visible	Marked
Xiphoid retractions	None	Just visible	Marked
Nasal flaring	None	Minimal	Marked
Expiratory grunting	None	Stethoscope only	Naked ear

- If the neonate remains cyanotic or exhibits severe pallor and is given supplemental O_2, assess the SpO_2, ideally via the right hand (preductal SpO_2). In healthy infants breathing room air immediately after birth, the preductal SpO_2 typically ranges from 60–70%. The SpO_2 may take 5–10 minutes to "normalize" (exceed 85%).
- After the infant has been adequately stabilized and transferred to the nursery, recommend a thorough exam (at 10–20 hours after birth) using the Ballard assessment to estimate gestational age and identify any potential developmental abnormalities.
- After stabilization, the newborn's respiratory status should be continuously observed for delayed development of respiratory distress or hypoxemia.

Respiratory distress can be evaluated using an objective system, such as the Silverman-Anderson scale (**Table 20-30**). A score of 0 on this index indicates no respiratory distress, scores of 1 to 6 indicate mild to moderate distress, and a score of 7 or higher indicates impending respiratory failure.

In terms of late development of hypoxemia, look for the appearance of central cyanosis in room air or a preductal SpO_2 that does not quickly normalize or falls back below 90%.

Treatment/Decision Making

- If a near-term baby (37 or more weeks' gestation) cries, begins breathing, and exhibits good muscle tone immediately after birth, there is no need for resuscitation. Instead, dry the infant, place in skin-to-skin contact with the mother, cover with dry linen to keep warm, and continue to observe breathing, activity, and color.
- If after clearing the airway, the newborn exhibits apnea, gasping, labored breathing, or a heart rate less than 100/min, immediately apply positive-pressure ventilation (PPV) via bag-valve-mask device or T-piece resuscitator.
- For meconium-stained babies:
  - With normal respiratory effort, muscle tone, and heart rate (> 100/min) do not intubate; instead, clear secretions and meconium from the mouth (*first*) and nose and continue to monitor.
  - With depressed respiratory effort, poor muscle tone, or a low heart rate (< 100/min), recommend ET intubation and tracheal suctioning immediately after delivery (ideally within 5 seconds); if no meconium is suctioned, do not repeat.
  - If meconium is retrieved via initial ET suctioning and the heart rate exceeds 100/min, recommend repeat suctioning. If the heart rate is less than 100/min, administer PPV and consider resuming suctioning later.
- During resuscitation, assess heart rate, respirations, and SpO_2, ideally via the right hand (preductal SpO_2).
- If supplemental O_2 is needed in the delivery room, target the following SpO_2 levels:

1 min ➜ 60–65%
2 min ➜ 65–70%
3 min ➜ 70–75%
4 min ➜ 75–80%
5 min ➜ 80–85%
10 min ➜ 85–95%

- If the heart rate is less than 60/min, initiate chest compressions, and recommend intubation (to coordinate compressions with PPV).
- Deliver compressions on the lower third of the sternum to a depth of about one-third the AP diameter of the chest.
- Maintain a 3:1 ratio of compressions to ventilations, giving 90 compressions and 30 breaths per minute (½ second per event, 120 events per minute).
- Continue chest compressions and ventilation until the heart rate is 60/min or greater.
- If the heart rate remains less than 60/min despite adequate ventilation with O_2 and chest compressions, recommend epinephrine administration.
- If after stabilization, an infant develops a Silverman-Anderson score greater than 5, recommend transfer to intensive care for further assessment and management.
- If after stabilization, an infant develops central cyanosis in room air or has a preductal Spo_2 that does not quickly normalize or falls back below 90%, recommend transfer to intensive care for further assessment and management.

Meconium Aspiration

Meconium consists of the thick, dark-green intestinal secretions of the fetus. Meconium normally is not passed out of the intestines until after birth. Common factors associated with meconium release into the amniotic fluid before birth include placental insufficiency, maternal hypertension, preeclampsia, maternal drug abuse, maternal infection, chorioamnionitis, and fetal hypoxic stress. Although sterile, when aspirated, meconium causes a severe chemical pneumonitis, variable degrees of airway obstruction/air trapping, and inactivation of surfactant. The resulting hypoxia and release of chemical mediators cause pulmonary vasoconstriction. In combination, these pathophysiologic events constitute the meconium aspiration syndrome (MAS).

MAS is defined as respiratory distress in an infant born through a meconium-stained amniotic fluid (MSAF) whose symptoms cannot be otherwise explained. Typically, the infant is born at or beyond full term ($\geq$ 37–39 weeks). The syndrome is considered mild if the infant requires less than 40% O_2 to maintain adequate oxygenation, moderate if more than 40% O_2 is needed, and severe if positive pressure ventilation is necessary to support life. MAS is often associated with persistent pulmonary hypertension of the newborn (PPHN).

Assessment/Information Gathering

- Diagnosis is based on a perinatal history of meconium-stained amniotic fluid combined with signs of respiratory distress in association with certain characteristic x-ray abnormalities.
- Evaluate for other perinatal factors associated with MAS: abnormal fetal heart rate patterns, fetal acidosis, cesarean delivery, and Apgar scores < 7.
- Be sure to closely monitor or to recommend monitoring any infant born through MSAF for any signs of respiratory distress for at least 24 hours.
- Assess for signs of respiratory distress consistent with MAS: tachypnea, cyanosis, intercostal retractions, grunting, alar/nasal flaring; in severe cases, a "barrel chest" (increased AP diameter) may also be observed, due to the presence of air trapping.
- Auscultate: breath sounds may reveal coarse bilateral rhonchi and crackles; in those with PPHN, a systolic murmur (indicating tricuspid regurgitation) may be heard over the heart.
- Recommend/assess x-ray, looking for diffuse or localized areas of overexpansion/hyperinflation and infiltration/atelectasis; air leaks (pneumothorax, pulmonary interstitial emphysema [PIE]) may also be evident; if present, cardiomegaly suggests coexisting PPHN.
- Recommend echocardiography to (1) rule out congenital heart disease, (2) assess cardiac function, and (3) determine the location and severity of right-to-left shunting and pulmonary hypertension.
- Laboratory evaluation—recommend the following:
  - ABG—may reflect primarily hypoxemia (mild to moderate MAS) or hypoxemia + respiratory and possibly metabolic acidosis (severe MAS)
  - CBC/differential

- ◦ Polycythemia may impair pulmonary blood flow/exacerbate MAS and PPHN.
- ◦ Thrombocytopenia increases the risk of neonatal hemorrhage.
- ◦ Neutropenia or neutrophilia may indicate infection.
- ◦ Hb and Hct levels—to assess for blood loss and adequacy of blood O_2 content

Treatment/Decision Making

At/After Birth

- • If the baby is meconium-stained with normal respiratory effort, muscle tone, and heart rate, *do not intubate*; instead, clear mouth (first!) and nose with a bulb syringe or suction catheter.
- • If the baby is meconium-stained with poor or no respiratory efforts, poor muscle tone, and heart rate < 100/min:
  - ◦ Intubate and suction the trachea immediately after delivery.
  - ◦ If meconium is retrieved and heart rate > 100/min, re-suction.
  - ◦ If the heart rate < 100/min, administer PPV and consider suctioning again later.
- • Recommend prophylactic surfactant replacement therapy using the INSURE method (*in*tubation, *sur*factant, *ex*tubation) with prompt extubation to nasal CPAP (can improve oxygenation, reduce pulmonary complications, and decrease the need for extracorporeal membrane oxygenation [ECMO] treatment).

General Management (Typically in a NICU)

Recommend the following:

- • Continuous monitoring of oxygenation, blood pressure, and perfusion via SpO_2 and umbilical arterial catheter
- • Maintenance of a neutral thermal environment (to prevent cold stress and minimize O_2 consumption)
- • Correction of any electrolyte and acid-base imbalances (can worsen PPHN)
- • Maintenance of normal blood glucose levels (hypoglycemia can worsen PPHN)
- • Maintenance of a normal Hb concentration (13–15 g/dL; *avoid polycythemia*)
- • Maintenance of mean systemic blood pressure > 45–50 mm Hg via fluid therapy and inotropes (e.g., dopamine; reduces right-to-left [R ➔ L] shunting)
- • Minimization of stimulation/handling and use of invasive procedures such as suctioning (stress causes catecholamine release, which increases PVR)
- • Provision of adequate sedation (to avoid stress response), typically via an opioid such as fentanyl, often in combination with a benzodiazepine

Respiratory Care

- • Oxygen therapy—provide O_2 as needed (via hood or ventilator) to maintain PaO_2 of 55–80 torr/SpO_2 of 88–95% (also acts as a pulmonary vasodilator).
- • Intubation and mechanical ventilation:
  - ◦ Recommend for infants with MAS, severe hypoxemia (PaO_2 < 50 torr on FiO_2 ≥ 0.60; P/F < 100), and respiratory acidosis (pH < 7.25).
  - ◦ The goal is to improve oxygenation while minimizing air trapping/overdistention, barotrauma/air-leak syndrome.
  - ◦ Depending on availability, can start with conventional or high-frequency ventilation (primarily high-frequency oscillation ventilation [HFOV]).
  - ◦ If inhaled nitric oxide (INO) is available and is likely to be used for PPHN, recommend starting it with HFOV (combined HFOV + INO is more effective than either alone).
- • Conventional ventilation:
  - ◦ Apply lung-protective ventilation: V_T 4–6 mL/kg (volume control [VC]) or peak inspiratory pressure (PIP) 25–28 cm H_2O (pressure control ventilation [PC]), rate 40–60/min, expiratory time (0.5-0.7 sec; I:E ≤ 1:1) sufficient to prevent air trapping, 4–7 cm H_2O PEEP.

- Aim for Pao_2 of 55–80 torr/Spo_2 88–95%, $Paco_2$ 40–60 torr, pH 7.3–7.4 (exception is to normalize $Paco_2$ and pH if coexisting PPHN).
- If air trapping/hyperinflation occurs, lower rate/increase expiratory time and decrease PEEP to 3–4 cm H_2O.
- If atelectasis is the primary problem or worsens, increase PEEP up to a maximum of 10 cm H_2O.
- Recommend switching to HFOV if two consecutive assessments over 3–6 hours reveal the following:
  - Fio_2 needs > 0.60
  - PIP > 30 cm H_2O
  - MAP > 15 cm H_2O
- Oxygenation index (OI) > 15–20 on H_2O (OI = [%O_2 × MAP]/Pao_2)
- High-frequency oscillation ventilation (HFOV):
  - To avoid the development or worsening of air trapping, set the frequency in the range of 6–8 Hz (no higher than 10 Hz).
  - The initial MAP may need to be higher than on conventional ventilation (up to 25 cm H_2O in some cases).
  - Use a stepwise incremental recruitment maneuver to set an "optimum" MAP.
  - Infants with prominent air-trapping and or PPHN may respond poorly to recruitment (fall in Pao_2/Sao_2 and BP, rise in PVR).
  - Once oxygenation has improved, reduce the MAP in a stepwise fashion (most infants with MAS can be stabilized with a MAP of 15–20 cm H_2O).
- Surfactant therapy: if a Fio_2 > 0.50 and MAP > 7 cm H_2O is required after intubation and conventional mechanical ventilation, recommend "rescue" surfactant therapy (maybe in addition to postpartum prophylaxis).
- If MAS is complicated with PPHN, recommend a pulmonary vasodilator, as follows:
  - If available, INO as follows:
    - Indication: persistent R ➔ L shunting, high PVR, OI > 20–25
    - Starting dose 20 ppm (therapeutic range is 5–20 ppm)
  - If INO is not available, a phosphodiesterase inhibitor, such as sildenafil or milrinone
- Extracorporeal membrane oxygenation (ECMO)
  - Recommend ECMO/transfer to ECMO center if OI > 40 despite optimized medical management, mechanical ventilation, and pulmonary vasodilator therapy.
  - Other criteria for ECMO include (1) > 34 weeks' gestation, (2) birth weight > 2000 g, (3) lack of major coagulopathy or active bleeding, (4) no major intracranial bleeding, (5) reversible lung disease, (6) duration of mechanical ventilation < 10–14 days.

Do Not Recommend

- Hyperventilation (has an adverse effect on cerebral circulation and can cause barotrauma)
- Corticosteroids (no consistent evidence of short-term benefit; may have adverse long-term effects)
- *Prophylactic* antibiotics (do not affect outcomes; only indicated if positive cultures)

Apnea of Prematurity

Apnea of prematurity is a developmental disorder affecting infants born at less than 37 weeks' gestation. Although likely caused by "physiologic immaturity" of respiratory control (central apnea), some premature infants also exhibit airway obstruction (obstructive apnea). By definition, the apnea episodes must be recurrent and either last for more than 20 seconds or be accompanied by cyanosis, a 4% or greater fall in Spo_2, or bradycardia. In general, the incidence of apnea of prematurity varies inversely with gestational age and birth weight, with nearly all infants born at less than 28 weeks' gestation or weighing less than 1000 g being affected. The incidence of apneas typically decreases over time, often resolving by 34–36 weeks' postconceptual age.

Assessment/Information Gathering

- Look for recurrent episodes of apnea with or without desaturation or bradycardia during the first 2 to 3 days after birth in any spontaneously breathing infant born at less than 37 weeks' gestational age (events are typically identified and recorded by cardiorespiratory monitors).
- Assess the infant and the record to rule out other common causes of apnea, including hypoxemia, anemia, sepsis, unstable thermal environment (hypothermia or hyperthermia), administration of opiates to the mother before birth or the infant postnatally, intracranial hemorrhage, congenital upper airway anomalies (e.g., choanal atresia), seizures, and electrolyte or acid-base disturbances.

Treatment/Decision Making

- Recommend that the infant be cared for in the prone position.
- Recommend continuous apnea monitoring for respiration and heart rate.
- Recommend continuous pulse oximetry if episodes of desaturation occur with the apnea.
- When a confirmed episode of apnea occurs, intervene immediately if the infant exhibits cyanosis or severe pallor; otherwise, wait 10 seconds to see if the apnea "self-corrects."
- If an apnea episode does not self-correct within 10 seconds of alarm notification, progressively follow these steps:
  1. Stimulate the infant by tickling or flicking the feet or stroking the abdomen.
  2. If there is no response, briefly suction the oropharynx, and then repeat the stimulation.
  3. If there is still no response, slightly extend the neck to minimize airway obstruction.
  4. If there is still no response, apply bag and mask ventilation using the O_2% that the infant was receiving before the episode (*not* 100%).
  5. If there is still no response, consider either intubation and mechanical ventilation or nasal NPPV.
- Recommend daily dosing of caffeine until the infant is at least 33 weeks' postconceptual age or has infrequent events that do not resolve spontaneously (apnea monitoring should continue for a further week after the medication is stopped).
- If the infant has frequent apnea episodes requiring stimulation despite caffeine administration, recommend or implement either nasal CPAP at 4–6 cm H_2O or a high-flow nasal cannula at 1–6 L/min, adjusted empirically to reduce the frequency of events.

Infant Respiratory Distress Syndrome

IRDS (previously called hyaline membrane disease) is a common disorder in premature infants. In these infants, the lungs have not yet completed development and, therefore, lack sufficient quantities of pulmonary surfactant. The lack of normal surfactant increases surface tension, making the alveoli prone to collapse. The resulting atelectasis causes shunting and severe hypoxemia that does not respond to O_2 therapy. The severe hypoxemia, in turn, causes pulmonary vasoconstriction and hypertension, which can lead to circulatory disturbances and extrapulmonary right-to-left shunting. The high surface tension also decreases lung compliance and increases the work of breathing.

Assessment/Information Gathering

- Assess the history, and look for evidence of prematurity (less than 37 weeks' gestation), low birth weight (less than 1500 g), and related maternal risk factors such as diabetes.
- Assess for prior measurement (at 35 weeks' gestation) of lecithin/sphingomyelin (L/S) ratio (less than 2) and absence of phosphatidylglycerol (PG) as indicators of pulmonary immaturity.
- Observe for signs of progressive respiratory distress shortly after birth, including tachypnea (more than 60 breaths/min), subcostal and intercostal retractions, expiratory grunting, decreased breath sounds, nasal flaring, and cyanosis in room air (signs may not appear for a few hours).

- Recommend a chest x-ray, looking for low lung volume with diffuse reticulogranular ("ground-glass") appearance and air bronchograms.
- Recommend an ABG, looking for respiratory acidosis with severe hypoxemia.
- In terms of the differential diagnosis, transient tachypnea of the newborn is generally seen in more mature infants (i.e., term or late preterm infants) compared to RDS.
- Recommend appropriate cultures to rule out an infectious cause, such as streptococcal pneumonia or sepsis.
- Recommend a hyperoxia test to rule out a CCHD as the cause of the cyanosis and respiratory distress.
- Recommend an echocardiogram if extrapulmonary shunting (e.g., PDA) is suspected.

Treatment/Decision Making

- For women at risk of giving birth between weeks 24 and 34 of pregnancy, recommend corticosteroid administration before birth ("antenatal steroids" enhance lung maturation and reduce the risk of RDS, brain hemorrhage, and death).
- For spontaneously breathing infants with clinical and x-ray findings indicating IRDS, recommend or implement early prophylactic surfactant therapy using the "intubation–surfactant–extubation" approach (i.e., the infant is briefly intubated after birth, is administered surfactant, and then is immediately extubated and placed on nasal CPAP at 4–6 cm H_2O).
- A high-flow nasal cannula at 1–6 L/min is an alternative to nasal CPAP; CPAP levels vary with flow and leakage and are judged empirically by patient response.
- Recommend maintenance of a neutral thermal environment using an incubator or radiant warmer.
- Provide sufficient FiO_2 to maintain the PaO_2 between 50 and 70 torr or the SpO_2 between 85% and 92%.
- Recommend intubation and mechanical ventilation for an infant less than 27 weeks' gestational age whose mother did not receive antenatal steroids or if the infant is apneic, is unable to maintain an adequate airway, exhibits increased work of breathing (grunting, retractions, flaring) on CPAP, or cannot maintain a pH higher than 7.25 on CPAP.
- When mechanical ventilation is required, to avoid volutrauma, recommend or implement permissive hypercapnia by using volume-controlled ventilation with low tidal volumes (4–5 mL/kg corrected) and letting the $PaCO_2$ rise as long as the pH remains higher than 7.20.
- Additionally, high-frequency modes of ventilation are used to further prevent alveolar damage and barotrauma caused by conventional modes.
- Aim for early extubation to nasal CPAP in the following circumstances:
  ○ The infant exhibits adequate respiratory drive.
  ○ Mean airway pressure is 7 cm H_2O or less.
  ○ Adequate oxygenation can be maintained on 35% O_2 or less.
- Do *not* recommend high-frequency ventilation (it does not offer any benefit over conventional ventilation).
- Do *not* recommend INO therapy unless the IRDS is accompanied by PPHN.

APPENDIX A | Test-Taking Tips and Techniques

Narciso E. Rodriguez and Albert J. Heuer

To perform well on the NBRC exams (the Therapist Multiple-Choice Examination or TMC and the Clinical Simulation Examination or CSE), you first must know the subject matter. However, to pass these exams, you also need good test-taking skills. **Figure A-1** offers our simple two-part "formula" for success on these exams.

Our simple formula reveals why many knowledgeable candidates fail their NBRC exams. Typically, such individuals do poorly because they lack the test-taking skills needed to translate their mastery of the subject matter into consistently correct answers. The common refrain "I'm no good at taking tests" is a symptom of this problem. Fortunately, this condition is treatable. With good guidance and practice, everyone can develop good test-taking skills. The purpose of this appendix is to help you become a better test-taker. By doing so, you will improve your odds of passing the NBRC exams.

How to Fail Your NBRC Exams

It might seem strange to begin with instructions on how to fail your test. However, knowing why people fail NBRC exams can help you avoid failure. Of course, the most common reason why candidates perform poorly on these exams is a lack of content knowledge. Other causes of failure include the following:

- Taking the test "cold" or unprepared
- Memorizing as many practice questions and answers as possible
- Reviewing everything you ever learned in school rather than a focused approach
- Cramming the night before the exam
- Letting anxiety get the best of you
- Not finishing the test
- Leaving questions unanswered
- Poor time management skills

It always amazes us how some candidates insist on taking the NBRC exams without proper preparation. Of course, some do it because they plan poorly and run out of time. Others take the test "cold" because they are overly confident. Last, and most foolish, are those who take these exams without preparation just to "see how they will do." By not preparing, you risk wasting both your time and your money should you fail. Although we do advocate "gambling" on specific test questions, taking an NBRC exam without any preparation is a very bad bet that you are likely to lose. As indicated in our formula for success, you cannot pass these tests without proper knowledge of their content. Moreover, a good understanding of the subject matter comes only with proper preparation, as provided in Chapters 1–17 of this text.

Another common cause of failure is the misguided strategy of memorizing hundreds of practice questions and answers. This strategy is a waste of time. Instead, you should use practice questions

| Passing the NBRC exam | = | Knowledge of subject matter | + | Good test-taking skills |

Figure A-1 Formula for Success on the NBRC Exams.

and answers to help identify concepts that you know and those on which you still need to review further.

We also know of candidates who prepare by surrounding themselves with all the books and lecture notes they acquired in school. Many of these candidates simply do not know where to begin, and most will feel overwhelmed by the sheer volume of study materials. Such a strategy typically causes anxiety and confusion, which lead to poor exam performance. You need to remember that the NBRC exams *do not* test for isolated facts or the "book knowledge" covered in school. Instead, *these exams assess your ability to analyze and apply related knowledge.* Thus, instead of reviewing everything taught in school, your time is better spent focusing on the specific test content as defined in the NBRC exam detailed content outline (DCO) and as covered in this text.

Cramming is probably the most common reason candidates fail NBRC exams. Lacking a good study plan and pressed for time, many folks put off preparation until the week before—*or even the night before*—their test date. Besides producing even worse anxiety than trying to review everything ever learned, cramming typically causes loss of sleep in the days leading up to the test. "Dazed and confused" best describes these candidates when they show up to take the test—and "disappointed" when they get their score reports!

Anxiety is another common cause of poor exam performance. More precisely, *overanxiety* can lead to failure. Some anxiety before taking a test is not only natural but can be beneficial. The stress associated with test-taking can help motivate you to excel and improve your exam performance.

Last, the surest way to fail any test is not to finish it because of poor time-management skills. Because every question on the NBRC multiple-choice exam that you do not answer counts against you, you cannot afford to throw away points by omitting answers or running out of time. To finish these exams in the allotted time, you will need to develop good pacing strategies (described subsequently in this appendix).

How to Pass Your NBRC TMC Exam

Based on our decades of experience working with NBRC candidates, we have developed a three-pronged strategy for passing the TMC exam. *First*, you must fully understand the structure and content of the TMC exam, an approach we call "know your enemy." *Second*, in studying for it, you need to prepare yourself as if "working" in the idealized setting we call the "NBRC hospital." *Third, and most important*, you need to develop good test-taking skills—that is, you must become "test-wise."

Know Your Enemy

A common strategy among generals planning a battle is to *know your enemy*. Thinking of your written exam as an adversary to be conquered can help you prepare for your upcoming "battle." In this case, knowing the enemy means understanding both the structure and the content of the exam you will take and applying this knowledge to your study plan.

The structure and content of the TMC exam are well defined in the current version of the NBRC's *Candidate Handbook and Application*. The current TMC exam consists of 160 multiple-choice questions (140 scored items and 20 pretest items) distributed among the three major content areas listed in the DCO. You have 3 hours to complete the examination. There are two established cut scores for this exam. Candidates attaining the lower score but scoring below the uppercut score will earn the CRT credential, whereas those meeting the higher cut score requirement will earn the CRT credential *and* become eligible to sit for the Clinical Simulation Examination (CSE) to earn the RRT credential.

The content of the exam is based on national survey data describing the essential knowledge, skills, and abilities required of entry-level respiratory therapists. Questions on the TMC exam fall into one of three major content sections: (I) Patient Data; (II) Troubleshooting and Quality Control of Devices, and Infection Control; and (III) Initiation and Modification of Interventions. Questions in the exam are written at three different cognitive levels: recall, application, and analysis. **Table A-1** shows the distribution of the exam questions by the number and level of items in each of the three major sections.

Table A-1 TMC Exam Question Structure

Section	Number of Questions	% of Total	% Recall	% Application	% Analysis
I	55	39%	22%	47%	31%
II	20	14%	35%	50%	15%
III	65	46%	18%	38%	44%
Total	140		22%	44%	34%

A careful review of Table A-1 demonstrates first that most of the questions (approximately 50%) assess your ability to initiate and modify interventions (section III). Second, more significant is the different level of cognitive questioning characterizing the TMC exam. Overall, almost 80% of the questions on the TMC exam are at the application or analysis level, with only 22% requiring recall of information.

To help understand the differences in the cognitive level of questions, we will look at three examples covering the same content area, with a checkmark (√) for the correct answer.

Recall Example

A-1. An otherwise healthy 25-year-old male patient who took an overdose of sedatives is being supported on a ventilator. Which of the following measures of total static compliance (lungs + thorax) would you expect in this patient?

    A. 100 mL/cm H_2O ✓
    B. 10 mL/cm H_2O
    C. 1 mL/cm H_2O
    D. 0.1 mL/cm H_2O

Comments: To evaluate and monitor a patient, you need to know what is normal and what is abnormal. This question tests your ability to recall normal static compliance.

Application Example

A-2. An adult patient receiving volume-control assist/control (VC, A/C) ventilation has a tidal volume of 700 mL, peak pressure of 50 cm H_2O, and a plateau pressure of 40 cm H_2O and is receiving 5 cm H_2O positive end-expiratory pressure (PEEP). What is this patient's static compliance?

    A. 200 mL/cm H_2O
    B. 20 mL/cm H_2O ✓
    C. 2 mL/cm H_2O
    D. 0.2 mL/cm H_2O

Comments: This item tests your ability to *apply* a formula to a clinical situation (most formula-type questions are at the application level). To answer it correctly, you need to enter the correct data into the formula for computing static compliance—that is, compliance (mL/cm H_2O) = tidal volume ÷ (plateau pressure – PEEP).

Analysis Example

A-3. A patient in the intensive care unit with congestive heart failure receiving assist/control ventilation with a set volume of 650 mL exhibits the following data on three consecutive patient-ventilator checks:

Time	Peak Pressure	Plateau Pressure	PEEP
9:00 am	40	25	8
10:00 am	50	35	8
11:00 am	60	45	8

The patient also exhibits diffuse crackles at the bases and some wheezing. Which of the following would you recommend for this patient?

A. A diuretic ✓
B. A bronchodilator
C. A mucolytic
D. A steroid

Comments: This item assesses your ability to *analyze* monitoring data and *apply* this information to *recommend* a treatment approach for this patient. *First*, you must analyze the data, which should reveal that the patient is suffering from a progressive decrease in compliance (rising plateau – PEEP pressure difference). *Second*, you need to recognize that in patients with congestive heart failure, the most common cause of a progressive decrease in compliance is the development of pulmonary edema. *Third*, you need to apply these data and your knowledge of pathophysiology and pharmacology to recommend the correct course of action—in this case, the administration of a diuretic such as furosemide (Lasix).

What conclusions can you gather from analysis of the NBRC TMC content outline in Table A-1? Key pointers include the following:

- Most test questions focus on therapeutic interventions (section III), so you should spend the bulk of your preparation time on this content (Chapters 9–17 of this text).
- Because one-fourth or fewer of the questions included on these exams are based on recall, *you cannot pass the TMC exam by merely memorizing facts.*
- When preparing for the TMC exam, you must stress *application and analysis* of patient data and use of that information to select, implement, or modify procedures.
- Because these exams focus on job-related skills, it can help to visualize and relate your experiences at the bedside while a student or entry-level therapist as you prepare for your test.

Working in the NBRC Hospital

Besides the structure and content of the exams, your study plan also should consider what we refer to as the "NBRC hospital." What is the NBRC hospital? *It is not a place but, rather, a state of mind.* You "enter" the NBRC hospital whenever you take an NBRC exam. This hospital may or may not resemble the clinical sites you rotated through as a student or the facility where you currently work. Instead, it represents the NBRC's perception of an idealized institution. What do we mean by *idealized?* We mean that the NBRC hospital's respiratory care department always relies on generally accepted standards in the field, based in part on current nationally recognized practice guidelines. Also, the NBRC hospital respiratory care department's "procedure manual" covers a wide variety of clinical skills performed by respiratory therapists (RTs) throughout the United States. For these reasons, when working in the NBRC hospital, you may be expected to know and do more or do things differently from the way they are done in your school or facility.

For example, in your facility, a separate electrocardiogram (ECG) department may be responsible for taking 12-lead ECGs and maintaining the related equipment. Perhaps ECG technicians, nurses, physician assistants, or residents are the ones responsible for obtaining 12-lead ECGs in your special care units or the emergency department. In the NBRC hospital, however, you should be able to obtain a 12-lead ECG, interpret the basic findings, and even troubleshoot the device should it not function properly.

Another potential distinction characterizing the NBRC hospital is the level of independent judgment you are expected to exercise. In many hospitals, RTs—especially new graduates—are limited in what they can do without physician approval. However, a quick review of the current TMC and CSE content outlines reveals that the single most important subsections in the therapeutic procedures section call for the RT to *independently* modify or recommend modifications to procedures based on the patient's response. Indeed, this expectation goes well beyond making adjustments to simple "floor therapy." For example, on both examinations, you will be asked to apply your knowledge to alter key mechanical ventilation parameters, such as the oxygen concentration (FiO_2) and the PEEP level. In these cases, the NBRC hospital typically gives you the freedom to make your own choices without being constrained by the need for physician approval. This is especially true if the scenario involves protocol-based care. Only if the question limits your discretion (as when a protocol boundary is reached) should you consider not exercising your independent judgment.

So, how do you prepare to "work" in the NBRC hospital? We recommend the following:

- Treat the NBRC exam content outlines as your departmental procedure manual, focusing in particular on those things you either do not do or do not frequently perform in your facility.
- Use the pre-test and post-test questions included in the online companion website to help you identify how the practices in the NBRC hospital differ from what you have learned in your training or experience.
- When given the opportunity, do not be afraid to exercise your independent judgment and modify a procedure when changes in the patient's status warrant it.

Develop Test Wisdom

Students and NBRC examination candidates who consistently do well on tests have two things going for them. First, *they know the content and are confident in that knowledge*. In addition, these high performers have a "secret weapon" in their back pocket—the ability to apply knowledge of test design and specific reasoning skills to improve their exam scores. We call this ability *test wisdom*.

How does test wisdom work? **Table A-2** demonstrates the difference between a test-unaware and a test-wise candidate on a hypothetical NBRC written exam. Both candidates are comfortable enough with the content to "know cold" or be sure about their answers to half the questions on the exam (70 items). Both must guess at the remaining 70 questions. Unfortunately, the test-unaware candidate does not do better by chance on these questions, getting about one in four correct, resulting in a failing score of 88/140, or 63%. In contrast, the test-wise candidate applies knowledge of test design and question reasoning skills to get half of these questions correct, resulting in an overall score of 105/140, or 75%—enough to reach the upper cut-score level and pass the exam.

Fortunately, test wisdom is a skill that most anyone can learn. It entails both techniques related to multiple-choice questions in general and specific rules of thumb applicable to NBRC-like items. By developing this skill, you not only will improve your exam scores but will also increase your command over testing situations in general. The added benefits are increased confidence and decreased anxiety when taking tests.

General Tips for Multiple-Choice Items

To become test-wise, you first must develop a good understanding of the structure of NBRC-type multiple-choice questions. Based on this knowledge, there are several general strategies that you can apply to increase your odds of correctly answering individual questions. Also, because so many candidates have concerns regarding the questions requiring computations, we discuss the special category of math problems.

Table A-2 Hypothetical Impact of Test Wisdom on Exam Performance

Candidate Response and Performance	Test-Unaware Candidate		Test-Wise Candidate	
	Questions Answered	Questions Correct	Questions Answered	Questions Correct
"Knows cold"	70	70	70	70
Guesses at	70	18	70	35
Raw score		88		105
Percentage		63%		75%
Result		FAIL!		PASS!

The Anatomy of Multiple-Choice Items

The TMC exam consists entirely of multiple-choice questions. Most of these are the simple "one best answer" type, but a few currently use the multiple-true format in the form of a table, also known as complex multiple-choice items.

The first skill in becoming test-wise is to understand the various parts of these questions and to use that knowledge to improve your odds of identifying the correct answer. **Table A-3** summarizes the key elements common to most NBRC written exam questions, with **Figure A-2** providing a "dissected" example.

Scenario

A question scenario briefly describes a clinical situation. We recommend that you thoroughly review the scenario before even looking at the stem or question options (note that sometimes the scenario and the stem are combined and must be reviewed together). When assessing the scenario, look for the following critical information:

- The location or setting (e.g., intensive care unit [ICU], outpatient clinic, patient's home)
- The available resources (e.g., equipment that is being used or is at hand)
- The patient's general characteristics (e.g., age, size, disease process, mental status)
- Any relevant objective data (e.g., from vital signs, arterial blood gases [ABGs], pulmonary function tests [PFTs])
- Any relevant subjective information (e.g., signs and symptoms)

Assume that all the information in the scenario is there for a reason. As you assess the scenario, note the patient's characteristics and any *abnormal* data or information, especially laboratory results.

Table A-3 Elements Common to NBRC Multiple-Choice Questions

Question Element	Description
Scenario	Brief description of the clinical situation
Stem	The statement that asks the question or specifies the problem
Options	Possible answers to the question or solution to the problem
Keyed response	The option that answers the question correctly (the correct answer)
Distractors	The remaining incorrect options

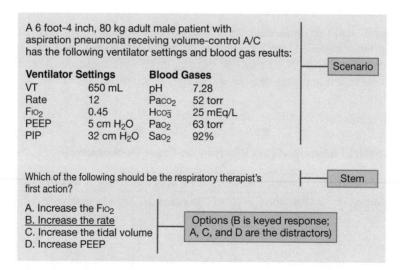

Figure A-2 The Key Elements in a Typical NBRC-Like Question. In this example, the scenario and the stem are separate. The scenario and stem may be combined in many cases.

As an example, based on your assessment of the scenario in Figure A-2, you should extract the following critical information:

1. The patient:
    a. Weighs 80 kg (about 176 lb), which is appropriate for his height (76 in.)
    b. Has aspiration pneumonia (often a cause of hypoxemia)
2. The equipment is a ventilator capable of volume control.
3. In terms of the objective data:
    a. The set tidal volume is about 8 mL/kg, toward the high end of the acceptable range.
    b. The peak inspiratory pressure (PIP) of 32 cm H_2O is also at the high end of the acceptable range for lung protection.
    c. The FiO_2 is at an acceptably safe level.
    d. The blood gas is abnormal:
        i. The primary/most severe problem is acute respiratory acidosis.
        ii. Oxygenation is adequate ($SaO_2 > 90\%$).

Stem

The stem asks the question or directs your action. In Figure A-2, the stem asks which action the RT should take *first*. As with the scenario, you always must read the stem carefully. The stem often contains keywords or phrases that may help you choose the correct answer. **Table A-4** describes common keywords or phrases that you should look for in question stems and suggests what to do when you encounter them.

In our sample question in Figure A-2, the stem contains the keyword *first*. This priority clue directs you to choose the action *most immediately* needed. Based on our analysis of the blood gas data, we identified the primary/most severe problem as being acute respiratory acidosis. The keyed response or right answer, therefore, should be one that best corrects this problem. Given that correction of respiratory acidosis requires an increase in the patient's minute ventilation, there are two possible options that would achieve that end—that is, increasing the rate or increasing the tidal volume. Which to choose? Based on analysis of the scenario, the choice should be clear. An increase in tidal volume would further increase the PIP and the risk of lung damage, making option B (*Increase the rate*) the best choice among the alternatives.

In addition to the general clues described in Table A-4, be on the lookout for other keywords or phrases. For example, compare the wording of the following two question stems related to endotracheal intubation:

Stem Wording A	Stem Wording B
Which of the following assessment procedures would help determine the proper positioning of an endotracheal tube in a patient's trachea?	Which of the following assessment procedures would confirm proper positioning of an endotracheal tube in a patient's trachea?

Table A-4 Keywords or Phrases Found in Question Stems

Type of Clue	What to Look For	What to Do
Priority	Words such as *first, initially, best, priority, safest, most,* and *least*	Put a value in each available option, and then place them in rank order.
Sequence	Words such as *before, after, during,* and *next*	Apply procedural knowledge or logic to place the option in a proper sequence.
Negative polarity	Words such as *not, except, contraindicated, unacceptable,* and *avoid*	Switch from being concerned with what is correct or true to what is false; consider each option to be a true/false question and select the false one.
Absolutes	Keywords such as *always* and *never*	Find the only option that would be correct in every case every time.
Verbal associations	Word or phrase in the stem that is identical or similar to a word in the correct answer	Select the option that includes wording identical to that found in the stem.

Note that the two stems are identical except for the verb. Question stem A specifies "help determine," whereas B specifies "confirm." This tiny variation in wording makes a huge difference in the likely best answer for these two questions. Whereas there are many potentially good answers for A (e.g., breath sounds, capnography, tube insertion length, an esophageal detection device, chest x-ray), there is only one consistently correct response for B (i.e., chest x-ray).

Although you should always be on the lookout for keywords or phrases in NBRC test items, we also recommend that you avoid reading too much into the exam questions. When you read too much into it or overthink a test item, you often end up selecting the wrong answer. Read all questions as is. Do *not* be led astray by either overanalyzing or oversimplifying any question. Last, avoid drawing any assumptions beyond those supported by the facts at hand. *The simplest interpretation is generally the correct one.*

You also might want to consider a useful strategy that many good test-takers employ. Good test-takers frequently paraphrase the question in their own words and then anticipate the answer—*before looking at the options available.* In the days of pencil-and-paper testing, this meant covering up each question's options with scratch paper or the test-taker's hand. Such a strategy can help minimize any confusion that a question's options may cause, especially the distractors. In general, this technique works best when you can quickly and confidently identify the answer in your head.

Options

Options are the possible answers to a question. The good news is that every NBRC exam item has only four options, labeled A through D. Also, good news for well-prepared candidates is that a substantial portion of these questions will be straightforward and relatively easy to answer. Indeed, if you understand and can apply the information being tested, you will often recognize the correct answer immediately.

The bad news is that not even the smartest candidate knows all the correct answers. Indeed, we believe that, on average, most candidates will be forced to guess on one-third to one-half of the exam questions. If the best you can do on these questions is to guess randomly at their answers, you will get only approximately 25% of them correct. To do better, you will need to apply our recommended option-selection strategies.

Option-Selection Strategies

To do well on the NBRC written exam, you need to examine each question's options carefully. *When you are sure of the correct response, select it, and move on.* In contrast, if the correct response is not immediately apparent to you, you will need to apply specific skills to analyze the available options before selecting an answer.

First, do not panic when you encounter questions that appear difficult or unfamiliar to you. All exam candidates will face dozens of such questions when they take this test. Instead of getting flustered, get resourceful. Whenever you encounter a difficult question, you need to rise to the challenge and use the strategies we provide here to select the most logical answer.

Useful general option selection strategies include the following:

- Always look for the *best option*, not just a correct one. As demonstrated in our previous example (see Figure A-2), two or more options may be correct, but one likely is the "most" correct in *the particular circumstances or with the specific patient described.*
- When you are unsure of the correct option, switch strategies from finding the right answer to using what you do know to identify the wrong answer(s).
- Eliminate options you know to be incorrect; each time you can eliminate a true distractor, you dramatically increase your chances of answering the question correctly.
- When in doubt, give each option a "true-false" test as compared with the stem (the true statement is usually the most plausible answer).
- Be wary of options that are unfamiliar to you; often, unfamiliar options are distractors.
- Avoid impulsively selecting an option only because it provides correct information; an option can provide correct information but still be the wrong choice because it does not answer the question asked.

If these selection strategies do not help, you will need to apply more specific reasoning skills to identify the correct answer. These skills involve identification of absolutes and qualifiers, dealing with equally plausible options, weighing two options that are opposite to each other, addressing duplicate facts appearing in options, finding the most general or global option, and dealing with a range of option values. Besides, if the question involves using basic math skills, a few key strategies can help you succeed whenever you need to perform computations.

Absolutes (Specific Determiners)

As with question stems, some options may include absolutes or specific determiners. You know an option contains a specific determiner when you find words such as *always, never, all, every, none,* and *only.* These keywords indicate that the option has no exceptions. Question A-4 provides an illustrative example.

A-4. Which of the following is true regarding patients in the early stages of an asthma attack?

    A. They all exhibit respiratory alkalosis.
    B. They always have moderate hypoxemia.
    C. They have decreased expiratory flows. ✓
    D. They never respond to β-adrenergic agents.

In this hypothetical example, options A, B, and D all contain specific determiners or absolutes. Often, options that use absolutes are false. Generally, you should avoid choosing an option that *must* be true or false every time, in every case, or without exception, as rarely is anything always a certain way, especially in health care. In this case, applying this strategy helps you quickly zero in on the correct answer (C), the only one not containing an absolute.

Because specific determiners are easy to identify, the NBRC minimizes their use on its exams. Thus, you should not expect to encounter these options frequently. Also note that some absolutes, especially those found in rules or standards, may be a correct choice. For example, most would agree that the statement "You always must properly identify the patient before treatment" holds without exception in general patient care situations. For this reason, if the scenario and stem are addressing policies, procedures, rules, or standards, you may need to allow for absolutes. In contrast, *if the question involves a patient in unique clinical circumstances, few, if any, absolutes pertain.*

Qualifiers

A qualifier is the opposite of a specific determiner. Qualifiers represent a conditional or "hedge" word or phrase such as *usually, probably, often, generally, may, frequently,* and *seldom.* Qualifiers may appear either in the question stem or in one or more options. Question A-5 is an excellent example of the use of qualifiers.

A-5. A patient's advanced directive:

    A. is usually obtained at the time of admission. ✓
    B. can be found in the physician's progress notes.
    C. represents a guideline, not a legal requirement.
    D. cannot be altered after it is written and signed.

Options that contain qualifiers usually represent good choices. In this example, only option A includes a qualifier and is, in fact, the correct option. As with absolutes, note that the NBRC minimizes the use of qualifiers in its exam questions, especially in question options. Nonetheless, you need to be on the lookout for these keywords and apply the appropriate strategy when needed.

Equally Plausible Options

As previously demonstrated (see Figure A-2), NBRC questions often contain two very similar or equivalent options. Question A-6 provides a different example.

A-6. An intubated patient is receiving volume-control ventilation. The patient's condition has not changed, but you observe higher peak inspiratory pressures than before. Which of the following is the most likely cause of this problem?

    A. There is a leak in the patient-ventilator system.
    B. The endotracheal tube cuff is deflated or burst.
    C. The endotracheal tube is partially obstructed. ✓
    D. The endotracheal tube is displaced into the pharynx.

Note that options A and B are equivalent because a deflated or burst endotracheal tube (ETT) cuff represents a leak in the patient-ventilator system. Usually, when two items are very similar to each other, and nothing in the scenario helps differentiate between them, they are distractors and should be eliminated from consideration. Then make your choice from among the remaining two options (in this case, option C is the correct choice). By doing so, you immediately improve your odds of correctly answering this question from 25% to 50%. As noted previously, this is precisely what test-wise candidates do.

What if three of the options are very similar to each other? In this case, apply the "odd man out" strategy, as applicable in answering Question A-7.

A-7. Over 3 hours, you note that a patient's plateau pressure has remained stable, but her peak pressure has been steadily increasing. Which of the following is the best explanation for this observation?

   A. The patient's airway resistance has increased. ✓
   B. The patient is developing atelectasis.
   C. The patient's compliance has decreased.
   D. The patient is developing pulmonary edema.

In this example, options B, C, and D are similar, in that they all correspond to a decrease in the patient's compliance. When this occurs, turn your attention to the different or "odd man out" option, which is most likely the correct one (option A in this example).

Opposite Options

Another very common way NBRC item writers create distractors is to include a pair of direct opposites among the options—what we call "mirror-image options." Question A-8 is an NBRC-like item with mirror-image options.

A-8. You are assisting with the oral intubation of an adult patient. After the ETT has been placed, you note that breath sounds are decreased on the left compared with the right lung. What is the most likely cause of this condition?

   A. The tip of the tube is in the right mainstem bronchus. ✓
   B. The cuff of the endotracheal tube has been overinflated.
   C. The endotracheal tube has been inserted into the esophagus.
   D. The tip of the tube is in the left mainstem bronchus.

In general, when you encounter two options that are opposites, the chances are good that the correct choice is one of the two. In this example, options A and D are mirror images of each other, and one of them is likely the correct answer. Referral back to the scenario (breath sounds decreased on the left compared to the right) should help you decide which of these two responses is correct (A).

It is important to note that there are exceptions to this strategy. Although you will encounter them less frequently, some questions may include mirror-image options as distractors, meaning that *both* are incorrect choices. In these cases, the item writer is using option opposites to divert your attention from the correct answer, as in Question A-9.

A-9. A patient receiving long-term ventilatory support exhibits a progressive weight gain and a reduction in the hematocrit. Which of the following is the most likely cause of this problem?

   A. Leukocytosis
   B. Chronic hypoxemia
   C. Water retention ✓
   D. Leukocytopenia

In this example, leukocytosis and leukocytopenia are opposites. Is one of them the correct choice, or are they both distractors? To make this decision often requires referring back to the scenario or the stem (they are combined in this question). Logically, both leukocytosis and leukocytopenia are more often the result of abnormal processes (such as infection) and less commonly the *cause* (a keyword in the stem) of such processes. Here, these two options are more likely both being used as distractors and should be eliminated. Now, by selecting from the two remaining two options, your odds of correctly answering this question have improved to 50-50. If you also remember that chronic hypoxemia tends to increase—and not decrease—the hematocrit, you can now be almost certain of selecting the correct option (C).

Duplicate Facts in Options

Item writers often create options that include two or more similar or identical statements among the choices. Question A-10 is a good example of this question design.

A-10. In reviewing the PFT results of a 67-year-old smoker with an admitting diagnosis of emphysema and chronic bronchitis, you would expect which of the following general findings?

    A. Increased airway resistance and decreased lung compliance
    B. Increased airway resistance and increased lung compliance ✓
    C. Decreased airway resistance and decreased lung compliance
    D. Decreased airway resistance and increased lung compliance

This question's options contain two contrasting sets of statements: increased/decreased resistance and increased/decreased compliance. When you encounter this type of question and are unsure of the answer, you should try to identify any statement that you know is *either* true or false. Once you do so, you usually can eliminate at least two options as being distractors. In this example, if you know that patients with emphysema and chronic bronchitis typically have high airway resistance, then you can immediately eliminate options C and D. Alternatively, if you know that patients with emphysema do *not* have decreased lung compliance, then you can eliminate options A and C. Either way, you have doubled the likelihood of selecting the correct answer (B).

Global Options

Question options often include a mix of general and specific statements, as in Question A-11.

A-11. In instructing a patient how to breathe during a small-volume nebulizer drug treatment, the respiratory therapist coaches the patient to hold his breath at the end of each inspiration. The purpose of this maneuver is to improve:

    A. drug delivery. ✓
    B. particle stability.
    C. aerosol penetration.
    D. inertial impaction.

In this example, option A is the most general or global alternative, whereas options B through D are much more specific. Candidates who are test-wise know that general statements are more likely to be the correct option than choices that are very specific or limited in focus—because the most global option usually includes the most information. In this question, particle stability, aerosol penetration, and inertial impaction are all factors that *fall under the broader concept of enhanced drug delivery*, making option A the best choice here.

Options Constituting a Range

Some test questions, especially those focusing on recall, provide options representing a range of values, typically from early to late, or from big to small. Question A-12 is a good example.

A-12. You obtain a SpO_2 measurement on a patient of 80%. Assuming this is an accurate measure of hemoglobin saturation, what is the patient's approximate PaO_2?

    A. 40 torr
    B. 50 torr ✓
    C. 60 torr
    D. 70 torr

When item writers create questions like this one, they often try to hide or mask the correct choice by placing it within a set of higher and lower values. In these cases, you should consider eliminating the highest and lowest values, choosing an option in the middle. Following this logic for this question would result in eliminating options A and D, giving you a 50-50 shot at the correct answer to this question (B). Of course, this strategy should be applied only when you do not know the answer. Those familiar with the "40-50-60/70-80-90" rule of thumb might recognize its application to this question and immediately know that 80% saturation roughly corresponds to a Pa_{O_2} of 50 torr.

Math Problems

Typically, the NBRC written exams will include a small number of questions that require a simple calculation to obtain the correct answer. To help you prepare for these questions, Appendix B reviews common cardiopulmonary calculations that are likely to appear on these exams. Here we provide more general guidance regarding selecting options when presented with questions involving math.

Because many candidates lack confidence in their math skills, they tend to panic when confronted with a question that requires computation. This response generally is unwarranted because the math skills tested on the NBRC exams are rather basic and typically involve no more than one or two computational steps. Thus, there is no reason to get anxious over these questions.

To improve your confidence in approaching math questions and help you consistently select the correct answers, we recommend the following:

- Always set up the problem before you begin to solve it; use the scratch paper provided at the testing center to write out the applicable formula, *being sure to set it up properly to solve for the value being requested*.
- After setting up the formula, try estimating or *ballparking* the answer without calculating it; prior estimation can help you avoid making formula or computational errors.
- After doing the computation, do it a second time to confirm that you get the same answer.
- Be careful to ensure the decimal point is correctly placed.
- Do not immediately select an answer that matches your calculation; most math question distractors are based on common computation errors. Instead, reread the problem, recheck your formula, and, if necessary, redo your math.
- If you are completely stumped, "choose from the means and not the extremes." If you do not know the applicable formula or cannot come up with a good estimate, toss out the high and low numbers and select one near the middle.
- If you find an obvious mathematical answer, fix it and ensure you select the answer matching your corrected calculation.

Question A-13 illustrates using math problem strategies to arrive at the correct answer.

A-13. A portable spirometer requires that you enter the patient's height in centimeters to derive normal values. The patient tells you that she is 5 feet, 6 inches tall. Which value would you enter into the device?

- **A.** 26 cm
- **B.** 66 cm
- **C.** 168 cm ✓
- **D.** 186 cm

First, you should set up the problem. This represents a straight unit conversion, from English to metric units (inches to centimeters). All such problems are based on a simple formula that requires knowledge of the applicable conversion factor:

$$\textbf{Measurement (X units)} \times \textbf{conversion factor} = \textbf{measurement (Y units)}$$

In this case, the X units are inches, the Y units are centimeters, and the conversion factor is 2.54 cm/inch. Thus, the proper setup of the formula for this problem is:

$$\textbf{Measurement (inches)} \times \textbf{2.54 cm/inch} = \textbf{measurement (cm)}$$

Slightly complicating this problem is your need to convert 5 feet 6 inches to inches. Because there are 12 inches to a foot, the patient is $(5 \times 12) + 6$, or 66 inches tall. Note that the numeric value 66 appears among the distractors. Including a value derived in an intermediate step as a distractor is a common ploy used by item writers. You can avoid succumbing to this ploy by completing all computations before comparing your answer to those provided.

Now that you are sure you have set up the correct formula to answer the question, estimate the answer before you compute it. The answer should be about 2½ times greater than the patient's height in inches, 66 inches. Twice 66 is *about* 130, and half of 66 is *about* 33, so the answer should be *about* 130 + 33 or 163 cm. Based on estimation alone, answer C, 168 cm, looks very good. Based on estimation, you also can eliminate option A because it is *less than* the patient's height in inches. Based on the setup of your formula, that would be impossible. Indeed, option A (26 cm) is lurking there to catch those who set up the formula improperly or use the wrong conversion factor. You would get 26 cm as the answer if you mistakenly *divided* the patient's height in inches by 2.54 instead of multiplying by this factor.

Last, after doing the initial computation, do not immediately select the answer. Instead, recompute the answer after rereading the question and rechecking the setup of your formula.

What if you do not know the exact formula or factor to use? Ideally, your estimated answer will allow you to eliminate at least some of the distractors and improve your odds of answering the question correctly. If elimination does not help, apply our last-ditch "choose from the means and not the extremes" strategy.

Specific Tips for Common NBRC-Type Items

Applying general option-selection strategies will go a long way toward improving your NBRC written exam score. To boost your score even more, we have developed several item-response guidelines that apply specifically to common NBRC question formats. By learning to apply these guidelines when you encounter these question formats, you will increase your likelihood of passing the exam!

The Triple S Rule

The "triple S" rule is the most basic of all principles we recommend you apply to answer NBRC-type questions. Put simply and as noted in earlier chapters of this text, if a patient gets worse when you are giving therapy, *stop, stabilize,* and *stay.* In other words, stop what you are doing, try to stabilize the patient, and stay until help arrives. Question A-14 is a good example of the triple S rule.

A-14. During postural drainage of the left lower lobe, a patient complains of acute chest pain. Which of the following should you do?

    A. Give the patient supplemental oxygen.
    B. Continue the treatment with the bed flat.
    C. Ask the nurse to administer pain medication.
    D. Discontinue the treatment, and monitor the patient. ✓

A corollary to the triple S rule is *never to start therapy* if the patient is exhibiting abnormal signs or symptoms that could be worsened by your action. Instead, as illustrated in Question A-15, you should always contact the physician.

A-15. A 45-year-old patient with asthma is prescribed 0.5 mL of albuterol (Proventil) in 3 mL normal saline via small-volume nebulizer. Before initiating therapy, you note from chart review that the patient is severely hypertensive and has been experiencing episodes of supraventricular tachycardia. Which of the following should you do?

    A. Administer the treatment as ordered.
    B. Postpone the treatment, and notify the physician. ✓
    C. Dilute the albuterol with extra normal saline.
    D. Decrease the amount of albuterol administered.

Act First, Ask Questions Later

With all the emphasis that teachers place on assessing patients, students often forget that sometimes you should act first and only then gather information. The best examples are always emergencies, where any delay for information gathering may cause harm to the patient. Question A-16 provides a good example of this principle.

A-16. A patient is admitted to the emergency department comatose with suspected smoke inhalation. After confirming airway patency, which of the following should you do *first?*

    A. Measure the SpO_2.
    B. Initiate 100% oxygen. ✓
    C. Obtain an arterial blood gas.
    D. Request a STAT chest x-ray.

In this scenario, getting more information is important, but the *priority* is to ensure adequate oxygenation. Given that the patient is suspected of having a smoke inhalation injury, 100% O_2 should be administered immediately, without waiting for more information.

Question A-17 also illustrates this principle, which emphasizes that your patient's safety and welfare must always be your *priority*.

A-17. You are called to the bedside of a patient by her ICU nurse to check the attached volume ventilator. You note that both the low-volume and high-pressure limit alarms are sounding on each breath. What should your first action be?

    A. Disconnect the patient, and manually ventilate with 100% O_2. ✓
    B. Call the attending physician for further patient information.
    C. Check the patient's chart for the original ventilator orders.
    D. Ask the nurse about how recently the patient was suctioned.

In this example, the patient is in danger, as evidenced by the ventilator alarms. Although options B, C, and D might help you understand the cause of the problem, they waste valuable time and ignore the immediate needs of the patient. Because your *priority* always must be the patient's safety and welfare, option A is the best answer to this question.

If It Ain't Broke, Don't Fix It!

Another of our "top 10" principles is to *leave well enough alone*—that is, "If it ain't broke, don't fix it!" Typically, this principle will show up on an NBRC exam as a situation in which patient data indicate normal parameters, but you are given the option to change things. *Don't.* Question A-18 illustrates the application of this item-response guideline.

A-18. A 60-kg (132-lb) COPD patient is receiving volume control SIMV with a V_T of 450 mL at a rate of 10/min and a FiO_2 of 0.35. Blood gases are as follows: pH = 7.36; $PaCO_2$ = 61 torr; HCO_3^- = 36 mEq/L; PaO_2 = 62 torr. Which of the following changes would you recommend at this time?

    A. Increase the SIMV rate.
    B. Increase the FiO_2.
    C. Maintain the current settings. ✓
    D. Increase V_T.

As previously emphasized, the scenario in this question includes vital information, specifically that the patient has COPD. As is common in such patients, the blood gas indicated *fully compensated respiratory acidosis*, so even though the PCO_2 is high, we don't want to alter ventilation. What about oxygenation, that is, the low PaO_2? That too is to be expected in patients with COPD. In fact, raising the FiO_2 could depress the patient's respiratory drive. *If it ain't broke, don't fix it*—maintain the current settings (option C).

Back Off Bad!

Exam candidates love to complain about NBRC questions with "two right answers." Of course, according to the NBRC, there is only one *best* answer to each question. One perfect example of this type of question is the "double effect" scenario. Typically, a patient who is receiving multiple therapies at the same time, either worsens or improves. At least two different changes could help the situation—which one do you choose? Question A-19 is a good example.

A-19. A 30-kg (66-lb) child is receiving volume-control SIMV. The following data are available:

Ventilator Settings	Blood Gases
Fio_2 0.45	pH 7.38
Mandatory rate 18	$Paco_2$ 42 torr
Total rate 23	Pao_2 150 torr
V_T 250 mL	HCO_3^- 23 mEq/L
PEEP 12 cm H_2O	BE 0 mEq/L

Based on these data, which of the following should you do?

> **A.** Decrease the tidal volume.
> **B.** Reduce the PEEP. ✓
> **C.** Decrease the rate.
> **D.** Lower the Fio_2.

In this scenario, the child's acid-base status and Pco_2 are normal, so no change in ventilation is warranted. The Pao_2 is above normal (hyperoxia) and can be safely lowered if the patient's hemoglobin is acceptable. You can lower the Pao_2 by either lowering the PEEP level *or* lowering the Fio_2. Both answers are right! Which do you choose?

There is only one correct answer. In this case, a Fio_2 of 0.45 presents little or no danger to the patient, but a PEEP of 12 cm H_2O is potentially hazardous. As a result, decrease the PEEP first! The lesson is that when confronted with two or more possible changes in therapy, both of which would have the same good effect, first change the treatment that poses the greatest potential harm to the patient—*back off bad!*

Data Just Don't Jibe

Given the number and variety of instruments used to measure and monitor a patient's physiologic status, it is no wonder that the NBRC will test your ability to recognize and deal with conflicting data—in other words, numbers that "just don't jibe" with each other. Question A-20 is a good example.

A-20. The following data are obtained for a patient:

Blood Gas Analyzer	CO-Oximeter
pH 7.35	Oxyhemoglobin 97%
$Paco_2$ 28 torr	Carboxyhemoglobin 1%
HCO_3^- 14 mEq/L	Methemoglobin 1%
BE –10 mEq/L	Hemoglobin 13.8 g/dL
Pao_2 40 torr	
Sao_2 73%	

You should do which of the following?

> **A.** Report the Sao_2 value as 73%.
> **B.** Report the Sao_2 value as 97%.
> **C.** Recommend the administration of bicarbonate.
> **D.** Recalibrate the instruments, and repeat the analysis. ✓

In this example, careful inspection of the data indicates a large discrepancy between the ABG analyzer's Pao_2 and Sao_2 (40 torr and 73%) and the actual oxyhemoglobin reported by the oximeter (97%). *One of these readings must be wrong.* Unfortunately, because no additional information is provided (patient or equipment status), the best option is to recalibrate the instruments and repeat the analysis. At the same time, you should probably give the patient supplemental oxygen (just to be sure) while re-analyzing the sample.

Errors, Errors Everywhere!

A little-known NBRC exam specification requires that candidates be able to "verify computations and note erroneous data." Usually, the NBRC will offer one or two questions that confirm your ability to "check your math" or to recognize incorrect data. Common math-error questions focus on equations you frequently use in clinical practice, such as the alveolar air equation and the calculation of compliance or airway resistance in ventilator patients. Also common are errors in reported lab values, as evident in Question A-21.

A-21. The results of an arterial blood gas analysis for a patient who is breathing 100% oxygen follow:

Blood Gases:
pH = 7.27
Pa_{CO_2} = 43 torr
HCO_3^- = 23 mEq/L
BE = +1
Pa_{O_2} = 598 torr
Sa_{O_2} = 100%

Which of the following is the likely problem?

A. Respiratory acidosis
B. Large physiologic shunt
C. Metabolic acidosis
D. Laboratory error ✓

Whenever one option (here D) includes the possibility of an error, check out the numbers! First, the Pa_{O_2} of 598 torr on 100% O_2 is not only possible but near normal (based on the alveolar air equation).

In contrast, the acid-base values are *not* consistent with the underlying relationship that determines pH (the Henderson-Hasselbalch equation). In this case, both the Pa_{CO_2} and HCO_3^- are normal. With both these values being within the normal range, the pH also would have to be close to normal, which it is not (pH = 7.27). The only possibility here is a laboratory error.

Don't Know What You're Missing!

In addition to using conflicting or erroneous data in its questions, the NBRC likes to give candidates questions with missing data. These questions are designed to "trap" those individuals who are inclined to act on insufficient information while rewarding those who carefully review the data. Question A-22 illustrates this type of question.

A-22. A doctor asks you to assess if a 75-kg (165-lb) patient with a neuromuscular disorder who is receiving volume control SIMV is ready for weaning. You obtain the following data during a bedside ventilatory assessment:

- Spontaneous tidal volume of 250 mL
- Minute ventilation 10 L/min
- Vital capacity of 750 mL
- Maximum inspiratory pressure (MIP) –28 cm H_2O

Based on this information, which of the following would you recommend?

A. Begin a spontaneous breathing T-piece trial.
B. Postpone weaning, and reevaluate the patient. ✓
C. Begin weaning using a pressure-support protocol.
D. Begin weaning by decreasing the SIMV rate.

In this question, many candidates would observe that the patient's vital capacity and MIP are borderline adequate and conclude that the patient is ready for weaning. *Wrong!* In this case, the minute ventilation and tidal volume data suggest a major problem, *but this becomes clear only after identifying and deriving the missing data*—the spontaneous breathing rate (spontaneous rate = 10 L/min

÷ 0.25 L/breath = 40 breaths/min). This yields a rapid shallow breathing index of 40/0.25 = 160, which is far above the threshold value of 100 that indicates a potential weaning problem and likely weaning failure. Based on the discovery and analysis of the missing data, you would recommend postponing weaning and reevaluating the patient.

This type of question should make it clear that when given a problem with numeric information, you should *always* review the numbers to see what, if anything, is missing. Then see if you can derive the missing data from the available numbers. This is often the key to solving these problems.

Jump Back, Jack!

Often, the NBRC presents you with a situation in which things go bad (e.g., the patient's condition worsens, equipment fails). Just as often, *your* action immediately preceded things going bad. In these cases, the corrective action is usually to reverse course and *undo* what you have done—*jump back, Jack!* Question A-23 illustrates this principle.

A-23. A surgeon orders an increase in PEEP from 6 to 10 cm H_2O for a postoperative patient receiving mechanical ventilation. After you adjust the PEEP setting, you note a rapid fall in the patient's arterial blood pressure. Which of the following actions would you recommend to the surgeon?

    A. Increase the Fio_2 by 10%.
    B. Administer a vasopressor.
    C. Return the PEEP to 6 cm H_2O. ✓
    D. Obtain a STAT blood gas.

One of the adverse effects of PEEP is decreased cardiac output (due to increased pleural pressure and decreased venous return). A rapid drop in a patient's blood pressure indicates decreased cardiac output. Whenever an adverse response to therapy occurs, your first consideration should be to stop the therapy and restore the patient to his or her prior state; in this case, return the PEEP to its initial level of 6 cm H_2O.

KISS It!

The KISS principle is straightforward: *K*eep *i*t *s*imple, *s*tupid! When taking an NBRC test, this means that the simplest solution to a problem is often the best and overthinking it is your enemy. Question A-24 is a good example of the KISS principle.

A-24. Manual ventilation of a patient with a self-inflating bag-valve-mask device fails to inflate the patient's chest adequately. You should do which of the following?

    A. Intubate and mechanically ventilate the patient.
    B. Switch to a gas-powered resuscitator with a mask.
    C. Reposition the patient's head, neck, and mask. ✓
    D. Insert a laryngeal mask airway (LMA).

In this sample troubleshooting question, most of the options might help resolve the problem. However, option C is the simplest and should at least be tried before moving on to more aggressive options. The lesson here is that whenever one of the options is relatively simple and could provide the solution to the problem at hand, it is probably the correct answer.

Gas Goes In; Gas Comes Out

Almost every NBRC exam includes two or more questions testing your ability to differentiate between leaks and obstructions in equipment, their sources, and their correction. A basic rule of thumb is that *leaks prevent pressure buildup, and obstructions cause pressure buildup*. The classic example is the simple bubble humidifier. Block the tubing outlet while gas is flowing, and the pressure pop-off should sound (an obstruction). If the pressure pop-off does not sound, there is a system leak. A similar example is the leak test you perform on a ventilator circuit.

Identifying sources of leaks is simple—any mechanical connection (e.g., tubing, nebulizer/humidifier caps, exhalation valves) is a potential source of leakage, as is the patient's airway (e.g., mouthpiece, mask, tracheal tube/cuff). To correct a leak, tighten the connection, fix or replace the component, or provide a better airway seal. Question A-25 provides a good example of a "leaky" question.

A-25. When checking a ventilator, you discover that the set PEEP level cannot be maintained.

Which of the following might be causing this problem?

	Leak in the Tubing	Faulty Exhalation Valve	Leak in the Airway Cuff	Loose Humidifier Connection
A.	YES	YES	NO	NO
B.	YES	NO	YES	NO
C.	NO	YES	NO	YES
D.	YES	YES	YES	YES

    A. A
    B. B
    C. C
    D. D ✓

According to our rule of thumb, this is definitely a leak scenario. Because any mechanical connection or the patient's airway can be the source of a leak, *all* of the cited problems could be the cause, making D the correct response.

Obstructions can be more challenging to identify, in part because an obstruction can be complete or partial and because "obstruction" during mechanical ventilation can involve any factor that raises airway pressure (increased resistance or decreased compliance). Correcting or overcoming an obstruction must address the underlying cause. Question A-26 illustrates this type of question.

A-26. At the bedside of a patient receiving volume-control A/C ventilation, you suddenly observe the simultaneous sounding of the high-pressure and low-volume alarms. Which of the following is the most likely cause of this problem?

    A. A leak in the ETT cuff
    B. A mucus plug in the ETT ✓
    C. Ventilator circuit disconnection
    D. Development of pulmonary edema

Because this scenario deals with volume-control ventilation, it is best to rely first on a tried-and-true alarm rule of thumb to identify this problem as being an obstruction:

If the Alarm Combination Is:	Then the Problem Is:
High pressure/low volume	An obstruction
Low pressure/low volume	A leak

The problem in Question A-26 is that two options involve "obstruction"—the mucus plug and the decreased compliance associated with the development of pulmonary edema. Which to choose? In this case, our prior advice on dissecting the question should help. Note the keyword *suddenly* in the stem. Although pulmonary edema can develop relatively quickly, it would not change airway pressures suddenly. In contrast, a mucus plug can cause a sudden rise in airway pressure, making B the best choice and correct answer.

Love Those Multiple Trues!

Students tend to hate multiple-true-type questions (the ones with all those answer combinations!). The fact is that most multiple-true questions are easier to answer than simple "ABCD" questions (probably the reason that the NBRC is slowly phasing them out). Why? Because more than any other type of question, multiple-trues improve your odds of being correct when you have only partial knowledge of the answer, because they often allow you to eliminate one or more options. Question A-27 demonstrates this important item-response concept.

A-27. Which of the following would facilitate the clearance of pulmonary secretions in a patient with cystic fibrosis?

	Pulmozyme (DNase)	Flutter Valve	Atropine Sulfate	Hypertonic Saline
A.	YES	NO	YES	NO
B.	NO	YES	NO	YES
C.	YES	YES	NO	YES
D.	NO	YES	YES	YES

   A. A
   B. B
   C. C ✓
   D. D

Most candidates will recognize the more obvious choice of Pulmozyme (DNase) as a proteolytic agent that might facilitate the clearance of pulmonary secretions. Based on this partial knowledge, you can eliminate options B and D because they do not include Pulmozyme. Alternatively, if based on your partial knowledge you recognize that atropine can dry airway secretions, you can eliminate options A and D because both include this drug. Note that either of these partial-knowledge approaches immediately improves your odds of getting this question correct from 1 out of 4 (for pure guessing) to 50-50. Then all you need to know is that either hypertonic saline *or* a flutter valve can also help, and you can be sure to get this item right!

Treat the Patient, Not the Monitor!

A favorite NBRC "trick" question is to place you in a scenario where patient and monitor data conflict, but an action is required. Common forms of this type question include (1) pulse oximetry data (good) versus bedside assessment of the patient's oxygenation (bad) and (2) ECG (good) versus bedside assessment of the patient's perfusion (bad). Question A-28 is a good example.

A-28. During a short pause from resuscitation of a child in the emergency department, you cannot palpate a carotid pulse but observe a regular rhythm on the ECG monitor (**Figure A-3**):
   Which of the following actions should you take at this time?

   A. Resume cardiac compressions and ventilation. ✓
   B. Discontinue compressions, and monitor the patient.
   C. Recommend cardioversion at 100 joules.
   D. Recommend epinephrine administration.

In Question A-28, the likely problem is a pulseless electrical activity (PEA). Remembering that the ECG represents only electrical activity and not mechanical action of the heart, thus, the fact that this patient with no pulse requires resuscitation should make this a "no-brainer." However, more than one-third of those candidates taking our practice exams decide to go against their better judgment (and their training) and instead treat the monitor. Test smart by not joining that group!

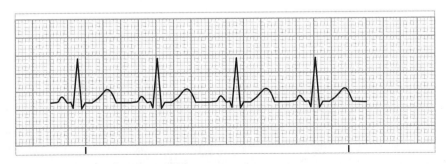

Figure A-3 ECG Rhythm Observed on Monitor.

Reproduced from Garcia T, Miller GT. *Arrhythmia recognition: the art of interpretation.* Sudbury, MA: Jones and Bartlett; 2004.

Order in the House

All NBRC entry-level exams assess your ability to sequence multiple therapies or coordinate your therapy with that of other health professionals. Most of these questions rely on simple common sense—for example, do not perform postural drainage immediately after a patient has eaten!

As a special case, you will often be asked in which order to perform combinations of therapy aimed at either getting drugs (e.g., steroids, antibiotics) in or getting secretions out of the airway. In these situations, apply the following rule of thumb:

1. Open 'em up.
2. Thin 'em down.
3. Clear 'em out.

"Open 'em up" means first open the airways, using a bronchodilator. "Thin 'em down" means you should next use hydrating or mucolytic agents (e.g., bland aerosols, Mucomyst, Pulmozyme, hypertonic saline) to decrease the viscosity of secretions. "Clear 'em out" means applying airway clearance methods to remove the secretions (e.g., directed coughing, postural drainage, suctioning). Last, administer any other drugs designed for pulmonary deposition (e.g., antibiotics, steroids). Question A-29 illustrates this approach.

A-29. A physician has ordered albuterol (Proventil), DNase (Pulmozyme), and tobramycin for inhalation (TOBI) for a patient with cystic fibrosis who also receives postural drainage three times a day. You should administer these therapies in which of the following sequences?

A. DNase, albuterol, tobramycin, postural drainage
B. Albuterol, DNase, postural drainage, tobramycin ✓
C. Postural drainage, albuterol, DNase, tobramycin
D. Tobramycin, DNase, albuterol, postural drainage

Give Me a V; Give Me an O!

Typically, the NBRC includes at least a half-dozen questions testing your ability to modify ventilator settings properly based on a blood gas report. You cannot afford to get many of these questions wrong.

First, you need to be able to interpret blood gases correctly. Just as critical, however, is the need to differentiate between problems of ventilation ("Give Me a V") and problems of oxygenation ("Give Me an O"). This is the secret for slam-dunking these questions.

To help you out in this area, we recommend that you draw a line or mark or circle to separate the blood gas report's ventilation/acid–base data from its oxygenation data. As an example:

Blood Gases
pH 7.22
$Paco_2$ 65 torr
HCO_3^- 26 mEq/L
BE +1

_____

Pao_2 70 torr
Sao_2 93%

Once you have drawn the line, *separately* assess (1) ventilation/acid–base status and then (2) the adequacy of oxygenation. In most cases, the NBRC will limit the problem to one or the other—that is, a problem of ventilation *or* a problem of oxygenation.

If the problem is mainly one of ventilation (as in the preceding data), either increase or decrease the ventilation, as appropriate. If the problem is primarily oxygenation, you will need to either raise or lower the Fio_2 or adjust PEEP/CPAP. Question A-30 is an example.

A-30. A 90-kg (198-lb) patient is being ventilated in the post-anesthesia care unit following upper abdominal surgery. Ventilator settings and arterial blood gas data are as follows:

Ventilator Settings		Blood Gases
Mode	Vol Ctrl SIMV	pH 7.51
V_T	600 mL	$Paco_2$ 31 torr
Set rate	14/min	HCO_3^- 24 mEq/L
Total rate	14/min	BE +1
Fio_2	0.40	Pao_2 115 torr
PEEP	5 cm H_2O	Sao_2 99%

Which of the following should you recommend?

A. Increase the Fio_2.
B. Decrease the rate. ✓
C. Decrease the tidal volume.
D. Discontinue the PEEP.

Here the problem is one of ventilation, *not* oxygenation. In this case, the patient is being hyperventilated (respiratory alkalosis), and the minute ventilation should be decreased. Because the tidal volume is acceptable (approximately 6–7 mL/kg), you should recommend lowering the rate.

Alternatively, you may identify the primary problem as one of oxygenation, as evident in Question A-31.

A-31. A 70-kg (154-lb) 45-year-old male with a diagnosis of bilateral pneumonia is receiving volume control SIMV. Ventilator settings and arterial blood gas data are as follows:

Ventilator Settings		Blood Gases
Mode	Vol Ctrl SIMV	pH 7.35
V_T	700 mL	$Paco_2$ 45 torr
Set rate	6/min	HCO_3^- 23 mEq/L
Total rate	10/min	BE –1
Fio_2	0.65	Pao_2 51 torr
PEEP	5 cm H_2O	Sao_2 86%

Which of the following should you recommend?

A. Increase PEEP. ✓
B. Increase the rate.
C. Increase the Fio_2.
D. Add an inspiratory plateau.

Because the Pao_2 is less than 60 torr and the Sao_2 is less than 90%, hypoxemia is present. Therefore, option A or C could potentially improve oxygenation (an excellent example of a "double-effect" item). Which option you choose depends on the underlying cause of the patient's hypoxemia.

To determine the cause and treatment of hypoxemia, we recommend you use the "60/60" rule, as described elsewhere in the text. In this case, the patient's Pao_2 is less than 60 torr, and the Fio_2 is greater than 0.60. According to the 60/60 rule, they are not responding appropriately to a moderately high Fio_2 and therefore, the cause of the patient's hypoxemia is physiologic shunting. When the cause of hypoxemia is physiologic shunting, increasing the Fio_2 will do little good and may potentially harm (oxygen toxicity). Instead, you need to open unventilated alveoli by adding or increasing PEEP/CPAP.

Who's in Charge Here?

Some questions check whether you know who prescribes respiratory care and who needs to be contacted if a change in care is needed, and no protocol exists to manage the patient. Question A-32 also tests your knowledge of what to do before initiating therapy for a patient.

A-32. A nurse tells you that his patient is scheduled to start chest physiotherapy four times a day this morning and that he would like you to get started before the patient goes to radiology for a CT scan. Which of the following should you do *first?*

    A. Auscultate and percuss the patient's chest.
    B. Initiate therapy after reviewing the x-ray.
    C. Interview the patient to obtain a history.
    D. Confirm the doctor's order in the chart. ✓

Similar questions will ask what to do if you believe a change in therapy is needed or if the patient asks specific questions regarding his or her diagnosis or prognosis (contact the doctor). Remember, all respiratory care is provided by physician prescription, and unless there is a pre-approved protocol in place, only the physician can change the order.

Taking Your Test

Good preparation for any test should also involve consideration of how to take the exam, that is, strategies to use just before and during actual test administration. Here we provide a few additional pointers specifically applicable to taking NBRC exams.

Be Familiar with the Exam Format

Our guideline of "know your enemy" applies not just to the content of the NBRC written exam, but also to the format. Fortunately, by the time most candidates sit for the TMC exam, they will have taken dozens of similar tests, usually in school. Indeed, most programs require that students pass a TMC-like exam to graduate. You probably already know most of what to expect on the real thing.

As most candidates are aware, all NBRC exams are administered by computer at selected testing centers throughout the United States. The NBRC test software presents one question at a time on the computer screen. As depicted in **Figure A-4**, each question appears at the top of the screen with the four answer options immediately below. A function bar appears below each question. This bar contains several important buttons and text boxes, and their functions are described in the figure.

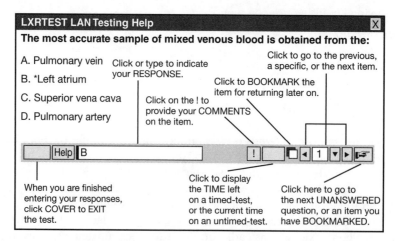

Figure A-4 NBRC Computer-Based Testing Screen.

Courtesy of the National Board for Respiratory Care.

If you choose to provide comments on specific test questions, the NBRC will apply this information when determining if test score adjustments are needed. For this reason, if you believe that the question you are trying to answer is flawed, be sure to provide a comment that explains why.

To select an option as your answer, you either click your mouse over the corresponding letter (A, B, C, or D) or type in that letter using the keyboard. To change your option choice, simply click on or key in a different letter. Your responses are not registered until you exit the exam for scoring so that you can change your answer to any question at any time during the exam period.

Strategies to Employ During the Test

The following strategies should help you perform at your best level when taking an NBRC written exam:

- Get comfortable.
- Answer all questions.
- Budget your time.
- Monitor your pace.
  - Answer easy questions first.
  - Bookmark difficult items, and return to them later.
  - Use all the available time.
- If in serious doubt, bookmark the question, and return to double-check as time allows.
- Correct any obvious errors discovered when checking your answers.

Getting comfortable might seem difficult when taking a high-stakes exam, but the preparation this text provides—especially the strategies reviewed in this chapter—should help allay your test anxiety. Moreover, just like an athlete with pre-game "butterflies in the stomach," once you get down to the task at hand, you will get into the needed rhythm.

Because your score on an NBRC written exam is based on the number of items you get correct, it is essential that you answer *all* questions. To do so, you need to develop a good pace and budget your time properly.

Budgeting your time is the single most crucial strategy when taking a test. On average, the NBRC gives you a little more than a minute for each question. To keep on pace, you need to be aware of your progress. However, rather than constantly checking the clock, we recommend that you check your progress every 20 to 30 minutes, to complete, on average, one question per minute. For example, if you check your progress at 1 hour into the exam, you should have completed about 60 questions.

To further maximize your use of time, you should answer the easy questions first and save the difficult ones for last. However, even if a question appears straightforward, do not rush through it. Spend enough time on each item to read it carefully, and apply the strategies we recommend here to select your answer. By the same token, you should not linger too long on any one question. In general, if you feel stumped on a question or know that more than a minute has elapsed, bookmark the item, and return to it later.

After completing all the easy questions, use the remaining time to review and answer all your bookmarked items. If you must guess, apply the option-selection strategies outlined in this chapter to better your odds of selecting the correct answer.

If time remains after you have answered all the questions, review those items about which you were most unsure. *If an answer was a guess, do not hesitate to reconsider your choice.* Note that this advice is contrary to what most students are taught (i.e., "your first guess is best"). Research consistently indicates that changing answers on multiple-choice exams is more likely to boost your score than to lower it.

After you finish the exam, clicking on the COVER button on the function bar will take you to a "cover page," which summarizes how many questions you have answered and how much time you have used. If you have completed all questions and are satisfied with your answers, you can EXIT the exam from this cover page. After exiting the exam, the testing center provides you with your score report. Due to new changes effective in 2020 your score report will only show your final grade. In order to obtain a more detailed report of your performance by areas of the examination you need to contact your program faculty or your former program director and request this report. If you have followed the guidance we provide throughout this text, we are confident you will receive a passing score.

Cardiopulmonary Calculations

Narciso E. Rodriguez and Albert J. Heuer

NBRC exams do not have a separate section assessing your computation skills. Instead, common calculations can be embedded anywhere throughout these tests. Typically, these calculations are few and require only basic math skills. Unfortunately, too many candidates simply "write off" these questions, assuming that without access to a calculator, they will get most of them wrong.

Giving up on *any* NBRC exam questions lowers your probability of passing. Even if you lack confidence in your math skills, you cannot afford to concede any questions involving computations. The good news is that the computations you will likely encounter on the NBRC exams are predictable and relatively simple. With the preparation we provide here, you should be able to answer these items correctly and pass the exam.

For organizational purposes, this appendix presents the most common calculations you may see on the NBRC exams by functional categories, such as computations involving ventilation or those related to oxygenation. For each calculation, we provide the applicable formula, an example computation, and one or more "ballpark rules." A ballpark rule is simply a way to help estimate the answer or the range within which the answer should fall. Our guidance is to always check your answer against the applicable rule before committing to it. If your answer is inconsistent with the ballpark rule, review the problem, the formula, and your computation.

Ventilation Calculations

Likely calculations regarding ventilation include the minute volume, tidal volume, physiologic deadspace, ratio of deadspace to tidal volume, and alveolar ventilation. Also possible are conversions between CO_2 percentages and partial pressures. **Table B-1** provides the formulas for these parameters, example calculations, and "ballpark" rules to help you estimate or verify your computations.

Table B-1 Computation Formulas and Example Problems for Ventilatory Parameters

Parameter/Formula	Example
Minute Volume ($\dot{V}E$)	
$$\dot{V}_E = f \times V_T$$ *Ballpark rule*: At normal rates of breathing, the computed minute volume for adults will generally be in the range of 4–10 L/min.	*Problem B.1* A patient has a tidal volume of 400 mL and is breathing at 14/min. What is the new minute volume? *Solution:* $\dot{V}_E = f \times V_T$ $\dot{V}_E = 14$ breaths/min $\times 400$ mL/breath $\dot{V}_E = 5600$ mL/min or 5.6 L/min

(continues)

Table B-1 Computation Formulas and Example Problems for Ventilatory Parameters (*Continued*)

Parameter/Formula	Example
Tidal Volume (V_T)	
$$V_T = \dot{V}_E \div f$$ *Ballpark rule*: If you obtain a $V_T < 200$ mL or > 1000 mL for an adult, recheck your calculations!	*Problem B.2* A patient has a minute volume of 8.25 L/min and is breathing at a rate of 22/min. What is his average tidal volume? *Solution*: $V_T = \dot{V}_E \div f$ $V_T = 8.25$ L/min $\div 22$ breaths/min $V_T = 0.375$ L/breath $= 375$ mL or 0.375 L
Physiologic Deadspace (V_D)	
$$V_D = V_T \times \frac{Pa_{CO_2} - P_{ECO_2}}{Pa_{CO_2}}$$ where V_D = physiologic deadspace, V_T = tidal volume, Pa_{CO_2} = arterial P_{CO_2}, and P_{ECO_2} = mixed expired P_{CO_2} *Ballpark rules*: (1) Unless the patient has a trach (which lowers V_D), V_D will be approximately 1 lb of PBW and usually less than 70% of the tidal volume; (2) large $Pa_{CO_2} - P_{ECO_2}$ differences ($> 15–20$ torr) indicate large deadspace volume.	*Problem B.3* A patient has a tidal volume of 450 mL, an arterial Pa_{CO_2} of 60 torr, and a P_{ECO_2} of 30 torr. What is the patient's deadspace? *Solution*: $V_D = V_T \times \dfrac{Pa_{CO_2} - P_{ECO_2}}{Pa_{CO_2}}$ $V_D = 450$ mL $\times [(60 - 30)/60]$ $V_D = 450$ mL $\times [30/60]$ $V_D = 225$ mL
Ratio of Deadspace to Tidal Volume (V_D/V_T)	
$$V_D/V_T = V_D \div V_T$$ or (if given V_D/V_T) $$V_D = V_D/V_T \times V_T$$ *Ballpark rule*: Unless the patient has a trach (which lowers V_D), V_D/V_T will generally be in the range of 0.30–0.70.	*Problem B.4* A 6-foot-tall, 170-lb patient with normal lungs has a tidal volume of 600 mL. What is his ratio of deadspace to tidal volume? *Solution*: With normal lungs, assume that V_D = 1 mL/lb predicted body weight (PBW). $V_D = 1$ lb $\times 170$ lb $= 170$ mL $V_D/V_T = 170 \div 600 = 0.28$ *Problem B.5* A 5-foot-tall, 105-lb patient has a ratio of deadspace to tidal volume of 0.40 and a tidal volume of 500 mL. What is her deadspace volume? *Solution*: $V_D = V_D/V_T \times V_T$ $V_D = 0.40 \times 500$ mL $= 200$ mL

Parameter/Formula	Example
Alveolar Ventilation ($\dot{V}_A$)	
$\dot{V}_A = f \times (V_T - V_D)$ *Ballpark rules:* (1) Unless otherwise stated, assume normal dead-space = 1 mL per lb of PBW; (2) $\dot{V}_A$ must always be less than the minute volume and in proportion to the V_D/V_T ratio.	*Problem B.5* A 6-foot, 4-inch-tall, 200-lb man with normal lungs has a tidal volume of 680 mL and is breathing at a rate of 15 breaths/min. What is his approximate alveolar ventilation? *Solution:* Assume normal deadspace of 1 mL/lb $\times$ 200 lb = 200 mL. $\dot{V}_A = f \times (V_T - V_D)$ $\dot{V}_A = 15 \times (680 - 200)$ $\dot{V}_A = 15 \times 480$ $\dot{V}_A = 7200$ mL/min or 7.2 L/min
Convert End-Tidal CO_2% ($Fetco_2$) to $Petco_2$	
$Petco_2 = Fetco_2 \times (P_B - 47)$ *Ballpark rule:* A normal $Fetco_2$ ranges between 4% and 6%; 5% $Fetco_2$ is equivalent to a $Petco_2$ of 36 to 40 torr.	*Problem B.6* A patient at sea level has an end-tidal CO_2 concentration ($Fetco_2$) of 0.043. What is her BTPS-corrected end-tidal Pco_2 ($Petco_2$)? *Solution:* Sea-level P_B = 760 mm Hg Correction for BTPS = –47 mm Hg $Petco_2 = Fetco_2 \times (P_B - 47)$ $Petco_2 = 0.043 \times (760 - 47)$ $Petco_2 = 0.043 \times 713$ $Petco_2 = 30.7$ mm Hg (torr)

Oxygenation Calculations

Likely calculations regarding oxygenation include the inspired and alveolar Po_2, A-a gradient, percent shunt, P/F ratio, and arterial O_2 content. **Table B-2** provides the formulas for these parameters, example calculations, and "ballpark" rules to help you estimate or verify your computations.

Table B-2 Computation Formulas and Example Problems for Oxygenation Parameters

Parameter/Formula	Example
Inspired Po_2 (Pio_2)	
$Pio_2 = Fio_2 \times P_B$ *Ballpark rule:* At sea level with an Fio_2 of 1.0, the Pio_2 = 760 torr; therefore, with an Fio_2 of 0.50, the $Pio_2 = 1/2 \times 760 = 380$ torr.	*Problem B.7* You are transporting a patient on 40% O_2 in an unpressurized airplane cabin at 8000-ft altitude (P_B = 565 mm Hg). What is his Pio_2? *Solution:* $Pio_2 = Fio_2 \times P_B$ $Pio_2 = 0.40 \times 565$ mm Hg $Pio_2 = 226$ mm Hg (torr)

(continues)

Table B-2 Computation Formulas and Example Problems for Oxygenation Parameters (*Continued*)

Parameter/Formula	Example
Alveolar P_{O_2} (P_{AO_2})	
$P_{AO_2} = F_{IO_2} \times (P_B - 47) - (1.25 \times P_{aCO_2})$ *Ballpark rules*: (1) Maximum P_{AO_2} at sea level breathing room air ≈ 130 torr and breathing 100% $O_2 \approx 680$ torr; (2) estimate normal P_{AO_2} as $6 \times O_2\%$—for example, you would expect a patient breathing 50% O_2 to have a P_{AO_2} of about 300 torr.	*Problem B.8* A patient breathing 60% O_2 at sea level has a P_{aCO_2} of 28 torr. What is her alveolar P_{O_2} (P_{AO_2})? *Solution*: Sea level $P_B = 760$ mm Hg $P_{AO_2} = F_{IO_2} \times (P_B - 47) - (1.25 \times P_{aCO_2})$ $P_{AO_2} = 0.60 \times (760 - 47) - (1.25 \times 28)$ $P_{AO_2} = 428 - 35$ $P_{AO_2} = 393$ mm Hg (torr)
A-a Gradient [$P(A\text{-}a)_{O_2}$]	
$P(A\text{-}a)_{O_2} = P_{AO_2} - P_{aO_2}$ *Ballpark rules*: (1) When breathing 100% O_2, the $P(A\text{-}a)_{O_2}$ typically ranges between 50 and 60 torr for normal subjects but may rise to more than 600 torr when severe shunting is present; (2) compare to % shunt, with about 5% shunt per 100 torr $P(A\text{-}a)_{O_2}$.	*Problem B.9* A patient breathing 100% O_2 at sea level has a P_{aO_2} of 250 torr and a P_{aCO_2} of 60 torr. What is her A-a gradient or $P(A\text{-}a)_{O_2}$? *Solution*: Sea level $P_B = 760$ mm Hg $P_{AO_2} = F_{IO_2} \times (P_B - 47) - (1.25 \times P_{aCO_2})$ $P_{AO_2} = 1.0 \times (760 - 47) - (1.25 \times 60)$ $P_{AO_2} = 713 - 75 = 638$ mm Hg (torr) $P(A\text{-}a)_{O_2} = P_{AO_2} - P_{aO_2}$ $P(A\text{-}a)_{O_2} = 638 - 250$ $P(A\text{-}a)_{O_2} = 388$ mm Hg (torr) ~20% physiologic shunt (see B.11))
Percent Shunt Estimate	
$\%\text{ shunt} = \dfrac{P(A\text{-}a)O_2 \times 0.003}{[P(A\text{-}a)O_2 \times 0.003] + 5}$ *Ballpark rule*: There is about a 5% shunt for every 100 torr $P(A\text{-}a)_{O_2}$.	*Problem B.10* What is the estimated percent shunt of the patient in Problem B.10? *Solution*: $\%\text{ shunt} = \dfrac{P(A\text{-}a)O_2 \times 0.003}{[P(A\text{-}a)O_2 \times 0.003] + 5}$ $\%\text{ shunt} = \dfrac{388 \times 0.003}{[388 \times 0.003] + 5}$ $\%\text{ shunt} = \dfrac{1.164}{6.164}$ $\%\text{ shunt} = 0.189 = 19\%$

Parameter/Formula	Example
Arterial Po$_2$ to Fio$_2$ Ratio (P/F Ratio)	
$\text{Pao}_2/\text{Fio}_2 = \text{Pao}_2 \div \text{Fio}_2$ *Ballpark rule*: Expect P/F ratios > 500 for patients with normal lung function; P/F ratios < 300 signify acute lung injury and abnormal gas exchange, and values less than 200 mm Hg indicate severe hypoxemia. Values < 100 are consistent with ARDS.	*Problem B.11* What is the P/F ratio of a patient breathing 50% O_2 with a Pao$_2$ of 68 torr? *Solution*: $\text{Pao}_2/\text{Fio}_2 = \text{Pao}_2 \div \text{Fio}_2$ $\text{Pao}_2/\text{Fio}_2 = 68 \div 0.50$ $\text{Pao}_2/\text{Fio}_2 = 136$
Arterial O$_2$ Content (Cao$_2$)	
$\text{Cao}_2 = (\text{dissolved O}_2) + (\text{O}_2 \text{ bound to Hb})$ $\text{Cao}_2 = (0.003 \times \text{Pao}_2) + (\text{total Hb} \times 1.36 \times \text{Sao}_2)$ *Ballpark rule*: If the Sao$_2$ > 75% (as is typically the case for arterial blood), the computed Cao$_2$ value in mL/dL will always be a bit larger than the total Hb present but never more than 40% larger—for example, with a total Hb of 8 g/dL and a Sao$_2$ of 90%, you would expect a Cao$_2$ between 8 and 11 mL/dL.	*Problem B.12* A patient has a hemoglobin concentration of 10 g/dL, a Pao$_2$ of 50 torr, and a Sao$_2$ of 80%. What is his total arterial O_2 content (Cao$_2$)? *Solution*: $\text{O}_2 \text{ bound to Hb} = (\text{total Hb} \times 1.36 \times \text{Sao}_2)$ $\text{O}_2 \text{ bound to Hb} = (10 \times 1.36 \times 0.80)$ $\text{O}_2 \text{ bound to Hb} = 10.9 \text{ mL/dL}$ $\text{Dissolved O}_2 = 0.003 \times \text{Pao}_2$ $\text{Dissolved O}_2 = 0.003 \times 50$ $\text{Dissolved O}_2 = 0.15 \text{ mL/dL}$ $\text{Cao}_2 = (\text{dissolved O}_2) + (\text{O}_2 \text{ bound to Hb})$ $\text{Cao}_2 = 0.15 + 10.9 = 11.05 \text{ mL/dL}$
Oxygen Index (OI)	
$\text{OI} = (\text{Fio}_2 \times \overline{\text{PAW}} \times 100) \div \text{Pao}_2$ *Ballpark rule*: Lower OI values tend to be better. An increasing OI suggests worsening oxygenation, and values greater than 40 are associated with severe IRDS/ARDS where ECMO is recommended.	*Problem B.13* Calculate the Oxygen Index (OI) for a patient who requires a mean airway pressure of 20 cm H_2O and a Fio$_2$ of 1.0 to obtain a Pao$_2$ of 50 torr. $\text{OI} = (1.0 \times 20 \times 100) \div 50$ $\text{OI} = 2000 \div 50$ $\text{OI} = 40$

Calculations Involving Pulmonary Mechanics

Likely calculations regarding pulmonary mechanics include the static compliance and airway resistance of patients receiving ventilatory support. **Table B-3** provides the formulas for these parameters, example calculations, and "ballpark" rules to help you verify your computations.

Table B-3 Computation Formulas and Example Problems for Pulmonary Mechanics Parameters

Parameter/Formula	Example
Static Compliance (C$_{LT}$)	
$$C_{LT} = \frac{V_T}{Pplat - PEEP}$$ where C$_{LT}$ = static compliance of the lungs and thorax, V$_T$ = the corrected tidal volume, P$_{plat}$ = the plateau pressure during a volume hold, and PEEP = the baseline airway pressure	*Problem B.14* A patient receiving VC ventilation with a tidal volume of 700 mL and 8 cm H$_2$O PEEP has a peak pressure of 42 cm H$_2$O and a plateau pressure of 35 cm H$_2$O. What is the static compliance? *Solution*:
Ballpark rule: Expect to see the C$_{LT}$ range from 100 mL/cm H$_2$O (normal) to 10 mL/cm H$_2$O (severe reduction in compliance, such as might occur in ARDS).	$$C_{LT} = \frac{V_T}{Pplat - PEEP}$$ C$_{LT}$ = 700/35 − 8 C$_{LT}$ = 26 mL/cm H$_2$O
Airway Resistance (R$_{AW}$)	
$$Raw = \frac{PIP - P_{plat}}{\dot{V}}$$ where R$_{AW}$ = airway resistance (cm H$_2$O/L/sec), PIP = peak inspiratory pressure, P$_{plat}$ = the plateau pressure during a volume hold, and $\dot{V}$ = inspiratory flow in liters/second.	*Problem B.15* A patient receiving VC ventilation with a tidal volume of 400 mL, an inspiratory flow of 75 L/min, and 6 cm H$_2$O PEEP has a peak pressure of 45 cm H$_2$O and a plateau pressure of 30 cm H$_2$O. What is the airway resistance? *Solution*: Convert 75 L/min to L/sec: 75 L ÷ 60 = 1.25 L/sec
Ballpark rule: Normal R$_{AW}$ for orally intubated patients ranges from 5 to 15 cm H$_2$O/L/sec; expect higher computed values in patients with airway obstruction.	$$Raw = \frac{PIP - P_{plat}}{\dot{V}}$$ R$_{AW}$ = (45 − 30)/1.25 R$_{AW}$ = 12 cm H$_2$O/L/sec

Pulmonary Function Calculations

Likely calculations related to pulmonary function testing include lung volumes and capacities, forced expiratory volume (time) as a percentage of forced vital capacity (FVC), the percent change in value, and the percent predicted compared to normal. **Table B-4** provides the formulas for these parameters, example calculations, and "ballpark" rules to help you estimate or verify your computations.

Table B-4 Computation Formulas and Example Problems for Selected Pulmonary Function Parameters

Parameter/Formula	Example
Volumes/Capacities	
Most common formulas: $VC = TLC - RV$ $VC = IRV + TV + ERV$ $TLC = FRC + IC$ $TLC = IRV + TV + ERV + RV$ $RV = FRC - ERV$ $RV = TLC - VC$ $FRC = RV + ERV$ $FRC = TLC - IC$	*Problem B.16* A patient has an FRC of 3800 mL, a tidal volume of 400 mL, and an expiratory reserve volume of 1300 mL. What is the residual volume? *Solution*: $RV = FRC - ERV$ $RV = 3800 - 1300$ $RV = 2500$ mL or 2.5 L
Ballpark rule: Verify the selected formula by drawing and labeling a graph of lung volumes and capacities before computation.	
Forced Expiratory Volume (Time) Percent	
$$FEV_t\% = \frac{FEV_t}{FVC} \times 100$$ where FEV_t = the forced expiratory volume at time t (typically 1, 3, or 6 seconds)	*Problem B.17* A patient has a forced vital capacity of 4.5 L and an FEV_3 of 4.0 L. What is the $FEV_3\%$? *Solution*: $$FEV_3\% = \frac{FEV_3}{FVC} \times 100$$
Ballpark rule: A patient with normal pulmonary function should have an $FEV_1\% > 75\%$ and a $FEV_3\% > 95\%$.	$FEV_3\% = 4.0/4.5 \times 100$ $FEV_3\% = 89\%$
Percent Change Value	
$$\%\,change = \frac{post - pre}{pre} \times 100$$ where *pre* is the pre-treatment value for the parameter being measured, and *post* is the post-treatment value.	*Problem B.18* A patient has an FEV_1 of 2.4 L before bronchodilator treatment and an FEV_1 of 2.7 L after treatment. What percent change in FEV_1 occurred? *Solution*: $$\%\,change = \frac{post - pre}{pre} \times 100$$
Ballpark rule: If post > pre, then computed % change must be positive; for FEV_1, and the PEFR the improvement must be at least 12–15% to be considered a significant response to bronchodilator therapy.	$$\%\,change = \frac{2.7 - 2.4}{2.4} \times 100$$ % change = 12.5%

(continues)

Table B-4 Computation Formulas and Example Problems for Selected Pulmonary Function Parameters (*Continued*)

Percent Predicted Value	
$\%\text{predicted} = \dfrac{\text{actual}}{\text{predicted}} \times 100$ where *actual* is the patient's measured value for that parameter and *predicted* is the patient's predicted normal value. *Note*: When monitoring for changes over time for some measures, such as peak flow, we substitute the patient's personal best value for the predicted value.	*Problem B.19* In the pulmonary lab, you measure a patient's forced vital capacity as 3.25 L. Her predicted normal FVC is 3.82 L. What percent of predicted normal is her FVC? *Solution*: $\%\text{predicted} = \dfrac{\text{actual}}{\text{predicted}} \times 10$
Ballpark rule: If actual < predicted, then computed % predicted must be < 100%.	$\%\text{predicted} = \dfrac{3.25}{3.82} \times 10$ % predicted = 85% of normal

Cardiovascular Calculations

Likely calculations regarding cardiovascular parameters include heart rate (from an ECG), pulse pressure, mean pressure, stroke volume, cardiac output, and cardiac index. **Table B-5** provides the formulas for these parameters, example calculations, and "ballpark" rules to help you estimate or verify your computations.

Table B-5 Computation Formulas and Example Problems for Cardiovascular Parameters

Parameter/Formula	Example
Heart Rate (from ECG)	
For regular rhythms: HR = 60 ÷ R-R (sec) where HR is the heart rate, and R-R is the R-to-R interval on an ECG rhythm strip.	*Problem B.20* On an ECG strip, a patient has a regular rhythm with an R-R interval of 10 mm (two large boxes). What is the heart rate?
Ballpark rule: Approximate HR = 300 ÷ R-R span in large (5-mm = 0.2-sec) boxes.	*Solution*: ECG recording speed = 25 mm/sec = 0.04 sec/mm 10 mm × 0.04 sec/mm = 0.40 sec 60 sec/min ÷ 0.40 sec = 150/min
Pulse Pressure	
Pulse pressure = systolic – diastolic	*Problem B.21*
Ballpark rules: (1) Compare to the normal resting value of about 40 mm Hg (up to 100 mm Hg is normal during exercise); (2) expect high values with atherosclerosis, hyperthyroidism, and aortic regurgitation; expect low values with CHF, cardiac tamponade, or cardiogenic shock.	A patient's arterial blood pressure is 165/90 mm Hg. What is her pulse pressure? *Solution*: Pulse pressure = systolic – diastolic Pulse pressure = 165 – 90 Pulse pressure = 75 mm Hg

Parameter/Formula	Example
Mean Blood Pressure Estimate	
Mean pressure = [systolic + (2 × diastolic)] ÷ 3	*Problem B.22*
Ballpark rule: For patients with relatively normal pulse pressure, the mean pressure will be a bit less than halfway between the systolic and diastolic pressures.	A patient's arterial blood pressure is 100/70 mm Hg. What is his mean arterial pressure?
	Solution:
	Mean pressure = [systolic + (2 × diastolic)] ÷ 3
	Mean pressure = [100 + (2 × 70)] ÷ 3
	Mean pressure = [100 + 140] ÷ 3
	Mean pressure = 80 mm Hg
Cardiac Output (CO)	
CO = (HR × SV) ÷ 1000	*Problem B.23*
where CO = cardiac output in L/min, HR = heart rate, and SV = average left ventricular stroke volume in mL.	A patient has a left ventricular stroke volume of 60 mL and a heart rate of 105 beats/min. What is the cardiac output?
Ballpark rules:	*Solution*:
(1) Compare to a "normal" output of 70 × 70 = 4900 or 4.9 L/min (HR = 70/min and SV = 70 mL);	CO = (HR × SV) ÷ 1000
	CO = (105 × 60) ÷ 1000
(2) for adult patients, expect to see the computed CO range between 3 and 10 L/min (normal 4–8 L/min).	CO = 6300 ÷ 1000
	CO = 6.3 L/min
Cardiac Index (CI)	
CI (L/min/m^2) = CO ÷ BSA	*Problem B.24*
where CO = cardiac output in L/min, and BSA = body surface area in m^2 (usually provided to you and based on the DuBois formula/nomogram).	A patient has a cardiac output of 6.1 L/min and a body surface area of 2.3 m^2. What is the cardiac index?
Ballpark rules:	*Solution*:
(1) For adults, the normal cardiac index will always be less than the cardiac output—about half as much for the average-size adult;	CI = CO ÷ BSA
	CI = 6.1 ÷ 2.3
(2) compare the computed value to the normal range of 2.5–5.0 L/min/m^2.	CI = 2.65 L/min/m^2
Stroke Volume (SV)	
SV = CO ÷ HR	*Problem B.25*
where SV = average left ventricular stroke volume in mL, CO = cardiac output in mL/min, and HR = heart rate.	A patient has a cardiac output of 4.0 L/min and a heart rate of 80. What is the stroke volume?
	Solution:
Ballpark rule: Compare to the normal range of 60–130 mL.	First convert CO in L/min to mL/min
	4.0 × 1000 = 4000 mL/min
	SV = CO ÷ HR
	SV = 4000 ÷ 80
	SV = 50 mL

Equipment Calculations

Likely calculations regarding equipment include cylinder duration of flow, air-entrainment ratios, total output flows for air-entrainment devices, suction catheter sizes, and pressure conversions. **Table B-6** provides the formulas for these parameters, example calculations, and "ballpark" rules to help you estimate or verify your computations.

Table B-6 Formulas and Example Problems for Equipment-Related Computations

Parameter/Formula	Example
Cylinder Duration of Flow	
$$\text{Time to empty (min)} = \frac{\text{psig} \times \text{factor}}{\text{flow}}$$ where *psig* is the cylinder pressure in pounds per square inch gauge, the *factor* is the cylinder factor (below), and *flow* is the flow in L/min. <table><tr><td>Gas</td><td>D</td><td>E</td><td>G</td><td>H/K</td></tr><tr><td>O_2, air</td><td>0.16</td><td>0.28</td><td>2.41</td><td>3.14</td></tr><tr><td>He/O_2</td><td>0.14</td><td>0.23</td><td>1.93</td><td>2.50</td></tr></table>	*Problem B.26* How long will an E cylinder of oxygen with a gauge pressure of 800 psi set to deliver 5 L/min take to become empty? *Solution:* $$\text{Time to empty (min)} = \frac{\text{psig} \times \text{factor}}{\text{flow}}$$ Time to empty (min) = $800 \times 0.28/5$ Time to empty (min) = 45 minutes
Ballpark rule: (1) A full E cylinder at 10 L/min will last about 1 hour; (2) a full H cylinder at 10 L/min will last about 10 times longer (10 hours).	*Note:* It is common practice to change out a cylinder at least 15–30 minutes before its contents are fully exhausted or when the cylinder content drops below 500 psi pressure.
Air-Entrainment Ratio (Air-to-O_2 Ratio)	
$$\text{Air:}O_2 \text{ ratio} = \frac{100 - \%O_2}{\%O_2 - 21}$$ *Note:* This formula is the same as the "magic box" that appears in many textbooks.	*Problem B.27* What is the air-to-O_2 ratio for a 35% air-entrainment mask? *Solution:* $$\text{Air:}O_2 \text{ ratio} = \frac{100 - \%O_2}{\%O_2 - 21}$$
Ballpark rule: 60% O_2 is achieved with an air-to-O_2 ratio of about 1:1; lower O_2% values mean higher ratios, and higher O_2% values mean lower ratios.	$$\text{Air:}O_2 \text{ ratio} = \frac{100 - 35}{35 - 21}$$ $$\text{Air:}O_2 \text{ ratio} = \frac{65}{14}$$ Air:O_2 ratio = 4.6:1 or 5:1
Air-Entrainment Device Total Output Flow	
Total flow = input flow $\times$ (air + O_2 ratio parts)	*Problem B.28*
Ballpark rule: For a given input flow, the lower the %O_2 setting of the air-entrainment device, the higher its total output flow. For example, with an input flow of 10 L/min, an air-entrainment nebulizer set to 60% O_2 (1:1 ratio) will deliver 20 L/min, but when set to 28% O_2 (10:1 ratio), it will deliver 110 L/min.	Assuming an input O_2 flow of 8 L/min for the air-entrainment mask in Problem B.27, what would be the total flow delivered to the patient? *Solution:* Total flow = input flow $\times$ (air + O_2 ratio parts) Total flow = $8 \times (5 + 1)$ Total flow = 48 L/min

Parameter/Formula	Example
Suction Catheter Size Estimation	
Catheter size (Fr) = 1.5 × ETT ID where catheter size is in French units (Fr), and endotracheal tube internal diameter (ETT ID) is in millimeters.	*Problem B.29* A patient has an 8-mm ID tracheostomy tube. Which size of suction catheter should you use? *Solution*:
Ballpark rule: Multiply the ETT ID by 2, and use the next-smallest-size French catheter.	Catheter size (Fr) = 1.5 × ETT ID Catheter size (Fr) = 1.5 × 8 = 12 Fr
Pressure Conversions	
The two conventional pressure units commonly used in respiratory care are cm H_2O and mm Hg (torr). A third unit is the kilopascal (kPa), which is the international system unit of pressure. To convert from a conventional unit to an alternative unit, *multiply it* by its conversion factor (see the following table). To convert from an alternative unit back to a conventional unit, *divide it* by the factor.	*Problem B.30* You record a patient's cuff pressure as 30 cm H_2O. What pressure is this in mm Hg? *Solution*: cm H_2O = 1.363 × mm Hg mm Hg = cm H_2O ÷ 1.36 mm Hg = 30 ÷ 1.36 = 22 mm Hg

Conventional Unit	Alternative Unit	Conversion Factor
mm Hg (torr)	cm H_2O	1.363
cm H_2O	kPa	0.098
mm Hg (torr)	kPa	0.133

Ballpark rule: 1 kilopascal equals about 10 cm H_2O or 10 mm Hg.

Formulas and Example Problems for Mechanical Ventilation Time and Flow Parameters

Likely calculations regarding mechanical ventilation involve time or flow parameters. In general, these calculations will apply only to volume- or pressure-control modes. **Table B-7** provides the formulas for these parameters, example calculations, and "ballpark" rules to help you estimate or verify your computations.

Table B-7 Common Mechanical Ventilation Time and Flow Parameters

Parameter/Formula	Example
Total Cycle Time (Seconds per Breath)	
$$\text{Total cycle time (sec)} = \frac{60}{f}$$ where f = set frequency or rate of breathing in breaths per minute.	*Problem B.31* An infant is receiving control-mode ventilation at a rate of 40 breaths per minute. What is the total cycle time? *Solution*:
Ballpark rule: Total cycle time also equals the sum of the inspiratory and expiratory times (if known).	$$\text{Total cycle time (sec)} = \frac{60}{f}$$ Total cycle time = 60/40 Total cycle time = 1.5 sec

(continues)

Table B-7 Common Mechanical Ventilation Time and Flow Parameters (*Continued*)

Parameter/Formula	Example
Ratio of Inspiratory to Expiratory Time (I:E Ratio)	
I:E ratio $= 1:\dfrac{T_E}{T_I}$ where T_E = the expiratory time in seconds, and T_I = the inspiratory time in seconds.	**Problem B.32** A patient on pressure-control ventilation has an inspiratory time of 2 seconds and an expiratory time of 3 seconds. What is his I:E ratio? *Solution:*
Ballpark rule: Unless the patient is receiving inverse-ratio ventilation ($T_I > T_E$), the I:E ratio normally will be less than 1:1 (e.g., 1:2, 1:3).	I:E ratio $= 1:\dfrac{T_E}{T_I}$ I:E ratio $= 1:3/2$ I:E ratio $= 1:1.5$
Inspiratory Time (T_I)	
T_I(seconds) = total cycle time $- T_E$ or T_I(seconds) $= \dfrac{\text{total cycle time}}{\text{sum of I:E ratio parts}}$	**Problem B.33** A patient on volume-control ventilation has an I:E ratio of 1:4 and a set rate of 20 per breaths/min. What is her inspiratory time? *Solution:*
Ballpark rule: When the I:E ratio is less than 1:1, T_I will always be shorter than T_E.	First compute total cycle time $= 60 \div 20 = 3$ seconds T_I(seconds) $= \dfrac{\text{total cycle time}}{\text{sum of I:E ratio parts}}$ T_I(seconds) $= 3/5 = 0.6$ seconds
Expiratory Time (T_E)	
T_E(seconds) = total cycle time $- T_I$	**Problem B.34** Compute the expiratory time of the patient in Problem B.33.
Ballpark rule: When the I:E ratio is less than 1:1, T_E will always be longer than T_I.	*Solution:* T_E(seconds) = total cycle time $- T_I$ T_E(seconds) $= 3 - 0.6 = 2.4$ seconds
Percent Inspiratory Time (%T_I or "Duty Cycle")	
$\%T_I = \dfrac{T_I}{\text{total cycle time}}$	**Problem B.35** *Solution:*
Ballpark rule: The %T_I and I:E ratio are related, as indicated in the following table. For I:E ratios less than 1:1, the %T_I = 100 ÷ (sum of I:E parts). <table><tr><th>I:E Ratio</th><th>%T_I</th></tr><tr><td>1:4</td><td>20%</td></tr><tr><td>1:3</td><td>25%</td></tr><tr><td>1:2</td><td>33%</td></tr><tr><td>1:1.5</td><td>40%</td></tr><tr><td>1:1</td><td>50%</td></tr><tr><td>1.5:1</td><td>60%</td></tr><tr><td>2:1</td><td>67%</td></tr></table>	Compute the %T_I of the patient in Problem B.33. *Solution:* $\%T_I = \dfrac{T_I}{\text{total cycle time}} \times 100$ $\%T_I = 0.6/3$ $\%T_I = 0.20 = 20\%$

Parameter/Formula	Example
Ventilator Flow (Volume Control Ventilation)	
$$\dot{V} = \frac{\dot{V}_E}{\%T_I}$$ where $\dot{V}$ is the inspiratory flow in L/min, $\dot{V}_E$ is the minute volume in L/min, and $\%T_I$ is the percent inspiratory time (as a decimal).	*Problem B.36* Which inspiratory flow is needed for a patient receiving volume-control ventilation at a rate of 15 breaths/min and an I:E ratio of 1:3, with a tidal volume of 600 mL? *Solution*: First compute the minute volume in L/min: $\dot{V}_E = 15 \times 600 = 9000$ mL $= 9.0$ L Next compute the $\%T_I$: $\%T_I = 100 \div (1+3) = 25\% = 0.25$ $\dot{V} = \frac{\dot{V}_E}{\%T_I} = 9.0/0.25$ $\dot{V} = 36$ L/min
Ballpark rule: A simple alternative that works as long as inverse-ratio ventilation is not being used is to multiply the sum of the I:E parts by the minute volume.	

Drug Calculations

Likely pharmacology-related calculations include dilution and dosage problems. **Table B-8** provides the generic formulas for these problems, example calculations, and "ballpark" rules to help you estimate or verify your computations.

Table B-8 Formulas and Example Problems for Drug Dilution and Dosage Computations

Formula	Example
Dilution	
$V_1 \times C_1 = V_2 \times C_2$ where V_1 is the original volume, C_1 is the original concentration, V_2 is the new volume, and C_2 is the new concentration.	*Problem B.37* A doctor orders 5 mL of 10% acetylcysteine (Mucomyst) via small-volume nebulizer TID for a patient with thick secretions. The pharmacy stocks only 20% acetylcysteine in multidose vials. How many milliliters of the 20% acetylcysteine would you administer to the patient for each treatment? *Solution*: $V_1 \times C_1 = V_2 \times C_2$ $V_2 = \frac{V_1 \times C_1}{C_2}$ $V_2 = \frac{5\,\text{mL} \times 10\%}{20\%}$ $V_2 = 2.5$ mL (mixed with 2.5 mL normal saline for total nebulizer volume of 5 mL)
Ballpark rule: Doubling the volume halves the concentration of the solute.	

(continues)

Table B-8 Formulas and Example Problems for Drug Dilution and Dosage Computations (*Continued*)

Formula	Example
Dosage Computations	
mg/mL = 10 × % concentration mg/mL $$\% \text{ concentration} = \frac{\text{mg/mL}}{10}$$ $$mL = \frac{\text{dosage(mg)}}{\text{concentration(mg/mL)}}$$	*Problem B.38* A doctor orders 2 mL of a 0.5% solution of a bronchodilator via SVN. How many milligrams of the drug are you administering? *Solution*: mg/mL = 10 × % concentration mg/mL = 10 × 0.5 mg/mL = 5 mg/mL 5 mg/mL × 2 mL = 10 mg
Ballpark rule: (1) A 1% solution contains 10 mg/mL of solute; (2) a 0.5% solution contains half as much (5 mg/mL); and (3) a 2% solution contains twice as much (20 mg/mL).	*Problem B.39* A doctor orders 40 mg of a 0.25% solution of a bronchodilator for continuous nebulization, to be diluted with 200 mL normal saline. How many milliliters of the bronchodilator solution would you mix with the saline solution? *Solution*: First, compute the mg/mL in the 0.25% bronchodilator solution: mg/mL = 10 × % concentration mg/mL = 10 × 0.25 mg/mL = 2.5 mg/mL Next, compute the mL bronchodilator solution required: $$mL = \frac{\text{dosage(mg)}}{\text{concentration(mg/mL)}}$$ mL = 40 mg/2.5 mg/mL mL = 16 mL

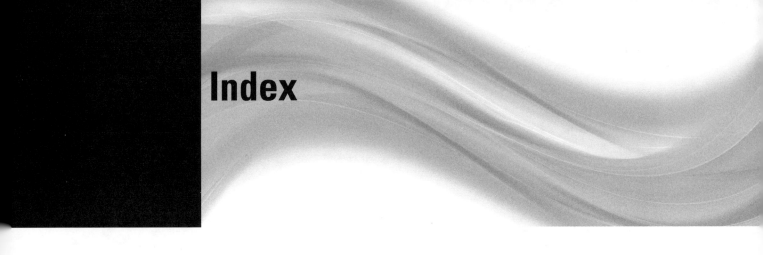

Index

Note: Page numbers followed by *b*, *f*, or *t* indicate material in boxes, figures, or tables, respectively.